# Molecular Biomarkers In Cardiology

# Molecular Biomarkers In Cardiology

Editor

**Pietro Scicchitano**

MDPI • Basel • Beijing • Wuhan • Barcelona • Belgrade • Manchester • Tokyo • Cluj • Tianjin

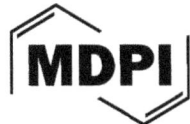

*Editor*
Pietro Scicchitano
Department of Cardiology—Hospital "F. Perinei" Altamura (BA)
Italy

*Editorial Office*
MDPI
St. Alban-Anlage 66
4052 Basel, Switzerland

This is a reprint of articles from the Special Issue published online in the open access journal *Biomolecules* (ISSN 2218-273X) (available at: https://www.mdpi.com/journal/biomolecules/special_issues/Biomolecular_Biomarkers_Cardiology#info).

For citation purposes, cite each article independently as indicated on the article page online and as indicated below:

LastName, A.A.; LastName, B.B.; LastName, C.C. Article Title. *Journal Name* **Year**, *Volume Number*, Page Range.

**ISBN 978-3-0365-0840-5 (Hbk)**
**ISBN 978-3-0365-0841-2 (PDF)**

© 2021 by the authors. Articles in this book are Open Access and distributed under the Creative Commons Attribution (CC BY) license, which allows users to download, copy and build upon published articles, as long as the author and publisher are properly credited, which ensures maximum dissemination and a wider impact of our publications.

The book as a whole is distributed by MDPI under the terms and conditions of the Creative Commons license CC BY-NC-ND.

# Contents

About the Editor . . . . . . . . . . . . . . . . . . . . . . . . . . . . . . . . . . . . . . . . . . . ix

Preface to "Molecular Biomarkers In Cardiology" . . . . . . . . . . . . . . . . . . . . . . . . . xi

Georgiana-Aura Giurgea, Katrin Zlabinger, Alfred Gugerell, Dominika Lukovic, Bonni Syeda, Ljubica Mandic, Noemi Pavo, Julia Mester-Tonczar, Denise Traxler-Weidenauer, Andreas Spannbauer, Nina Kastner, Claudia Müller, Anahit Anvari, Jutta Bergler-Klein and Mariann Gyöngyösi
Multimarker Approach to Identify Patients with Coronary Artery Disease at High Risk for Subsequent Cardiac Adverse Events: The Multi-Biomarker Study
Reprinted from: *Biomolecules* **2020**, *10*, 909, doi:10.3390/biom10060909 . . . . . . . . . . . . . . . 1

Meenashi Vanathi Balashanmugam, Thippeswamy Boreddy Shivanandappa, Sivagurunathan Nagarethinam, Basavaraj Vastrad and Chanabasayya Vastrad
Analysis of Differentially Expressed Genes in Coronary Artery Disease by Integrated Microarray Analysis
Reprinted from: *Biomolecules* **2020**, *10*, 35, doi:10.3390/biom10010035 . . . . . . . . . . . . . . . 13

Javier Angeles-Martínez, Rosalinda Posadas-Sánchez, Eyerahi Bravo-Flores, María del Carmen González-Salazar and Gilberto Vargas-Alarcón
Common Variants in *IL-20* Gene are Associated with Subclinical Atherosclerosis, Cardiovascular Risk Factors and IL-20 Levels in the Cohort of the Genetics of Atherosclerotic Disease (GEA) Mexican Study
Reprinted from: *Biomolecules* **2020**, *10*, 75, doi:10.3390/biom10010075 . . . . . . . . . . . . . . . 35

Ibrahim T. Fazmin, Zakaria Achercouk, Charlotte E. Edling, Asri Said and Kamalan Jeevaratnam
Circulating microRNA as a Biomarker for Coronary Artery Disease
Reprinted from: *Biomolecules* **2020**, *10*, 1354, doi:10.3390/biom10101354 . . . . . . . . . . . . . . . 49

Salwa A. Elgebaly, Robert H. Christenson, Hossam Kandil, Nashwa El-Khazragy, Laila Rashed, Beshoy Yacoub, Heba Eldeeb, Mahmoud Ali, Roshanak Sharafieh, Ulrike Klueh and Donald L. Kreutzer
Nourin-Dependent miR-137 and miR-106b: Novel Early Inflammatory Diagnostic Biomarkers for Unstable Angina Patients
Reprinted from: *Biomolecules* **2021**, *11*, 368, doi:10.3390/biom11030368 . . . . . . . . . . . . . . . 71

Gabriel Herrera-Maya, Gilberto Vargas-Alarcón, Oscar Pérez-Méndez, Rosalinda Posadas-Sánchez, Felipe Masso, Teresa Juárez-Cedillo, Galileo Escobedo, Andros Vázquez-Montero and José Manuel Fragoso
The Ser290Asn and Thr715Pro Polymorphisms of the *SELP* Gene Are Associated with A Lower Risk of Developing Acute Coronary Syndrome and Low Soluble P-Selectin Levels in A Mexican Population [†]
Reprinted from: *Biomolecules* **2020**, *10*, 270, doi:10.3390/biom10020270 . . . . . . . . . . . . . . . 87

Surendra Kumar, Vijay Kumar and Jong-Joo Kim
Sarcomeric Gene Variants and Their Role with Left Ventricular Dysfunction in Background of Coronary Artery Disease
Reprinted from: *Biomolecules* **2020**, *10*, 442, doi:10.3390/biom10030442 . . . . . . . . . . . . . . . 99

Valerie Samouillan, Ignacio Miguel Martinez de Lejarza Samper, Aleyda Benitez Amaro, David Vilades, Jany Dandurand, Josefina Casas, Esther Jorge, David de Gonzalo Calvo, Alberto Gallardo, Enrique Lerma, Jose Maria Guerra, Francesc Carreras, Ruben Leta and Vicenta Llorente Cortes
Biophysical and Lipidomic Biomarkers of Cardiac Remodeling Post-Myocardial Infarction in Humans
Reprinted from: *Biomolecules* **2020**, *10*, 1471, doi:10.3390/biom10111471 . . . . . . . . . . . . . . . 115

Gilberto Vargas-Alarcon, Oscar Perez-Mendez, Julian Ramirez-Bello, Rosalinda Posadas-Sanchez, Hector Gonzalez-Pacheco, Galileo Escobedo, Betzabe Nieto-Lima, Elizabeth Carreon-Torres and Jose Manuel Fragoso
The c.*52 *A/G* and c.*773 *A/G* Genetic Variants in the UTR'3 of the *LDLR* Gene Are Associated with the Risk of Acute Coronary Syndrome and Lower Plasma HDL-Cholesterol Concentration
Reprinted from: *Biomolecules* **2020**, *10*, 1381, doi:10.3390/biom10101381 . . . . . . . . . . . . . . . 135

Yuliya I. Ragino, Ekaterina M. Stakhneva, Yana V. Polonskaya and Elena V. Kashtanova
The Role of Secretory Activity Molecules of Visceral Adipocytes in Abdominal Obesity in the Development of Cardiovascular Disease: A Review
Reprinted from: *Biomolecules* **2020**, *10*, 374, doi:10.3390/biom10030374 . . . . . . . . . . . . . . . 149

Akira Hara, Masayuki Niwa, Tomohiro Kanayama, Kei Noguchi, Ayumi Niwa, Mikiko Matsuo, Takahiro Kuroda, Yuichiro Hatano, Hideshi Okada and Hiroyuki Tomita
Galectin-3: A Potential Prognostic and Diagnostic Marker for Heart Disease and Detection of Early Stage Pathology
Reprinted from: *Biomolecules* **2020**, *10*, 1277, doi:10.3390/biom10091277 . . . . . . . . . . . . . . . 167

Valeria Conti, Graziamaria Corbi, Maria Vincenza Polito, Michele Ciccarelli, Valentina Manzo, Martina Torsiello, Emanuela De Bellis, Federica D'Auria, Gennaro Vitulano, Federico Piscione, Albino Carrizzo, Paola Di Pietro, Carmine Vecchione, Nicola Ferrara and Amelia Filippelli
Sirt1 Activity in PBMCs as a Biomarker of Different Heart Failure Phenotypes
Reprinted from: *Biomolecules* **2020**, *10*, 1590, doi:10.3390/biom10111590 . . . . . . . . . . . . . . . 185

Maria-Mădălina Bostan, Cristian Stătescu, Larisa Anghel, Ionela-Lăcrămioara Șerban, Elena Cojocaru and Radu Sascău
Post-Myocardial Infarction Ventricular Remodeling Biomarkers—The Key Link between Pathophysiology and Clinic
Reprinted from: *Biomolecules* **2020**, *10*, 1587, doi:10.3390/biom10111587 . . . . . . . . . . . . . . . 199

Jianli Bi, Vidu Garg and Andrew R. Yates
Galectin-3 and sST2 as Prognosticators for Heart Failure Requiring Extracorporeal Life Support: Jack n' Jill
Reprinted from: *Biomolecules* **2021**, *11*, 166, doi:10.3390/biom11020166 . . . . . . . . . . . . . . . 221

Alessia Giarraputo, Ilaria Barison, Marny Fedrigo, Jacopo Burrello, Chiara Castellani, Francesco Tona, Tomaso Bottio, Gino Gerosa, Lucio Barile and Annalisa Angelini
A Changing Paradigm in Heart Transplantation: An Integrative Approach for Invasive and Non-Invasive Allograft Rejection Monitoring
Reprinted from: *Biomolecules* **2021**, *11*, 201, doi:10.3390/biom11020201 . . . . . . . . . . . . . . . 231

**Luca Sgarra, Alessandro Santo Bortone, Maria Assunta Potenza, Carmela Nacci, Maria Antonietta De Salvia, Tommaso Acquaviva, Emanuela De Cillis, Marco Matteo Ciccone, Massimo Grimaldi and Monica Montagnani**
Endothelial Dysfunction May Link Interatrial Septal Abnormalities and MTHFR-Inherited Defects to Cryptogenic Stroke Predisposition
Reprinted from: *Biomolecules* **2020**, *10*, 861, doi:10.3390/biom10060861 . . . . . . . . . . . . . . . . **249**

# About the Editor

**Pietro Scicchitano** Medical Doctor at Cardiology Unit, Hospital "F Perinei" Altamura (BA) Italy.

PhD course degree in Biomolecular, Pharmaceutical and Medical Sciences in 23/02/2021 with maximum votes acum Laude Specialization Course in Cardiovascular Diseases in 25/06/2014 with maximum votes cum Laude.

Degree in Medicine and Surgery in 22/10/2008 with maximum votes cum Laude.

Degree of Instructor in Basic Life Support and Defibrillation obtained in 26/05/2007.

From 01/2013, member of the directive nucleo of Hypertension, Prevention and Rehabilitation Group of Italian Society of Cardiology.

From 12/2012, member of the Membership Working Group on Peripheral Circulation—European Society of Cardiology and of member of the Working Group on Atherosclerosis and Vascular Biology—European Society of Cardiology.

From 02/2012, member of the Working Group on Acute Cardiac Care—European Society of Cardiology.

From 03/01/2011 to 28/02/2011 Internship in Universitares Herzzentrum Hamburg—Klinik und Poliklinik fur Allgemeine und Interventionelle Kardiologie, Cardiovascular Ultrasound Imaging and Echocardiography Laboratory.

Peer reviewer and Editorial Board Member of several international journals.

Author of: 130 full article in International Scientific Journals; 260 abstracts published in International Journals; 4 chapters of scientific book.

# Preface to "Molecular Biomarkers In Cardiology"

It is a great pleasure to introduce the "Molecular Biomarkers In Cardiology" book.

The aim is to offer readers the best overview of the current state of knowledge of biomolecular biomarkers in cardiovascular diseases.

Cardiovascular diseases still represent the leading cause of death worldwide. The need to prevent the acute onset of such diseases and predict their occurrence is the major goal of medicine. By succeeding in preventing the negative consequences of cardiovascular diseases, physicians can prevent both the mortality and morbidity of the patients. Therefore, the improvement in the quality of life and the reduction in the financial burden of health due to the reduced impact of chronic comorbidities related to cardiovascular diseases will also improve the economics of the nations.

The use of biomarkers is key to conquering the tip of this target mountain.

Indeed, the ideal biomarkers should be sensitive and specific, able to detect the onset of pathologies early and in time to allow physicians to counteract the progression of the disease.

Biomolecular approaches for the early identification of cardiovascular diseases before their onset are an attractive field in cardiology. There is little evidence regarding a perfect biomarker able to identify the unstable atherosclerotic plaque, the occurrence of aortic dissection, or the incipient onset of heart failure.

The papers which had been included in this book focus on genetic and molecular aspects of coronary artery and cerebrovascular diseases. The authors concentrated on possible methods of the early identification of conditions and individual predisposition to atherosclerosis consequences.

The aim is to develop a possible model for individualizing the approach to each, single subject, thus promoting targeted preventive strategies and therapies.

**Pietro Scicchitano**
*Editor*

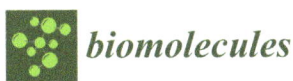 

Article

# Multimarker Approach to Identify Patients with Coronary Artery Disease at High Risk for Subsequent Cardiac Adverse Events: The Multi-Biomarker Study

Georgiana-Aura Giurgea [1], Katrin Zlabinger [2], Alfred Gugerell [2], Dominika Lukovic [2], Bonni Syeda [2], Ljubica Mandic [2], Noemi Pavo [2], Julia Mester-Tonczar [2], Denise Traxler-Weidenauer [2], Andreas Spannbauer [2], Nina Kastner [2], Claudia Müller [2], Anahit Anvari [2], Jutta Bergler-Klein [2] and Mariann Gyöngyösi [2,*]

- [1] Department of Angiology, Internal Medicine II, Medical University of Vienna, 1090 Vienna, Austria; georgiana-aura.giurgea@meduniwien.ac.at
- [2] Department of Cardiology, Internal Medicine II, Medical University of Vienna, 1090 Vienna, Austria; katrin.zlabinger@meduniwien.ac.at (K.Z.); alfred.gugerell@meduniwien.ac.at (A.G.); dominika.lukovic@meduniwien.ac.at (D.L.); b.syeda@internist-nord.at (B.S.); ljubica.mandic@gmail.com (L.M.); noemi.pavo@meduniwien.ac.at (N.P.); julia.mester-tonczar@meduniwien.ac.at (J.M.-T.); denise.traxler-weidenauer@meduniwien.ac.at (D.T.-W.); andreas.spannbauer@meduniwien.ac.at (A.S.); nina.kastner@meduniwien.ac.at (N.K.); claudia.mueller@meduniwien.ac.at (C.M.); anahit.anvari@meduniwien.ac.at (A.A.); jutta.bergler-klein@meduniwien.ac.at (J.B.-K.)
- \* Correspondence: mariann.gyongyosi@meduniwien.ac.at; Tel.: +43-1-40400-46140

Received: 8 May 2020; Accepted: 10 June 2020; Published: 15 June 2020

**Abstract:** In our prospective non-randomized, single-center cohort study ($n$ = 161), we have evaluated a multimarker approach including S100 calcium binding protein A12 (S100A1), interleukin 1 like-receptor-4 (IL1R4), adrenomedullin, copeptin, neutrophil gelatinase-associated lipocalin (NGAL), soluble urokinase plasminogen activator receptor (suPAR), and ischemia modified albumin (IMA) in prediction of subsequent cardiac adverse events (AE) during 1-year follow-up in patients with coronary artery disease. The primary endpoint was to assess the combined discriminatory predictive value of the selected 7 biomarkers in prediction of AE (myocardial infarction, coronary revascularization, death, stroke, and hospitalization) by canonical discriminant function analysis. The main secondary endpoints were the levels of the 7 biomarkers in the groups with/without AE; comparison of the calculated discriminant score of the biomarkers with traditional logistic regression and C-statistics. The canonical correlation coefficient was 0.642, with a Wilk's lambda value of 0.78 and $p < 0.001$. By using the calculated discriminant equation with the weighted mean discriminant score (centroid), the sensitivity and specificity of our model were 79.4% and 74.3% in prediction of AE. These values were higher than that of the calculated C-statistics if traditional risk factors with/without biomarkers were used for AE prediction. In conclusion, canonical discriminant analysis of the multimarker approach is able to define the risk threshold at the individual patient level for personalized medicine.

**Keywords:** multimarker approach; adverse event; risk prediction; canonical discriminant analysis; C-statistics; coronary artery disease

## 1. Introduction

Cardiovascular mortality or morbidity risk scores are essential in primary and secondary prevention of cardiovascular adverse events (AE), and are mostly based on traditional cardiovascular risk factors, such as hypertension, diabetes mellitus, hyperlipidemia, smoking, and family history. Risk scores are created and calculated for patients with acute coronary syndrome: Thrombolysis in

Myocardial Infarction (TIMI), Platelet Glycoprotein IIb/IIIa in Unstable Angina: Receptor Suppression Using Integrilin (PURSUIT), the Global Registry of Acute Coronary Events (GRACE) [1], for stable angina pectoris: Framingham Risk Score [2], Vienna and Ludwigshafen Coronary Artery Disease (VILCAD) score [3], or for general patient population, such as the SCORE-European High Risk Chart [4]. Previous studies suggested, that biomarkers of inflammation, fibrinolysis or fibrin formation, endothelial function, oxidative stress, or renal or heart function parameter enhance the value of risk prediction and enable early intervention and prevention of subsequent cardiovascular adverse events (AE) [5]. Adding of routinely used biomarkers, such as troponin T or NT-pro-brain natriuretic peptide (pro-BNP) or blood cholesterol level to the traditional risk factors enhanced moderately the risk prediction in the individual patients [6]. Single or combined new biomarkers, such as copeptin, neutrophil gelatinase-associated lipocalin (NGAL), or soluble urokinase plasminogen activator receptor (suPAR) have been tested and validated in larger cohorts of patients, anticipating prognostic values of these biomarkers [7–9]. However, statistical association between biomarkers and onset of AEs in a large patient cohort is not necessarily useful for personalized risk stratification [10]. In contrast with single blood marker analysis, the multi-biomarker approach by using traditional or new circulating proteins might have the potential to enhance the risk stratification in individual patients.

We have selected 7 non-traditional biomarkers of different classes, possessing diagnostic or prognostic significance in forecasting of cardiovascular AEs, and combined them in a multi-biomarker approach to yield prognostic value for a single patient. The selected biomarkers were as follows: S100 calcium binding protein A12 (S100A1) and interleukin 1 like-receptor-4 (ST2, IL1R4) (markers of inflammation), adrenomedullin and copeptin (vasoactive markers), NGAL (tissue injury marker), suPAR (fibrinolysis marker), and ischemia modified albumin (IMA) (oxidative stress marker).

S100A12 protein is released from activated macrophages and has been proposed to contribute to the acceleration of atherosclerosis [11,12]. Midregional pro-adrenomedullin (MR-proADM, adrenomedullin) is a potent vasodilatatory peptide, and a marker of hemodynamic stress [13,14]. Copeptin, the C-terminal portion of the vasopressin prohormone, is released stoichiometrically with vasopressin in the neurohypophysis, and in combination with troponin T, improved the early risk stratification of patients presenting with acute chest pain [15]. NGAL is a marker of acute kidney injury but has also been associated with different cardiovascular diseases and elevated in patients with heart failure after myocardial infarction [16]. The suPAR is a plasma marker of low-grade inflammation that has been associated with cardiovascular risk [17,18]. IL1R4 is up-regulated in conditions with increased myocardial strain [19–23]. IMA is a sensitive biomarker of myocardial ischemia after percutaneous coronary intervention (PCI), or during coronary artery bypass surgery (CABG), and used for risk stratification tool for suspected acute coronary syndrome or as a prognostic marker in patients with cardiopulmonary resuscitation [24,25]. All of these biomarkers have been associated with cardiovascular events in patients with coronary artery disease (CAD).

The aim of the multi-biomarker study was to evaluate the multimarker approach for personalized medicine including the selected biomarkers S100A1, adrenomedullin, copeptin, NGAL, suPAR, IL1R4, and IMA in prediction of subsequent cardiac AEs during 1-year follow-up (FUP) in patients with CAD.

## 2. Materials and Methods

### 2.1. Study Design

The multi-biomarker study and biobank is a prospective non-randomized, single-center cohort study, including patients with either stable CAD or subacute myocardial infarction (AMI)—including ST-segment elevation myocardial infarction (STEMI) or non-STEMI (NSTEMI). Blood samples were taken to assess the discriminatory values of the single or multi-biomarker approach for prediction of major cardiac AE during the 1-year FUP period. The study was conducted at the Department of Cardiology, Medical University of Vienna in accordance with the Declaration of Helsinki (1975) and approved by the Ethics Committee of the Medical University of Vienna (EK Nr: 2011/1091 and 1276/2019). Written informed consent was obtained from all patients.

*2.2. Patient Population, Inclusion and Exclusion Criteria*

Patients with stable CAD and recent AMI were included. Stable CAD was defined as previously angiographical documented CAD, with/without previous PCI, AMI, CABG, with no angina pectoris or inducible myocardial ischemia at the time of the study inclusion, recruited in the outpatient clinic. Recent AMI was defined as current STEMI or NSTEMI after primary PCI, recruited in the internal ward before hospital discharge post-AMI. The mean time of blood collection in the AMI group was $2.4 \pm 0.3$ days post AMI-onset.

Inclusion criteria were proven CAD (stable CAD or recent AMI) in patients older than 19 years, and willing to participate in the study.

Exclusion criteria were known cancer, acute or chronic infective or auto-immune inflammatory diseases, hemodynamically significant valvular diseases, hypertrophic or restrictive cardiomyopathy, congenital heart disease, previous acute renal failure, major surgery within the last 3 months, liver diseases requiring treatment, inability or unwillingness to comply with the study protocol, and chronic renal failure with glomerular filtration rate (GFR) $\leq 40$.

*2.3. Endpoints of the Study*

The primary endpoint of the study was to assess the combined discriminatory predictive value of the biomarkers S100A1, adrenomedullin, copeptin, NGAL, suPAR, IL1R4, and IMA in prediction of cardiac AE, defined as recurring myocardial infarction, coronary revascularization by PCI or CABG, death, stroke, hospitalization due to angina pectoris without revascularization or heart failure and implantation of pacemaker or automatic implantable cardioverter defibrillator /AICD/ due to malignant arrhythmias, in comparison with the usual logistic regression or C-statistics.

The secondary endpoints of the study were the levels of the 7 selected biomarkers in the subgroups of stable CAD (group CAD) and recent AMI (group AMI), association between the new biomarkers and NT-proBNP.

*2.4. Clinical Data Collection*

Baseline medical history (age, gender, presence of atherosclerotic risk factors, such as hypertension, diabetes mellitus, hyperlipidemia, smoking, previous AMI, PCI, CABG, peripheral and/or carotid artery disease), current medical treatment (daily regular dose of aspirin, clopidogrel, beta-blocker, ACE inhibitor or ARB), and transthoracic echocardiography (TTE) data (global left ventricular function expressed as wall motion score index) were recorded at the study inclusion and at the 1-year control clinical investigation.

At 1-year FUP, patients were invited to medical examination and TTE. The follow-up clinical history was documented, including the AEs.

*2.5. Laboratory Procedures*

Fasting venous blood samples were obtained into commercially available tubes. Serum and plasma aliquots were stored at $-80\ °C$ until biomarker assay. Troponin T, N-terminal-proBNP (NT-proBNP), and creatine kinase MB fraction (CK-MB) were assessed using a routine diagnostic analyzer in the hospital laboratory.

Biomarker concentrations in samples were measured by commercially available enzyme-linked immunosorbent assays (ELISA): S100A12 and copeptin from Cloud-Clone Corp. (Houston, TX, USA); suPAR, adrenomedullin and IMA from MyBioSource Inc. (San Diego, CA, USA); NGAL (Lipocalin 2) from ABCAM (Cambridge, UK) and IL1R4/ST2 from Sigma-Aldrich Co (St. Louis, MO, USA). All assays were performed according to the manufacturer's instructions.

## 2.6. Statistics

The statistical analysis was performed using SPSS® version 23 (SPSS Inc, Chicago, IL). Continuous parameters with normal or non-normal distribution were expressed as mean ± standard deviations or median with interquartile range, respectively. Categorical variables were listed as number and percentages. For all tests, two-sided analyses were used and the significance level was set at $p < 0.05$.

The predictive power of the biomarkers in classification of AEs was calculated by using canonical discriminant function analysis. The predictor (independent) variables were the 7 selected biomarkers and NT-proBNP. Wilk's lambda test was used to test the significance between the groups with/without AEs. Parameters with discriminatory function <0.3 (non-significant correlation with the other parameter with low discriminatory function between the groups) were stepwise excluded from the further discriminant function model. A discriminant score was calculated by using weighted combination of the biomarkers with >3 discriminatory function. The means and SDs of the discriminant scores and the weighted mean score cut-off values between the groups (event yes/no) were calculated and described as centroid. Sensitivity and specificity of the discriminatory score were determined from the classification results. To confirm the correctness of the scoring, individual patient discriminant scores were calculated, and the mean scores of the groups (AE or non-AE) were compared by 2-sided Student $t$-test.

Multivariate binary logistic regression analysis was performed to analyze the traditional risk factors, supplemented with the biomarkers predictive for subsequent cardiac AE. Continuous parameters were transformed to binary parameter using the quadratic difference between supposed predictive value (75% interquartile value) and observed binary outcome (0 for no event, 1 for event) for each patient. The following parameters were included into the analysis: male gender, age, presence of atherosclerotic risk factors (diabetes mellitus, hypertension, smoking, hyperlipidemia), all 7 selected biomarkers, and NT-proBNP. C-statistics was performed to predict risk and sensitivity and specificity of all included clinical and biomarker risk factors.

Linear regression analysis was used to search association between NT-proBNP (as established prognostic marker) and the 7 selected biomarkers: S100A1, adrenomedullin, copeptin, NGAL, suPAR, IL1R4, and IMA.

## 3. Results

A total of 181 patients were included in the study. Due to comorbidities possibly or definitively influencing the blood levels of the selected 7 biomarkers, such as moderate to severe acute or chronic renal failure, or malignant or other chronic disease diagnosed after study inclusion, 20 patients were excluded from the biomarker measurement study. Therefore, blood levels of the 7 selected biomarkers were measured in 161 patients and these 161 patients were included in the further analyses.

### 3.1. Clinical Events during the 1-Year FUP

In total, 48 cardiac AEs occurred. Four patients died, 8 patients experienced re-AMI, and 23 patients were hospitalized for heart failure or angina pectoris, or implantation of pacemaker or automatic implantable cardioverter defibrillator. Coronary revascularization was performed in 13 patients.

Table 1 lists the patient characteristics, and the baseline blood levels of biomarkers in all patients, and the groups AE and non-AE. Patients with adverse event at the follow-up had more often diabetes mellitus and previous bypass surgery, and more patients were smokers. NGAL, suPAR, and IL1R4 were significantly higher in group AE, however, large scatter of the data was observed.

**Table 1.** Clinical and laboratory parameters of patients with coronary artery disease with/without cardiac adverse events (AE) during the 1-year follow-up.

| Clinical and Laboratory Parameter | All Patients $n = 161$ | Group AE $n = 48$ | Group Non-AE $n = 113$ | p Value between Groups |
|---|---|---|---|---|
| Male gender n (%) | 126 (78.3%) | 35 (72.9%) | 91 (80.5%) | 0.301 |
| Age (y; mean ± SD) | 67.0 ± 11.9 | 70.4 ± 11.1 | 65.6 ± 12.0 | 0.017 |
| Diabetes mellitus n (%) | 41 (25.5%) | 18 (37.5%) | 23 (20.4%) | 0.030 |
| Hypertension n (%) | 129 (80.1%) | 41 (85.4%) | 88 (77.9%) | 0.388 |
| Hyperlipidemia n (%) | 117 (72.7%) | 37 (77.1%) | 80 (70.8%) | 0.447 |
| Smoking n (%) | 58 (36.0%) | 26 (55.3%) | 32 (28.3%) | 0.011 |
| Previous MI n (%) | 83 (51.6%) | 29 (60.4%) | 54 (47.8%) | 0.295 |
| Previous PCI n (%) | 85 (52.8%) | 22 (45.8%) | 63 (55.8%) | 0.301 |
| Previous CABG n (%) | 31 (19.3%) | 17 (35.4%) | 14 (12.4%) | 0.002 |
| PAD n (%) | 20 (12.4%) | 9 (18.8%) | 11 (9.7%) | 0.123 |
| Carotid artery disease n (%) | 28 (17.4%) | 9 (18.8%) | 19 (17.0%) | 0.822 |
| Aspirin (%) | 161 (100%) | 48 (100%) | 113 (100%) | 1 |
| Clopidogrel n (%) | 132 (82.0%) | 38 (79.2%) | 94 (83.2%) | 0.408 |
| Beta-blocker n (%) | 152 (94.4%) | 43 (89.6%) | 109 (96.4%) | 0.398 |
| ACE-inhibitor/ARB n (%) | 146 (90.7%) | 42 (87.5%) | 104 (92.0%) | 0.780 |
| NT-proBNP (median; Q) (pg/mL) | 280 (232; 335) | 282 (243; 507) | 279 (232; 309) | 0.224 |
| Troponin T (ng/L) (median; Q) (ng/mL) | 0.01 (0.01; 0.41) | 0.01 (0.01; 0.04) | 0.01 (0.01; 0.08) | 0.313 |
| Creatine kinase (U/L) (median; Q) | 116 (66; 188) | 88 (67; 177) | 118 (66; 106) | 0.541 |
| Baseline WMSI (mean ± SD) | 1.31 ± 0.46 | 1.22 ± 0.45 | 1.34 ± 0.47 | 0.115 |
| Follow-up WMSI (mean ± SD) | 1.31 ± 0.51 | 1.28 ± 0.51 | 1.32 ± 0.51 | 0.651 |
| **Selected biomarkers (Median, 25% and 75% Quartiles)** | | | | |
| S100A1(ng/mL) | 5504 (0; 11858) | 5311 (0; 14462) | 5674 (0; 11327) | 0.724 |
| Adrenomedullin (ng/mL) | 189 (146; 328) | 178 (144; 279) | 194 (150; 343) | 0.187 |
| Copeptin (pg/mL) | 1049 (817; 1049) | 938 (731; 1049) | 1049 (844; 1049) | 0.058 |
| NGAL (pg/mL) | 18.5 (11.0; 39.0) | 40.3 (16.5; 57.7) | 16.2 (9.9; 27.6) | <0.05 |
| suPAR (ng/mL) | 5.37 (3.70; 8.51) | 9.18 (3.58; 11.99) | 4.94 (3.70; 6.95) | <0.05 |
| IL1R4 (pg/mL) | 347 (211; 616) | 542 (222; 769) | 318 (193; 548) | <0.05 |
| IMA (ng/mL) | 167 (53; 219) | 156 (34; 211) | 178 (76; 221) | 0.120 |

MI: myocardial infarction; PCI: percutaneous coronary intervention; CABG: coronary artery bypass graft surgery; PAD: peripheral artery disease; ACE: angiotensin converting enzyme; ARB: angiotensin receptor blocker; NT-proBNP: N-terminal pro-brain natriuretic peptide; WMSI: wall motion score index, S100A1: S100 calcium binding protein A12; NGAL: neutrophil gelatinase-associated lipocalin; suPAR: soluble urokinase plasminogen activator receptor; IL1R4: interleukin 1 like-receptor-4; IMA: ischemia modified albumin. Q: 25% and 75% quartiles.

### 3.2. Multimarker Approach for Prediction of Adverse Events

The structure matrix of the canonical discriminant analysis including all selected 7 biomarkers showed low (<0.3) Pearson correlation between S100A1, adrenomedullin, copeptin, and IMA and the other biomarkers, with a low sensitivity of 43.5% and high specificity of 94.5% in prediction of AE. In order to increase the sensitivity of the multiple biomarker testing, we have stepwise excluded biomarkers with low level of correlation between the other markers. Finally, including the factors with the strongest discriminant predictive power, NGAL, suPAR, and IL1R4, the canonical correlation coefficient was 0.496, with a Wilk's lambda value of 0.001, resulting in a discriminant model of:

$$\text{Discriminant score} = -2.01 + 0.025 \times \text{NGAL}_i + 0.130 \times \text{suPAR}_i + 0.001 \times \text{IL1R4}_i,$$

where i: individual value of the same patient.

The weighted mean discriminant score (cutting point, centroid) was 0.225 (Figure 1), resulting in a sensitivity of 79.4% and specificity of 74.3% in prediction of adverse event, if the calculated discriminant equation was used. Accordingly, 76.9% of patients have been correctly classified to groups AE or non-AE if the calculated scores were used in the individual patient level. Patients with AEs had significantly higher discriminant value (calculated from the discriminant equation) as compared with patients without events (Figure 1).

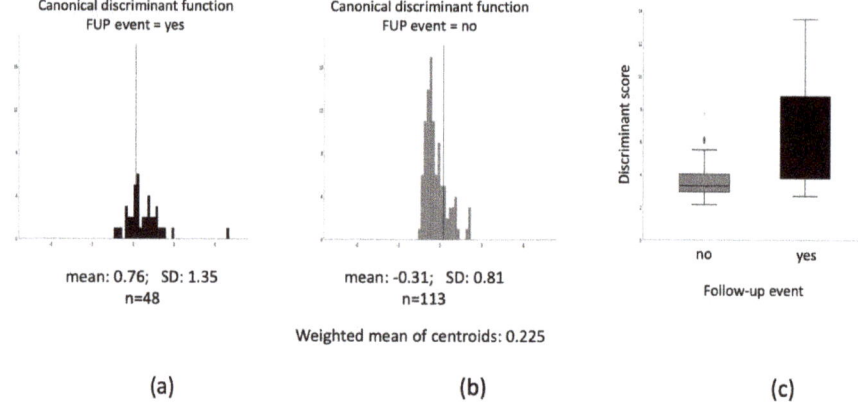

**Figure 1.** Discriminant scores, weighted mean of centroids, and C-statistics of patients experiencing cardiovascular adverse events. (**a**) and (**b**) discriminant score values of patients with (**a**) or without (**b**) adverse events at the 1-year follow-up (FUP); (**c**) mean (SD) discriminant scores of patients with or without adverse events at the FUP.

Interestingly, including NT-proBNP into the model did not enhance the power of the analysis, e.g., it did not increase the sensitivity/specificity values of the event prediction, most probably due to the significant association between NT-proBNP and NGAL or suPAR or IL1R4, respectively (Figure 2).

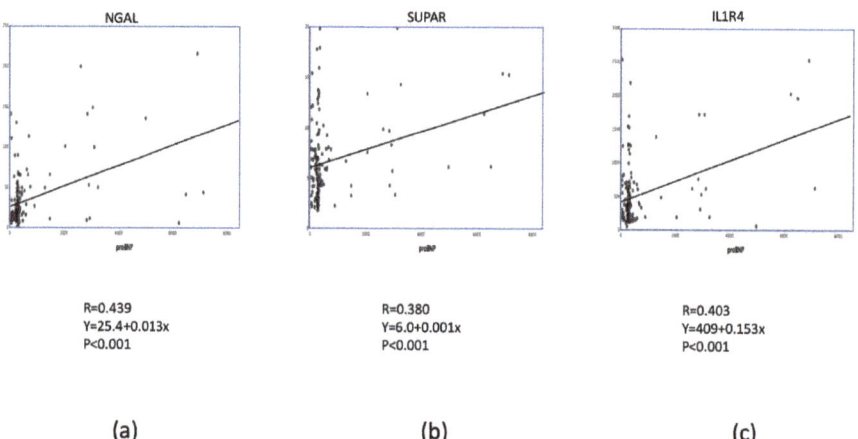

**Figure 2.** Significant correlation between N-terminal-pro-brain natriuretic peptide (NT-proBNP) (pg/mL) and new biomarkers with (**a**) neutrophil gelatinase-associated lipocalin (NGAL) (pg/mL); (**b**) soluble urokinase plasminogen activator receptor (SUPAR) (ng/mL); (**c**) interleukin 1 like-receptor-4 (ST2, IL1R4) (pg/mL).

### 3.3. Risk Prediction Including Clinical Variables by Using Logistic Regression and C-Statistics

Binary logistic regression analysis including the traditional risk factors (age, male gender, diabetes, hypertension, hyperlipidemia, and smoking) could not reveal any significant predictors for adverse events. C-statistics revealed a C value (area under the curve of ROC analysis) of 0.58, with no significant prediction value for AEs (Figure 3).

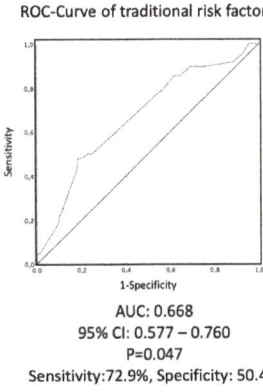
ROC-Curve of traditional risk factors
AUC: 0.668
95% CI: 0.577 – 0.760
P=0.047
Sensitivity:72.9%, Specificity: 50.4%

(a)

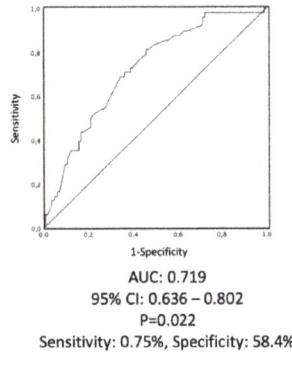
ROC-Curve of traditional risk factors + biomarkers
AUC: 0.719
95% CI: 0.636 – 0.802
P=0.022
Sensitivity: 0.75%, Specificity: 58.4%

(b)

**Figure 3.** C-statistics and receiver operator characteristics (ROC) curves of predictive adverse events of patients experiencing cardiovascular adverse events. (**a**) ROC curve analysis if traditional risk factors (male gender, older age, diabetes, hypertension, hyperlipidemia, and smoking) were included into the analysis; (**b**) ROC curve if 7 biomarkers and NT-proBNP were additionally included into the analysis of traditional risk factors.

Entering of the selected 7 biomarkers and NT-proBNP into the logistic regression analysis containing also the traditional risk factors did not result in any significant predictors. However, adding the 8 biomarkers increased moderately but significantly the prediction of AEs by a C value of 0.668 ($p = 0.047$) (Figure 3) in the C-statistics, with an optimized sensitivity and specificity values of 72.9% and 50.4%.

*3.4. Diagnostic Value of Selected Biomarkers in Recent AMI*

Patients were classified into subgroups CAD ($n = 39$) and AMI ($n = 42$). Table 2 lists the baseline clinical variables of the subgroups. Patients in the group CAD had a higher incidence of previous AMI and PCI. Patients in the AMI group had higher NT-proBNP, CK, and TnT 2.4 ± 0.3 days post AMI onset.

**Table 2.** Clinical and laboratory parameters of subgroup of patients with stable coronary artery disease (subgroup CAD) or with recent acute myocardial infarction (subgroup AMI).

| Clinical and Laboratory Parameter | Subgroup CAD $n = 111$ | Subgroup AMI $n = 50$ | $p$ Value between the Groups |
|---|---|---|---|
| Male gender n (%) | 89 (80.2%) | 37 (74.0%) | 0.412 |
| Age (y; mean ± SD) | 68.4 ± 11.5 | 64.0 ± 12.3 | 0.036 |
| Diabetes mellitus n (%) | 34 (30.6%) | 7 (14.0%) | 0.031 |
| Hypertension n (%) | 92 (82.9%) | 37 (74.0%) | 0.205 |
| Hyperlipidemia n (%) | 77 (69.4%) | 40 (80.0%) | 0.185 |
| Smoking n (%) | 34 (30.6%) | 24 (48.0%) | 0.167 |
| Previous MI n (%) | 71 (64.0%) | 12 (24.0%) | <0.001 |
| Previous PCI n (%) | 74 (66.7%) | 11 (22.0%) | <0.001 |
| Previous CABG n (%) | 25 (22.5%) | 6 (12.0%) | 0.135 |
| PAD n (%) | 15 (13.5%) | 5 (10.0%) | 0.614 |
| Carotid artery disease n (%) | 23 (20.7%) | 5 (10%) | 0.117 |
| Aspirin n (%) | 111 (100%) | 50 (100%) | 1 |
| Clopidogrel n (%) | 92 (82.9%) | 40 (80.0%) | 0.666 |
| Beta-blocker n (%) | 102 (91.9%) | 50 (100%) | 0.863 |
| ACE-inhibitor/ARB n (%) | 102 (91.9%) | 44 (88.0%) | 0.814 |

Table 2. Cont.

| Clinical and Laboratory Parameter | Subgroup CAD n = 111 | Subgroup AMI n = 50 | p Value between the Groups |
|---|---|---|---|
| NT-proBNP (median; Q) (pg/mL) | 278 (241; 301) | 359 (182; 881) | 0.029 |
| Troponin T (ng/L) (median; Q) (ng/mL) | 0.01 (0.01; 0.01) | 0.26 (0.04; 2.33) | <0.001 |
| Creatine kinase (U/L) (median; Q) | 85 (55; 137) | 248 (131; 569) | <0.001 |
| Baseline WMSI (mean ± SD) | 1.29 ± 0.43 | 1.34 ± 0.54 | 0.611 |
| Follow-up WMSI (mean ± SD) | 1.29 ± 0.46 | 1.34 ± 0.64 | 0.716 |
| FUP events n (%) | 30 (27.0%) | 18 (36.0%) | 0.268 |
| Hospitalization n (%) | 16 (14.4%) | 7 (14.0%) | |
| Acute MI n (%) | 6 (5.4%) | 2 (4.0%) | |
| Revascularization n (%) | 6 (5.4%) | 7 (14%) | |
| Death n (%) | 2 (1.8%) | 2 (4.0%) | |

MI: myocardial infarction; PCI: percutaneous coronary intervention; ACBP: aorto-coronary bypass surgery; PAD: peripheral artery disease; ACE: angiotensin converting enzyme; ARB: angiotensin receptor blocker; NT-proBNP: N-terminal pro-brain natriuretic peptide; WMSI: wall motion score index; Q: 25% and 75% quartiles.

Table 2 and Figure 4 shows the blood levels of biomarkers. Beside the significantly elevated NT-proBNP value in the AMI group, from the 7 new biomarkers, only suPAR showed a trend towards higher value in the AMI group.

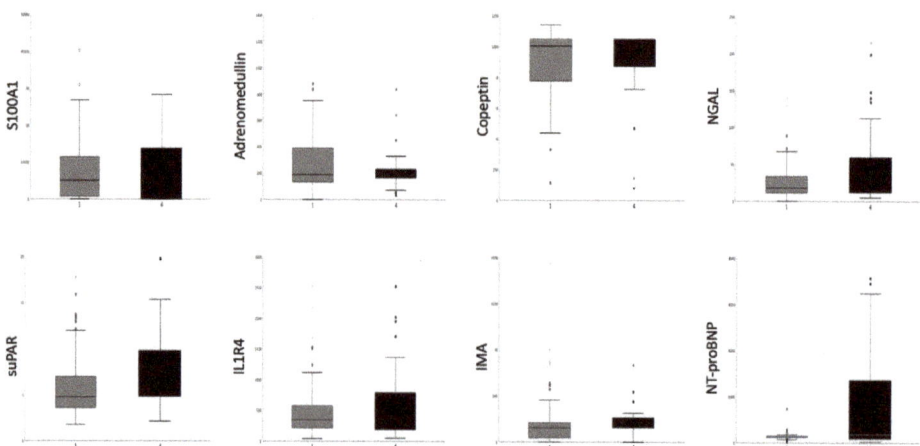

**Figure 4.** Blood levels of biomarkers of patients with stable coronary artery disease (subgroup CAD) or with recent acute myocardial infarction (subgroup AMI). S100 calcium binding protein A12 (S100A1) (ng/mL), adrenomedullin (ng/mL), copeptin (pg/mL), neutrophil gelatinase-associated lipocalin (NGAL) (pg/mL), soluble urokinase plasminogen activator receptor (suPAR) (ng/mL), interleukin 1 like-receptor-4 (ST2, IL1R4) (pg/mL), ischemia modified albumin (IMA) ng/mL), N-terminal-pro-brain natriuretic peptide (NT-proBNP) (pg/mL). No significant differences between the subgroups.

## 4. Discussion

To our knowledge, this is the first study to use the multi-biomarker approach by using the absolute values of the blood biomarkers, by using canonical discriminant analysis. Our study demonstrated, that (1) canonical discriminant analysis of the multimarker approach is able to define risk threshold in the individual single patient level; (2) the weighted mean discriminant score (cutting point, centroid) resulted in a sensitivity of 79.4% and specificity of 74.3% in prediction of adverse event, if calculated discriminant equation was used, with 76.9% of patients classified correctly to groups AE or non-AE; (3) classical C-statistics for adverse event prediction including the traditional risk factors (age, male gender, diabetes, hypertension, hyperlipidemia, and smoking) and 8 biomarkers revealed a C value of 0.719 ($p = 0.022$), with a sensitivity and specificity values of 75.0% and 58.4%; (4) canonical discriminant analysis using the absolute values of biomarkers of coronary artery disease has a better sensitivity and specificity in prediction of adverse events than the usual logistic regression or C-statistics in a single patient level. Additionally, our study revealed low diagnostic value of the selected 7 biomarkers in patients with recent AMI.

We have selected different class biomarkers (inflammation, vasoactive, fibrinolysis, oxidative stress, and tissue injury), since the biomarker of the same or similar classes may have coincidental information, failing to give additive values in event prediction. Additionally, a limited number of non-correlative markers may better improve the risk stratification than a larger number of biomarkers acting in the similar biological pathway. Most probably, this might be the reason, why the additive biomarker NT-proBNP did not improve the sensitivity/specificity values in our study, since NT-proBNP showed a significant correlation with all 3 biomarkers entered into the discriminant equation.

Previous studies investigating the role of multiple biomarkers in patients with or without CAD have demonstrated only modest improvement in predictive accuracy, by using C-statistic, if biomarkers were added to traditional clinical risk factors [26,27]. C-statistics are commonly applied to quantify and evaluate the risk score in patients with predefined AEs [28]. In C-statistics, a receiver operating characteristic (ROC) curve displays the diagnostic capacity of a binary classification system. In contrast discriminant analysis, it is allowed to utilize the continuous absolute values of the measured parameters without compulsory transformation of the continuous variables to categorical ones. Therefore, this analysis type may separate the groups by the most exact way and discard parameters mathematically which have less prediction value in the group classification. We did not include the established clinical risk factors into our discriminant model, because (1) dichotomy variables might weaken the prediction of AEs in our mathematical model; (2) the control of the cardiovascular risk factors via first and second prevention and guided therapies modify the course of heart diseases, effectively balancing the pre-existing risk; and (3) presence of multiple risk factors influences the co-incident risk factors, such as diabetic nephropathy results in hypertension, or male patients have higher risk for event in younger age than woman in similar age.

The sensitivity and specificity values of our discriminant model were 79.4.% and 74.3%, below the expected prediction values of over 80%, even if Wilk's lambda statistic value was significant. This is probably due to the heterogeneous patient population. We recognized a large scatter of the blood levels of the individual biomarkers, raising methodological concerns of the available ELISA kits.

The usual multivariate binary logistic regression model including the traditional risk factors did not reveal any significant predictors, even not, if the biomarkers (7 selected and NT-proBNP) were included into the model with mandatory transformation of the continuous variables to categorical ones. In contrast, C-statistics presented non-significant predictor values of the traditional risk factors, but adding the 8 biomarkers to the model improved the prediction significantly, albeit moderately. However, this latter approach still presented a less predictive accuracy with less optimal sensitivity and specificity values. The discrepancies between the outcomes of the logistic regression and C-statistics indicate the inconsistencies in statistical results, if individual patient risk prediction is required.

Our study has some limitations. There are several biomarkers associated with autoimmune diseases (such as copeptin with multiple sclerosis, NGAL, and systemic lupus erythematosus), therefore we have excluded patients with autoimmune disorders from our study [29,30]. We have also excluded patients with moderate or severe renal failure, because circulating levels of several biomarkers (copeptin, NT-proBNP, NGAL) are influenced by chronic kidney disease, independent from the coronary artery disease. Most of the assumptions needed for the correct calculation of the discriminant analysis were fulfilled, e.g., independent cases, within-group variance-co-variance matrices are equal across the groups; categorical parameter is used for group variable. However, some predictor variables do not have multivariate normal distribution, but our analysis including 161 patients is robust enough to overcome this assumption, and has high sensitivity and specificity to balance the outliers. As usual, in academic studies, our patient collective is heterogeneous, with a relatively small effect size in terms of AEs. However, a multimarker approach with calculated discriminant scores might be helpful for individual patient stratification, and improves the risk calculation at the individual patient level. Measuring more biomarkers would definitively increase in cost, with eventually only minor additive value in risk prediction.

## 5. Conclusions

Our canonical discriminatory model with multimarker approach is able to define a risk threshold at the individual patient level, additive to the conventional risk stratifications as part of personalized medicine in cardiology.

**Author Contributions:** Conceptualization, G.-A.G., B.S., J.B.-K., and M.G.; methodology, A.G., D.L., L.M., J.M.-T., and N.K.; validation, G.-A.G., N.P., D.T.-W., and J.B.-K.; formal analysis, K.Z., A.G., L.M., J.M.-T., D.T.-W., A.S., N.K., C.M., A.A., and M.G.; investigation, A.-G.G., B.S., L.M., J.B.-K., and M.G.; data curation, A.-G.G., K.Z., D.L., B.S., L.M., J.B.-K., C.M., A.A., and M.G.; writing—original draft preparation, G.-A.G., J.B.-K., and M.G.; writing—review and editing, K.Z., A.G., A.S., D.L., B.S., L.M., N.P., J.M.-T., D.T.-W., and N.K.; supervision, A.S.; project administration, G.-A.G., B.S., C.M., A.A., and L.M. All authors have read and agreed to the published version of the manuscript.

**Funding:** This research received no external funding.

**Conflicts of Interest:** The authors declare no conflict of interest.

## References

1. Morrow, D.A. Cardiovascular risk prediction in patients with stable and unstable coronary heart disease. *Circulation* **2010**, *121*, 2681–2691. [CrossRef]
2. Schnabel, R.B.; Sullivan, L.M.; Levy, D.; Pencina, M.J.; Massaro, J.M.; D'Agostino, R.B., Sr.; Newton-Cheh, C.; Yamamoto, J.F.; Magnani, J.W.; Tadros, T.M.; et al. Development of a risk score for atrial fibrillation (Framingham Heart Study): A community-based cohort study. *Lancet* **2009**, *373*, 739–745. [CrossRef]
3. Goliasch, G.; Kleber, M.E.; Richter, B.; Plischke, M.; Hoke, M.; Haschemi, A.; Marculescu, R.; Endler, G.; Grammer, T.B.; Pilz, S.; et al. Routinely available biomarkers improve prediction of long-term mortality in stable coronary artery disease: The Vienna and Ludwigshafen Coronary Artery Disease (VILCAD) risk score. *Eur. Heart J.* **2012**, *33*, 2282–2289. [CrossRef] [PubMed]
4. Conroy, R.M.; Pyörälä, K.; Fitzgerald, A.P.; Sans, S.; Menotti, A.; De Backer, G.; De Bacquer, D.; Ducimetière, P.; Jousilahti, P.; Keil, U.; et al. SCORE project group. Estimation of ten-year risk of fatal cardiovascular disease in Europe: The SCORE project. *Eur. Heart J.* **2003**, *24*, 987–1003. [CrossRef]
5. Meeuwsen, J.A.L.; Wesseling, M.; Hoefer, I.E.; de Jager, S.C.A. Prognostic value of circulating inflammatory cells in patients with stable and acute coronary artery disease. *Front. Cardiovasc. Med.* **2017**, *4*, 44. [CrossRef] [PubMed]
6. Tang, W.H. Contemporary challenges in translating biomarker evidence into clinical practice. *J. Am. Coll. Cardiol.* **2010**, *55*, 2077–2079. [CrossRef]
7. Reichlin, T.; Hochholzer, W.; Stelzig, C.; Laule, K.; Freidank, H.; Morgenthaler, N.G.; Bergmann, A.; Potocki, M.; Noveanu, M.; Breidthardt, T.; et al. Incremental value of copeptin for rapid rule out of acute myocardial infarction. *J. Am. Coll. Cardiol.* **2009**, *54*, 60–68. [CrossRef]
8. Nakada, Y.; Kawakami, R.; Matsui, M.; Ueda, T.; Nakano, T.; Takitsume, A.; Nakagawa, H.; Nishida, T.; Onoue, K.; Soeda, T.; et al. Prognostic value of urinary neutrophil gelatinase-associated lipocalin on the first day of admission for adverse events in patients with acute decompensated heart failure. *J. Am. Heart Assoc.* **2017**, *6*. [CrossRef] [PubMed]
9. Sehestedt, T.; Lyngbaek, S.; Eugen-Olsen, J.; Jeppesen, J.; Andersen, O.; Hansen, T.W.; Linneberg, A.; Jørgensen, T.; Haugaard, S.B.; Olsen, M.H.; et al. Soluble urokinase plasminogen activator receptor is associated with subclinical organ damage and cardiovascular events. *Atherosclerosis* **2011**, *216*, 237–243. [CrossRef]
10. Wang, T.J. Multiple biomarkers for predicting cardiovascular events: Lessons learned. *J. Am. Coll. Cardiol.* **2010**, *55*, 2092–2095. [CrossRef]

11. Mori, Y.; Kosaki, A.; Kishimoto, N.; Kimura, T.; Iida, K.; Fukui, M.; Nakajima, F.; Nagahara, M.; Urakami, M.; Iwasaka, T.; et al. Increased plasma S100A12 (EN-RAGE) levels in hemodialysis patients with atherosclerosis. *Am. J. Nephrol.* **2009**, *29*, 18–24. [CrossRef] [PubMed]
12. Shiotsu, Y.; Mori, Y.; Nishimura, M.; Sakoda, C.; Tokoro, T.; Hatta, T.; Maki, N.; Iida, K.; Iwamoto, N.; Ono, T.; et al. Plasma S100A12 level is associated with cardiovascular disease in hemodialysis patients. *Clin. J. Am. Soc. Nephrol.* **2011**, *6*, 718–723. [CrossRef]
13. Khan, S.Q.; O'Brien, R.J.; Struck, J.; Quinn, P.; Morgenthaler, N.; Squire, I.; Davies, J.; Bergmann, A.; Ng, L.L. Prognostic value of midregional pro-adrenomedullin in patients with acute myocardial infarction: The LAMP (Leicester Acute Myocardial Infarction Peptide) study. *J. Am. Coll. Cardiol.* **2007**, *49*, 1525–1532. [CrossRef]
14. Wild, P.S.; Schnabel, R.B.; Lubos, E.; Zeller, T.; Sinning, C.R.; Keller, T.; Tzikas, S.; Lackner, K.J.; Peetz, D.; Rupprecht, H.J.; et al. Midregional proadrenomedullin for prediction of cardiovascular events in coronary artery disease: Results from the AtheroGene study. *Clin. Chem.* **2012**, *58*, 226–236. [CrossRef] [PubMed]
15. Keller, T.; Tzikas, S.; Zeller, T.; Czyz, E.; Lillpopp, L.; Ojeda, F.M.; Roth, A.; Bickel, C.; Baldus, S.; Sinning, C.R.; et al. Copeptin improves early diagnosis of acute myocardial infarction. *J. Am. Coll. Cardiol.* **2010**, *55*, 2096–2106. [CrossRef] [PubMed]
16. Yndestad, A.; Landro, L.; Ueland, T.; Dahl, C.P.; Flo, T.H.; Vinge, L.E.; Espevik, T.; Frøland, S.S.; Husberg, C.; Christensen, G.; et al. Increased systemic and myocardial expression of neutrophil gelatinase-associated lipocalin in clinical and experimental heart failure. *Eur. Heart J.* **2009**, *30*, 1229–1236. [CrossRef] [PubMed]
17. Eugen-Olsen, J.; Andersen, O.; Linneberg, A.; Ladelund, S.; Hansen, T.W.; Langkilde, A.; Petersen, J.; Pielak, T.; Møller, L.N.; Jeppesen, J.; et al. Circulating soluble urokinase plasminogen activator receptor predicts cancer, cardiovascular disease, diabetes and mortality in the general population. *J. Intern. Med.* **2010**, *268*, 296–308. [CrossRef]
18. Koller, L.; Stojkovic, S.; Richter, B.; Sulzgruber, P.; Potolidis, C.; Liebhart, F.; Mörtl, D.; Berger, R.; Goliasch, G.; Wojta, J.; et al. Soluble urokinase-type plasminogen activator receptor improves risk prediction in patients with chronic heart failure. *JACC Heart Fail.* **2017**, *5*, 268–277. [CrossRef]
19. Dieplinger, B.; Mueller, T. Soluble ST2 in heart failure. *ClinChimActa* **2015**, *443*, 57–70. [CrossRef]
20. Sabatine, M.S.; Morrow, D.A.; Higgins, L.J.; MacGillivray, C.; Guo, W.; Bode, C.; Rifai, N.; Cannon, C.P.; Gerszten, R.E.; Lee, R.T.; et al. Complementary roles for biomarkers of biomechanical strain ST2 and N-terminal prohormone B-type natriuretic peptide in patients with ST-elevation myocardial infarction. *Circulation* **2008**, *117*, 1936–1944. [CrossRef] [PubMed]
21. Dhillon, O.S.; Narayan, H.K.; Quinn, P.A.; Squire, I.B.; Davies, J.E.; Ng, L.L. Interleukin 33 and ST2 in non-ST-elevation myocardial infarction: Comparison with Global Registry of Acute Coronary Events Risk Scoring and NT-proBNP. *Am. Heart J.* **2011**, *161*, 1163–1170. [CrossRef] [PubMed]
22. Eggers, K.M.; Armstrong, P.W.; Califf, R.M.; Simoons, M.L.; Venge, P.; Wallentin, L.; James, S.K. ST2 and mortality in non-ST-segment elevation acute coronary syndrome. *Am. Heart J.* **2010**, *159*, 788–794. [CrossRef]
23. Dieplinger, B.; Egger, M.; Haltmayer, M.; Kleber, M.E.; Scharnagl, H.; Silbernagel, G.; de Boer, R.A.; Maerz, W.; Mueller, T. Increased soluble ST2 predicts long-term mortality in patients with stable coronary artery disease: Results from the Ludwigshafen risk and cardiovascular health study. *Clin. Chem.* **2014**, *60*, 530–540. [CrossRef] [PubMed]
24. Turedi, S.; Gunduz, A.; Mentese, A.; Dasdibi, B.; Karahan, S.C.; Sahin, A.; Tuten, G.; Kopuz, M.; Alver, A. Investigation of the possibility of using ischemia-modified albumin as a novel and early prognostic marker in cardiac arrest patients after cardiopulmonary resuscitation. *Resuscitation* **2009**, *80*, 994–999. [CrossRef] [PubMed]
25. Kanko, M.; Yavuz, S.; Duman, C.; Hosten, T.; Oner, E.; Berki, T. Ischemia-modified albumin use as a prognostic factor in coronary bypass surgery. *J. Cardiothorac. Surg.* **2012**, *7*, 3. [CrossRef] [PubMed]
26. Kim, H.C.; Greenland, P.; Rossouw, J.E.; Manson, J.E.; Cochrane, B.B.; Lasser, N.L.; Limacher, M.C.; Lloyd-Jones, D.M.; Margolis, K.L.; Robinson, J.G. Multimarker prediction of coronary heart disease risk. *J. Am. Coll. Cardiol.* **2010**, *55*, 2080–2091. [CrossRef] [PubMed]
27. Wang, T.J.; Gona, P.; Larson, M.G.; Tofler, G.H.; Levy, D.; Newton-Cheh, C.; Jacques, P.F.; Rifai, N.; Selhub, J.; Robins, S.J.; et al. Multiple biomarkers for the prediction of first major cardiovascular events and death. *N. Engl. J. Med.* **2006**, *355*, 2631–2639. [CrossRef] [PubMed]
28. Uno, H.; Cai, T.; Pencina, M.J.v.; D'Agostino, R.B.; Wei, L.J. On the C-statistics for evaluating overall adequacy of risk prediction procedures with censored survival data. *Stat. Med.* **2011**, *30*, 1105–1117. [CrossRef]

29. Baranowska-Bik, A.; Kochanowski, J.; Uchman, D.; Litwiniuk, A.; Kalisz, M.; Martynska, L.; Wolinska-Witort, E.; Baranowska, B.; Bik, W. Association of copeptin and cortisol in newly diagnosed multiple sclerosis patients. *J. Neuroimmunol.* **2015**, *282*, 21–24. [CrossRef] [PubMed]
30. Gómez-Puerta, J.A.; Ortiz-Reyes, B.; Urrego, T.; Vanegas-García, A.L.; Muñoz, C.H.; González, L.A.; Cervera, R.; Vásquez, G. Urinary neutrophil gelatinase-associated lipocalin and monocyte chemoattractant protein 1 as biomarkers for lupus nephritis in Colombian SLE patients. *Lupus* **2018**, *27*, 637–646. [CrossRef]

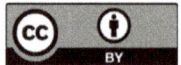

© 2020 by the authors. Licensee MDPI, Basel, Switzerland. This article is an open access article distributed under the terms and conditions of the Creative Commons Attribution (CC BY) license (http://creativecommons.org/licenses/by/4.0/).

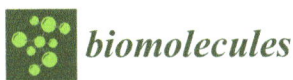 

Article

# Analysis of Differentially Expressed Genes in Coronary Artery Disease by Integrated Microarray Analysis

Meenashi Vanathi Balashanmugam [1], Thippeswamy Boreddy Shivanandappa [1], Sivagurunathan Nagarethinam [1], Basavaraj Vastrad [2] and Chanabasayya Vastrad [3,*]

1. Department of Biomedical Sciences, College of Pharmacy, Shaqra University, Al Dawadmi 11911, Saudi Arabia; meenashivanathi@gmail.com (M.V.B.); t_swamy@hotmail.com (T.B.S.); sivagurunathann@gmail.com (S.N.)
2. Department of Pharmaceutics, SET'S College of Pharmacy, Dharwad, Karnataka 580002, India; basavarajmv@gmail.com
3. Biostatistics and Bioinformatics, Chanabasava Nilaya, Bharthinagar, Dharwad 580001, Karanataka
* Correspondence: channu.vastrad@gmail.com; Tel.: +91-9480-073398

Received: 16 November 2019; Accepted: 20 December 2019; Published: 25 December 2019

**Abstract:** Coronary artery disease (CAD) is a major cause of end-stage cardiac disease. Although profound efforts have been made to illuminate the pathogenesis, the molecular mechanisms of CAD remain to be analyzed. To identify the candidate genes in the advancement of CAD, microarray dataset GSE23766 was downloaded from the Gene Expression Omnibus database. The differentially expressed genes (DEGs) were identified, and pathway and gene ontology (GO) enrichment analyses were performed. The protein-protein interaction network was constructed and the module analysis was performed using the Biological General Repository for Interaction Datasets (BioGRID) and Cytoscape. Additionally, target genes-miRNA regulatory network and target genes-TF regulatory network were constructed and analyzed. There were 894 DEGs between male human CAD samples and female human CAD samples, including 456 up regulated genes and 438 down regulated genes. Pathway enrichment analyses revealed that DEGs (up and down regulated) were mostly enriched in the superpathway of steroid hormone biosynthesis, ABC transporters, oxidative ethanol degradation III and Complement and coagulation cascades. Similarly, geneontology enrichment analyses revealed that DEGs (up and down regulated) were mostly enriched in the forebrain neuron differentiation, filopodium membrane, platelet degranulation and blood microparticle. In the PPI network and modules (up and down regulated), MYC, NPM1, TRPC7, UBC, FN1, HEMK1, IFT74 and VHL were hub genes. In the target genes-miRNA regulatory network and target genes—TF regulatory network (up and down regulated), TAOK1, KHSRP, HSD17B11 and PAH were target genes. In conclusion, the pathway and GO ontology enriched by DEGs may reveal the molecular mechanism of CAD. Its hub and target genes, MYC, NPM1, TRPC7, UBC, FN1, HEMK1, IFT74, VHL, TAOK1, KHSRP, HSD17B11 and PAH were expected to be new targets for CAD. Our finding provided clues for exploring molecular mechanism and developing new prognostics, diagnostic and therapeutic strategies for CAD.

**Keywords:** coronary artery disease; differentially expressed genes; hub genes; protein-protein interaction network; pathway enrichment analyses

## 1. Introduction

Coronary artery disease (CAD), the most common type of heart disease, is considered a complicated disease. CAD is caused due to narrowing or blockage of the coronary arteries due to buildup of cholesterol and fatty deposits on the inner walls of the arteries [1]. The causes of CAD consist of genetic risk and environmental influence [2–4]. Compared with histological classification, genes play many key roles in the diagnosis, treatment, and prognosis of CAD [5]. Alteration in genes such as ABCA1 [6] and human paraoxonase/arylesterase (HUMPONA) [7] were associated with development of CAD. Polymorphism in genes such as β fibrinogen [8] apolipoprotein A-I [9] heme oxygenase-1 [10], PON1 and PON2 [11], PAI-1 [12], MMP-2, MMP-3, MMP-9 and MMP-12 [13], NADH/NADPH oxidase [14] and angiotensin II type 1 receptor [15] were responsible for the progression of CAD. To date, the precise molecular mechanisms of CAD are still unknown, it is extremely important to uncover the underlying genes contributed to CAD.

With the rapid development of microarray technology, some high throughput platforms for analysis of gene expression are widely used to explore the differentially expressed genes (DEGs) during progression of cardiac diseases and molecular mechanisms of cardiovascular drugs [16,17]. However, the DEGs diagnosed with microarray dependon the sample size, gender, grading, and ethnic group, etc. The genes obtained from microarrays might be more representative.

In the current study, messenger RNA (mRNA) microarray datasets (GSE23766) were downloaded from the Gene Expression Omnibus (GEO) database, which were subsequently analyzed to obtain overlapping DEGs. Pathway and gene ontology (GO) enrichment analysis and PPI network construction, module analysis, target genes-miRNA regulatory network construction and target genes-TF regulatory network construction were applied to diagnose the important genes linked with CAD.

## 2. Materials and Methods

### 2.1. Microarray Data and Data Processing

Flowchart of materials and methods is shown in Figure 1. The gene expression profile GSE23766 was downloaded from the GEO database (http://www.ncbi.nlm.nih.gov/geo/), which were all based on GPL6480 Agilent-014850 Whole Human Genome Microarray 4 × 44K G4112F (AGILENT TECHNOLOGIES, INC, 5301 Stevens Creek Blvd, Santa Clara, CA 95051, USA). The GSE23766 dataset contained 16 male human CAD samples and 16 female human CAD samples. Series Matrix text files of the dataset were obtained. Subsequently, background correction, quartile normalization and probe summarization were performed with the limma R package [18,19].

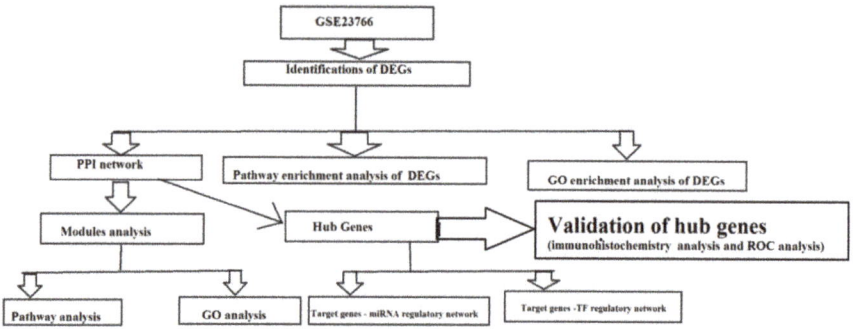

**Figure 1.** Study design (flow diagram of study).

### 2.2. Identification of DEGs between Male CAD and Female CAD Samples

In this study, we used an empirical Bayes t-test (eBayes) to identify the DEGs between male human CAD samples and female human CAD samples with cutoff value |log2(Fold Change)| > 0.1694 for up regulated genes, |log2(Fold Change)| > 0.229 for down regulated genes and adjusted $p$-value < 0.05.

## 2.3. Pathway Enrichment Analysis of DEGs

The pathway enrichment of candidate DEGs were analyzed using multiple online databases. ToppGene (ToppFun) (https://toppgene.cchmc.org/enrichment.jsp) [20] is a website for gene annotation and visualization with an integrated discovery function and can, therefore, provide the biological meaning of genes, including gene annotations and visualization. Pathway enrichment analysis of DEGs was carried out using the Kyoto Encyclopedia of Genes and Genomes (KEGG; http://www.genome.jp/kegg/) [21], Pathway Interaction Database (PID, http://pid.nci.nih.gov/) [22], Reactome (https://reactome.org/PathwayBrowser/) [23], Molecular signatures database (MSigDB, http://software.broadinstitute.org/gsea/msigdb/) [24], GenMAPP (http://www.genmapp.org/) [25], Pathway Ontology (https://bioportal.bioontology.org/ontologies/PW) [26] and PantherDB (http://www.pantherdb.org/) [27] websites, with $p < 0.05$ as the cutoff value.

## 2.4. GO Enrichment Analysis of DEGs

GO (http://www.geneontology.org/) [28] analysis is a common genes analysis method, which can contribute functional classification for genomic data, with categories of biological processes (BP), cellular component (CC), and molecular function (MF). ToppGene (ToppFun) (https://toppgene.cchmc.org/enrichment.jsp) [20] is an online tool for gene functional classification, which can systematic and integrative analysis of large gene lists.

## 2.5. Comprehensive Analysis of PPI Network and Modules

We used Biological General Repository for Interaction Datasets (BioGRID) (https://thebiogrid.org/) to assess protein–protein interaction (PPI) information [29]. In addition, in order to explore the relationship between DEGs, we used the BioGRID which is integrated with various protein interaction database partners such as Molecular INTeraction Database (MINT, https://mint.bio.uniroma2.it/) [30], IntAct (https://www.ebi.ac.uk/intact/) [31], Database of Interacting Proteins (DIP, https://dip.doe-mbi.ucla.edu/dip/Main.cgi) [32], Pathway Commons (http://www.pathwaycommons.org/) [33], iRefIndex (http://irefindex.org/wiki/index.php?title=iRefIndex) [34], STRING (https://string-db.org/) [35], MatrixDB (http://matrixdb.univ-lyon1.fr/) [36], MPIDB (https://www.jcvi.org/mpidb/about.php) [37], InnateDB (https://www.innatedb.com/) [38], iRefWeb (http://wodaklab.org/iRefWeb/search/index) [39], I2D (http://ophid.utoronto.ca/ophidv2.204/) [40] and converted the results visually by using Cytoscape software (http://www.cytoscape.org/) [41]. Topological properties of PPI network such as node degree [42], betweenness [43], stress [44], closeness [45] and clustering coefficient [46] were calculated. Furthermore, module analysis was performed by using the PEWCC1 [47] plugin (version 1.3) to explore the most important clustering modules in the huge PPI network (degree cutoff = 5, k-core = 2, node score cutoff = 0.2, and max. Depth rom Seed: 100).

## 2.6. Construction of Target Genes-miRNA Regulatory Network

The miRNAs of target genes were predicted by two established miRNA target prediction databases such as DIANA-TarBase (http://diana.imis.athena-innovation.gr/DianaTools/index.php?r=tarbase/index) [48] and miRTarBase (http://mirtarbase.mbc.nctu.edu.tw/php/download.php) [49]. The miRNAs predicted by online tool NetworkAnalyst (https://www.networkanalyst.ca/) [50] were selected as the miRNAs of target genes. A network based on correlation analysis of target genes and miRNAs linked with CAD was constructed by Cytoscape software (http://www.cytoscape.org/, version 3.7.2, National Institutes of Health, Bethesda, MD, USA) [41]. In the network, a green (up regulated) and red (down regulated) circular node represented the target genes and a white and blue diamond shape node represented the miRNA, their interaction was represented by a line. The numbers of lines in the networks indicated the contribution of one miRNA to the surrounding target genes, and the higher the degree, the more central the target gene was within the network.

## 2.7. Construction of Target Genes-TF Regulatory Network

The transcription factors (TFs) of target genes were predicted by established TF target prediction databases such as JASPAR (http://jaspar.genereg.net/) [51]. The miRNAs predicted by online tool Network Analyst (https://www.networkanalyst.ca/) [50] were selected as the TFs of target genes. A network based on correlation analysis of target genes and TFs linked with CAD was constructed by Cytoscape software (http://www.cytoscape.org/) [41]. In the network, a green (up regulated) and red (down regulated) circular node represented the target genes and a gray and blue triangle shape node represented the TF, their interaction was represented by a line. The numbers of lines in the networks indicated the contribution of one TF to the surrounding target genes, and the higher the degree, the more central the target gene was within the network.

## 2.8. Hub Gene Expression Levels in CAD

The Human Protein Atlas (HPA) (https://www.proteinatlas.org/) was used to validate the expression level of the hub genes [52].

## 2.9. Receiver Operating Characteristic Curve Analysis

Receiver operating characteristic curve (ROC) analysis was performed using R package "pROC" [53] to distinguish male CAD samples from female CAD tissues. In GSE23766, we worked out the AUC to distinguish male CAD samples from female CAD tissues. After that, we compared the expression levels of candidate hub genes in male CAD and female CAD tissues using GSE23766.

## 3. Results

### 3.1. Identification of DEGs

After quality control, normalization and batch effect adjustment, gene expression profiles from CAD samples with male and female were compared. The boxplot proved good normalization of the GSE23766 data (Figure 2A,B). A total of 894 significant DEGs (adjusted $p$-value < 0.05, |log2(Fold Change)| > 0.1694 for up regulated genes, |log2(Fold Change)| > 0.229 for down regulated genes), including 456 up regulated and 438 down regulated genes, were identified from GSE23766 dataset (Table S1). The volcano plot of each gene expression profile data was shown in Figure 3. Hierarchical clustering analysis showed the expression pattern of DEGs among samples, which suggested that the expression of genes in CAD with male significantly differ from those in adjacent CAD with female (Figures 4 and 5).

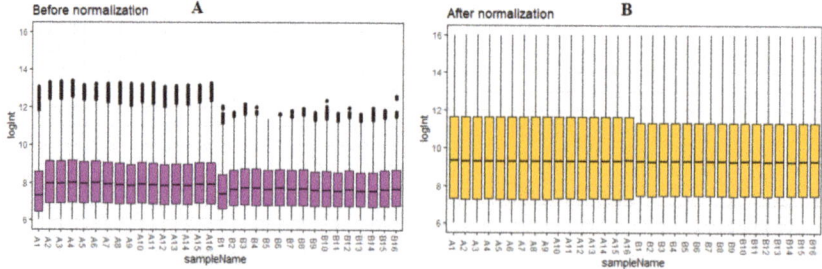

**Figure 2.** Box plots of the gene expression data before (**A**) and after normalization (**B**). Horizontal axis represents the sample symbol and the vertical axis represents the gene expression values. The black line in the box plot represents the median value of gene expression. (A1–A16 = male human CAD samples; B1–B16 = female human CAD samples).

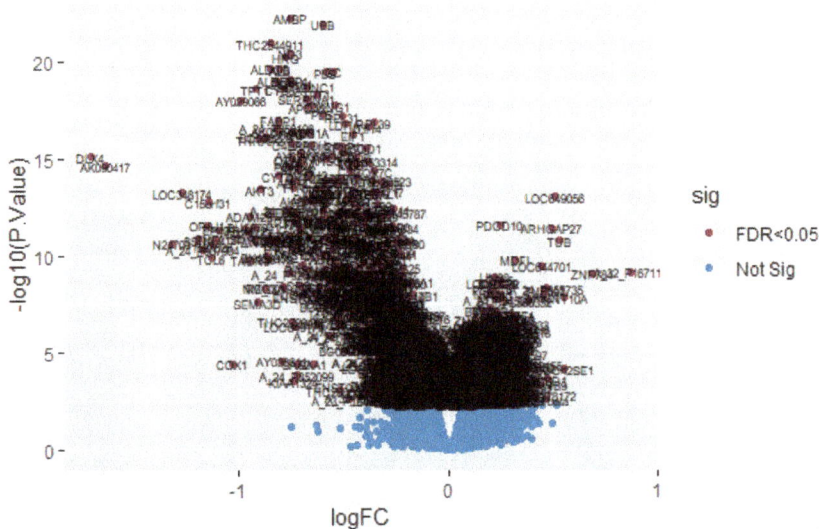

**Figure 3.** Volcano plot of differentially expressed genes. Genes with a significant change of more than two-fold were selected.

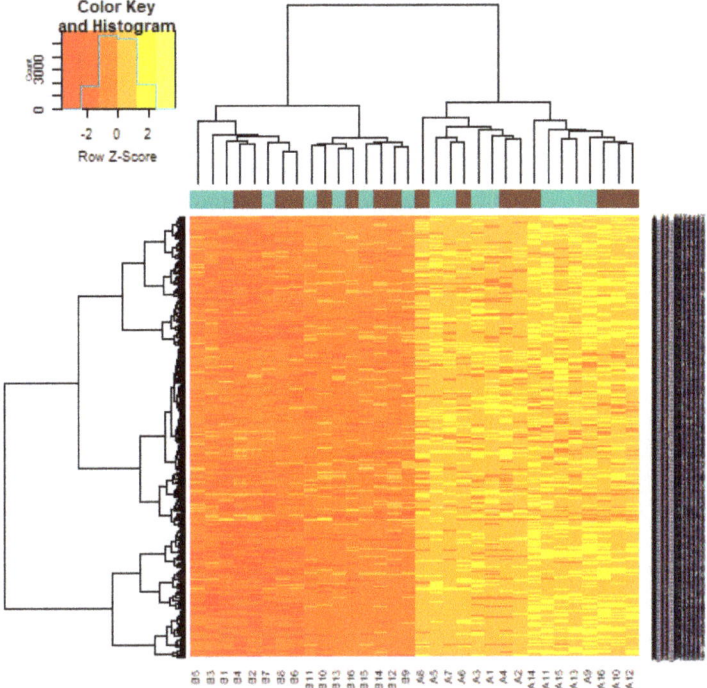

**Figure 4.** Heat map of up regulated differentially expressed genes. Legend on the top left indicate log fold change of genes. (A1, A2, A3, A4, A5, A6, A7, A8, A9, A10, A11, A12, A13, A14, A15, A16 = male human CAD samples; B1, B2, B3, B4, B5, B6, B7, B8, B9, B10, B11, B12, B13, B14, B15, B16 = female human CAD samples).

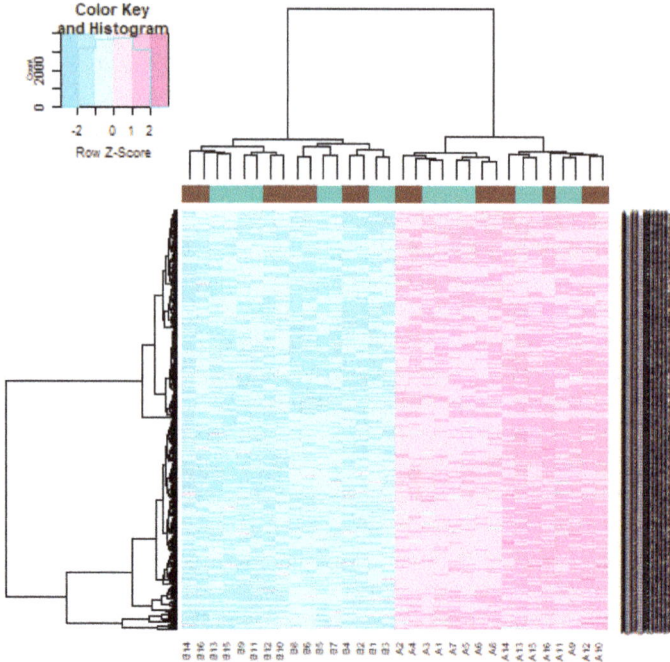

**Figure 5.** Heat map of down regulated differentially expressed genes. Legend on the top left indicate log fold change of genes. (A1, A2, A3, A4, A5, A6, A7, A8, A9, A10, A11, A12, A13, A14, A15, A16 = male human CAD samples; B1, B2, B3, B4, B5, B6, B7, B8, B9, B10, B11, B12, B13, B14, B15, B16 = female human CAD samples).

*3.2. Pathway Enrichment Analysis*

To gain further insight into the identified DEGs (up and down regulated genes), pathway and GO enrichment analyses were conducted using ToppGene and are given in Tables S2 and S3. Pathway enrichment analysis showed that up regulated genes were mainly involved in PABC transporters, BARD1 signaling events, androgen/estrogene/progesterone biosynthesis and multidrug resistance-associated protein mediated transport, while down regulated genes were mainly involved to complement and coagulation cascades, FOXA2 and FOXA3 transcription factor networks, fatty acid metabolism and fibrinolysis pathway. Gene ontology (GO) enrichment analysis showed that up regulated genes were mainly associated in biological processes (BP), cellular component (CC) and molecular function (MF), including forebrain neuron differentiation, filopodium membrane and DNA binding, bending, while down regulated genes were mainly associated in biological processes (BP), cellular component (CC) and molecular function (MF), including platelet degranulation, blood microparticle and peptidase regulator activity.

*3.3. GO Enrichment Analysis of DEGs*

Enrichment analyses for the up regulated and down regulated genes were performed by ToppGene. The up regulated genes were mainly enriched in forebrain neuron differentiation and negative regulation of immune system process by BP, filopodium membrane and nucleolus by CC and DNA binding, bending and protein dimerization activity by MF, respectively (Table S4). Meanwhile, down regulated genes were mainly enriched in platelet degranulation and response to inorganic substance by BP, blood microparticle and extracellular space by CC and peptidase regulator activity and endopeptidase inhibitor activity by MF, respectively (Table S5).

## 3.4. Comprehensive Analysis of PPI Network and Modules

The PPI network of up regulated genes consisted of 5840 nodes and 16,142 edges (Figure 6). Hub genes with high node degree such as MYC (degree = 998), NPM1 (degree = 820), UBE2D3 (degree = 488), TERF1 (degree = 429) and PSMA3 (degree = 403) were listed in Table S6. R square = 0.724 and correlation coefficient = 0.986 for node degree (Figure 7A). Hub genes with high betweenness such as MYC (betweenness = 0.15430897), NPM1 (betweenness = 0.11756148), TERF1 (betweenness = 0.06992938), PSMA3 (betweenness = 0.05585022) and MDFI (betweenness = 0.055025) were listed in Table S6. R square = 0.473 and correlation coefficient = 0.170 for betweenness (Figure 7B). Hub genes with high stress such as MYC (stress = 168499346), NPM1 (stress = 107362468), PSMA3 (stress = 49381886), MDFI (stress = 39487556) and TERF1 (stress = 32105062) were listed in Table S6. R square = 0.017 and correlation coefficient = −0.032 for stress (Figure 7C). Hub genes with high closeness such as NPM1 (closeness = 0.38413706), MYC (closeness = 0.37588193), TERF1 (closeness = 0.36795083), CCT6A (closeness = 0.36512827) and RPS14 (closeness = 0.36450945) were listed in Table S6. R square = 0.286 and correlation coefficient = 0.183 for closeness (Figure 7D). Hub genes with low clustering coefficient such as TRPC7 (clustering coefficient = 0), TNFRSF11B (clustering coefficient = 0), ABCB4 (clustering coefficient = 0), DPY19L2 (clustering coefficient = 0) and ABCG5 (clustering coefficient = 0) were listed in Table S6. R square = 0.471 and correlation coefficient = 0.790 for clustering coefficient (Figure 7E). The PPI network of down regulated genes consisted of 4014 nodes and 8815 edges (Figure 8). Hub genes with high node degree such as UBC (degree = 799), FN1 (degree = 718), VHL (degree = 587), HSPA8 (degree = 576) and SOD1 (degree = 245) were listed in Table S6. R square = 0.710 and correlation coefficient = 0.974 for node degree (Figure 9A). Hub genes with high betweenness such as FN1 (betweenness = 0.32861508), UBC (betweenness = 0.21817265), HSPA8 (betweenness = 0.17366877), VHL (betweenness = 0.09640801) and SOD1 (betweenness = 0.0712639) were listed in Table S6. R square = 0.394 and correlation coefficient = 0.172 for betweenness (Figure 9B). Hub genes with high stress such as UBC (stress = 75534956), FN1 (stress = 48390654), HSPA8 (stress = 48349874), VHL (stress = 18147816) and SOD1 (stress = 17465716) were listed in Table S6. R square = 0.282 and correlation coefficient = 0.015 for stress (Figure 9C). Hub genes with high closeness such as FN1 (closeness = 0.437081), HSPA8 (closeness = 0.39532803), UBC (closeness = 0.39232515), VHL (closeness = 0.37550751) and SOD1 (closeness = 0.36971275) were listed in Table S6. R square = 0.106 and correlation coefficient = 0.224 for closeness (Figure 9D). Hub genes with low clustering coefficient such as HEMK1 (clustering coefficient = 0), ADH1C (clustering coefficient = 0), CYSLTR2 (clustering coefficient = 0), CYP2E1 (clustering coefficient = 0) and COX7C (clustering coefficient = 0) were listed in Table S6. R square = 0.651 and correlation coefficient = 0.940 for clustering coefficient (Figure 9E).

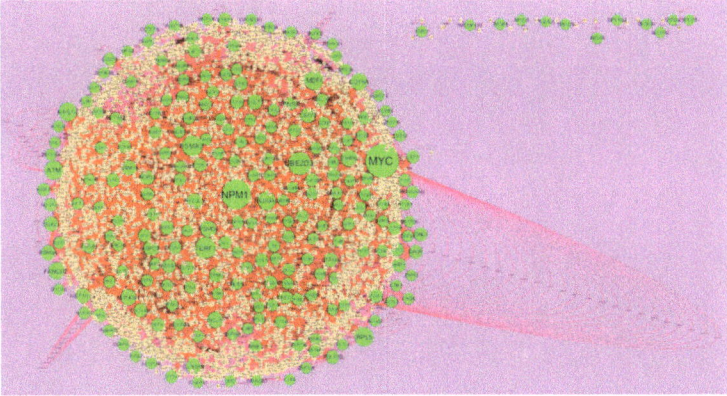

**Figure 6.** Protein–protein interaction network of up regulated genes. Green nodes denotes up regulated genes.

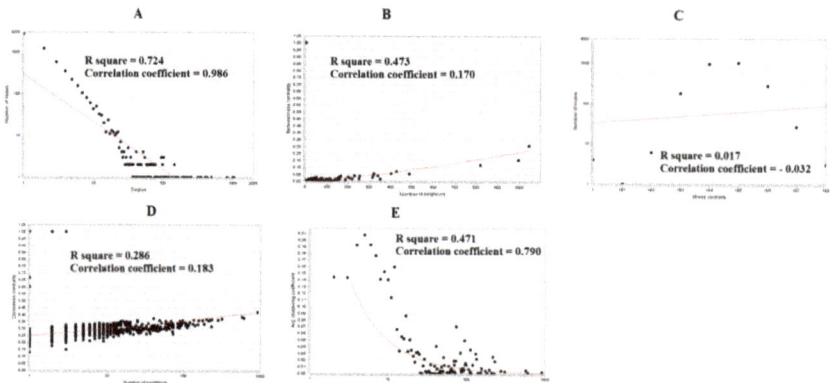

**Figure 7.** Regression diagrams for up regulated genes (**A**) Node degree; (**B**) Betweenness centrality; (**C**) Stress centrality; (**D**) Closeness centrality; (**E**) Clustering coefficient.

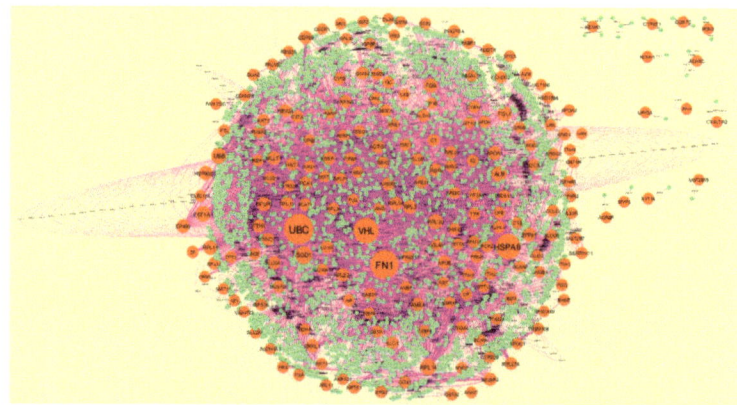

**Figure 8.** Protein–protein interaction network of down regulated genes. Orange nodes denotes down regulated genes.

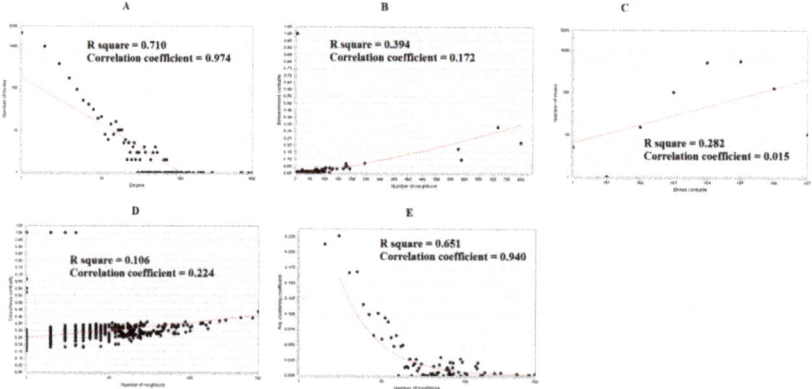

**Figure 9.** Regression diagrams for down regulated genes (**A**) Node degree; (**B**) Betweenness centrality; (**C**) Stress centrality; (**D**) Closeness centrality; (**E**) Clustering coefficient.

After cluster analysis, according to the given parameters, four significant modules (module 4, module 5, module 12 and module 14) were obtained from PPI network for up regulated genes (Figure 10), while four significant modules (module 2, module 4, module 8 and module 13) were obtained from PPI network for down regulated genes (Figure 11). Pathway and GO enrichment analysis showed that up regulated genes in module 4, module 5, module 12 and module 14 were closely related to signaling pathways regulating pluripotency of stem cells, platinum drug resistance, negative regulation of immune system process and protein dimerization activity, while down regulated genes in module 2, module 4, module 8 and module 13 were closely related to amb2 Integrin signaling, hypoxia-inducible factor in the cardiovascular system, platelet degranulation and response to inorganic substance.

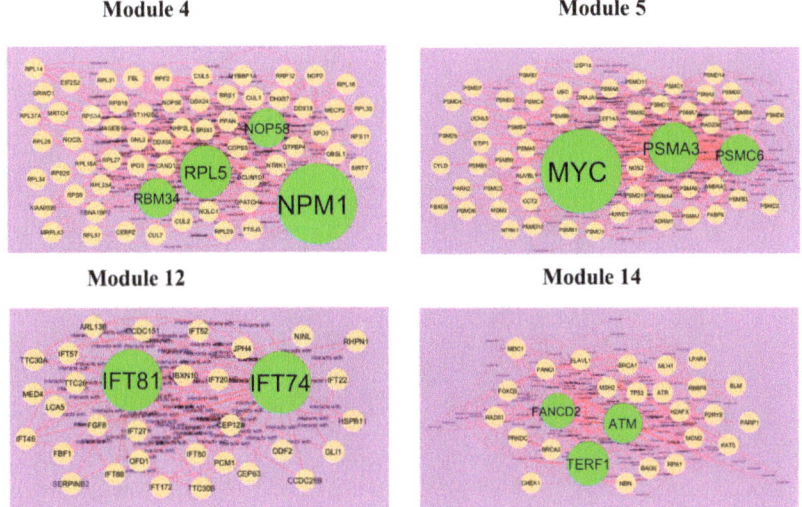

**Figure 10.** Modules in protein–protein interaction (PPI) network. The green nodes denote the up regulated genes.

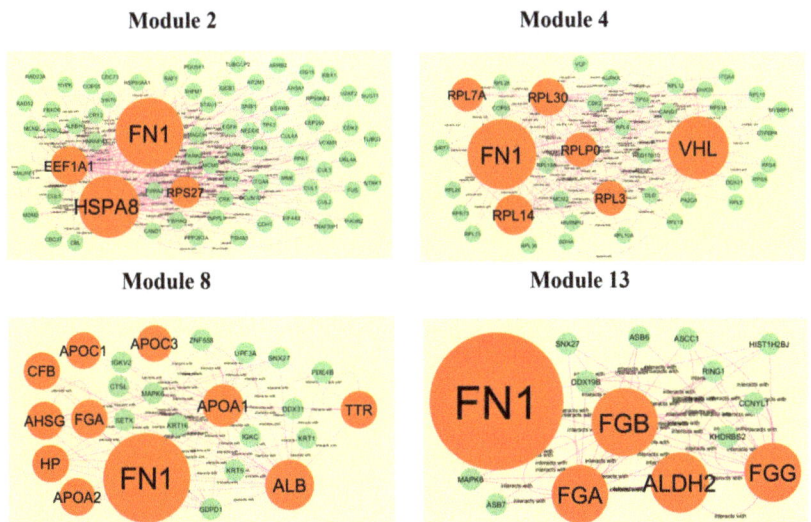

**Figure 11.** Modules in PPI network. The orange nodes denote the down regulated genes.

## 3.5. Construction of Target Genes-miRNA Regulatory Network

MicroRNAs (miRNAs) expressions were responsible for progression of CAD [54]. The miRNAs that may control the up and down regulated target genes are shown in Figures 12 and 13. Top five up regulated target genes such as TAOK1 interacts with 222 miRNAs (ex, hsa-mir-3941), HMGB1 interacts with 143 miRNAs (ex, hsa-mir-1183), ZNF708 interacts with 104 miRNAs (ex, hsa-mir-6832-5p), MYC interacts with 103 miRNAs (ex, hsa-mir-4662b) and ZNF101 interacts with 91 miRNAs (ex, hsa-mir-3187-3p) are listed in Table S7. Top five down regulated target genes such as KHSRP interacts with 178 miRNAs (ex, hsa-mir-548ac), TRIM72 interacts with 123 miRNAs (ex, hsa-mir-6890-3p), MLLT1 interacts with 95 miRNAs (ex, hsa-mir-5681a), C3 interacts with 93 miRNAs (ex, hsa-mir-3135b) and DDIT4 interacts with 82 miRNAs (ex, hsa-mir-3607-3p) are listed in Table S7.

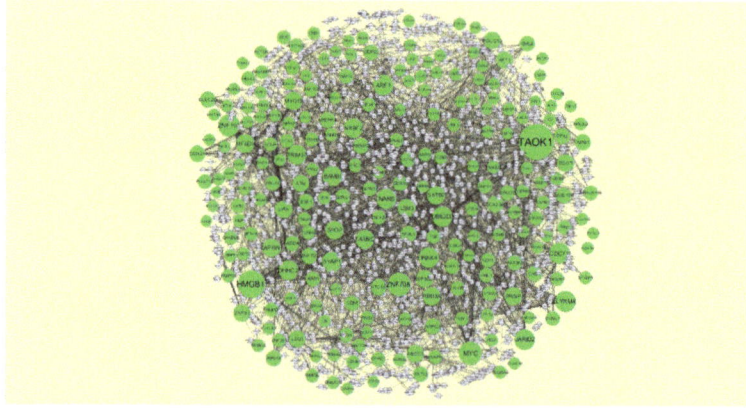

**Figure 12.** The network of up regulated genes and their related miRNAs. The green circles nodes are the up regulated genes, and white diamond nodes are the miRNAs.

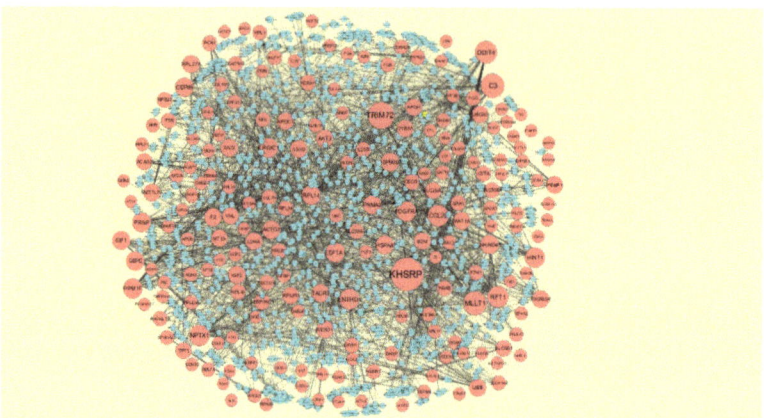

**Figure 13.** The network of down- regulated genes and their related miRNAs. The red circles nodes are the down regulated genes, and blue diamond nodes are the miRNAs.

## 3.6. Construction of Target Genes–TF Regulatory Network

Transcription factors (TFs) expressions were responsible for progression of CAD [55]. The TFs that may control the up and down regulated target genes are shown in Figures 14 and 15. Top five up regulated target genes such as HSD17B11 interacts with 166 TFs (ex, FOXC1), HEPACAM2 interacts with 128 TFs (ex, GATA2), CACYBP interacts with 88 TFs (ex, FOXL1), NAPG interacts with 76 TFs (ex, YY1) and PSMA3 interacts with 59 TFs (ex, USF2) are listed in Table S8. Top five down regulated target genes such as PAH interacts with 149 TFs (ex, FOXC1), CYP3A4 interacts with 118 TFs (ex, GATA2), CP interacts with 76 TFs (ex, YY1), COX7C interacts with 66 TFs (ex, SRF) and TTTY10 interacts with 59 TFs (ex, FOXL1) are listed in Table S8.

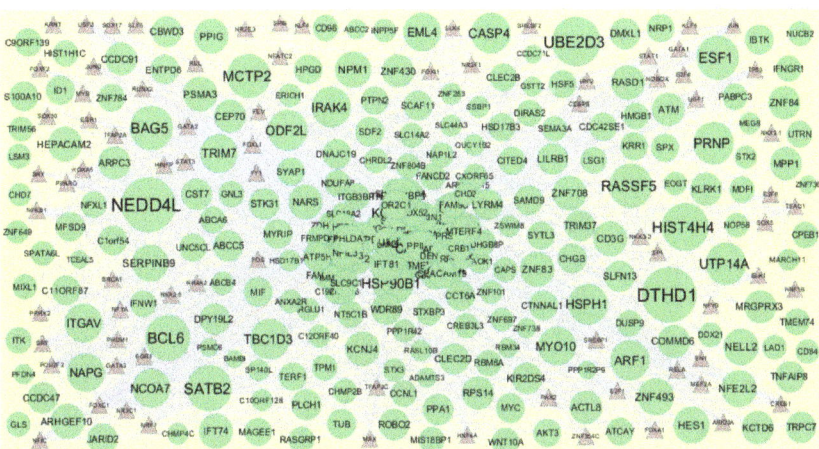

**Figure 14.** The network of up regulated genes and their related TFs. The green circles nodes are the up regulated genes, and brown triangle nodes are the TFs.

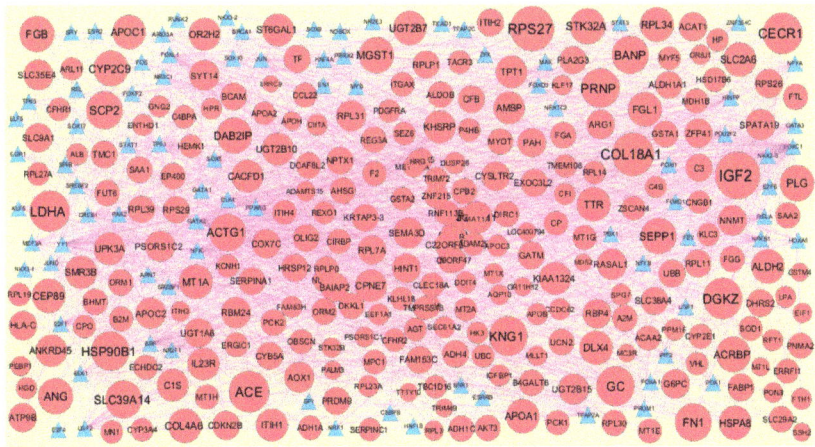

**Figure 15.** The network of down regulated genes and their related TFs. The green circles nodes are the down regulated genes, and blue triangle nodes are the TFs.

*3.7. Validation of Hub Genes by Immunohistochemistry from HPA Database and Receiver Operating Characteristic Curve analysis*

The analysis from The Human Protein Atlas indicated that the expression of hub genes (up regulated) such as NPM1, ATM, TRIP6, HSP90B1 and HIST1H1C are enhanced in CAD smooth muscle tissue (Figure 16), whereas, the expression of hub genes (down regulated) such as UBC, FN1, RPL14, UBB and EEF1A1 are reduced in CAD smooth muscle tissue (Figure 17). The results of ROC curve indicated that NPM1, TRIP6, HSP90B1, UBC, FN1, RPL14, UBB and EEF1A1 could distinguish male CAD samples from female CAD tissues best, among all the up and down regulated hub genes (NPM1: AUC = 1; ATM: AUC = 0.875; TRIP6: AUC = 1; HSP90B1: AUC = 1, HIST1H1C: AUC = 0.938; UBC: AUC = 1; FN1: AUC = 1; RPL14: AUC = 1; UBB: AUC = 1; EEF1A1: AUC = 1) (Figure 18).

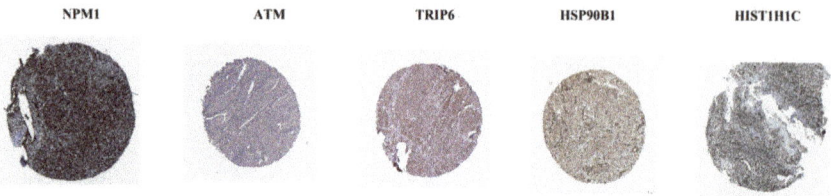

**Figure 16.** Validation of the hub genes (up regulated) with immunohistochemistry from HPA database. Hub genes NPM1, ATM, TRIP6, HSP90B1 and HIST1H1C were high expressed in CAD.

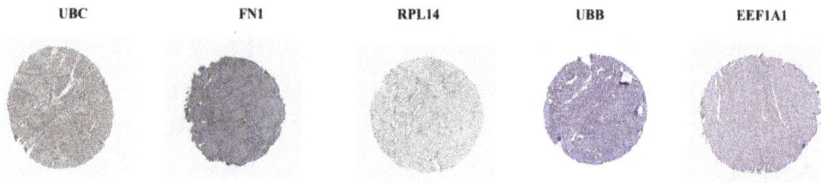

**Figure 17.** Validation of the hub genes (up regulated) with immunohistochemistry from HPA database. Hub genes UBC, FN1, RPL14, UBB and EEF1A1 were low expressed in CAD.

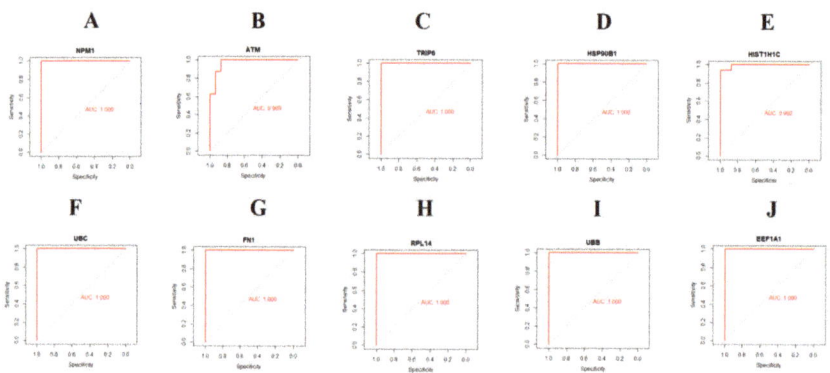

**Figure 18.** Receiver operating characteristic (ROC) curves and area under the curve (AUC) statistics to evaluate the diagnostic efficiency of the hub genes in GSE23766. (**A**) NPM1 (**B**) ATM (**C**) TRIP6 (**D**) HSP90B1 (**E**) HIST1H1C (**F**) UBC (**G**) FN1 (**H**) RPL14 (**I**) UBB (**J**) EEF1A1.

## 4. Discussion

The majority of patients with CAD are diagnosed at advanced stages and have poor overall survival [56]. However, the molecular mechanisms associated in the development of CAD remain unclear.

In the current study, the raw gene expression data of GSE23766 was obtained from the GEO and a total of 894 important DEGs were identified in male CAD samples compared with female CAD samples, including 456 up regulated genes and 438 down regulated genes. Low expression of LIN28 was associated with progression of cardiac ischaemia [57], but this gene may be linked with development of CAD. DUSP9 was involved in progression of cardiac hypertrophy [58], but this gene may be responsible for progression of CAD. Mutation in PSMC6 was important for progression of type 1 diabetes [59], but variation in this gene may be associated with the development of CAD. Decrease expression of ATP5H was liable for progression of mitochondrial dysfunction in cardiomyocytes [60], but low expression of this gene may be linked with the advancement of CAD. Genes such as IRAK4 [61], albumin (ALB) [62] and plasminogen (PLG) [63] were involved in progression of CAD. Alteration in SEPP1 was important for development of peripheral arterial disease [64], but modification in this gene may be liable for advancement of CAD. Polymorphism in ALDH2 was liable for development of CAD [65]. Modification in SERPINA1 was diagnosed with development of large artery stroke [66], but this altered gene may be liable for progression of CAD.

In pathway enrichment analysis, up regulated genes were enriched in various pathway databases such as superpathway of steroid hormone biosynthesis, ABC transporters, BARD1 signaling events, ABC-family proteins mediated transport, methionine metabolism, telomeres, telomerase, cellular aging, and immortality, androgen/estrogen/progesterone biosynthesis, multidrug resistance-associated protein mediated transport and lysosomal acid lipase deficiency (Wolman Disease). Mutation in HSD17B3 was linked with development of type 2 diabetes [67], but this variant gene may be responsible for progression of CAD. ABCG5 was linked with progression of CAD [68]. Mutation in ataxia telangiectasia mutated (ATM) was responsible for progression of CAD in male [69]. ABCC5 was expressed in heart disease [70], but this gene may be associated with advancement of CAD. Lysosomal acid, cholesterol esterase (LIPA) was important for development of CAD [71]. In these pathways genes such as HSD17B11, ABCB4, ABCC2, ABCA6, FANCD2, UBE2D3, NPM1, PSMA3, methionyl-tRNA synthetase (MARS), 5-methyltetrahydrofolate-homocysteine methyltransferase (MTR), v-myc myelocytomatosis viral oncogene homolog (avian) (MYC) and TERF1 were predicted as novel prognostic or diagnostic biomarkers and new therapeutic target in CAD. Up regulated genes such as ABCB4, ABCC2, ABCG5, ABCC5 and ABCA6 were involved in centralized pathway of ABC transporters was associated with pathogenesis of CAD [72]. Down regulated genes were enriched in various pathway databases such as oxidative ethanol degradation III, complement and coagulation cascades, FOXA2 and FOXA3 transcription factor networks, metallothioneins bind metals, fatty acid metabolism, fibrinolysis pathway, plasminogen activating cascade, altered lipoprotein metabolic and enoxaparin pathway. Polymorphism in fibrinogen alpha chain (FGA) was liable for progression of myocardial infarction [73], but this polymorphic gene may be involved in pathogenesis of CAD. Fibrinogen gamma chain (FGG) was diagnosed with progression of ischemic stroke [74], but this gene may be identified with development of CAD. Increased expression of genes such as CPB2 was liable for advancement of myocardial infarction [75], but elevated expression of this gene may be associated with progression of CAD. Over expression of complement component 3 (C3) was responsible for advancement of CAD in female [76]. Low expression of C4B was culpable for pathogenesis of myocardial infarction [77], but decrease expression of this gene may be involved in progression of CAD. Genes such as APOA1 [78] IGFBP1 [79], ACAT1 [80], apolipoprotein B (APOB) [81] and APOC1 [82] were important for pathogenesis of CAD. Genes such as PCK1 [83] and ALDH1A1 [84] were associated with development of diabetes and obesity, but these genes may be linked with progression of CAD. Polymorphism in genes such as MT1A [85], MT2A [86], CYP2C9 [87], CYP3A4 [88], fibrinogen beta chain (FGB) [89], ADH1C [90], lipoprotein, Lp(a) (LPA) [91] and APOC3 [92] were liable for advancement of CAD. Alteration in APOC2 was involved in progression of hypertriglyceridaemia [93], but this gene may be responsible for the development of CAD. Down regulated genes such as ACAT1, ADH1A, ADH1C, ADH4, ACAA2, ALDH1A1, ALDH2, CYP2C9, CYP2E1, CYP3A4 were involved in centralized pathway of fatty acid metabolism was associated with pathogenesis of CAD [94]. In these pathways genes such as CYP2E1, A2M, coagulation factor II (thrombin) (F2), complement factor I (CFI), SERPINC1, integrin, alpha X (complement component 3 receptor 4 subunit) (ITGAX), complement factor B (CFB), C1S, C4BPA, KNG1, transthyretin (prealbumin, amyloidosis type I) (TTR) aldolase B, fructose-bisphosphate (ALDOB), G6PC, MT1B, MT1E, MT1F, MT1G, MT1H, MT1M, MT1X, ADH1A,

ADH4 and ACAA2 were predicted as novel prognostic or diagnostic biomarkers and new therapeutic targets in CAD.

In GO enrichment analysis, up regulated genes were enriched in all GO categories such as forebrain neuron differentiation, filopodium membrane and DNA binding, bending. SEMA3A was responsible for progression of myocardial infarction [95], but this gene may be associated with pathogenesis of CAD. Genes such as HES1 [96] and NRP1 [97] were important for progression of cardiac ischemia, but these genes may be linked with CAD. Loss of utrophin (UTRN) was involved in the advancement of cardiomyopathy [98], but this gene may be liable for progression of CAD. Increased expression of HMGB1 was answerable for progression of CAD [99]. In these GO categories, genes such as PHLDA1, SATB2, ROBO2, LEF1, MYO10 and integrin, alpha V (ITGAV) were predicted as novel prognostic or diagnostic biomarkers and new therapeutic target in CAD. Down regulated genes were enriched in all GO categories such as platelet degranulation, blood microparticle and peptidase regulator activity. Polymorphism in apolipoprotein H (APOH) was linked with progression of hypercholesterolemia [100], but this polymorphic gene may be liable for development of CAD. Genes such as IGF2 [101], ITIH4 [102], haptoglobin (HP) [103] and ceruloplasmin (ferroxidase) (CP) [104] were important for advancement of CAD. High expression of SOD1 was involved in the progression of CAD [105]. ITIH3 was answerable for advancement of myocardial infarction [106], but this gene may be associated with development of CAD. Transferrin (TF) was identified with progression of acute stroke [107], but this gene may be linked with development of CAD. Loss of CFHR1 was important for progression of hypertension [108], but loss this gene may be responsible for advancement of CAD. Polymorphism in genes such as angiotensinogen (AGT) [109] and HSPA8 [110] were important for theadvancement of CAD. In these GO categories genes such as alpha-2-HS-glycoprotein (AHSG), histidine-rich glycoprotein (HRG), FN1, ORM1, ORM2, TMPRSS13, ACTG1, haptoglobin-related protein (HPR), alpha-1-microglobulin/bikunin precursor (AMBP), APOA2, group-specific component (GC), ITIH1, ITIH2, acrosin binding protein (ACRBP) and PEBP1 were predicted as novel prognostic or diagnostic biomarkers and new therapeutic target in CAD.

In PPI network, up regulated genes such as MYC, NPM1, UBE2D3, TERF1, PSMA3, MDFI, CCT6A and RPS14 were identified as hub genes showing the highest node degree, betweenness, stress and closeness. Up regulated genes such as TRPC7, TNFRSF11B, ABCB4, DPY19L2 and ABCG5 were identified as hub genes showing the lowest clustering coefficient. TRPC7 was linked with development of CAD [111]. Polymorphism in TNFRSF11B was identified with development of ischemic stroke [112], but this gene may be important for progression of CAD. In this PPI network genes such as myoD family inhibitor (MDFI), CCT6A, RPS14 and DPY19L2 were predicted as novel prognostic or diagnostic biomarkers and new therapeutic target in CAD. Down regulated genes such as UBC, FN1, VHL, HSPA8 and SOD1 were identified as hub genes showing the highest node degree, betweenness, stress and closeness. Down regulated genes such as HEMK1, ADH1C, CYSLTR2, CYP2E1 and COX7C were identified as hub genes showing the lowest clustering coefficient. In this PPI network genes such as ubiquitin C (UBC), VHL (von Hippel-Lindau tumor suppressor), HEMK1, CYSLTR2 and COX7C were predicted as novel prognostic or diagnostic biomarkers and new therapeutic target in CAD.

In module analysis, up regulated genes such as NPM1, RPL5, NOP58, RBM34, MYC, PSMA3, PSMC6, IFT74 and IFT8 were identified as hub genes showing the highest node degree in all four significant modules. In these modules genes such as RPL5, NOP58, RBM34, IFT74 and IFT8 were predicted as novel prognostic or diagnostic biomarkers and new therapeutic target in CAD. Down regulated genes such as FN1, HSPA8, EEF1A1, RPS27, VHL, RPL7A, RPL30, RPLP0, RPL3, RPL14, ALB, TTR, APOA1, APOC3, APOC1, CFB, AHSG, FGA, HP, APOA2, FGB, FGG, ALDH2 and FGA were identified as hub genes showing the highest node degree in all four significant modules. In these modules genes such as EEF1A1, RPS27, RPL7A, RPL30, RPLP0, RPL3 and RPL14 were predicted as novel prognostic or diagnostic biomarkers and new therapeutic target in CAD.

In target gene-miRNA network, up regulated genes such as TAOK1, HMGB1, ZNF708, MYC and ZNF101 were identified as target genes showing the highest number of integration with miRNAs.

In this network gene such as TAOK1, ZNF708 and ZNF101 along with miRNA such as hsa-mir-3941, hsa-mir-1183, hsa-mir-6832-5p, hsa-mir-4662b and hsa-mir-3187-3p were predicted as novel prognostic or diagnostic biomarkers and new therapeutic target in CAD. Whereas, down regulated genes such as KHSRP, TRIM72, MLLT1, C3 and DDIT4 were identified as target genes showing the highest number of integration with miRNAs. Low expression of TRIM72 was responsible for development of cardiovascular diseases [113], but loss of this gene may be linked with progression of CAD. In this network down regulated genes such as KH-type splicing regulatory protein (FUSE binding protein 2) (KHSRP), MLLT1 and DDIT4 along with miRNA such as hsa-mir-548ac, hsa-mir-6890-3p, hsa-mir-5681a, hsa-mir-3135b and hsa-mir-3607-3p were predicted as novel prognostic or diagnostic biomarkers and new therapeutic target in CAD.

In the target gene-TF network, up regulated genes such as HSD17B11, HEPACAM2, CACYBP, NAPG and PSMA3 were identified as target genes showing the highest number of integration with TFs. In this network genes such as HEPACAM2, calcyclin binding protein (CACYBP) and N-ethylmaleimide-sensitive factor attachment protein, gamma (NAPG) along TFs such as FOXC1, FOXL1, YY1 and USF2 were predicted as novel prognostic or diagnostic biomarkers and new therapeutic target in CAD. Transcription factor GATA2 was linked with pathogens of CAD [114]. Down regulated genes such as PAH, CYP3A4, CP, COX7C and TTTY10 were identified as target genes showing the highest number of integration with TFs. Phenylalanine hydroxylase (PAH) was associated with development of cardiovascular diseases [115], but this gene may be identified with advancement of CAD. In this network down regulated gene TTTY10 along transcription factor SRF (serum response factor) were predicted as novel prognostic or diagnostic biomarkers and new therapeutic target in CAD.

In conclusion, the present study identified 13 hub genes (up regulated) and 10 hub genes (down regulated) that may be associated in the progression of CAD. Among them, 12 hub genes (up regulated) and 7 hub genes (down regulated) are closely related to the prognosis of CAD. Also identified 10 miRNA and 10 TFs may be associated in the progression of CAD. These hub genes may be regarded as diagnostic and prognostic biomarkers, and could become potential therapeutic target for future CAD therapeutic strategies. However, bioinformatics only plays a predictive role; the function of these hub genes in CAD needs further study to elucidate the biological characteristics.

**Supplementary Materials:** The following are available online at http://www.mdpi.com/2218-273X/10/1/35/s1.

**Author Contributions:** M.V.B. was associated with project administration and acquisition of resources. T.B.S. was associated with methodology and formal analysis. S.N. was associated with review and editing, and visualization. B.V. was participated in writing original draft and investigation, C.V. was performed software, supervision, formal analysis and validation. All authors have read and agreed to the published version of the manuscript.

**Funding:** This research received no external funding.

**Acknowledgments:** I thank David J. Waxman, Boston University, Department of Biology and Bioinformatics Program, 5 Cummington Mall, Boston, MA, USA, very much, the author who deposited their microarray dataset, GSE23766, into the public GEO database.

**Conflicts of Interest:** The authors declare no conflict of interest.

**Ethical Approval:** This article does not contain any studies with human participants or animals performed by any of the authors.

**Informed Consent:** No informed consent because this study does not contain human or animals participants.

**Availability of Data and Materials:** The datasets supporting the conclusions of this article are available in the GEO (Gene Expression Omnibus) (https://www.ncbi.nlm.nih.gov/geo/) repository. [(GSE23766) (https://www.ncbi.nlm.nih.gov/geo/query/acc.cgi?acc=GSE23766)].

**Consent for Publication:** Not applicable.

## References

1. Diamond, G.A.; Forrester, J.S. Analysis of probability as an aid in the clinical diagnosis of coronary-artery disease. *N. Engl. J. Med.* **1979**, *300*, 1350–1358. [CrossRef] [PubMed]

2. Ghassibe-Sabbagh, M.; Platt, D.E.; Youhanna, S.; Abchee, A.B.; Stewart, K.; Badro, D.A.; Haber, M.; Salloum, A.K.; Douaihy, B.; el Bayeh, H. Genetic and environmental influences on total plasma homocysteine and its role in coronary artery disease risk. *Atherosclerosis* **2012**, *222*, 180–186. [CrossRef] [PubMed]
3. Howson, J.M.; Zhao, W.; Barnes, D.R.; Ho, W.K.; Young, R.; Paul, D.S.; Waite, L.L.; Freitag, D.F.; Fauman, E.B.; Salfati, E.L.; et al. Fifteen new risk loci for coronary artery disease highlight arterial-wall-specific mechanisms. *Nat. Genet.* **2017**, *49*, 1113–1119. [CrossRef] [PubMed]
4. Aceña, Á.; Pello, A.M.; Carda, R.; Lorenzo, Ó.; Gonzalez-Casaus, M.L.; Blanco-Colio, L.M.; Martín-Ventura, J.L.; Palfy, J.; Orejas, M.; Rábago, R.; et al. Parathormone Levels Are Independently Associated with the Presence of Left Ventricular Hypertrophy in Patients with Coronary Artery Disease. *J. Nutr. Health Aging* **2016**, *20*, 659–664. [CrossRef] [PubMed]
5. Samani, N.J.; Erdmann, J.; Hall, A.S.; Hengstenberg, C.; Mangino, M.; Maye, R.B.; Dixon, R.J.; Meitinger, T.; Braund, P.; Wichmann, H.E.; et al. Genomewide association analysis of coronary artery disease. *N. Engl. J. Med.* **2007**, *357*, 443–453. [CrossRef] [PubMed]
6. Clee, S.M.; Zwinderman, A.H.; Engert, J.C.; Zwarts, K.Y.; Molhuizen, H.O.; Roomp, K.; Jukema, J.W.; van Wijland, M.; van Dam, M.; Hudson, T.J.; et al. Common genetic variation in ABCA1 is associated with altered lipoprotein levels and a modified risk for coronary artery disease. *Circulation* **2001**, *103*, 1198–1205. [CrossRef]
7. Serrato, M.; Marian, A.J. A variant of human paraoxonase/arylesterase (HUMPONA) gene is a risk factor for coronary artery disease. *J. Clin. Investig.* **1995**, *96*, 3005–3008. [CrossRef]
8. Behague, I.; Poirier, O.; Nicaud, V.; Evans, A.; Arveiler, D.; Luc, G.; Cambou, J.P.; Scarabin, P.Y.; Bara, L.; Green, F.; et al. Beta fibrinogen gene polymorphisms are associated with plasma fibrinogen and coronary artery disease in patients with myocardial infarction. The ECTIM Study. Etude Cas-Temoins sur l'Infarctus du Myocarde. *Circulation* **1996**, *93*, 440–449. [CrossRef]
9. Ordovas, J.M.; Schaefer, E.J.; Salem, D.; Ward, R.H.; Glueck, C.J.; Vergani, C.; Wilson, P.W.; Karathanasis, S.K. Apolipoprotein A-I gene polymorphism associated with premature coronary artery disease and familial hypoalphalipoproteinemia. *N. Engl. J. Med.* **1986**, *314*, 671–677. [CrossRef]
10. Kaneda, H.; Ohno, M.; Taguchi, J.; Togo, M.; Hashimoto, H.; Ogasawara, K.; Aizawa, T.; Ishizaka, N.; Nagai, R. Heme oxygenase-1 gene promoter polymorphism is associated with coronary artery disease in Japanese patients with coronary risk factors. *Arterioscler. Thromb. Vasc. Biol.* **2002**, *22*, 1680–1685. [CrossRef]
11. Sanghera, D.K.; Aston, C.E.; Saha, N.; Kamboh, M.I. DNA polymorphisms in two paraoxonase genes (PON1 and PON2) are associated with the risk of coronary heart disease. *Am. J. Hum. Genet.* **1998**, *62*, 36–44. [CrossRef] [PubMed]
12. Margaglione, M.; Cappucci, G.; Colaizzo, D.; Giuliani, N.; Vecchione, G.; Grandone, E.; Pennelli, O.; Di Minno, G. The PAI-1 gene locus 4G/5G polymorphism is associated with a family history of coronary artery disease. *Arterioscler. Thromb. Vasc. Biol.* **1998**, *18*, 152–156. [CrossRef] [PubMed]
13. Lamblin, N.; Bauters, C.; Hermant, X.; Lablanche, J.M.; Helbecque, N.; Amouyel, P. Polymorphisms in the promoter regions of MMP-2, MMP-3, MMP-9 and MMP-12 genes as determinants of aneurysmal coronary artery disease. *J. Am. Coll. Cardiol.* **2002**, *40*, 43–48. [CrossRef]
14. Inoue, N.; Kawashima, S.; Kanazawa, K.; Yamada, S.; Akita, H.; Yokoyama, M. Polymorphism of the NADH/NADPH oxidase p22 phox gene in patients with coronary artery disease. *Circulation* **1998**, *97*, 135–137. [CrossRef] [PubMed]
15. Amant, C.; Hamon, M.; Bauters, C.; Richard, F.; Helbecque, N.; McFadden, E.P.; Escudero, X.; Lablanche, J.M.; Amouyel, P.; Bertrand, M.E. The angiotensin II type 1 receptor gene polymorphism is associated with coronary artery vasoconstriction. *J. Am. Coll. Cardiol.* **1997**, *29*, 486–490. [CrossRef]
16. Ma, J.; Liew, C.C. Gene profiling identifies secreted protein transcripts from peripheral blood cells in coronary artery disease. *J. Mol. Cell. Cardiol.* **2003**, *35*, 993–998. [CrossRef]
17. Archacki, S.R.; Angheloiu, G.; Tian, X.L.; Tan, F.L.; DiPaola, N.; Shen, G.Q.; Moravec, C.; Ellis, S.; Topol, E.J.; Wang, Q. Identification of new genes differentially expressed in coronary artery disease by expression profiling. *Physiol. Genom.* **2003**, *15*, 65–74. [CrossRef]
18. Carvalho, B.S.; Irizarry, R.A. A framework for oligonucleotide microarray preprocessing. *Bioinformatics* **2010**, *6*, 2363–2367. [CrossRef]
19. Ritchie, M.E.; Phipson, B.; Wu, D.; Hu, Y.; Law, C.W.; Shi, W.; Smyth, G.K. limma powers differential expression analyses for RNA-sequencing and microarray studies. *Nucleic Acids Res.* **2015**, *43*, e47. [CrossRef]

20. Chen, J.; Bardes, E.E.; Aronow, B.J.; Jegga, A.G. ToppGene Suite for gene list enrichment analysis and candidate gene prioritization. *Nucleic Acids Res.* **2009**, *37*, W305–W311. [CrossRef]
21. Aoki-Kinoshita, K.F.; Kanehisa, M. Gene annotation and pathway mapping in KEGG. *Methods. Mol. Biol.* **2007**, *396*, 71–91. [CrossRef] [PubMed]
22. Schaefer, C.F.; Anthony, K.; Krupa, S.; Buchoff, J.; Day, M.; Hannay, T.; Buetow, K.H. PID: The Pathway Interaction Database. *Nucleic Acids Res.* **2009**, *37*, D674–D679. [CrossRef] [PubMed]
23. Croft, D.; O'Kelly, G.; Wu, G.; Haw, R.; Gillespie, M.; Matthews, L.; Caudy, M.; Garapati, P.; Gopinath, G.; Jassal, B.; et al. Reactome: A database of reactions, pathways and biological processes. *Nucleic Acids Res.* **2011**, *39*, D691–D697. [CrossRef] [PubMed]
24. Liberzon, A.; Subramanian, A.; Pinchback, R.; Thorvaldsdóttir, H.; Tamayo, P.; Mesirov, J.P. Molecular signatures database (MSigDB) 3.0. *Bioinformatics* **2011**, *27*, 1739–1740. [CrossRef]
25. Dahlquist, K.D.; Salomonis, N.; Vranizan, K.; Lawlor, S.C.; Conklin, B.R. GenMAPP, a new tool for viewing and analyzing microarray data on biological pathways. *Nat. Genet.* **2002**, *31*, 19–20. [CrossRef]
26. Petri, V.; Jayaraman, P.; Tutaj, M.; Hayman, G.T.; Smith, J.R.; De Pons, J.; Laulederkind, S.J.; Lowry, T.F.; Nigam, R.; Wang, S.J.; et al. The pathway ontology-updates and applications. *J. Biomed. Semant.* **2014**, *5*, 7. [CrossRef]
27. Mi, H.; Muruganujan, A.; Thomas, P.D. PANTHER in 2013: Modeling the evolution of gene function, and other gene attributes, in the context of phylogenetic trees. *Nucleic Acids Res.* **2013**, *41*, D377–D386. [CrossRef]
28. Harris, M.A.; Clark, J.; Ireland, A.; Lomax, J.; Ashburner, M.; Foulger, R.; Eilbeck, K.; Lewis, S.; Marshall, B.; Mungall, C.; et al. The Gene Ontology (GO) database and informatics. *Nucleic Acids Res.* **2004**, *32*, D258–D261. [CrossRef]
29. Oughtred, R.; Stark, C.; Breitkreutz, B.J.; Rust, J.; Boucher, L.; Chang, C.; Kolas, N.; O'Donnell, L.; Leung, G.; McAdam, R.; et al. The BioGRID interaction database: 2019 update. *Nucleic Acids Res.* **2019**, *47*, D529–D541. [CrossRef]
30. Licata, L.; Briganti, L.; Peluso, D.; Perfetto, L.; Iannuccelli, M.; Galeota, E.; Sacco, F.; Palma, A.; Nardozza, A.P.; Santonico, E.; et al. MINT, the molecular interaction database: 2012 update. *Nucleic Acids Res.* **2012**, *40*, D857–D861. [CrossRef]
31. Orchard, S.; Kerrien, S.; Abbani, S.; Aranda, B.; Bhate, J.; Bidwell, S.; Bridge, A.; Briganti, L.; Brinkman, F.S.; Chatr-Aryamontri, A.; et al. Protein interaction data curation: The International Molecular Exchange (IMEx) consortium. *Nat. Methods* **2012**, *9*, 345–350. [CrossRef] [PubMed]
32. Salwinski, L.; Miller, C.S.; Smith, A.J.; Pettit, F.K.; Bowie, J.U.; Eisenberg, D. The Database of Interacting Proteins: 2004 update. *Nucleic Acids Res.* **2004**, *32*, D449–D451. [CrossRef] [PubMed]
33. Cerami, E.G.; Gross, B.E.; Demir, E.; Rodchenkov, I.; Babur, O.; Anwar, N.; Schultz, N.; Bader, G.D.; Sander, C. Pathway Commons, a web resource for biological pathway data. *Nucleic Acids Res.* **2011**, *39*, D685–D690. [CrossRef] [PubMed]
34. Razick, S.; Magklaras, G.; Donaldson, I.M. iRefIndex: A consolidated protein interaction database with provenance. *BMC Bioinform.* **2008**, *9*, 405. [CrossRef] [PubMed]
35. Szklarczyk, D.; Gable, A.L.; Lyon, D.; Junge, A.; Wyder, S.; Huerta-Cepas, J.; Simonovic, M.; Doncheva, N.T.; Morris, J.H.; Bork, P.; et al. STRING v11: Protein-protein association networks with increased coverage, supporting functional discovery in genome-wide experimental datasets. *Nucleic Acids Res.* **2019**, *47*, D607–D613. [CrossRef]
36. Clerc, O.; Deniaud, M.; Vallet, S.D.; Naba, A.; Rivet, A.; Perez, S.; Thierry-Mieg, N.; Ricard-Blum, S. MatrixDB: Integration of new data with a focus on glycosaminoglycan interactions. *Nucleic Acids Res.* **2019**, *47*, D376–D381. [CrossRef]
37. Goll, J.; Rajagopala, S.V.; Shiau, S.C.; Wu, H.; Lamb, B.T.; Uetz, P. MPIDB: The microbial protein interaction database. *Bioinformatics* **2008**, *24*, 1743–1744. [CrossRef]
38. Breuer, K.; Foroushani, A.K.; Laird, M.R.; Chen, C.; Sribnaia, A.; Lo, R.; Winsor, G.L.; Hancock, R.E.; Brinkman, F.S.; Lynn, D.J. InnateDB: Systems biology of innate immunity and beyond–recent updates and continuing curation. *Nucleic Acids Res.* **2013**, *41*, D1228–D1233. [CrossRef]
39. Turner, B.; Razick, S.; Turinsky, A.L.; Vlasblom, J.; Crowdy, E.K.; Cho, E.; Morrison, K.; Donaldson, I.M.; Wodak, S.J. iRefWeb: Interactive analysis of consolidated protein interaction data and their supporting evidence. *Database* **2010**, *2010*, baq023. [CrossRef]

40. Kotlyar, M.; Pastrello, C.; Sheahan, N.; Jurisica, I. Integrated interactions database: Tissue-specific view of the human and model organism interactomes. *Nucleic Acids Res.* **2016**, *44*, D536–D541. [CrossRef]
41. Shannon, P.; Markiel, A.; Ozier, O.; Baliga, N.S.; Wang, J.T.; Ramage, D.; Amin, N.; Schwikowski, B.; Ideker, T. Cytoscape: A software environment for integrated models of biomolecular interaction networks. *Genome Res.* **2003**, *3*, 2498–2504. [CrossRef] [PubMed]
42. Przulj, N. Biological network comparison using graphlet degree distribution. *Bioinformatics* **2007**, *23*, e177–e183. [CrossRef] [PubMed]
43. Yang, Q.; Lonardi, S. A parallel edge-betweenness clustering tool for Protein-Protein Interaction networks. *Int. J. Data Min. Bioinform.* **2007**, *1*, 241–247. [CrossRef] [PubMed]
44. Bi, D.; Ning, H.; Liu, S.; Que, X.; Ding, K. Gene expression patterns combined with network analysis identify hub genes associated with bladder cancer. *Comput. Biol. Chem.* **2015**, *56*, 71–83. [CrossRef] [PubMed]
45. Xiao, Q.; Wang, J.; Peng, X.; Wu, F.X.; Pan, Y. Identifying essential proteins from active PPI networks constructed with dynamic gene expression. *BMC Genom.* **2015**, *16*. [CrossRef] [PubMed]
46. Asur, S.; Ucar, D.; Parthasarathy, S. An ensemble framework for clustering protein-protein interaction networks. *Bioinformatics* **2007**, *23*, i29–i40. [CrossRef]
47. Zaki, N.; Efimov, D.; Berengueres, J. Protein complex detection using interaction reliability assessment and weighted clustering coefficient. *BMC Bioinform.* **2013**, *14*, 163. [CrossRef]
48. Vlachos, I.S.; Paraskevopoulou, M.D.; Karagkouni, D.; Georgakilas, G.; Vergoulis, T.; Kanellos, I.; Anastasopoulos, I.L.; Maniou, S.; Karathanou, K.; Kalfakakou, D.; et al. DIANA-TarBase v7.0: Indexing more than half a million experimentally supported miRNA:mRNA interactions. *Nucleic Acids Res.* **2015**, *43*, D153–D159. [CrossRef]
49. Chou, C.H.; Shrestha, S.; Yang, C.D.; Chang, N.W.; Lin, Y.L.; Liao, K.W.; Huang, W.C.; Sun, T.H.; Tu, S.J.; Lee, W.H.; et al. miRTarBase update 2018: A resource for experimentally validated microRNA-target interactions. *Nucleic Acids Res.* **2018**, *46*, D296–D302. [CrossRef]
50. Zhou, G.; Soufan, O.; Ewald, J.; Hancock, R.E.W.; Basu, N.; Xia, J. NetworkAnalyst 3.0: A visual analytics platform for comprehensive gene expression profiling and meta-analysis. *Nucleic Acids Res.* **2019**. [CrossRef]
51. Khan, A.; Fornes, O.; Stigliani, A.; Gheorghe, M.; Castro-Mondragon, J.A.; van der Lee, R.; Bessy, A.; Chèneby, J.; Kulkarni, S.R.; Tan, G.; et al. JASPAR 2018: Update of the open-access database of transcription factor binding profiles and its web framework. *Nucleic Acids Res.* **2018**, *46*, D260–D266. [CrossRef] [PubMed]
52. Uhlen, M.; Oksvold, P.; Fagerberg, L.; Lundberg, E.; Jonasson, K.; Forsberg, M.; Zwahlen, M.; Kampf, C.; Wester, K.; Hober, S.; et al. Towards a knowledge-based Human Protein Atlas. *Nat. Biotechnol.* **2010**, *28*, 1248–1250. [CrossRef]
53. Robin, X.; Turck, N.; Hainard, A.; Tiberti, N.; Lisacek, F.; Sanchez, J.C.; Müller, M. pROC: An open-source package for R and S+ to analyze and compare ROC curves. *BMC Bioinform.* **2011**, *12*, 77. [CrossRef] [PubMed]
54. Zhong, Z.; Hou, J.; Zhang, Q.; Zhong, W.; Li, B.; Li, C.; Liu, Z.; Yang, M.; Zhao, P. Circulating microRNA expression profiling and bioinformatics analysis of dysregulated microRNAs of patients with coronary artery disease. *Medicine* **2018**, *97*, e11428. [CrossRef] [PubMed]
55. Bhagavatula, M.R.; Fan, C.; Shen, G.Q.; Cassano, J.; Plow, E.F.; Topol, E.J.; Wang, Q. Transcription factor MEF2A mutations in patients with coronary artery disease. *Hum. Mol. Genet.* **2004**, *13*, 3181–3188. [CrossRef]
56. Detrano, R.; Janosi, A.; Steinbrunn, W.; Pfisterer, M.; Schmid, J.J.; Sandhu, S.; Guppy, K.H.; Lee, S.; Froelicher, V. International application of a new probability algorithm for the diagnosis of coronary artery disease. *Am. J. Cardiol.* **1989**, *64*, 304–310. [CrossRef]
57. Joshi, S.; Wei, J.; Bishopric, N.H. A cardiac myocyte-restricted Lin28/let-7 regulatory axis promotes hypoxia-mediated apoptosis by inducing the AKT signaling suppressor PIK3IP1. *Biochim. Biophys. Acta* **2016**, *1862*, 240–251. [CrossRef]
58. Singh, G.B.; Raut, S.K.; Khanna, S.; Kumar, A.; Sharma, S.; Prasad, R.; Khullar, M. MicroRNA-200c modulates DUSP-1 expression in diabetes-induced cardiac hypertrophy. *Mol. Cell. Biochem.* **2017**, *424*, 1–11. [CrossRef]
59. Sjakste, T.; Paramonova, N.; Osina, K.; Dokane, K.; Sokolovska, J.; Sjakste, N. Genetic variations in the PSMA3, PSMA6 and PSMC6 genes are associated with type 1 diabetes in Latvians and with expression level of number of UPS-related and T1DM-susceptible genes in HapMap individuals. *Mol. Genet. Genom.* **2016**, *291*, 891–903. [CrossRef]

60. Wang, H.W.; Zhao, W.P.; Liu, J.; Tan, P.P.; Tian, W.S.; Zhou, B.H. ATP5J and ATP5H Proactive Expression Correlates with Cardiomyocyte Mitochondrial Dysfunction Induced by Fluoride. *Biol. Trace Elem. Res.* **2017**, *180*, 63–69. [CrossRef]
61. Rekhter, M.; Staschke, K.; Estridge, T.; Rutherford, P.; Jackson, N.; Gifford-Moore, D.; Foxworthy, P.; Reidy, C.; Huang, X.D.; Kalbfleisch, M.; et al. Genetic ablation of IRAK4 kinase activity inhibits vascular lesion formation. *Biochem. Biophys. Res. Commun.* **2008**, *367*, 642–648. [CrossRef] [PubMed]
62. Gorinstein, S.; Caspi, A.; Libman, I.; Katrich, E.; Lerner, H.T.; Trakhtenberg, S. Fresh israeli jaffa sweetie juice consumption improves lipid metabolism and increases antioxidant capacity in hypercholesterolemic patients suffering from coronary artery disease: Studies in vitro and in humans and positive changes in albumin and fibrinogen fractions. *J. Agric. Food. Chem.* **2004**, *52*, 5215–5222. [CrossRef] [PubMed]
63. Schaefer, A.S.; Bochenek, G.; Jochens, A.; Ellinghaus, D.; Dommisch, H.; Güzeldemir-Akçakanat, E.; Graetz, C.; Harks, I.; Jockel-Schneider, Y.; Weinspach, K.; et al. Genetic evidence for PLASMINOGEN as a shared genetic risk factor of coronary artery disease and periodontitis. *Circ. Cardiovasc. Genet.* **2015**, *8*, 159–167. [CrossRef] [PubMed]
64. Strauss, E.; Oszkinis, G.; Staniszewski, R. SEPP1 gene variants and abdominal aortic aneurysm: Gene association in relation to metabolic risk factors and peripheral arterial disease coexistence. *Sci. Rep.* **2014**, *4*, 7061. [CrossRef] [PubMed]
65. Guo, Y.J.; Chen, L.; Bai, Y.P.; Li, L.; Sun, J.; Zhang, G.G.; Yang, T.L.; Xia, J.; Li, Y.J.; Chen, X.P. The ALDH2 Glu504Lys polymorphism is associated with coronary artery disease in Han Chinese: Relation with endothelial ADMA levels. *Atherosclerosis* **2010**, *211*, 545–550. [CrossRef] [PubMed]
66. Malik, R.; Dau, T.; Gonik, M.; Sivakumar, A.; Deredge, D.J.; Edeleva, E.V.; Götzfried, J.; van der Laan, S.W.; Pasterkamp, G.; Beaufort, N.; et al. Common coding variant in SERPINA1 increases the risk for large artery stroke. *Proc. Natl. Acad. Sci. USA* **2017**, *114*, 3613–3618. [CrossRef]
67. Rotroff, D.M.; Pijut, S.S.; Marvel, S.W.; Jack, J.R.; Havener, T.M.; Pujol, A.; Schluter, A.; Graf, G.A.; Ginsberg, H.N.; Shah, H.S.; et al. Genetic Variants in HSD17B3, SMAD3, and IPO11 Impact Circulating Lipids in Response to Fenofibrate in Individuals with Type 2 Diabetes. *Clin. Pharmacol.* **2018**, *103*, 712–721. [CrossRef]
68. Yu, X.H.; Qian, K.; Jiang, N.; Zheng, X.L.; Cayabyab, F.S.; Tang, C.K. ABCG5/ABCG8 in cholesterol excretion and atherosclerosis. *Clin. Chim. Acta* **2014**, *428*, 82–88. [CrossRef]
69. Schiekofer, S.; Bobak, I.; Kleber, M.E.; Maerz, W.; Rudofsky, G.; Dugi, K.A.; Schneider, J.G. Association between a gene variant near ataxia telangiectasia mutated and coronary artery disease in men. *Diabetes Vasc. Dis. Res.* **2014**, *11*, 60–63. [CrossRef]
70. Dazert, P.; Meissner, K.; Vogelgesang, S.; Heydrich, B.; Eckel, L.; Böhm, M.; Warzok, R.; Kerb, R.; Brinkmann, U.; Schaeffeler, E.; et al. Expression and localization of the multidrug resistance protein 5 (MRP5/ABCC5), a cellular export pump for cyclic nucleotides, in human heart. *Am. J. Pathol.* **2003**, *163*, 1567–1577. [CrossRef]
71. Wild, P.S.; Zeller, T.; Schillert, A.; Szymczak, S.; Sinning, C.R.; Deiseroth, A.; Schnabel, R.B.; Lubos, E.; Keller, T.; Eleftheriadis, M.S.; et al. A genome-wide association study identifies LIPA as a susceptibility gene for coronary artery disease. *Circ. Cardiovasc. Genet.* **2011**, *4*, 403–412. [CrossRef] [PubMed]
72. Westerterp, M.; Bochem, A.E.; Yvan-Charvet, L.; Murphy, A.J.; Wang, N.; Tall, A.R. ATP-binding cassette transporters, atherosclerosis, and inflammation. *Circ. Res.* **2014**, *114*, 157–170. [CrossRef] [PubMed]
73. Jacquemin, B.; Antoniades, C.; Nyberg, F.; Plana, E.; Müller, M.; Greven, S.; Salomaa, V.; Sunyer, J.; Bellander, T.; Chalamandaris, A.G.; et al. Common genetic polymorphisms and haplotypes of fibrinogen alpha, beta, and gamma chains affect fibrinogen levels and the response to proinflammatory stimulation in myocardial infarction survivors: The AIRGENE study. *J. Am. Coll. Cardiol.* **2008**, *52*, 941–952. [CrossRef] [PubMed]
74. Cheung, E.Y.; Uitte de Willige, S.; Vos, H.L.; Leebeek, F.W.; Dippel, D.W.; Bertina, R.M.; de Maat, M.P. Fibrinogen gamma' in ischemic stroke: A case-control study. *Stroke* **2008**, *39*, 1033–1035. [CrossRef]
75. Leenaerts, D.; Bosmans, J.M.; van der Veken, P.; Sim, Y.; Lambeir, A.M.; Hendriks, D. Plasma levels of carboxypeptidase U (CPU, CPB2 or TAFIa) are elevated in patients with acute myocardial infarction. *J. Thromb. Haemost* **2015**, *13*, 2227–2232. [CrossRef]
76. Széplaki, G.; Prohászka, Z.; Duba, J.; Rugonfalvi-Kiss, S.; Karádi, I.; Kókai, M.; Kramer, J.; Füst, G.; Kleiber, M.; Romics, L.; et al. Association of high serum concentration of the third component of complement (C3) with pre-existing severe coronary artery disease and new vascular events in women. *Atherosclerosis* **2004**, *177*, 383–389. [CrossRef]

77. Blaskó, B.; Kolka, R.; Thorbjornsdottir, P.; Sigurdarson, S.T.; Sigurdsson, G.; Rónai, Z.; Sasvári-Székely, M.; Bödvarsson, S.; Thorgeirsson, G.; Prohászka, Z.; et al. Low complement C4B gene copy number predicts short-term mortality after acute myocardial infarction. *Int. Immunol.* **2008**, *20*, 31–37. [CrossRef]
78. Shanker, J.; Perumal, G.; Rao, V.S.; Khadrinarasimhiah, N.B.; John, S.; Hebbagodi, S.; Mukherjee, M.; Kakkar, V.V. Genetic studies on the APOA1-C3-A5 gene cluster in Asian Indians with premature coronary artery disease. *Lipids Health Dis.* **2008**, *7*, 33. [CrossRef]
79. Heald, A.H.; Cruickshank, J.K.; Riste, L.K.; Cade, J.E.; Anderson, S.; Greenhalgh, A.; Sampayo, J.; Taylor, W.; Fraser, W.; White, A.; et al. Close relation of fasting insulin-like growth factor binding protein-1 (IGFBP-1) with glucose tolerance and cardiovascular risk in two populations. *Diabetologia* **2001**, *44*, 333–339. [CrossRef]
80. Miyazaki, A.; Sakashita, N.; Lee, O.; Takahashi, K.; Horiuchi, S.; Hakamata, H.; Morganelli, P.M.; Chang, C.C.; Chang, T.Y. Expression of ACAT-1 protein in human atherosclerotic lesions and cultured human monocytes-macrophages. *Arterioscler. Thromb. Vasc. Biol.* **1998**, *18*, 1568–1574. [CrossRef]
81. Thompson, A.; Danesh, J. Associations between apolipoprotein B, apolipoprotein AI, the apolipoprotein B/AI ratio and coronary heart disease: A literature-based meta-analysis of prospective studies. *J. Intern. Med.* **2006**, *259*, 481–492. [CrossRef] [PubMed]
82. Chang, C.T.; Liao, H.Y.; Chang, C.M.; Chen, C.Y.; Chen, C.H.; Yang, C.Y.; Tsai, F.J.; Chen, C.J. Oxidized ApoC1 on MALDI-TOF and glycated-ApoA1 band on gradient gel as potential diagnostic tools for atherosclerotic vascular disease. *Clin. Chim. Acta* **2013**, *420*, 69–75. [CrossRef] [PubMed]
83. Beale, E.G.; Harvey, B.J.; Forest, C. PCK1 and PCK2 as candidate diabetes and obesity genes. *Cell Biochem. Biophys.* **2007**, *48*, 89–95. [CrossRef] [PubMed]
84. Landrier, J.F.; Kasiri, E.; Karkeni, E.; Mihály, J.; Béke, G.; Weiss, K.; Lucas, R.; Aydemir, G.; Salles, J.; Walrand, S.; et al. Reduced adiponectin expression after high-fat diet is associated with selective up-regulation of ALDH1A1 and further retinoic acid receptor signaling in adipose tissue. *FASEB J.* **2017**, *31*, 203–211. [CrossRef] [PubMed]
85. Giacconi, R.; Bonfigli, A.R.; Testa, R.; Sirolla, C.; Cipriano, C.; Marra, M.; Muti, E.; Malavolta, M.; Costarelli, L.; Piacenza, F.; et al. +647 A/C and +1245 MT1A polymorphisms in the susceptibility of diabetes mellitus and cardiovascular complications. *Mol. Genet. Metab.* **2008**, *94*, 98–104. [CrossRef]
86. Yang, X.Y.; Sun, J.H.; Ke, H.Y.; Chen, Y.J.; Xu, M.; Luo, G.H. Metallothionein 2A genetic polymorphism and its correlation to coronary heart disease. *Eur. Rev. Med. Pharmacol. Sci.* **2014**, *18*, 3747–3753.
87. Ercan, B.; Ayaz, L.; Çiçek, D.; Tamer, L. Role of CYP2C9 and CYP2C19 polymorphisms in patients with atherosclerosis. *Cell. Biochem. Funct.* **2008**, *26*, 309–313. [CrossRef]
88. He, B.X.; Shi, L.; Qiu, J.; Tao, L.; Li, R.; Yang, L.; Zhao, S.J. A functional polymorphism in the CYP3A4 gene is associated with increased risk of coronary heart disease in the Chinese Han population. *Basic. Clin. Pharmacol. Toxicol.* **2011**, *108*, 208–213. [CrossRef]
89. Li, Y.Y.; Wu, X.Y.; Xu, J.; Qian, Y.; Zhou, C.W.; Wang, B. Apo A5 -1131T/C, FgB -455G/A, -148C/T, and CETP TaqIB gene polymorphisms and coronary artery disease in the Chinese population: A meta-analysis of 15,055 subjects. *Mol. Biol. Rep.* **2013**, *40*, 1997–2014. [CrossRef]
90. Ebrahim, S.; Lawlor, D.A.; Shlomo, Y.B.; Timpson, N.; Harbord, R.; Christensen, M.; Baban, J.; Kiessling, M.; Day, I.; Gaunt, T.; et al. Alcohol dehydrogenase type 1C (ADH1C) variants, alcohol consumption traits, HDL-cholesterol and risk of coronary heart disease in women and men: British Women's Heart and Health Study and Caerphilly cohorts. *Atherosclerosis* **2008**, *196*, 871–878. [CrossRef]
91. Clarke, R.; Peden, J.F.; Hopewell, J.C.; Kyriakou, T.; Goel, A.; Heath, S.C.; Parish, S.; Barlera, S.; Franzosi, M.G.; Rust, S.; et al. Genetic variants associated with Lp(a) lipoprotein level and coronary disease. *N. Engl. J. Med.* **2009**, *361*, 2518–2528. [CrossRef]
92. Russo, G.T.; Meigs, J.B.; Cupples, L.A.; Demissie, S.; Otvos, J.D.; Wilson, P.W.; Lahoz, C.; Cucinotta, D.; Couture, P.; Mallory, T.; et al. Association of the Sst-I polymorphism at the APOC3 gene locus with variations in lipid levels, lipoprotein subclass profiles and coronary heart disease risk: The Framingham offspring study. *Atherosclerosis* **2001**, *158*, 173–181. [CrossRef]
93. Siguel, E.N.; Lerman, R.H. Altered fatty acid metabolism in patients with angiographically documented coronary artery disease. *Metabolism* **1994**, *43*, 982–993. [CrossRef]
94. Surendran, R.P.; Visser, M.E.; Heemelaar, S.; Wang, J.; Peter, J.; Defesche, J.C.; Kuivenhoven, J.A.; Hosseini, M.; Péterfy, M.; Kastelein, J.J.; et al. Mutations in LPL, APOC2, APOA5, GPIHBP1 and LMF1 in patients with severe hypertriglyceridaemia. *J. Intern. Med.* **2012**, *272*, 185–196. [CrossRef] [PubMed]

95. Rienks, M.; Carai, P.; Bitsch, N.; Schellings, M.; Vanhaverbeke, M.; Verjans, J.; Cuijpers, I.; Heymans, S.; Papageorgiou, A. Sema3A promotes the resolution of cardiac inflammation after myocardial infarction. *Basic Res. Cardiol.* **2017**, *112*, 42. [CrossRef]
96. Yu, L.; Li, Z.; Dong, X.; Xue, X.; Liu, Y.; Xu, S.; Zhang, J.; Han, J.; Yang, Y.; Wang, H. Polydatin Protects Diabetic Heart against Ischemia-Reperfusion Injury via Notch1/Hes1-Mediated Activation of Pten/Akt Signaling. *Oxid. Med. Cell. Longev.* **2018**, *2018*, 2750695. [CrossRef]
97. Wang, Y.; Cao, Y.; Yamada, S.; Thirunavukkarasu, M.; Nin, V.; Joshi, M.; Rishi, M.T.; Bhattacharya, S.; Camacho-Pereira, J.; Sharma, A.K.; et al. Cardiomyopathy and Worsened Ischemic Heart Failure in SM22-α Cre-Mediated Neuropilin-1 Null Mice: Dysregulation of PGC1α and Mitochondrial Homeostasis. *Arterioscler. Thromb. Vasc. Biol.* **2015**, *35*, 1401–1412. [CrossRef]
98. Chun, J.L.; O'Brien, R.; Berry, S.E. Cardiac dysfunction and pathology in the dystrophin and utrophin-deficient mouse during development of dilated cardiomyopathy. *Neuromuscul. Disord.* **2012**, *22*, 368–379. [CrossRef]
99. Yan, X.X.; Lu, L.; Peng, W.H.; Wang, L.J.; Zhang, Q.; Zhang, R.Y.; Chen, Q.J.; Shen, W.F. Increased serum HMGB1 level is associated with coronary artery disease in nondiabetic and type 2 diabetic patients. *Atherosclerosis* **2009**, *205*, 544–548. [CrossRef]
100. Takada, D.; Ezura, Y.; Ono, S.; Iino, Y.; Katayama, Y.; Xin, Y.; Wu, L.L.; Larringa-Shum, S.; Stephenson, S.H.; Hunt, S.C.; et al. Apolipoprotein H variant modifies plasma triglyceride phenotype in familial hypercholesterolemia: A molecular study in an eight-generation hyperlipidemic family. *J. Atheroscler. Thromb.* **2003**, *10*, 79–84. [CrossRef]
101. Rodríguez, S.; Gaunt, T.R.; O'Dell, S.D.; Chen, X.H.; Gu, D.; Hawe, E.; Miller, G.J.; Humphries, S.E.; Day, I.N. Haplotypic analyses of the IGF2-INS-TH gene cluster in relation to cardiovascular risk traits. *Hum. Mol. Genet.* **2004**, *13*, 715–725. [CrossRef] [PubMed]
102. Xu, H.; Shang, Q.; Chen, H.; Du, J.; Wen, J.; Li, G.; Shi, D.; Chen, K. ITIH4: A New Potential Biomarker of "Toxin Syndrome" in Coronary Heart Disease Patient Identified with Proteomic Method. *Evid. Based. Complement. Alternat. Med.* **2013**, *2013*, 360149. [CrossRef] [PubMed]
103. Cahill, L.E.; Levy, A.P.; Chiuve, S.E.; Jensen, M.K.; Wang, H.; Shara, N.M.; Blum, S.; Howard, B.V.; Pai, J.K.; Mukamal, K.J.; et al. Haptoglobin genotype is a consistent marker of coronary heart disease risk among individuals with elevated glycosylated hemoglobin. *J. Am. Coll. Cardiol.* **2013**, *61*, 728–737. [CrossRef] [PubMed]
104. Hammadah, M.; Fan, Y.; Wu, Y.; Hazen, S.L.; Tang, W.H. Prognostic value of elevated serum ceruloplasmin levels in patients with heart failure. *J. Card. Fail.* **2014**, *20*, 946–952. [CrossRef] [PubMed]
105. Tanaka, M.; Mokhtari, G.K.; Terry, R.D.; Balsam, L.B.; Lee, K.H.; Kofidis, T.; Tsao, P.S.; Robbins, R.C. Overexpression of human copper/zinc superoxide dismutase (SOD1) suppresses ischemia-reperfusion injury and subsequent development of graft coronary artery disease in murine cardiac grafts. *Circulation* **2004**, *110*, II200–II206. [CrossRef] [PubMed]
106. Ebana, Y.; Ozaki, K.; Inoue, K.; Sato, H.; Iida, A.; Lwin, H.; Saito, S.; Mizuno, H.; Takahashi, A.; Nakamura, T.; et al. A functional SNP in ITIH3 is associated with susceptibility to myocardial infarction. *J. Hum. Genet.* **2007**, *52*, 220–229. [CrossRef]
107. Altamura, C.; Squitti, R.; Pasqualetti, P.; Gaudino, C.; Palazzo, P.; Tibuzzi, F.; Lupoi, D.; Cortesi, M.; Rossini, P.M.; Vernieri, F. Ceruloplasmin/Transferrin system is related to clinical status in acute stroke. *Stroke* **2009**, *40*, 1282–1288. [CrossRef]
108. Gan, W.; Wu, J.; Lu, L.; Xiao, X.; Huang, H.; Wang, F.; Zhu, J.; Sun, L.; Liu, G.; Pan, Y.; et al. Associations of CFH polymorphisms and CFHR1-CFHR3 deletion with blood pressure and hypertension in Chinese population. *PLoS ONE* **2012**, *7*, e42010. [CrossRef]
109. Renner, W.; Nauck, M.; Winkelmann, B.R.; Hoffmann, M.M.; Scharnagl, H.; Mayer, V.; Boehm, B.O.; März, W. Association of angiotensinogen haplotypes with angiotensinogen levels but not with blood pressure or coronary artery disease: The Ludwigshafen Risk and Cardiovascular Health Study. *J. Mol. Med.* **2005**, *83*, 235–239. [CrossRef]
110. He, M.; Guo, H.; Yang, X.; Zhou, L.; Zhang, X.; Cheng, L.; Zeng, H.; Hu, F.B.; Tanguay, R.M.; Wu, T. Genetic variations in HSPA8 gene associated with coronary heart disease risk in a Chinese population. *PLoS ONE* **2010**, *5*, e9684. [CrossRef]

111. Peppiatt-Wildman, C.M.; Albert, A.P.; Saleh, S.N.; Large, W.A. Endothelin-1 activates a $Ca^{2+}$-permeable cation channel with TRPC3 and TRPC7 properties in rabbit coronary artery myocytes. *J. Physiol.* **2007**, *580*, 755–764. [CrossRef] [PubMed]
112. Biscetti, F.; Straface, G.; Giovannini, S.; Santoliquido, A.; Angelini, F.; Santoro, L.; Porreca, C.F.; Pecorini, G.; Ghirlanda, G.; Flex, A. Association between TNFRSF11B gene polymorphisms and history of ischemic stroke in Italian diabetic patients. *Hum. Genet.* **2013**, *132*, 49–55. [CrossRef] [PubMed]
113. Zhao, J.; Lei, H. Tripartite Motif Protein 72 Regulates the Proliferation and Migration of Rat Cardiac Fibroblasts via the Transforming Growth Factor-β Signaling Pathway. *Cardiology* **2016**, *134*, 340–346. [CrossRef] [PubMed]
114. Muiya, N.P.; Wakil, S.; Al-Najai, M.; Tahir, A.I.; Baz, B.; Andres, E.; Al-Boudari, O.; Al-Tassan, N.; Al-Shahid, M.; Meyer, B.F.; et al. A study of the role of GATA2 gene polymorphism in coronary artery disease risk traits. *Gene* **2014**, *544*, 152–158. [CrossRef] [PubMed]
115. Murr, C.; Grammer, T.B.; Meinitzer, A.; Kleber, M.E.; März, W.; Fuchs, D. Immune activation and inflammation in patients with cardiovascular disease are associated with higher phenylalanine to tyrosine ratios: The ludwigshafen risk and cardiovascular health study. *J. Amino Acids* **2014**, *2014*, 783730. [CrossRef]

© 2019 by the authors. Licensee MDPI, Basel, Switzerland. This article is an open access article distributed under the terms and conditions of the Creative Commons Attribution (CC BY) license (http://creativecommons.org/licenses/by/4.0/).

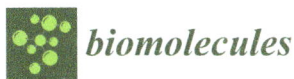 

Article

# Common Variants in *IL-20* Gene are Associated with Subclinical Atherosclerosis, Cardiovascular Risk Factors and IL-20 Levels in the Cohort of the Genetics of Atherosclerotic Disease (GEA) Mexican Study

Javier Angeles-Martínez [1,†], Rosalinda Posadas-Sánchez [2,†], Eyerahi Bravo-Flores [3], María del Carmen González-Salazar [2] and Gilberto Vargas-Alarcón [1,*]

1. Department of Molecular Biology, Instituto Nacional de Cardiología Ignacio Chávez, Mexico City 14080, Mexico; jabojangeles@yahoo.com.mx
2. Department of Endocrinology, Instituto Nacional de Cardiología Ignacio Chávez, Mexico City 14080, Mexico; rossy_posadas_s@yahoo.it (R.P.-S.); telesforo_13@yahoo.com.mx (M.d.C.G.-S.)
3. Department of Immunobiochemistry, Instituto Nacional de Perinatología Isidro Espinosa de los Reyes, Mexico City 11000, Mexico; eyerahiqfb@yahoo.com.mx
* Correspondence: gvargas63@yahoo.com; Tel.: +52-55-5573-2911 (ext. 20134)
† The contributions of J. Angeles-Martínez and R. Posadas-Sánchez are equal and the order of authorship is arbitrary.

Received: 27 November 2019; Accepted: 28 December 2019; Published: 3 January 2020

**Abstract:** Inflammation has been involved in the development of atherosclerosis, type 2 diabetes mellitus, insulin resistance, and obesity. Interleukin 20 is a pro-inflammatory cytokine encoded by a polymorphic gene located in chromosome 1. The aim of the study was to evaluate the association of two *IL-20* polymorphisms (rs1400986 and rs1518108) with subclinical atherosclerosis (SA), cardiovascular risk factors and IL-20 levels in a cohort of Mexican individuals. The polymorphisms were determined in 274 individuals with SA and 672 controls. Under different models, rs1400986 (OR = 0.51, $P_{codominant1}$ = 0.0001; OR = 0.36, $P_{codominant2}$ = 0.014; OR = 0.49, $P_{dominant}$ = 0.0001 and OR = 0.55, $P_{additive}$ = 0.0001) and rs1518108 (OR = 0.62, $P_{codominant2}$ = 0.048 and OR = 0.79, $P_{additive}$ = 0.048) were associated with a lower risk of SA. These polymorphisms were associated with cardiovascular risk factors in individuals with SA and controls. Controls with the rs1400986 *TT* genotype presented high levels of IL-20 ($p$ = 0.031). In individuals with the rs1400986 *CC* genotype, we observed a negative correlation between IL-20 levels and total abdominal tissue (TAT), visceral abdominal tissue (VAT) and subcutaneous abdominal tissue (SAT). Our results indicate that the *IL-20* rs1400986 and rs1518108 polymorphisms were associated with decreased risk of developing SA and with some cardiovascular risk factors in individuals with SA and healthy controls. Negative correlation between BMI and VAT/SAT ratio in individuals with rs1400986 *CC* genotype and among IL-20 levels and TAT, VAT and SAT was observed.

**Keywords:** cardiovascular risk factors; genetic association; inflammation; interleukin 20; polymorphisms; subclinical atherosclerosis

## 1. Introduction

Cardiovascular disease, principally coronary artery disease (CAD) is the leading cause of preventable death worldwide [1]. A major reason for this trend is the ongoing epidemic of type 2 diabetes mellitus (T2DM) and obesity-induced insulin resistance (IR) [2]. Substantial evidence shows that IR is associated with CAD risk factors and is likely a common ground for the diabetic atherogenic milieu [3]. Further, IR and T2DM are thought to be mechanistically linked to CAD via subclinical atherosclerosis (SA) [4]. SA develops over several decades and often remains asymptomatic until the occurrence of an acute, life-threatening event. Two subclinical measures of atherosclerosis have been used to predict CAD. One is carotid intima-media thickness (cIMT), a measure of the intimal and medial layers of the carotid artery walls and the other is coronary artery calcification (CAC), a marker of subclinical coronary atherosclerosis [5,6]. Visceral adipose tissue (VAT) accumulation is clearly associated with a higher risk of T2DM and CAD and is positively associated with cardiovascular risk factors [7–9]. It is well known that inflammation plays an important role in the development of T2DM, IR, obesity and CAD [10–12]. IL-20 is a pro-inflammatory cytokine produced preferentially by monocytes [13]. It belongs to the IL-10 family, which also includes IL-19, IL-22, IL-24, IL-26, IL-28 and IL-29 [14]. This cytokine acts stimulating the angiogenic activity through the induction of vascular endothelial growth factor (VEGF) and IL-8 production. Chen et al. [15] analyzed the expression of IL-20 and its receptor complex in human and mice (apolipoprotein E-deficient) atherosclerotic lesions. The results of this study suggest that IL-20 is a proatherogenic cytokine that contribute to the progression of the disease. The *IL-20* gene is located in chromosome 1 and two polymorphisms (rs1400986 and rs1518108) have been associated with inflammatory diseases, such as, psoriasis and ulcerative colitis [14,15]. Also, these polymorphisms were associated with chronic hepatitis B infection in African-Americans [16]. On the other hand, an "in silico" analysis that we made showed that the rs1400986 polymorphism modify a binding site for the MZF1 transcriptional factor, having a possible functional effect. Despite the important role of this cytokine in the inflammatory process and in consequence in the development of atherosclerosis [15,17], at the present, there are not studies that analyzed the association of the polymorphisms located in the gene that encodes this cytokine with the presence of atherosclerosis and cardiovascular risk factors. Thus, the aim of the present study was to evaluate the association of rs1400986 and rs1518108 *IL-20* polymorphisms with SA and cardiovascular risk factors in a Mexican population.

## 2. Materials and Methods

### 2.1. Study Population

The study complies with the Declaration of Helsinki and was approved by the Ethics Committee of the Instituto Nacional de Cardiología Ignacio Chávez (INCICH). All participants provided written informed consent. Study participants were a subset of the Genetics of Atherosclerotic Disease (GEA) Mexican Study ($n$ = 946) population. To be included in the study, volunteers were apparently healthy and asymptomatic without family history of premature CAD. Participants were recruited from blood bank donors and through brochures posted in social services centers. Computed tomography (CT) scans of the chest and abdomen were performed using a 64-channel multidetector helical computed tomography system (Somatom Cardiac Sensation, 64, Forcheim, Germany) and interpreted by experienced radiologists. Scans were read to assess and quantify various parameters: (a) total abdominal tissue (TAT), subcutaneous abdominal tissue (SAT) and visceral abdominal tissue (VAT) areas as previously reported by Kvist et al. (1988) [18]; (b) liver to spleen attenuation ratio (L:SAR) as described by Longo et al. (1993) [19]; and (c) coronary arterial calcification (CAC) score using the Agatston method [20]. Fatty liver was defined as L:SAR ≤ 1.0. In all individuals, clinical, demographic, anthropometric and biochemical parameters were evaluated as previously described [21–23]. Exclusion criteria were congestive heart failure, liver, renal, thyroid or oncological disease and premature CAD.

### 2.2. Definition of Subclinical Atherosclerosis

CAC quantified by the Agatston score has been known to be an excellent biomarker of atherosclerosis, independently predicting clinical outcomes, such as coronary heart disease [24–26]. In our group, after performing the computed tomography scans, 274 individuals were classified into the SA group (individuals with a CAC score > 0), while 672 participants comprised the healthy control group (CAC score = 0).

## 2.3. Quantification of IL-20 Concentration

In a subsample of 106 control individuals, IL-20 plasma concentrations were quantified. For the determination of the IL-20 levels, we designed a panel, which also included the IL-19 and IL-22 cytokines (Bio-Rad, Hercules, CA, USA). The levels were detected using Luminex multi-analyte technology (Bio-Plex ProTM, Bio-Rad, Hercules, CA, USA) according to the manufacturer's instruction. Before starting the bioassay, the samples were thawed on ice and once ready for use, they were centrifuged at 10,000 rpm for 4 min. Samples were incubated with antibodies immobilized on color-coded microparticles, washed to remove unbound material and then incubated with biotinylated antibodies to the molecules of interest. After further washing, the streptavidin-phycoerythrin conjugate that binds to the biotinylated antibodies was added before the final washing step. The Luminex analyzer was used to determine the magnitude of the phycoerythrin-derived signal in a microparticle-specific manner. The data were analyzed using Bio-Plex Manager software. Data were expressed in pg/mL.

## 2.4. Genetic Analysis

Genomic DNA from whole blood containing ethylenediamine-tetra-acetic acid was isolated with a no enzymatic method [27]. According to the manufacturer's instructions (Applied Biosystems, Foster City, CA, United States), the rs1400986 (C___1747382_10) and rs1518108 (C___1747381_10) IL-20 polymorphisms were determined in genomic DNA using 5' exonuclease TaqMan genotyping assays on an ABI Prism 7900HT Fast Real-Time polymerase chain reaction (PCR) system. Ten percent of the samples were determined twice in order to corroborate the assignment of the genotypes.

## 2.5. Statistical Analysis

Data are expressed as the mean (standard deviation), median (interquartile range) or frequencies. Normality of distribution was tested by the Kolmogorov-Smirnov test. The differences in continuous variables between groups were assessed with t-Student's test and Mann-Whitney U test, as appropriate. Nominal variables were analyzed using the chi-squared test. The analysis was made using the SPSS version 20.0 statistical package (SPSS, Chicago, Il, USA). The associations of the polymorphisms with SA and cardiovascular risk factors were analyzed using logistic regression under the following inheritance models: additive (add-major allele homozygotes vs. heterozygotes vs. minor allele homozygotes), codominant 1 (cod1-major allele homozygotes vs. heterozygotes), codominant 2 (cod2-major allele homozygotes vs. minor allele homozygotes), dominant (dom-major allele homozygotes vs. heterozygotes+minor allele homozygotes) and recessive (rec-major allele homozygotes+heterozygotes vs. minor allele homozygotes). When the association with SA was tested, the models were adjusted for age, gender, body mass index, current smoking status, alanine aminotransferase, aspartate aminotransferase and uric acid. To evaluate the association with cardiovascular risk factors, the models were adjusted for age, gender and BMI. Bonferroni correction was used for multiple testing due to the increased risk of Type I error (0.05 divided by 5; $P < 0.01$). Statistical power to detect associations of polymorphisms with SA exceeded 0.80 as estimated with QUANTO software (http://hydra.usc.edu/GxE/). Genotype frequencies did not deviate from Hardy-Weinberg equilibrium in any case (HWE, $p > 0.05$). Pairwise linkage disequilibrium (LD, D') estimations between polymorphisms and haplotype reconstruction were performed with Haploview version 4.1 (https://www.broadinstitute.org/haploview/haploview) (Broad Institute of Massachusetts Institute of Technology and Harvard University, Cambridge, MA, USA).

## 3. Results

### 3.1. Study Samples Characteristics

Table 1 summarizes the baseline characteristics of the study groups. After all the experiments and the data compilation, 274 individuals with SA (199 males and 75 females) and 672 healthy controls (257 males and 415 females) were included in the final analysis. Descriptive statistics of the study participants and differences in median by clinical features for each predictor variable are provided in Tables 1 and 2. In comparison with the healthy control group, individuals with SA exhibited higher levels of systolic and diastolic blood pressure, VAT, SAT, total-cholesterol (TC), low density lipoprotein-cholesterol (LDL-C), triglycerides, non-high density lipoprotein-cholesterol (non-HDL-C), gamma-glutamyl transpeptidase (GGT), apolipoprotein B, glucose, homeostasis model assessment of insulin resistance (HOMA-IR), creatinine, adiponectin, uric acid and albumin (Table 1).

Table 1. Clinical and metabolic characteristics of the studied groups.

|  | Control (n = 672) | SA (n = 274) | p |
|---|---|---|---|
| Age (years) | 52 ± 9 | 59 ± 8 | <0.0001 |
| Gender (% male) | 38.2 | 72.6 | <0.0001 |
| Body Mass Index (kg/m$^2$) | 27.9 (25.4–30.9) | 28.1 (25.6–31.3) | 0.219 |
| Waist Circumferences (cm) | 93.4 ± 11.7 | 97.4 ± 11.1 | <0.0001 |
| Systolic Blood Pressure (mmHg) | 115 (106–126) | 124 (113–137) | <0.0001 |
| Diastolic Blood Pressure (mmHg) | 72 (66–78) | 77 (70–83) | <0.0001 |
| Total Adipose Fat (cm$^3$) | 443 (350–542) | 442 (353–569) | 0.391 |
| Visceral Adipose fat (cm$^3$) | 146 (105–188) | 180 (141–230) | <0.0001 |
| Subcutaneous Adipose fat (cm$^3$) | 286 (218–371) | 260 (193–340) | 0.002 |
| Total Cholesterol (mg/dL) | 190 (168–209) | 198 (171–221) | 0.002 |
| HDL-C (mg/dL) | 47 (37–57) | 43 (36–50) | <0.0001 |
| LDL-C (mg/dL) | 115.6 (96.2–133.2) | 124.4 (102.3–145.2) | <0.0001 |
| Triglycerides (mg/dL) | 141 (107–194) | 158 (118–206) | 0.007 |
| Non-HDL-Cholesterol (mg/dL) | 140 (120–162) | 153 (129–175) | <0.0001 |
| ALT (IU/L) | 23 (17–32) | 22 (17–32) | 0.819 |
| AST (IU/L) | 25 (21–30) | 25 (21–31) | 0.542 |
| GGT (IU/L) | 24 (17–41) | 29 (21–41) | 0.001 |
| Alkaline Phosphatase (IU/L) | 81 (68–98) | 77 (65–93) | 0.013 |
| Apo B (mg/dL) | 86 (72–106) | 96 (79–119) | <0.0001 |
| Apo A1 (mg/dL) | 132 (113–157) | 133 (113–157) | 0.81 |
| Apo-B/Apo-A | 0.65 (0.51–0.84) | 0.7 (0.6–0.9) | 0.001 |
| Glucose (mg/dL) | 90 (84–97) | 95 (87–107) | <0.0001 |
| Insulin (μIU/mL) | 18 (13–24) | 19 (13–25) | 0.212 |
| HOMA-IR | 3.9 (2.7–5.8) | 4.7 (3.1–6.8) | <0.0001 |
| hsCRP (mg/dL) | 1.69 (0.87–3.46) | 1.71 (0.89–3.45) | 0.76 |
| Creatinine (mg/dL) | 0.8 (0.7–0.9) | 0.9 (0.7–1.1) | <0.0001 |
| Adiponectin (μg/mL) | 8.4 (5–12.9) | 6.4 (4.2–10.2) | <0.0001 |
| Uric Acid (mg/dL) | 5.4 (4.4–6.4) | 5.9 (4.9–6.9) | <0.0001 |
| Albumin (μg/mL) | 6.3 (2.9–12) | 7.2 (2.9–19) | 0.026 |
| Free Fatty Acid (mEq/L) | 0.5 (0.4–0.7) | 0.6 (0.4–0.7) | 0.631 |
| IR of the Adipose Tissue | 9.7 (6.2–14.5) | 10.2 (6.6–13.9) | 0.629 |

Data are shown as mean ±SD, median (interquartile range) or percentage. Comparisons were made using Student's t-test or Mann-Whitney U test, as appropriate, for continuous variables and by Chi square analysis for categorical variables. SA: Subclinical atherosclerosis; IR: Insulin resistance; hsCRP: High sensitivity C reactive protein; HOMA: Homeostasis model assessment of insulin resistance; GGT: Gamma Glutamyl transpeptidase; AST: Aspartate aminotransferase; HDL-C: High density lipoprotein-cholesterol; LDL-C: Low density lipoprotein-cholesterol; ALT: Alanine aminotransferase.

Additionally, in comparison with the control group, participants in the SA group showed a higher prevalence of hypercholesterolemia, LDL-C > 130 mg/dL, hypertriglyceridemia, T2DM, IR, metabolic syndrome, hypertension, high VAT, fatty liver and hyperuricemia (Table 2).

**Table 2.** Cardiovascular factors prevalence in the study population.

|  | Control (n = 672) | SA (n = 274) | * P |
|---|---|---|---|
| Total Cholesterol >200 mg/dL (%) | 35.4 | 47.1 | 0.001 |
| LDL-Cholesterol > 130 mg/dL (%) | 29.3 | 42.9 | <0.0001 |
| Hypoalphalipoproteinemia (%) | 47.7 | 45.3 | 0.518 |
| Hypertriglyceridemia (%) | 45.2 | 53.5 | 0.022 |
| Non-HDL-Cholesterol > 160 mg/dL (%) | 25.9 | 42 | <0.0001 |
| Overweight (%) | 45.8 | 47.4 | 0.114 |
| Obesity (%) | 31.1 | 33.9 | 0.083 |
| Abdominal Obesity (%) | 79.6 | 82.1 | 0.417 |
| Type 2 Diabetes Mellitus (%) | 10.6 | 23 | <0.0001 |
| Hyperinsulinemia (%) | 55.4 | 62.8 | 0.023 |
| Insulin resistance (%) | 57.5 | 67.9 | 0.002 |
| Metabolic Syndrome (%) | 40.6 | 54 | <0.0001 |
| Hypertension (%) | 29.2 | 49.6 | <0.0001 |
| High Total Abdominal Tissue (%) | 55.4 | 61.7 | 0.045 |
| High Subcutaneous Abdominal Tissue (%) | 50 | 54.7 | 0.106 |
| High Visceral Abdominal Tissue (%) | 58.8 | 73.7 | <0.0001 |
| Fatty Liver (%) | 32.1 | 39.3 | 0.024 |

Data is shown as percentage. * Comparisons were made using Chi square analysis. SA: Subclinical atherosclerosis, LDL: Low density lipoprotein and HDL: High density lipoprotein.

### 3.2. Association of Polymorphisms with SA

Genotype distribution of the polymorphisms in individuals with SA and controls were in accordance with the HWE expectation ($p > 0.05$). Genotype distribution in the study groups is presented in Table 3. Under several inheritance models, adjusted by age, gender, body mass index, current smoking status, alanine aminotransferase, aspartate aminotransferase and uric acid, the rs1400986 polymorphism was significantly associated with a low risk of developing SA (OR = 0.51, 95% CI: 0.36–0.73, $P_{cod1}$ = 0.0001; OR = 0.36, 95% CI: 0.16–0.81, $P_{cod2}$ = 0.014; OR = 0.49, 95% CI: 0.35–69, $P_{dom}$ = 0.0001 and OR = 0.55, 95% CI: 0.41–0.73, $P_{add}$ = 0.0001). In addition, the rs1518108 polymorphism showed a marginally significant association with a low risk of developing SA (OR = 0.62, 95% CI: 0.39–99, $P_{cod2}$ = 0.048 and OR = 0.79, 95% CI: 0.63–99, $P_{add}$ = 0.048). Thus, both polymorphisms were independently associated with a lower risk of developing SA.

**Table 3.** Association between IL-20 gene polymorphisms and subclinical atherosclerosis.

| SNP | Model | Genotypes and Alleles | SA n | Control n | p | OR | 95% CI |
|---|---|---|---|---|---|---|---|
| rs1400986 |  | CC | 177 | 336 |  |  |  |
|  |  | CT | 87 | 293 |  |  |  |
|  |  | TT | 10 | 43 |  |  |  |
|  |  | C | 441 | 965 | 0.0001 | 0.61 | 0.48–0.78 |
|  |  | T | 107 | 379 |  |  |  |
|  | codominant1 | CC | 177 | 336 | 0.0001 | 0.51 | 0.36–0.73 |
|  |  | CT | 87 | 293 |  |  |  |
|  | codominant2 | CC | 177 | 336 | 0.014 | 0.36 | 0.16–0.81 |
|  |  | TT | 10 | 43 |  |  |  |
|  | dominant | CC | 177 | 336 | 0.0001 | 0.49 | 0.35–0.69 |
|  |  | CT + TT | 97 | 336 |  |  |  |
|  | recessive | CC + CT | 264 | 629 | 0.063 | 0.47 | 0.21–1.04 |
|  |  | TT | 10 | 43 |  |  |  |
|  | additive | – | – | – | 0.0001 | 0.55 | 0.41–0.73 |
| rs1518108 |  | CC | 79 | 181 |  |  |  |
|  |  | CT | 140 | 336 |  |  |  |
|  |  | TT | 55 | 155 |  |  |  |
|  |  | C | 298 | 698 | 0.229 | 0.89 | 0.75–1.06 |

Table 3. Cont.

| SNP | Model | Genotypes and Alleles | SA n | Control n | p | OR | 95% CI |
|---|---|---|---|---|---|---|---|
| | | T | 250 | 646 | | | |
| | codominant1 | CC | 79 | 181 | 0.246 | 0.79 | 0.54–1.16 |
| | | CT | 140 | 336 | | | |
| | codominant2 | CC | 79 | 181 | 0.048 | 0.62 | 0.39–0.99 |
| | | TT | 55 | 155 | | | |
| | dominant | CC | 79 | 181 | 0.102 | 0.74 | 0.51–1.06 |
| | | CT + TT | 195 | 491 | | | |
| | recessive | CC + CT | 219 | 517 | 0.110 | 0.72 | 0.49–1.07 |
| | | TT | 55 | 155 | | | |
| | additive | – | – | – | 0.0480 | 0.79 | 0.63–0.99 |

Models were adjusted for age, gender, body mass index, current smoking status, alanine aminotransferase, aspartate aminotransferase and uric acid. SA: Subclinical atherosclerosis.

### 3.3. Association of the IL-20 Polymorphisms with Cardiovascular Risk Factors

Table 4 shows the association of IL-20 polymorphisms with some cardiovascular risk factors in (i) controls and (ii) SA individuals. In healthy controls, rs1400986 was significantly associated with high levels of inflammation (hsCRP ≥ 3mg/L, OR = 1.45, 95% CI: 1.01–2.10, $P_{cod1}$ = 0.047) and with low levels of GGT > p75 (OR = 0.41, 95% CI: 0.19–0.88, $P_{cod2}$ = 0.023 and OR = 0.42, 95% CI: 0.19–0.89, $P_{rec}$ = 0.024). The rs1518108 polymorphism was associated with risk of hypertension (OR = 1.83, 95% CI: 1.16–2.86, $P_{cod1}$ = 0.008 and OR = 1.68, 95% CI: 1.10–2.59, $P_{dom}$ = 0.016), high levels of inflammation (hsCRP ≥ 3mg/L, OR = 1.73, 95% CI: 1.03–2.89, $P_{cod2}$ = 0.037 and OR = 1.31, 95% CI: 1.01–1.70, $P_{rec}$ = 0.036) and levels of TAT > p75 (OR = 1.69, 95% CI: 1.07–2.69, $P_{cod1}$ = 0.025 and OR = 1.54, 95% CI: 1.004–2.37, $P_{dom}$ = 0.048). In SA individuals, under different models, the rs1518108 polymorphism was associated with levels of GGT > p75 (OR = 0.51, 95% CI: 0.28–0.91, $P_{cod1}$ = 0.023; OR = 0.35, 95% CI: 0.16–0.74, $P_{cod2}$ = 0.006; OR = 0.46, 95% CI: 0.26–0.79, $P_{dom}$ = 0.006 and OR = 0.58, 95% CI: 0.40–0.99, $P_{add}$ = 0.004) and alkaline phosphatase (ALP) > p75 (OR = 0.46, 95% CI: 0.26–0.84, $P_{cod1}$ = 0.011; OR = 0.48, 95% CI: 0.28–0.83, $P_{dom}$ = 0.010 and OR = 0.68, 95% CI: 0.47–0.99, $P_{add}$ = 0.046) (Table 4). In summary, in SA individuals, the rs1518108 was associated with high levels of GGT and ALP, whereas in controls, this polymorphism was associated with inflammation, hypertension and high levels of TAT. In controls, also the rs1400986 was associated with inflammation and low levels of GGT.

Table 4. Association among IL-20 gene polymorphisms and cardiovascular risk factors in controls and SA individuals.

| SNP | Model | Genotypes | Variable | | p | OR | 95% CI |
|---|---|---|---|---|---|---|---|
| (i) Controls | | | | | | | |
| rs1400986 | | | Inflammation | | | | |
| | | | Yes n = 203 | No n = 469 | | | |
| | codominant1 | CC | 91 | 245 | 0.047 | 1.45 | 1.01–2.10 |
| | | CT | 101 | 192 | | | |
| | | | GGT > 75 | | | | |
| | | | Yes n = 267 | No n = 400 | | | |
| | codominant2 | CC | 140 | 196 | 0.023 | 0.41 | 0.19–0.88 |
| | | TT | 10 | 32 | | | |
| | recessive | CC + CT | 257 | 368 | 0.024 | 0.42 | 0.19–0.89 |
| | | TT | 10 | 32 | | | |

**Table 4.** Cont.

| SNP | Model | Genotypes | Variable | | p | OR | 95% CI |
|---|---|---|---|---|---|---|---|
| rs1518108 | | | Hypertension | | | | |
| | | | Yes<br>n = 196 | No<br>n = 476 | | | |
| | codominant1 | CC | 38 | 143 | 0.008 | 1.83 | 1.16–2.86 |
| | | CT | 113 | 223 | | | |
| | dominant | CC | 38 | 143 | 0.016 | 1.68 | 1.10–2.59 |
| | | CT + TT | 158 | 333 | | | |
| | | | Inflammation | | | | |
| | | | Yes<br>n = 203 | No<br>n = 469 | | | |
| | codominant2 | CC | 43 | 138 | 0.037 | 1.73 | 1.03–2.89 |
| | | TT | 51 | 104 | | | |
| | recessive | CC + CT | 152 | 365 | 0.036 | 1.31 | 1.01–1.70 |
| | | TT | 51 | 104 | | | |
| | | | Total abdominal tissue >75 | | | | |
| | | | Yes<br>n = 360 | No<br>n = 290 | | | |
| | codominant1 | CC | 96 | 79 | 0.025 | 1.69 | 1.07–2.69 |
| | | CT | 179 | 146 | | | |
| | dominant | CC | 96 | 79 | 0.048 | 1.54 | 1.004–2.37 |
| | | CT + TT | 264 | 211 | | | |
| (ii) SA | | | | | | | |
| rs1518108 | | | GGT > 75 | | | | |
| | | | Yes<br>n = 111 | No<br>n = 163 | | | |
| | codominant1 | CC | 43 | 36 | 0.023 | 0.51 | 0.28–0.91 |
| | | CT | 51 | 88 | | | |
| | codominant2 | CC | 43 | 36 | 0.006 | 0.35 | 0.16–0.74 |
| | | TT | 17 | 39 | | | |
| | dominant | CC | 43 | 36 | 0.006 | 0.46 | 0.26–0.79 |
| | | CT + TT | 68 | 127 | | | |
| | additive | - | - | - | 0.004 | 0.58 | 0.40–0.99 |
| | | | ALP > 75 | | | | |
| | | | Yes<br>n = 91 | No<br>n = 183 | | | |
| | codominant1 | CC | 36 | 43 | 0.011 | 0.46 | 0.26–0.84 |
| | | CT | 38 | 101 | | | |
| | dominant | CC | 36 | 43 | 0.01 | 0.48 | 0.28–0.83 |
| | | CT + TT | 55 | 140 | | | |
| | additive | - | - | - | 0.046 | 0.68 | 0.47–0.99 |

Table shows the model with significant associations. Models were adjusted for age, gender and body mass index. Inflammation was considered when hsCRP ≥ 3mg/L.

### 3.4. Association of the rs1400986 Genotypes with IL-20 Levels

Levels of IL-20 were determined in 106 control participants (34 with CC, 36 with CT and 36 with TT genotypes). Individuals with extreme outlier's values were not included in the analysis (1 participant). SNP rs1400986 was associated with IL-20 levels. Figure 1 shows that individuals with TT genotype have significantly higher IL-20 levels than individuals with CC + CT genotypes (4.9 (3.1–10.7) pg/mL versus 3.6 (1.8–7.1) pg/mL respectively, $P = 0.0313$).

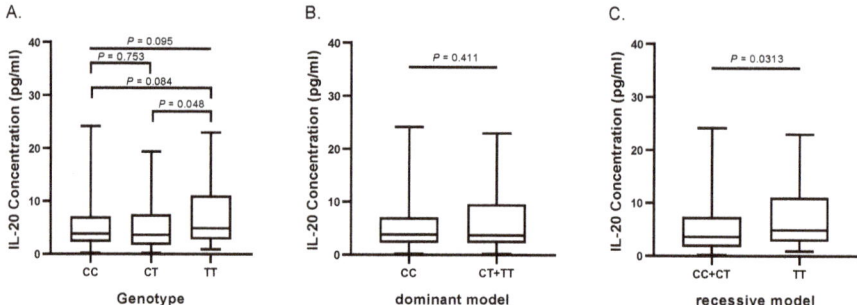

**Figure 1.** Association of the rs1400986 genotypes with IL-20 concentrations in control individuals. (**A**) Individuals with *TT* genotype have significantly higher IL-20 concentrations that those individuals with *CT* genotype (4.9 (3.1–10.7) pg/m vs. 3.8 (1.8–7.1) pg/mL, respectively, $P = 0.048$). (**B**) IL-20 concentrations in individuals with *CC* vs *CT* + *TT* genotypes (dominant model). No differences were observed. (**C**) IL-20 concentrations in individuals with *CC* + *CT* vs. *TT* genotypes (recessive model). Individuals with *TT* genotype have significantly higher IL-20 concentrations that those individuals with *CC* + *CT* genotype (4.9 (3.1–10.7) pg/m vs. 3.6 (1.8–7.1) pg/mL, respectively, $P = 0.0313$). Lines into bars indicate median; interquartile range (IQR 25–75) is shown in graphic representation. *P*: Kruskal-Wallis test and Mann-Whitney *U*-test.

### 3.5. Correlation of rs1400986 Genotypes with IL-20 Levels and Adipose Tissue

As for body–mass index (BMI) and the VAT/SAT ratio, the individuals with *CC* genotypes showed a statistically significant negative correlation between these parameters ($r^2 = 0.021$; $P = 0.0087$) and no such association was found in relation to *CT* + *TT* genotypes ($P = 0.579$) (Figure 2A). In order to better understand whether adipose tissue levels may impact the IL-20 concentration according to the genotypes of the rs1400986 polymorphism, we performed a correlation analysis in 106 control participants (*CC n* = 34, *CT n* = 36 and *TT n* = 36). Among individuals with the *CC* genotype, the IL-20 concentrations were negatively correlated with TAT ($r^2 = 0.23$; $P = 0.0037$, Figure 2B), VAT ($r^2 = 0.12$; $P = 0.0427$, Figure 2C) and SAT ($r^2 = 0.21$; $P = 0.006$, Figure 2D). These correlations were not found in individuals with *CT* + *TT* genotypes. Thus, negative correlation between BMI and VAT/SAT ratio in individuals with rs1400986 *CC* genotype and among IL-20 levels and TAT, VAT and SAT was observed.

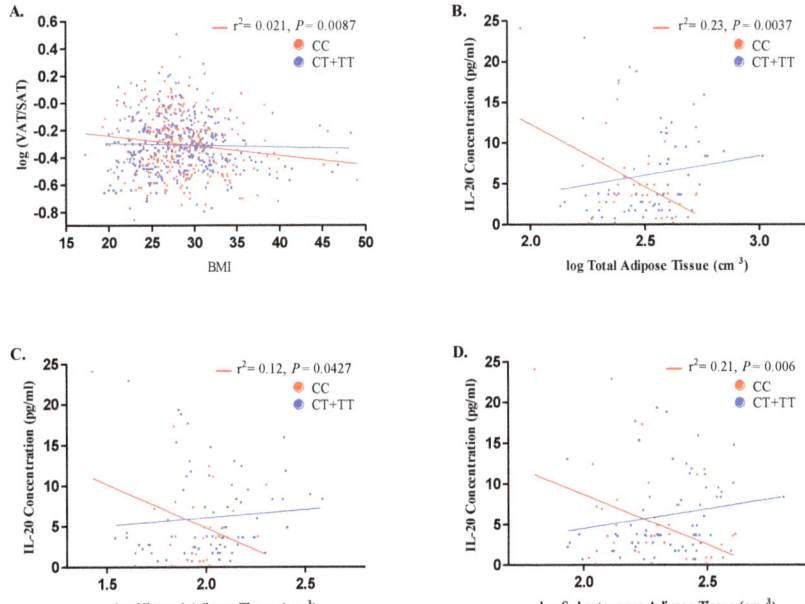

**Figure 2.** Correlation between adipose tissue distributions, body mass index and IL-20 concentrations according to rs1400986 genotypes in control individuals. Lines represent simple linear regression: blue lines represent CT + TT genotypes carriers and red represent CC genotype carriers. (**A**) Overall, body mass index (BMI) was negatively correlated with visceral to subcutaneous adipose tissue ratio (VAT/SAT) in individuals with CC genotypes but not in individuals with CT + TT genotypes. On adipose tissue stratification, a negatively and significant correlation of IL-20 levels and log TAT (**B**), log VAT (**C**) and log SAT (**D**) was observed in individuals with CC genotypes.

### 3.6. Haplotypes Analysis

The IL-20 polymorphisms were not in linkage disequilibrium (D′ > 0.048 and $r^2$ > 0.09). In fact, 4 different haplotypes were observed; one of these haplotypes (TT) was significantly associated with a lower risk of SA (OR = 0.63, 95% CI: 0.50–0.80, P = 0.00016) (Table 5).

**Table 5.** IL-20 haplotype frequencies in SA and healthy controls.

| Haplotypes | SA (n = 274) | | Control (n = 672) | | $X^2$ | P | OR | 95% CI |
|---|---|---|---|---|---|---|---|---|
| | n | % | n | % | | | | |
| CC | 134 | 48.9 | 298 | 44.4 | 3.88 | 0.077 | 1.19 | 1.01–1.42 |
| CT | 87 | 31.6 | 184 | 27.4 | 3.376 | 0.066 | 1.22 | 1.00–1.48 |
| TT | 39 | 14.2 | 139 | 20.7 | 10.684 | 0.00016 | 0.63 | 0.50–0.80 |
| TC | 14 | 5.4 | 51 | 7.6 | 2.94 | 0.086 | 0.69 | 0.48–0.99 |

The order of the alleles in the haplotypes is according to the positions of the polymorphisms in the chromosome (rs1400986 and rs1518108). SA: subclinical atherosclerosis; OR: odds ratio.

## 4. Discussion

The results of the study are the first demonstration of the association between *IL-20* polymorphisms and SA. Here, we provide genetic evidence that the rs1400986 and rs1518108 polymorphisms occurring in the *IL-20* gene were independently associated with a lower risk of developing SA. When these polymorphisms were analyzed as a haplotype, the association remaining significant. Associations with cardiovascular risk factors were observed in both studied groups. In AS individuals, the rs1518108 was associated with high levels of GGT and ALP, whereas in controls, this polymorphism was associated with high levels of hsCRP and TAT and with hypertension. In controls, also the rs1400986 was associated with high levels of hsCRP and low levels of GGT. High levels of IL-20 were observed in control individuals with rs1400986 *TT* genotype. Negative correlation between BMI and VAT/SAT ratio in individuals with rs1400986 *CC* genotype and among IL-20 levels and TAT, VAT and SAT was observed. Chen et al., [15] shown that IL-20 and its receptors are expressed in the human and experimental atherosclerosis plaque. More importantly, the authors demonstrated that systemic delivery of IL-20 accelerates atherogenesis in the apolipoprotein E-knockout mouse model. Our current study supports an important role of the *IL-20* polymorphisms in SA and in some cardiovascular risk factors.

It was found that IL20 cytokine has been involved in the developing of atherosclerosis [15,17], however, at the present, there are not studies that analyzed the association of the polymorphisms located in the gene that encodes this cytokine with the presence of atherosclerosis. The association of these polymorphisms with some inflammatory diseases has been reported, specifically in psoriasis and ulcerative colitis [28,29]. In African Americans, the rs1400986 and rs1518108 polymorphisms were associated with chronic hepatitis B infection [16]. Galimova et al., [30] analyzed 48 polymorphisms in 377 patients with psoriasis and 403 healthy controls and reported that the rs1400986 *T* allele was associated with decreased risk of psoriasis and that the combination of *IL10* rs1554286 and *IL20* rs1518108 was associated also with a reduced risk of presenting this disease. In these studies, were only compared the three different genotypes in each polymorphism, they did not use an analysis considering the inheritance models like in our study. In our study these polymorphisms were associated with lower risk of SA under different inheritance models. The rs1400986 was associated under the five models analyzed (cod1, cod2, dom, rec and add), whereas the rs1518108 was associated under two models (cod2 and add). This result corroborates the association, principally of the rs1400986 polymorphism with SA. An in-silico analysis showed that the rs1400986 polymorphism modify a binding site for the MZF1 transcriptional factor. MZF1 is a transcriptional regulator of several proteins; one of them is the SERPINA3 (serine proteinase inhibitor A3), protein that has been recently suggested as a potential predictive marker of clinical outcomes in myocardial infarction [31]. The association of the rs1400986 polymorphism with SA that we detected in our study could be related with the effect of the MZF2 transcriptional factor in the IL-20 levels.

In our study, the rs1518108 polymorphism was associated with high levels of GGT in SA individuals. High concentrations of GGT have been associated with cardiovascular diseases [32] and with non-alcoholic fatty liver disease (NAFLD) [33]. Is well known that fatty liver is an important condition associated with the developing of atherosclerosis [34]. In a previous study, increased expression of IL-20 was detected in obese patients with NAFLD [35].

Both IL-20 polymorphisms were associated with high levels of hsCRP in control individuals corroborating an inflammatory effect of this cytokine in these individuals. The rs1400986 *TT* genotype was associated with decreased risk of SA, however in control individuals this genotype was associated with high levels of IL-20, which is a pro-inflammatory cytokine. This contradictory result could be explained considering that the production of IL-20 and other molecules is a complex mechanism that involves not only changes at DNA level but also epigenetics modifications. Moreover, it is important, to considered that in our study, the levels of IL-20 were measured in circulating blood and only in a small group of control individuals. Unfortunately, these levels were not measured in SA individuals. The panel used for the determination of the IL-20 levels was designed by us and also included the IL-19 and IL-22 cytokines, both members of the IL-10 family. Associations of the levels of these cytokines with specific polymorphisms located in its respective genes are currently being analyzed.

It is important to mention, that the genotypes of *IL-20* rs1400986 polymorphism presented a negative correlation with TAT, VAT and SAT in control individuals. Thus, in individuals with rs1400986 *CC* genotype, the levels of the IL-20 cytokine decreased when the levels of TAT, VAT or SAT increase. Recently, Tanaka et al. [36] analyzed the impact of the VAT and SAT distribution on coronary plaque scores. They reported that high SAT and low VAT correlated inversely with the extent and severity of coronary artery plaques.

Our study presents some strengths: The group of individuals that we analyzed belong to the GEA project that was designed to examine the genetic bases of premature CAD and SA and its association with emerging and traditional cardiovascular risk factors in the Mexican population. This is a large cohort that was characterized from demographic, anthropometric, biochemical, clinical and tomographic point of view. Also, in the whole group of individuals, ancestry markers were determined and the distribution of Amerindian, European and African ancestry was similar in the groups included, thus the study has no ethnic bias [23]. Despite this, there are some limitations to consider. The results were not replicated in an independent set of patients and controls. Considering that this is the first time that polymorphisms located within the IL-20 gene are associated with SA and cardiovascular risk factors, replication in another cohort of patients is necessary to confirm these results. The IL-20 levels were only determined in a small sample of control individuals and not in the SA individuals. The study included only individuals with SA defined as CAC > 0.0, thus the association of these polymorphisms with coronary artery disease is mandatory.

## 5. Conclusions

In summary, our results indicate that the rs1400986 and rs1518108 polymorphisms in the *IL-20* gene were associated (independently or as a haplotype) with decreased risk of developing SA. These polymorphisms were also associated with some cardiovascular risk factors in individuals with SA and healthy controls. Healthy controls with the rs1400986 *TT* genotype presented high levels of IL-20. Negative correlation between BMI and VAT/SAT ratio in individuals with rs1400986 *CC* genotype and among IL-20 levels and TAT, VAT and SAT was observed. To the best of our knowledge, this is the first study that evaluates the association of *IL-20* polymorphisms with SA, cardiovascular risk factors and IL-20 levels. For this reason, the detected associations are not yet definitive and replicate studies in independent populations are warranted to confirm these findings.

**Author Contributions:** Conceptualization, G.V.-A. and J.A.-M.; Methodology, G.V.-A. and R.P.-S.; Formal analysis, J.A.-M. and E.B.-F.; Resources, G.V.-A. and R.P.-S.; Visualization, J.A.-M. and G.V.-A.; Supervision, E.B.-F. and M.d.C.G.-S.; Project administration, G.V.-A. and R.P.-S.; Funding acquisition, G.V.-A.; Data curation, J.A.-M., E.B.-F. and R.P.-S.; Writing—original draft preparation, J.A.-M., G.V.-A., R.P.-S., E.B.-F. and M.d.C.G.-S.; Writing—review and editing, G.V.-A. and J.A.-M. All authors have read and agreed to the published version of the manuscript.

**Funding:** This work was supported in part by grants from the Consejo Nacional de Ciencia y Tecnología, México (Projects No. CB-156911 and FC-1958).

**Acknowledgments:** Javier Angeles-Martínez is a doctoral student in the Programa de Doctorado en Ciencias Biomédicas, Universidad Nacional Autónoma de México (UNAM). The authors are grateful to Angel Rene López-Uribe for his technical assistance.

**Conflicts of Interest:** The authors declare that there is no conflict of interests regarding the publication of this paper.

## References

1. Nowbar, A.N.; Gitto, M.; Howard, J.P.; Francis, D.P.; Al-Lamee, R. Mortality From Ischemic Heart Disease: Analysis of Data From the World Health Organization and Coronary Artery Disease Risk Factors From NCD Risk Factor Collaboration. *Circ. Cardiovasc. Qual. Outcomes* **2019**, *12*, e005375. [CrossRef] [PubMed]
2. Chobot, A.; Górowska-Kowolik, K.; Sokołowska, M.; Jarosz-Chobot, P. Obesity and diabetes-Not only a simple link between two epidemics. *Diabetes Metab. Res. Rev.* **2018**, *34*, 3042. [CrossRef] [PubMed]
3. Cho, Y.-R.; Ann, S.H.; Won, K.-B.; Park, G.-M.; Kim, Y.-G.; Yang, D.H.; Kang, J.-W.; Lim, T.-H.; Kim, H.-K.; Choe, J.; et al. Association between insulin resistance, hyperglycemia and coronary artery disease according to the presence of diabetes. *Sci. Rep.* **2019**, *9*, 6129. [CrossRef] [PubMed]
4. Fakhrzadeh, H.; Sharifi, F.; Alizadeh, M.; Arzaghi, S.M.; Tajallizade-Khoob, Y.; Tootee, A.; Alatab, S.; Mirarefin, M.; Badamchizade, Z.; Kazemi, H. Relationship between insulin resistance and subclinical atherosclerosis in individuals with and without type 2 diabetes mellitus. *J. Diabetes Metab. Disord.* **2015**, *15*, 41. [CrossRef]

5. Newman, A.B.; Naydeck, B.L.; Sutton-Tyrrell, K.; Edmundowicz, D.; O'Leary, D.; Kronmal, R.; Burke, G.L.; Kuller, L.H. Relationship between coronary artery calcification and other measures of subclinical cardiovascular disease in older adults. *Arterioscler. Thromb. Vasc. Biol.* **2002**, *22*, 1674–1679. [CrossRef]
6. Wagenknecht, L.E.; Langefeld, C.D.; Carr, J.J.; Riley, W.; Freedman, B.I.; Moossavi, S.; Bowden, D.W. Race-specific relationships between coronary and carotid artery calcification and carotid intimal medial thickness. *Stroke* **2004**, *35*, 97–99. [CrossRef]
7. Haberka, M.; Skilton, M.; Biedroń, M.; Szóstak-Janiak, K.; Partyka, M.; Matla, M.; Gąsior, Z. Obesity, visceral adiposity and carotid atherosclerosis. *J. Diabetes Complicat.* **2019**, *33*, 302–306. [CrossRef]
8. Baloglu, I.; Turkmen, K.; Selcuk, N.; Tonbul, H.; Ozcicek, A.; Hamur, H.; Iyısoy, S.; Akbas, E. The Relationship between Visceral Adiposity Index and Epicardial Adipose Tissue in Patients with Type 2 Diabetes Mellitus. *Exp. Clin. Endocrinol. Diabetes* **2019**. [CrossRef]
9. Gruzdeva, O.; Borodkina, D.; Uchasova, E.; Dyleva, Y.; Barbarash, O. Localization of fat depots and cardiovascular risk. *Lipids Health Dis.* **2018**, *17*, 218. [CrossRef]
10. Lontchi-Yimagou, E.; Sobngwi, E.; Matsha, T.E.; Kengne, A.P. Diabetes Mellitus and Inflammation. *Curr. Diab. Rep.* **2013**, *13*, 435–444. [CrossRef]
11. Wu, H.; Ballantyne, C.M. Skeletal muscle inflammation and insulin resistance in obesity. *J. Clin. Investig.* **2017**, *127*, 43–54. [CrossRef] [PubMed]
12. Poston, R.N. Atherosclerosis: Integration of its pathogenesis as a self-perpetuating propagating inflammation: A review. *Cardiovasc. Endocrinol. Metab.* **2019**, *8*, 51–61. [PubMed]
13. Wolk, K.; Kunz, S.; Asadullah, K.; Sabat, R. Cutting edge: Immune cells as sources and targets of the IL-10 family members? *J. Immunol.* **2002**, *168*, 5397–5402. [CrossRef] [PubMed]
14. Pestka, S.; Krause, C.D.; Sarkar, D.; Walter, M.R.; Shi, Y.; Fisher, P.B. Interleukin -10 and R elated C ytokines and R eceptors. *Annu. Rev. Immunol.* **2004**, *22*, 929–979. [CrossRef] [PubMed]
15. Chen, W.-Y.; Cheng, B.-C.; Jiang, M.-J.; Hsieh, M.-Y.; Chang, M.-S. IL-20 is expressed in atherosclerosis plaques and promotes atherosclerosis in apolipoprotein E-deficient mice. *Arterioscler. Thromb. Vasc. Biol.* **2006**, *26*, 2090–2095. [CrossRef]
16. Truelove, A.L.; Oleksyk, T.K.; Shrestha, S.; Thio, C.L.; Goedert, J.J.; Donfield, S.M.; Kirk, G.D.; Thomas, D.L.; O'Brien, S.J.; Smith, M.W. Evaluation of IL10, IL19 and IL20 gene polymorphisms and chronic hepatitis B infection outcome. *Int. J. Immunogenet.* **2008**, *35*, 255–264. [CrossRef]
17. Caligiuri, G.; Kaveri, S.V.; Nicoletti, A. IL-20 and atherosclerosis: Another brick in the wall. *Arterioscler. Thromb. Vasc. Biol.* **2006**, *26*, 1929–1930. [CrossRef]
18. Kvist, H.; Chowdhury, B.; Grangård, U.; Tylén, U.; Sjöström, L. Total and visceral adipose-tissue volumes derived from measurements with computed tomography in adult men and women: Predictive equations. *Am. J. Clin. Nutr.* **1988**, *48*, 1351–1361. [CrossRef]
19. Longo, R.; Ricci, C.; Masutti, F.; Vidimari, R.; Crocé, L.S.; Bercich, L.; Tiribelli, C.; Dalla Palma, L. Fatty infiltration of the liver. Quantification by 1H localized magnetic resonance spectroscopy and comparison with computed tomography. *Investig. Radiol.* **1993**, *28*, 297–302. [CrossRef]
20. Mautner, G.C.; Mautner, S.L.; Froehlich, J.; Feuerstein, I.M.; Proschan, M.A.; Roberts, W.C.; Doppman, J.L. Coronary artery calcification: Assessment with electron beam CT and histomorphometric correlation. *Radiology* **1994**, *192*, 619–623. [CrossRef]
21. Posadas-Sánchez, R.; Ocampo-Arcos, W.A.; López-Uribe, A.R.; González-Salazar, M.C.; Cardoso-Saldaña, G.; Mendoza-Pérez, E.; Medina-Urrutia, A.; Jorge-Galarza, E.; Posadas-Romero, C. Asociación del ácido úrico con factores de riesgo cardiovascular y aterosclerosis subclínica en adultos mexicanos. *Rev. Mex. Endocrinol. Metab. Nutr.* **2014**, *1*, 14–21.
22. Medina-Urrutia, A.; Posadas-Romero, C.; Posadas-Sánchez, R.; Jorge-Galarza, E.; Villarreal-Molina, T.; González-Salazar, M.D.C.; Cardoso-Saldaña, G.; Vargas-Alarcón, G.; Torres-Tamayo, M.; Juárez-Rojas, J.G. Role of adiponectin and free fatty acids on the association between abdominal visceral fat and insulin resistance. *Cardiovasc. Diabetol.* **2015**, *14*, 20. [CrossRef] [PubMed]
23. Posadas-Sánchez, R.; Pérez-Hernández, N.; Rodríguez-Pérez, J.M.; Coral-Vázquez, R.M.; Roque-Ramírez, B.; Llorente, L.; Lima, G.; Flores-Dominguez, C.; Villarreal-Molina, T.; Posadas-Romero, C.; et al. Interleukin-27 polymorphisms are associated with premature coronary artery disease and metabolic parameters in the Mexican population: The genetics of atherosclerotic disease (GEA) Mexican study. *Oncotarget* **2017**, *8*, 64459–64470. [CrossRef] [PubMed]

24. Faggiano, P.; Dasseni, N.; Gaibazzi, N.; Rossi, A.; Henein, M.; Pressman, G. Cardiac calcification as a marker of subclinical atherosclerosis and predictor of cardiovascular events: A review of the evidence. *Eur. J. Prev. Cardiol.* **2019**, *26*, 1191–1204. [CrossRef] [PubMed]
25. Detrano, R.; Guerci, A.D.; Carr, J.J.; Bild, D.E.; Burke, G.; Folsom, A.R.; Liu, K.; Shea, S.; Szklo, M.; Bluemke, D.A.; et al. Coronary Calcium as a Predictor of Coronary Events in Four Racial or Ethnic Groups. *N. Engl. J. Med.* **2008**, *358*, 1336–1345. [CrossRef] [PubMed]
26. Greenland, P.; LaBree, L.; Azen, S.P.; Doherty, T.M.; Detrano, R.C. Coronary artery calcium score combined with Framingham score for risk prediction in asymptomatic individuals. *JAMA* **2004**, *291*, 210–215. [CrossRef] [PubMed]
27. Lahiri, D.K.; Nurnberger, J.I. A rapid non-enzymatic method for the preparation of HMW DNA from blood for RFLP studies. *Nucleic Acids Res.* **1991**, *19*, 5444. [CrossRef]
28. Kingo, K.; Kõks, S.; Nikopensius, T.; Silm, H.; Vasar, E. Polymorphisms in the interleukin-20 gene: Relationships to plaque-type psoriasis. *Genes Immun.* **2004**, *5*, 117–121. [CrossRef]
29. Yamamoto-Furusho, J.K.; De-León-Rendón, J.L.; de la Torre, M.G.; Alvarez-León, E.; Vargas-Alarcón, G. Genetic polymorphisms of interleukin 20 (IL-20) in patients with ulcerative colitis. *Immunol. Lett.* **2013**, *149*, 50–53. [CrossRef]
30. Galimova, E.; Rätsep, R.; Traks, T.; Kingo, K.; Escott-Price, V.; Kõks, S. Interleukin-10 family cytokines pathway: Genetic variants and psoriasis. *Br. J. Dermatol.* **2017**, *176*, 1577–1587. [CrossRef]
31. Zhao, L.; Zheng, M.; Guo, Z.; Li, K.; Liu, Y.; Chen, M.; Yang, X. Circulating Serpina3 levels predict the major adverse cardiac events in patients with myocardial infarction. *Int. J. Cardiol.* **2019**. [CrossRef] [PubMed]
32. Chung, H.S.; Lee, J.S.; Kim, J.A.; Roh, E.; Lee, Y.B.; Hong, S.H.; Yoo, H.J.; Baik, S.H.; Kim, N.H.; Seo, J.A.; et al. γ-Glutamyltransferase Variability and the Risk of Mortality, Myocardial Infarction and Stroke: A Nationwide Population-Based Cohort Study. *J. Clin. Med.* **2019**, *8*, 832. [CrossRef] [PubMed]
33. Bobrus-Chociej, A.; Flisiak-Jackiewicz, M.; Daniluk, U.; Wojtkowska, M.; Kłusek-Oksiuta, M.; Tarasów, E.; Lebensztejn, D. Estimation of gamma-glutamyl transferase as a suitable simple biomarker of the cardiovascular risk in children with non-alcoholic fatty liver disease. *Acta Biochim. Pol.* **2018**, *65*, 539–544. [CrossRef] [PubMed]
34. Gaggini, M.; Morelli, M.; Buzzigoli, E.; DeFronzo, R.A.; Bugianesi, E.; Gastaldelli, A. Non-alcoholic fatty liver disease (NAFLD) and its connection with insulin resistance, dyslipidemia, atherosclerosis and coronary heart disease. *Nutrients* **2013**, *5*, 1544–1560. [CrossRef] [PubMed]
35. Estep, J.M.; Goodman, Z.; Sharma, H.; Younossi, E.; Elarainy, H.; Baranova, A.; Younossi, Z. Adipocytokine expression associated with miRNA regulation and diagnosis of NASH in obese patients with NAFLD. *Liver Int.* **2015**, *35*, 1367–1372. [CrossRef] [PubMed]
36. Tanaka, T.; Kishi, S.; Ninomiya, K.; Tomii, D.; Koseki, K.; Sato, Y.; Okuno, T.; Sato, K.; Koike, H.; Yahagi, K.; et al. Impact of abdominal fat distribution, visceral fat and subcutaneous fat on coronary plaque scores assessed by 320-row computed tomography coronary angiography. *Atherosclerosis* **2019**, *287*, 155–161. [CrossRef]

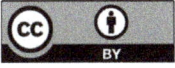

© 2020 by the authors. Licensee MDPI, Basel, Switzerland. This article is an open access article distributed under the terms and conditions of the Creative Commons Attribution (CC BY) license (http://creativecommons.org/licenses/by/4.0/).

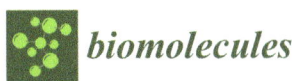 

*Review*

# Circulating microRNA as a Biomarker for Coronary Artery Disease

Ibrahim T. Fazmin [1,2], Zakaria Achercouk [1], Charlotte E. Edling [1], Asri Said [3] and Kamalan Jeevaratnam [1,*]

1. Faculty of Health and Medical Science, University of Surrey, Guildford GU2 7AL, UK; itf21@cam.ac.uk (I.T.F.); za270@cam.ac.uk (Z.A.); c.edling@surrey.ac.uk (C.E.E.)
2. School of Clinical Medicine, University of Cambridge, Cambridge CB2 1TN, UK
3. School of Medicine, University Malaysia Sarawak, Kota Samarahan 94300, Sarawak, Malaysia; sasri@unimas.my
* Correspondence: drkamalanjeeva@gmail.com; Tel.: +44-1483-682395

Received: 7 August 2020; Accepted: 19 September 2020; Published: 23 September 2020

**Abstract:** Coronary artery disease (CAD) is the leading cause of sudden cardiac death in adults, and new methods of predicting disease and risk-stratifying patients will help guide intervention in order to reduce this burden. Current CAD detection involves multiple modalities, but the consideration of other biomarkers will help improve reliability. The aim of this narrative review is to help researchers and clinicians appreciate the growing relevance of miRNA in CAD and its potential as a biomarker, and also to suggest useful miRNA that may be targets for future study. We sourced information from several databases, namely PubMed, Scopus, and Google Scholar, when collating evidentiary information. MicroRNAs (miRNA) are short, noncoding RNAs that are relevant in cardiovascular physiology and pathophysiology, playing roles in cardiac hypertrophy, maintenance of vascular tone, and responses to vascular injury. CAD is associated with changes in miRNA expression profiles, and so are its risk factors, such as abnormal lipid metabolism and inflammation. Thus, they may potentially be biomarkers of CAD. Nevertheless, there are limitations in using miRNA. These include cost and the presence of several confounding factors that may affect miRNA profiles. Furthermore, there is difficulty in the normalisation of miRNA values between published studies, due to pre-analytical variations in samples.

**Keywords:** coronary artery disease; biomarkers; noncoding RNA; microRNA

---

## 1. Introduction

Coronary artery disease (CAD) is a significant cause of morbidity and mortality in the elderly. It is a complex, chronic pathological process in the intima of coronary arteries, yielding atherosclerotic lesions that restrict blood flow to the myocardium and may be associated with a degree of inflammation. Whilst the disease can remain stable, acute plaque rupture followed by coronary artery thrombosis can be a fatal event. Early detection of this disease will allow for early management and intervention, reducing morbidity and mortality.

Biomarkers are defined as characteristics that may be measured as indicators of normal biological processes or pathogenic processes [1]. Biomarkers may involve several modalities, such as substances measured in the blood and other bodily fluids, as well as imaging results and technologies like electrocardiography; in particular, multi-biomarker approaches may be promising approaches for the better detection of pathophysiology [2]. Currently, CAD detection involves several modalities. Functional tests, such as stress electrocardiograms, and anatomical imaging, such as angiography, provide clinicians with indications of CAD severity [3]. Numerous studies have assessed the validity of these modalities. Their reliability, whilst being generally suitable, varies depending on context [4].

A potential reason for this is variations between heterogenous study populations; however, simultaneous consideration of different biomarkers may improve reliability [4].

Recently, microRNAs (miRNA) have been proposed as a potential biomarker for use in various clinical contexts. They are major effectors of gene silencing through post-transcriptional repression and mRNA degradation [5]. This review aims to discuss the potential utility of microRNA (miRNA), as a diagnostic and prognostic tool for clinicians to detect CAD.

## 2. Localisation of miRNA

MiRNA are short RNAs (18–25 nts) that engage in the sequence specific inactivation of mRNA (Figure 1). They are encoded by their own non-protein coding genes located across the genome, though they also occur in the introns and exons of other genes [6,7]. MiRNAs are predominantly located intracellularly, although a proportion of them can be detected in the extracellular environment (ECmiRNA), including in plasma and various other body fluids [8–10]. They occur freely circulating or associated with other molecules, including within extracellular vesicles, such as exosomes and microvesicles, and can also be complexed with lipoproteins [11–15].

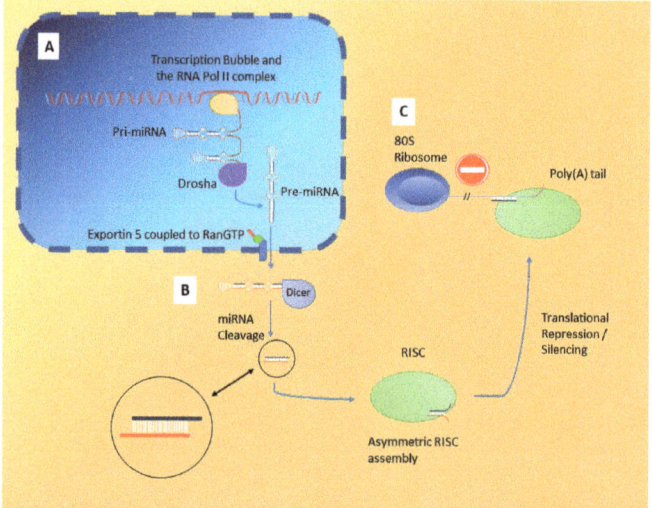

**Figure 1.** MiRNA biogenesis and their means of transcriptional silencing. RNA Pol II: RNA polymerase II; miRNA: microRNA; RanGTP: Ran coupled to guanosine triphosphate; RISC: RNA-induced silencing complex; Poly(A) tail: poly-adenosine tail; 80S ribosome: eukaryotic ribosome. (**A**) Within the nucleus (blue area), miRNA are initially transcribed (e.g., from an miRNA gene) from DNA by RNA polymerase II (yellow) in the form of primary miRNA, or pri-miRNA, which contain stem-loop structures. The enzyme Drosha (purple) proceeds to cleave these stem–loop structures from the rest of the transcript, and these structures are now defined as precursor miRNA, or pre-miRNA. These are then exported from the nucleus via exportin 5 coupled to the Ran cycle. (**B**) Once in the cytosol (yellow area), the enzyme Dicer recognises pre-miRNA and cleaves them to produce mature miRNA molecules with two nucleotide overhangs on their 3′ ends. This molecule is then incorporated into an RNA-induced silencing complex (RISC, green) and the passenger strand (red backbone) is destroyed. This results in an active RISC complex. (**C**) The active RISC complex uses the guide strand of the miRNA (blue backbone) to target mRNA transcripts, specifically those that are complementary to the seed sequence of the guide strand. Through translational repression and RNA decay, miRNA reduce the expression of certain genes through RISC. Also note that the poly(A) tail is shown in pink. Ago2: Argonaute 2; DGCR8: DiGeorge syndrome critical region 8.

Microvesicles and exosomes are both types of extracellular vesicles with multiple roles in normal cell physiology. One of their major functions is intercellular communication through the carriage of signalling molecules, including proteins, mRNAs, and miRNAs amongst others, to targets of variable distance from the cell of origin [16,17]. Exosomes have a size range of 30–100 nm, and themselves originate from organelles of the endocytic pathway, the multivesicular bodies [16,17]. A multivesicular body is produced by the invagination of an endosome to produce intraluminal vesicles, into which specific molecules are sorted. Multivesicular bodies are trafficked to and subsequently fuse with the plasma membrane, at which point the intraluminal vesicles, now labelled as exosomes, are released into the extracellular space [16,17]. Microvesicles have a size range of 0.1–1.0 µm and are produced from the plasma membrane directly through outward blebbing [17,18]. Specific molecular cargo is transported towards regions of the plasma membrane where local alterations in the lipid composition reduce the rigidity of the membrane and facilitate further curvature [17,18]. The assembly of contractile machinery in these regions produce cytoskeletal rearrangements that pinch off nascent microvesicles [17,18]. The membrane budding that produces microvesicles differs from the blebbing process that produces apoptotic bodies, which is a less specific process [17,18]. These extracellular vesicles can then be trafficked through autocrine, paracrine, and endocrine paths (Figure 2). The multiple forms of endocytosis are the typical forms of vesicle uptake, though membrane fusion between microvesicles and the target cell plasma membrane has also been observed [17]. The mechanism utilised is likely dependent on the recipient cell type and the suitable expression of receptors compatible with the vesicle [17].

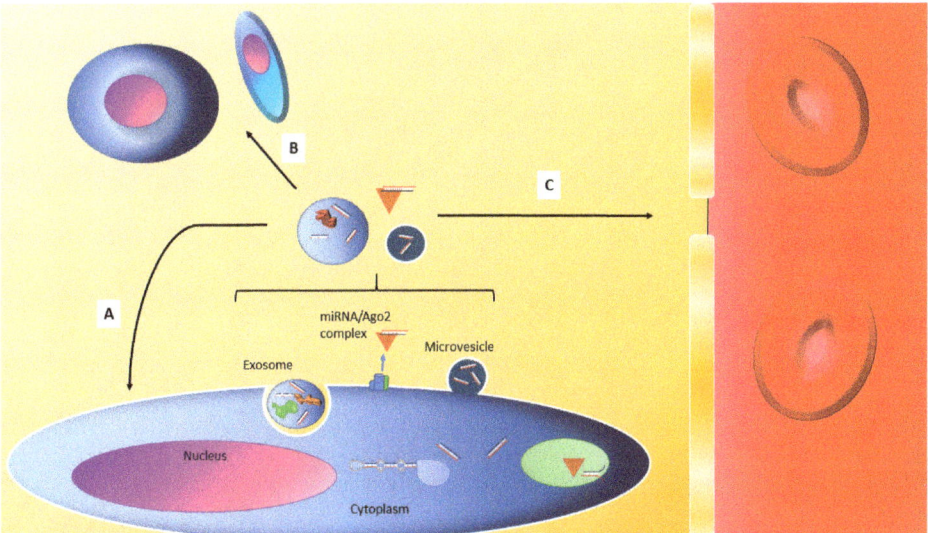

**Figure 2.** Export pathways for miRNA and means of interaction with other cells/cell of origin as a potential means of signalling. (**A**) The autocrine pathway, whereby extracellular miRNAs re-enter the cell from which they originated. (**B**) The paracrine pathway, whereby extracellular miRNAs are transported towards and enter cells of the same or different type to the miRNA's cell of origin. (**C**) The endocrine pathway, whereby extracellular miRNAs enter the circulation and are thus transported to cells in other tissues/organs. Ago2: Argonaute 2; miRNA: microRNA.

Research suggests that miRNA occur within exosomes, not on their surface membranes or associated with surface structures [11,19]. Additionally, a significant number of transcripts in the exosomes are not present in the donor cells from which they are derived; this profiling suggests that the miRNA profile of exosomes does not directly reflect the transcriptional status of the donor cell [11,19].

Exosomes have therefore been proposed to be a means of cell type-specific intercellular paracrine communication through delivering RNAs, which would affect the recipient cell's proteome, and this has been demonstrated in several in vitro models involving both animal and human cells [11,19–23].

While the principles of miRNA transfer by microvesicles are similar to that by exosomes, there are some notable differences [13]. For one, microvesicles (MVs) are synthesised from the plasma membranes of donor cells, and so the profile of the membrane proteins on them reflects the donor cell type. It seems probable that miRNA secretion via this mechanism is independent of the donor cell's transcriptional status [24]. Known cell types that produce miRNA-loaded MVs include endothelial cells, mesenchymal stem cells, and cancer cells [12]. Finally, ECmiRNA are also found complexed with HDLs, and these have been of interest as biomarkers of CAD [25,26]. However, recent studies cast doubt on the exact role of exosomes and microvesicles as carriers of miRNA. One important criticism has been that extracellular vesicles may co-purify miRNA found in culture and supplement media, such as foetal bovine serum, potentially confounding results [27]. Newer techniques, such as high-resolution density gradient fractionation and direct immunoaffinity capture, suggest that the secretion of DNA and RNA products is independent of extracellular vesicles, perhaps through a proposed model of autophagy or multivesicular-endosome-dependent but exosome-independent mechanism [28]. Furthermore, only a small fraction of in vitro, human lymphocyte-derived extracellular vesicles have been found to carry miRNA, and the binding of extracellular vesicles to cell membranes has not been observed. This may be due to a short exposure time and variability in conditions from physiological conditions [29]. Thus, there is a requirement for further investigation in this domain, although microvesicle RNA biology has been successfully translated to use in clinical settings in the diagnosis of haematological and oncological disorders [30].

Freely-circulating miRNA have been demonstrated by PCR miRNA assays conducted on fractionated, filtered, and ultracentrifuged plasma obtained from peripheral blood samples [14,15]. The miRNA may be bound to Argonaute (Ago2), an extracellular miRNA binding protein, and together they form a stable nucleoprotein complex. These stable complexes exist intracellularly, so it may be plausible that a certain proportion of ECmiRNA are released following cell death processes, e.g., necrosis and apoptosis, though it remains a possibility that miRNA/Ago2 complexes are/can be directly released from cells in order to communicate with others [14,15].

## 3. Physiological Roles of miRNA and Their Clinical Relevance

The significance of miRNA is made evident by the defective organogenesis and embryonic lethality that is found in murine models of tissue-specific or germline Dicer knockouts, respectively [31,32]. Dysregulation of miRNA is linked to the aetiology or pathogenesis of viral infections, cancer, and metabolic diseases [33]. Notable cardiovascular examples are miR-208, miR-143/145, and miR-21. MiR-208 is derived from an intron of the α-MHC (myosin heavy chain) gene, which is uniquely expressed in the myocardium and encodes an isoform of myosin heavy chain [34]. It acts within a network to upregulate the expression of β-MHC in response to stress, but its absence does not result in the absence of myocardium, therefore yielding viable mice [35].

The miR-143/145 cluster regulates the expression of cytoskeletal genes in vascular smooth muscle cells (VSMCs), and although murine knockouts are still viable, they show reduced vascular tone and significantly reduced capacity for migration in the process of neointima formation following vascular injury [36,37]. Stress-induced hypertrophy of cardiomyocytes is, at least in part, facilitated by miR-21-mediated silencing of two target proteins [38]. Indeed, miRNA have a wide range of cardiovascular functions, and their absence induces many abnormal phenotypes [7]. A recently compiled database of extracellular vesicle miRNA describes their potential roles as biomarkers in various diseases, including myocardial infarctions [39–42].

Thus, miRNA may either have a causative role or are a consequence of pathology. In the case of the former, the relevant miRNA could be operating as an initiator or maintainer of the condition (i.e., is a necessary component of a particular disease process), or could simply yield susceptibility (i.e., could potentially be sufficient to produce the disease phenotype, for example by yielding a substrate that enables the disease to precipitate). In the case of the latter, the measured changes in miRNA levels may be due to unregulated secretion from injured/stressed cells, or as a homeostatic response to the insult, with the communication between the cells occurring at the paracrine or the endocrine level [43].

Hence, for both of these, by measuring the changes in the miRNA signatures in an individual before, during, and after recovery from a particular pathology, we may be able to identify how the miRNA are behaving with respect to aetiology and pathogenesis (i.e., whether changes in miRNA behaviour affect susceptibility, are an outright cause, or more simply are products of the disease process). These signatures themselves may be detected in biopsies or peripheral blood samples, and are defined by the identity of the specific miRNAs that are detected, as well as by their concentrations. There already exists diagnostic miRNA tests based on either an miRNA panel or single miRNA quantification for diseases like certain cancers, indicating a successful proof of concept for the use of miRNA as biomarkers in disease [44,45].

## 4. Coronary Artery Disease (CAD) Pathophysiology

To better appreciate and evaluate the potential of miRNA as biomarkers in CAD, it is necessary to first consider the pathology of CAD. The pathogenesis of coronary artery plaques in CAD involves endothelial cell activation and the subsequent infiltration of the tunica intima by oxidised lipoproteins and monocytes. These monocytes go on to differentiate into macrophages and transform into foam cells as they consume these lipoproteins [46,47]. Consequently, a chronic inflammatory response is produced, whereby the macrophages begin the secretion of cytokines and chemoattractant factors that promotes the activation of the endothelium, which beckons further adhesion and infiltration (diapedesis) of more monocytes/other leukocytes [48]. This leads to the development of a raised lesion with a fibrous cap (from the myofibroblasts) and a lipid-rich interior (from lysed foam cells). The "shoulder" of the cap is found to have both of these cell types in addition to T-lymphocytes (although their role is not entirely understood) [49].

Angiogenesis may occur within the plaque and contribute to the expansion of the plaque through haemorrhaging of the new vessels forming at the shoulder into the less dense, lipid-rich core. The plaque may subsequently rupture, which can lead to thrombosis as coagulation factors and thrombocytes adhere to the lesion, as well as embolisation of plaque fragments. Other complications include calcification, or the formation of an aneurysm as the tunica media weakens from the arterial remodelling [50]. Endothelial cells are also induced to produce a pro-inflammatory response, which propagates the further infiltration of monocytes and degeneration of the elastic laminae in the media [51]. This weakened area of vessel wall can dilate in response to pressure applied to it. CAD pathophysiology therefore has the potential to give rise to measurable circulating biomarkers, due to the close involvement of disease with the circulating vasculature. Established surrogates that are commonly used, such as circulating LDL, HDL, troponin, and creatinine kinase, are associated with different stages in their pathophysiology: LDL and HDL being more relevant upstream as risk factors, and troponin and creatinine kinase more relevant downstream as a consequence of sufficiently advanced disease. Thus, there may be other biomarkers that may be of use in either a prognostic or diagnostic capacity. miRNA may be one such class.

## 5. CAD Biomarkers and miRNA

Current standard molecular biomarkers include proteins, lipids, and other metabolites. Cardiac troponins are well-established and are commonly used indicators of adverse cardiac events [52]. Creatinine kinase is also used in the same context, although it is less specific due to its presence in skeletal muscle and cerebral tissue. However, troponins and creatinine kinase involve the terminal series of events in CAD: ischaemic damage to the myocardium arising as a result of acute coronary syndrome [9,53].

Novel serum biomarkers, and more recently urinary biomarkers for CAD, are of increasing interest. For example, high-sensitivity C-reactive protein and high-sensitivity troponin I assays have been proposed as biomarkers of coronary artery disease and its progression [54–56]. They pose the advantages of being non-invasive, compared to percutaneous coronary angiography, and without the radiation exposure of CT coronary angiography [57]. In a study that tested over 100 different serum biomarkers in over 1000 patients, four biomarkers in combination (adiponectin, apolipoprotein C-I, midkine, and kidney injury molecule-1 (KIM-1)) were found to predict incidence of severe CAD [58].

Alongside these novel biomarkers, numerous studies have tried to identify miRNA, which may distinguish between individuals with different cardiovascular health statuses (Table 1) [59–61]. These miRNAs may be considered at local sites, such as at plaques or sites of endothelial injury, or freely circulating in serum. There is a vast constellation of research, and several candidate miRNAs have been identified, although this is complicated by a lack of correlation between studies. This may be due to experimental design variation, as studies involve different experimental models, time courses (acute vs. chronic disease), and quantification methodologies.

## 5.1. Localised Changes in miRNA Profiles

At the tissue level, specific miRNAs are expressed at the sites of myocardial injury/ischaemia or at the site of the atherosclerotic lesion. This expression may be in vascular tissue, myocardium, or plaque cells. Vessel wall biology changes drastically as atherogenesis progresses, and the changes in miRNA expression reflect this (Figure 3). In vascular smooth muscle cells. miRNA-1, -10a, -21, -100, -133, -143, -145, and -204 have been characterised with their standard contractile phenotype [62,63]. This is contrasted with a myofibroblast phenotype that VSMCs differentiate into during plaque development, which is instead associated with miRNA-24, -26a, -31, -146a, -208, and -221 [62,63]. The latter set of miRNA directs VSMCs to a secretory phenotype, with increased proliferative and migratory activity [63–68].

In the case of miRNA-21, however, there is evidence of the inverse, whereby this miRNA, which is elevated in CAD, may promote VSMC proliferation and indicate the progression of atherosclerosis [69]. Through the inhibition of FOXP1 and ZDHHC14 expression, respectively, miRNA-206 and -574-5p also act to do the same, and are demonstrated to be elevated in CAD patients, although the former seems to actually be anti-atherogenic [70].

Endothelial cells produce a baseline level of miRNA-155 and miRNA-126-5p under healthy conditions, whereas miRNA-21, miRNA-34a, and miRNA-210 are featured more in the endothelium of atherosclerotic lesions (Figure 3) [63]. These are due to increased shear stress from altered tissue morphology, interrupted cell cycle control, and hypoxia, respectively, all of which occur in atherosclerotic plaques. However, the downregulation of miRNA-126-5p removes a significant promoter of endothelial cell repair and maintenance, which further enables atherogenesis [71].

Endothelial progenitor cells (EPCs) are mobilised to give rise to endothelial cells in angiogenic atherosclerotic lesions, in a process marked by changes in the miRNA. In particular, miRNA-361-5p and miRNA-206, which are upregulated in CAD patients, are potentially responsible for controlling the expression of vascular endothelial growth factor in EPCs, as well as EPC activity [72,73]. Connections have been made with further miRNA, though only in the broad scope of these lesions as a whole (Table 1).

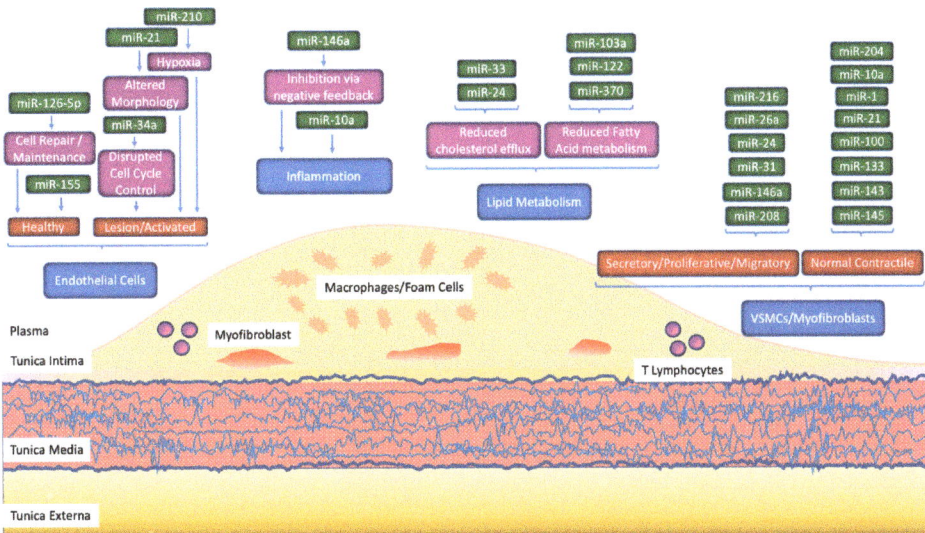

**Figure 3.** Associations between miRNA in different cells and constituent pathways in coronary artery disease (CAD) pathogenesis. Pathological alterations in the phenotypes of particular cells of the circulatory system, in addition to normal homeostatic processes, are core to the development of CAD (shown in blue, phenotypes in red, pathophysiological processes in purple). Various miRNAs have been identified as being associated with these pathological developments (shown in green), with previous studies showing that they may be implicated in particular contributing mechanisms. VSMC: vascular smooth muscle cell.

## 5.2. Changes in Circulating miRNA

Certain miRNA will be released from cells as either a homeostatic response to CAD or following cell death (Figure 3). Therefore, miRNAs that are linked to such insults, such as miRNA-499, miRNA-208, and miRNA-1 [74–77], could plausibly be released from ischaemic cardiomyocytes as they necrose. Muscle-enriched miR-133a, together with miR-1, shows a steeper and earlier increase than cardiac-enriched miRNA (miR-499 and miR-208b) upon myocardial injury [42]. Alternatively, cell death within the atherosclerotic lesion itself can produce circulating miRNA. A fraction of endothelial cells in atherosclerotic plaques undergo apoptosis, and thus release apoptotic bodies that have been found to contain miRNA-126 (Figure 3) [14]. In actuality, this miRNA acts through CXCL12 to stabilise plaques and protect the vessel wall structure from further damage under atherogenesis (Table 1).

In terms of homeostatic responses, leukocytes, such as peripheral blood mononuclear cells (PBMCs), demonstrate altered miRNA profiles in CAD patients relative to healthy controls. One study reported differences in the levels of miRNA-147, which was downregulated, and miRNA-135a, which was upregulated, in these cells [78]. Another group observed that CAD patients' PBMCs also had an increased expression of miRNA-146a/b under inflammatory stimuli associated with CAD, and lowered expression of let-7i [79,80].

In another study comparing the expression levels of multiple circulating miRNAs between eight CAD patients and eight healthy volunteers, all of the miRNA primarily expressed in the endothelium—miRNA-126, -17, -20a, -92a, -221, -199a-5p, -27a, -130a, and -21, as well as let-7d—had significantly lower levels in the circulation in CAD patients [61] (note, however, that miRNA-126 is also highly enriched in platelets [81]). This was in contrast to the miRNAs that were specifically expressed in striated muscle, of which only one (miRNA-208b) was found to have a significant difference, and was instead elevated in CAD patients [61].

Determining the cell type of origin, as well as the precise roles of both of these types of miRNA, would further define the underlying communications and transformations that lead to plaque formation. However, it may be suggested that circulating miRNA are the most feasible candidates as biomarkers, due to the comparative ease of extraction

## 6. miRNA in CAD Pathophysiology

The relevance of miRNAs as biochemical precursors to the more macroscopic cellular and histological events that comprise atherogenesis is becoming increasingly evident [82,83]. As discussed above, lipid metabolism and inflammatory changes are key aspects of this process. Therefore, here we discuss miRNA in these contexts and highlight the changes that occur in pathological processes.

### 6.1. Lipid Metabolism

LDLs, mainly in their oxidised form, are the primary carriers of the cholesterol and triglycerides that are found in atherosclerotic lesions. Implicated in the synthesis of these molecules are miRNA-24, -33, -103a, and -122, all of which are found to have been significantly increased in the PBMCs of CAD patients [84,85]. Further investigations of miRNA-33 have reported that it suppresses the cholesterol efflux mechanism in cells, at least in part by inhibiting the expression of ATP-binding cassette transporter A1 [86,87]. Likewise, the expression miRNA-370 is also significantly raised in CAD patients [88]. This miRNA downregulates the expression of a carnitine palmitoyl transferase protein that is required for the trafficking of fatty acids into the mitochondria for β-oxidation, and is also higher in CAD patients [87]. In addition, these individuals can be identified from increased miRNA-486, -92a, -208a, -122, -93, and -17-5p [86,87].

### 6.2. Inflammation

Endothelial vulnerability to pathological inflammatory activity may, in part, be regulated by miRNA-10a, which is also reduced in CAD patients compared to healthy controls [71,82,89,90]. miRNA-155 shows the same trend, though there is contrasting evidence when the miRNA's levels in the plasma and plaques of individuals with atherosclerosis were investigated [89,90]. Li et al. [90] have also shown that miRNA-155 reduces the expression of calcium-regulated heat stable protein 1 and promotes TNF-α expression in macrophages, suppressing foam cell formation [71,89,90].

Furthermore, miRNA-22 is known to repress the chemokine CCL2 in PBMCs, which modulates intercellular communication in inflamed tissues [82,91]. In CAD patients, the levels of these miRNAs in PBMCs are reduced. In addition to this, miRNA-146a is also reduced in CAD patients [91]. This miRNA is induced by pro-inflammatory cytokines to inhibit the nuclear factor-κB pathway in a negative feedback loop to resolve inflammation in its later stages [82,91]. MiRNA, therefore, plays a role in inflammatory processes that may form one component of the complex pathophysiology of atherosclerosis, and may represent potential biomarker candidates early in the disease process [82].

## 7. Pitfalls in Assessing miRNA as Biomarker Targets

### 7.1. Confounding Factors

When considering the utility of miRNA as biomarkers, one needs to consider any variances in their expression not relating to pathological processes alone. One such source of variation may be population-level changes. Thus, studies has shown geographical/ethnic differences in the expression levels of miRNA [92,93].

Age and sex are other factors that correlate with the frequency of different miRNA in circulation [94]. This has been demonstrated in an analysis of platelet-derived mRNA and miRNA [95]. However, in terms of cardiac-specific miRNA, there is limited data on CAD-associated miRNAs and their variation with the sex and ethnicity of a patient. Discrepancies in miRNA levels with respect to age have been reported in a few studies, which is a further confounder, as ageing is a critical risk factor of cardiovascular health. For example, with miRNA-149, -424, and -765, the former two are downregulated and the latter upregulated in middle-aged (aged 49–57) CAD patients [96]. Another study showed that miRNA-126-3p expression is greater in senescent endothelial cells than in younger cells, and their quantity in circulation is also increased [97].

Furthermore, cardiac fibroblasts increase their expression of miRNA-21 and miRNA-22 with age, which can lead to increased fibrosis and progression towards senescence, respectively [98]. Cardiomyocytes show the same change in miRNA-22, whereby they have been demonstrated to have a suppressive effect on autophagy in aged cardiomyocytes, producing an improved functional recovery of myocardium post-infarct in elderly mice, though not in younger mice [99].

Moreover, the level of miRNA-155, in addition to actually being higher in human females, decreases with age. Other miRNA have been implicated in cardiac ageing and associated dysfunction in addition to CAD, including the miRNA-17-92 cluster, miRNA-18, miRNA-19, and miRNA-17-3p [98,100–102]. Therefore, since not all studies investigating these miRNA have adjusted their results to control for these factors, any reported variation in miRNA may partially be explained by factors other than CAD [103].

*7.2. Measuring Serum and Plasma miRNA*

Of the published studies that analyse circulating miRNA, the general trend seems to concentrate on using plasma-based samples. This specification is critical, as the difference in the molecular profile between serum and plasma results in a difference between the recorded miRNA levels as the sample is being prepared, as serum holds a higher concentration of RNA than plasma [104]. Further to this point is that coagulation increases variability in serum miRNA concentrations [104]. Hence, we must recognise the difficulty of normalising miRNA values due to pre-analytical variations, including blood cell counts and the miRNA load of the cells and platelets in circulation.

Furthermore, any haemolysis releasing the miRNA contained within blood cells will affect the total miRNA concentration and profile that we identify from serum, though cellular contamination would cause the same changes in plasma and serum samples. Thus, care should be taken when preparing samples to prevent distorted results [104–106], and it may be best to produce a standard operating procedure (SOP) for acquiring miRNA data, based on currently existing SOPs for collecting such samples.

## 8. Validity of miRNA as Biomarkers

When addressing the feasibility/validity of miRNA as a biomarker, a few critical points must first be considered. Firstly, ease of access is not a concern, as miRNAs occur in peripheral blood so whole blood samples can be taken. However, it should be noted that the majority of miRNA in peripheral blood will likely be derived primarily from well-vascularised tissues, e.g., lungs and kidneys, in addition to blood cells themselves (platelets are a major contributor to the circulating RNA pool [107]), so the relative quantities of particular miRNAs should be taken into account.

Secondly, cost is likely a significant concern, due to the processes required to prepare the miRNA: RNA purification, reverse transcription–polymerase and quantitative polymerase chain reaction/microarrays/sequencing, controlling RNase activity, etc. [108,109]

Thirdly is timing/storage. MiRNA/Ago2 complexes have remarkable biologic stability and occur both in microvesicles and freely in plasma, though miRNA integrity is also maintained in tissues that have been fixed in formalin and embedded in paraffin, as is done with biopsies [108,109]. This protects the original samples, though preparation of purified miRNA must still be done carefully, and regular monitoring and appropriate storage are necessary. Control of the temperature and RNase activity are crucial to prevent degradation.

Lastly is content/criterion validity [110]. Major efforts have been and are currently being invested into establishing the reliability of miRNA as a diagnostic for a diverse range of human diseases (i.e., carrying indicative or predictive value), as well as into developing diagnostic tests for them and trying to understand their contribution to the disease's manifestation, as mentioned [43,111–114]. Prognostic information and severity assessments also stand to be improved through the use of miRNA [115].

While the quantification and normalisation methodologies are still being developed, stability, accessibility, and disease specificity still lend miRNAs significant value as biomarkers, and evidence of this continues to grow [116,117].

Given that there are several miRNAs, it is likely to be beneficial to assay these particular biomarkers in a panel of tests. When considering the levels of all of those that are tested for, we gain a better understanding of the pathology's context. Some groups support this notion, with the suggestion that using a panel of select miRNA "may have a greater target-organ specificity and better diagnostic value than a single miRNA or well-established clinical biomarker" [116]. This is easily demonstrated by the range of miRNAs that are found to be involved in a singular disease, and a singular miRNA may be involved in multiple diseases, producing a web of interaction [116]. A gene can have sequences complementary to different miRNA seed sequences, and an miRNA may target multiple genes, so this is a feasible paradigm.

**Table 1.** miRNAs as active factors/potential biomarkers in CAD and associated pathologies. Methodologies of miRNA identification, quantification, sample location, experimental model, and time course of disease pathology are indicated. Where the quoted reference is a review article synthesizing several sources of evidence, this has been indicated.

| References | miRNA | Quantitative Effect | Outcome | Sample Type | miRNA Identification/Quantification Method | Cell Lines/Study Population | Acute/Chronic Disease Status |
|---|---|---|---|---|---|---|---|
| Wang et al., 2016 [18] | miRNA-146a | Upregulated | This miRNA may be a potential biomarker for poor coronary collateral circulation in CAD patients. | Plasma | qRT-PCR | Human patients | Chronic (1-month cut-off) |
| Li et al., 2017 [19] | miRNA-155-5p miRNA-483-5p miRNA-451a | miRNA-155-5p and miRNA-483-5p are upregulated; miRNA-451a is down-regulated | Potential biomarkers for the early detection of atherosclerotic plaque rupture. | Plasma | qRT-PCR | Human patients | Stable CAD |
| Zhao et al., 2015 [7] | miRNA-143 miRNA-145 | Contested | Altered in CAD. Potentially released from vascular walls. | Plasma | (Review article) | (Review article) | (Review article) |
| Li et al., 2017 [20] | miRNA-122 miRNA-140-3p miRNA-720 miRNA-2861 miRNA-3149 | Upregulated | Elevated during the early stages of ACS. | Plasma | qRT-PCR | Bama male minipigs and human patients | Minipigs: normal and acute MI. Human patients: Stable angina, unstable angina and acute MI. |
| Jansen et al., 2017 [21] | miRNA-21 miRNA-126-3p miRNA-222 | Upregulated | These miRNAs increased in concentration following periods of cardiac stress in patients with stenosed coronary arteries. | Plasma | qRT-PCR | Human patients | Stable CAD |
| Soeki et al., 2015 [22] | miRNA-100 | - | Associated with coronary plaque instability. Potentially released from plaques. | Plasma | qRT-PCR | Human patients | Unknown |
| Liu et al., 2017 [23] | miRNA-29a | Upregulated | Moderate expression of miRNAs of extracellular matrix proteins. Associated with atherosclerosis and intima-media thickness of carotid arteries. | Plasma | qRT-PCR | Human patients | Unknown |
| Wang et al., 2017 [24] | miRNA-126 | Downregulated | A potential biomarker for CAD. Inversely correlated to placenta growth factor. | Plasma | qRT-PCR | Human patients | CAD for 15–24 months |
| Al-Kafaji et al., 2017 [125] | miRNA-126 | Downregulated | A potential biomarker for CAD. Inversely correlated with LDL concentration. | Plasma | qRT-PCR | Human patients | Type 2 diabetics, some with CAD diagnoses |
| Al-Muhtaresh et al., 2019 [126] | miRNA-1 miRNA-133 | Upregulated | Potential biomarkers. Both correlate with LDL-C levels; miR-1 is known to negatively regulate Bcl2 [127]. | Plasma | qRT-PCR | Human patients | Type 2 diabetics, some with CAD diagnoses |
| Zernecke et al., 2009 [14] | miRNA-126 | - | Released from apoptotic bodies derived from endothelial cells from atherosclerotic plaques. Reduces inflammatory activity/plaque development. | Plasma/Plaque | qRT-PCR | Human aortic smooth muscle cell culture. Human atherosclerotic plaques. ApoE-/- murine endothelial cell cultures. HUVEC cell line | Unknown |
| Wang et al., 2014 [128] | miRNA-31 miRNA-720 | Downregulated | Potential biomarkers for early CAD. | Plasma/endothelial progenitor cells | qRT-PCR | Human patients | Unknown CAD |
| Zhang et al., 2017 [129] | miRNA-208a | - | Significant association with Gensini score, and by extension the severity of atherosclerosis. Potential biomarker for CAD severity. | Plasma | qRT-PCR | Human patients | Unknown CAD |
| Jansen et al., 2014 [11] | miRNA-126 miRNA-199a | - | The levels of these miRNA, which occur in circulating microvesicles, are potentially prognostic for major adverse cardiovascular events in patients with stable CAD. | Plasma | qRT-PCR | Human patients | Stable CAD |

Table 1. Cont.

| References | miRNA | Quantitative Effect | Outcome | Sample Type | miRNA Identification/Quantification Method | Cell Lines/Study Population | Acute/Chronic Disease Status |
|---|---|---|---|---|---|---|---|
| Han et al., 2015 [130] | miRNA-21, miRNA-23a, miRNA-30a, miRNA-34a, miRNA-106b | Upregulated | These miRNAs occur at higher levels in ApoE-/- mice, which models hypercholesterolaemia. MiRNA-21, -23a, and -34a are potential biomarkers for CAD. MiRNA-21 has been linked to CAD-derived ACS. | Plasma | qRT-PCR and miRNA microarrays | ApoE-/- mice and human CAD patients | Unknown |
| Zhou et al., 2016 [70] | miRNA-206, miRNA-564-5p | Upregulated | Potential biomarkers for CAD | Plasma | qRT-PCR and miRNA microarrays | Human patients | Unknown |
| Sayed et al., 2015 [96] | miRNA-149, miRNA-424, miRNA-765 | MiRNA-149 and miRNA-424 were upregulated, miRNA-765 was downregulated | Potential biomarkers for CAD in middle-aged patients | Plasma | qRT-PCR | Human patients | Stable and unstable CAD |
| Gao et al., 2015 [131] | miRNA-145 | Downregulated | This miRNA regulates VSMC fate, inhibiting proliferation. It is the modal miRNA in healthy vessel walls, though in atherosclerotic plaques it may not even be detected. Plasma concentration levels are significantly reduced in CAD patients, and those with three-vessel disease have a significantly lower quantity as well. Potential biomarker for CAD. | Plasma/plaque | qRT-PCR | Human patients | Unknown (patients diagnosed with CAD for more than a year) |
| Ren et al., 2013 [132] | miRNA-106b/25 cluster, miRNA-17/92a cluster, miRNA-21/590-5p cluster, miRNA-126, miRNA-451 | Upregulated in patients with unstable angina, though there is evidence that miRNA-17/92a was actually downregulated in CAD patients [63]. | These miRNAs are elevated in CAD patients relative to those with stable AP. MiRNA-17/92a is involved in angiogenesis, which further complicates plaques. Increased miRNA-21 can yield increased MMP activity, which can hinder plaque progression. Potential biomarkers for CAD. | Plasma | qRT-PCR | Human patients | CAD and unstable angina |
| Chen et al., 2015 [133] | miRNA-17-5p | Upregulated | Potential biomarker for early CAD. | Plasma | qRT-PCR | Human patients | Unknown |
| Faccini et al., 2017 [89] | miRNA-155, miRNA-145, let-7c | Downregulated | Potential biomarkers for CAD | Plasma | qRT-PCR and miRNA microarrays | Human patients | Unknown |
| Koroleva et al., 2017 [51] | miRNA-21, miRNA-100, miRNA-127, miRNA-133, miRNA-143/145, miRNA-221/222, miRNA-494 | All upregulated apart from miRNA-221/222, which was downregulated | The expression of these miRNA may influence plaque stability: miRNA-21, -143, and -221 are pro-stability; miRNA-100, -127, -133, and -494 are pro-instability. | Plaque | (Review article) | (Review article) | (Review article) |
| Lin et al., 2016 [134] | miRNA-365 | Downregulated | Regulation of the inflammatory response, specifically IL-6 activity, such that IL-6 expression increases as miRNA-365 expression decreases. | Plaque, serum, and circulating monocytes | qRT-PCR | Human patients | Unknown (patients with atherosclerosis) |
| Cipollone et al., 2011 [35] | miRNA-100, miRNA-127, miRNA-145, miRNA-133a/b | Upregulated | The expression of these miRNA varies with plaque stability. MiRNA-133 is relevant to stroke-related proteins and is thought to be vascular smooth muscle-specific. | Plaque | qRT-PCR | Human patients | Unknown |

Table 1. Cont.

| References | miRNA | Quantitative Effect | Outcome | Sample Type | miRNA Identification/Quantification Method | Cell Lines/Study Population | Acute/Chronic Disease Status |
|---|---|---|---|---|---|---|---|
| Kumar et al., 2014 [136] | miRNA-712 miRNA-205 | Upregulated in atherosclerosis | These miRNA target and reduce expression of metalloproteinase inhibitor 3 (TIMP3), increasing the activity of matrix metalloproteinases (MMPs), which affects inflammatory processes and VSMC/leukocyte migration in atherosclerosis. | Endothelial cells (Plaque) | Review (qRT-PCR, microarrays, and fluorescent in situ hybridisation) | Review (mice (C57Bl/6 and ApoE$^{-/-}$)) | Review (unknown) |
| Tian et al., 2014 [137] | miRNA-155 | Upregulated | Raised inflammatory response and foam cell differentiation. | Monocytes (plaque) | qRT-PCR | ApoE$^{-/-}$ mice | Unknown |
| Horie et al., 2012 [138] | miRNA-33 | - | Deficiency in ApoE knockout mice suppressed atherogenesis/plaque progression. | Monocytes/macrophages (plaque) | qRT-PCR | ApoE$^{-/-}$ mice | Unknown |
| Fang et al., 2010 [139] | miRNA-10a | Downregulated | Expression levels were reduced in endothelial cells that are thought to be pre-atherosclerotic, affecting inflammation signalling. | Endothelial cells (plaque) | qRT-PCR, miRNA microarrays, and fluorescent in situ hybridisation | Adult pigs | Unknown |
| Zernecke et al., 2009 [41] | miRNA-126 | - | Released from apoptotic bodies derived from endothelial cells from atherosclerotic plaques. MiRNAs reduce inflammatory activity/plaque development. | Plasma/plaque | qRT-PCR | Human aortic smooth muscle cell culture. Human atherosclerotic plaques. ApoE$^{-/-}$ murine endothelial cell cultures. HUVEC cell line. | Unknown |
| Raitoharju et al., 2011 [62] | miRNA-21 miRNA-34a miRNA-146a miRNA-146b-5p miRNA-210 | Upregulated | These miRNAs were upregulated in plaques compared to left internal thoracic arteries that were not atherosclerotic. This has been linked to VSMC changes seen in atherogenesis. | Plaque | miRNA microarrays and qRT-PCR | Human patients | Unknown |
| Shan et al., 2015 [40] | miRNA-223 | Upregulated | This miRNA seems to be secreted from cells in the circulation. Their levels are elevated in the serum and atherosclerotic lesions in apolipoprotein-E knockout mice. | Plaque serum/blood cells | qRT-PCR | Sprague–Dawley rat VSMC cultures and C67Bl/6 murine platelets | Unknown |
| Bidzhekov et al., 2012 [141] | miRNA-26b miRNA30e-5p miRNA-105 miRNA125a-5p miRNA-520b | MiRNA-26b, -30e-5p, and -125a-5p were upregulated. MiRNA-105 and miRNA-520b were downregulated. | These miRNAs had altered expression in CAD patients relative to healthy controls. | Plaque, monocytes | qRT-PCR and miRNA microarrays | Human patients | Unknown |
| Jansen et al., 2013 [142] | miRNA-126 | Downregulated | Circulating levels of miRNA-126 decreased in CAD patients. | Circulating microparticles | qRT-PCR | Mice and human patients | Stable CAD since 2003 |
| Schulte et al., 2015 [143] | miRNA-197 miRNA-223 | - | Strong prognostic value in CAD patients for cardiac death. | Serum | qRT-PCR | Human patients | Unknown CAD |
| Hulsmans et al., 2012 [144] | miRNA-181a | Downregulated | Potential biomarker for CAD, as well as metabolic syndrome | Monocytes | qRT-PCR and miRNA microarrays | Human patients | Unknown |

ACS: acute coronary syndrome, ApoE: Apolipoprotein E, CAD: coronary artery disease, HUVEC: human umbilical vein endothelial cells, MI: myocardial infarction, qRT-PCR: quantitative real time polymerase chain reaction.

## 9. Conclusions

The field of miRNA biomarkers is still relatively young, although it shows significant promise for diagnostics, including for CAD. Many candidate biomarkers have been investigated which characterise different aspects of this vascular disease. There are still challenges, both in the scientific understanding of their roles in CAD and in normalising their measured values across samples and accounting for natural variation in the healthy population.

**Author Contributions:** Conceptualization, K.J.; writing—original draft preparation, I.T.F. and Z.A.; writing—review and editing, I.T.F., Z.A., C.E.E., and A.S.; supervision, A.S. and K.J.; funding acquisition, K.J. All authors have read and agreed to the published version of the manuscript.

**Funding:** This research was funded by the Research England Global Challenge Research Fund, and the APC was funded by the University of Surrey.

**Conflicts of Interest:** The authors declare no conflict of interest. The funders had no role in the design of the study; in the collection, analyses, or interpretation of data; in the writing of the manuscript, or in the decision to publish the results.

## References

1. 2016 Diagnostic Biomarkers. In *BEST (Biomarkers, EndpointS, and other Tools) Resource*; Food and Drug Administration (US): Silver Spring, MD, USA; National Institutes of Health (US): Bethesda, MD, USA, 2018; pp. 3–5.
2. Salzano, A.; Marra, A.M.; D'Assante, R.; Arcopinto, M.; Bossone, E.; Suzuki, T.; Cittadini, A. Biomarkers and Imaging: Complementary or Subtractive? *Heart Fail. Clin.* **2019**, *15*, 321–331. [CrossRef] [PubMed]
3. Mordi, I.R.; Badar, A.A.; John Irving, R.; Weir-McCall, J.R.; Houston, J.G.; Lang, C.C. Efficacy of noninvasive cardiac imaging tests in diagnosis and management of stable coronary artery disease. *Vasc. Health Risk Manag.* **2017**, *13*, 427–437. [CrossRef] [PubMed]
4. Vogel, R.A. Biomarkers of High-Grade Coronary Stenosis: Searching for Seventies. *J. Am. Coll. Cardiol.* **2017**, *69*, 1157–1159. [CrossRef] [PubMed]
5. Carthew, R.W.; Sontheimer, E.J. Origins and Mechanisms of miRNAs and siRNAs. *Cell* **2009**, *136*, 642–655. [CrossRef] [PubMed]
6. Rodriguez, A.; Griffiths-Jones, S.; Ashurst, J.L.; Bradley, A. Identification of mammalian microRNA host genes and transcription units. *Genome Res.* **2004**, *14*, 1902–1910. [CrossRef] [PubMed]
7. Bartel, D.P. MicroRNAs: Genomics, Biogenesis, Mechanism, and Function. *Cell* **2004**, *116*, 281–297. [CrossRef]
8. Arroyo, J.D.; Chevillet, J.R.; Kroh, E.M.; Ruf, I.K.; Pritchard, C.C.; Gibson, D.F.; Mitchell, P.S.; Bennett, C.F.; Pogosova-Agadjanyan, E.L.; Stirewalt, D.L.; et al. Argonaute2 complexes carry a population of circulating microRNAs independent of vesicles in human plasma. *Proc. Natl. Acad. Sci. USA* **2011**, *108*, 5003–5008. [CrossRef]
9. Cortez, M.A.; Bueso-Ramos, C.; Ferdin, J.; Lopez-Berestein, G.; Sood, A.K.; Calin, G.A. MicroRNAs in body fluids–the mix of hormones and biomarkers. *Nat. Rev. Clin. Oncol.* **2011**, *8*, 467–477. [CrossRef]
10. Weber, J.A.; Baxter, D.H.; Zhang, S.; Huang, D.Y.; Huang, K.H.; Lee, M.J.; Galas, D.J.; Wang, K. The microRNA spectrum in 12 body fluids. *Clin. Chem.* **2010**, *56*, 1733–1741. [CrossRef]
11. Valadi, H.; Ekström, K.; Bossios, A.; Sjöstrand, M.; Lee, J.J.; Lötvall, J.O. Exosome-mediated transfer of mRNAs and microRNAs is a novel mechanism of genetic exchange between cells. *Nat. Cell Biol.* **2007**, *2*, 1000. [CrossRef]
12. Sohel, M.H. Extracellular/Circulating MicroRNAs: Release Mechanisms, Functions and Challenges. *ALS* **2016**, *10*, 175–186. [CrossRef]
13. Yuan, A.; Farber, E.L.; Rapoport, A.L.; Tejada, D.; Deniskin, R.; Akhmedov, N.B.; Farber, D.B. Transfer of microRNAs by embryonic stem cell microvesicles. *PLoS ONE* **2009**, *4*, e4722. [CrossRef] [PubMed]
14. Zernecke, A.; Bidzhekov, K.; Noels, H.; Shagdarsuren, E.; Gan, L.; Denecke, B.; Hristov, M.; Köppel, T.; Jahantigh, M.N.; Lutgens, E.; et al. Delivery of MicroRNA-126 by Apoptotic Bodies Induces CXCL12-Dependent Vascular Protection. *Sci. Signal* **2009**, *2*, 81. [CrossRef] [PubMed]
15. Turchinovich, A.; Weiz, L.; Langheinz, A.; Burwinkel, B. Characterization of extracellular circulating microRNA. *Nucleic Acids Res.* **2011**, *39*, 7223–7233. [CrossRef] [PubMed]

16. Hessvik, N.P.; Llorente, A. Current knowledge on exosome biogenesis and release. *Cell. Mol. Life Sci.* **2018**, *75*, 193–208. [CrossRef] [PubMed]
17. Ståhl, A.L.; Johansson, K.; Mossberg, M.; Kahn, R.; Karpman, D. Exosomes and microvesicles in normal physiology, pathophysiology, and renal diseases. *Pediatr. Nephrol.* **2019**, *34*, 11–30. [CrossRef] [PubMed]
18. Tricarico, C.; Clancy, J.; D'Souza-Schorey, C. Biology and biogenesis of shed microvesicles. *Small GTPases* **2017**, *8*, 220–232. [CrossRef]
19. Pegtel, D.M.; Cosmopoulos, K.; Thorley-Lawson, D.A.; Van Eijndhoven, M.A.J.; Hopmans, E.S.; Lindenberg, J.L.; De Gruijl, T.D.; Würdinger, T.; Middeldorp, J.M. Functional delivery of viral miRNAs via exosomes. *Proc. Natl. Acad. Sci. USA* **2010**, *107*, 6328–6333. [CrossRef]
20. Stoorvogel, W. Functional transfer of microRNA by exosomes. *Blood* **2012**, *119*, 646–648. [CrossRef]
21. Pfeffer, S.; Zavolan, M.; Grässer, F.A.; Chien, H.; Russo, J.J.; Ju, J.; John, B.; Enright, A.J.; Marks, D.; Sander, C.; et al. Identification of Virus-Encoded MicroRNAs. *Science (80-)* **2004**, *304*, 734–736. [CrossRef]
22. Xia, T.; O'Hara, A.; Araujo, I.; Barreto, J.; Carvalho, E.; Sapucaia, J.B.; Ramos, J.C.; Luz, E.; Pedroso, C.; Manrique, M.; et al. EBV microRNAs in primary lymphomas and targeting of CXCL-11 by ebv-mir-BHRF1-3. *Cancer Res.* **2008**, *68*, 1436–1442. [CrossRef] [PubMed]
23. Buck, A.H.; Coakley, G.; Simbari, F.; Mcsorley, H.J.; Quintana, J.F.; Le, T.; Kumar, S.; Abreu-goodger, C.; Lear, M.; Harcus, Y.; et al. Exosomes secreted by nematode parasites transfer small RNAs to mammalian cells and modulate innate immunity. *Nat. Commun.* **2014**, *5*, 5488. [CrossRef] [PubMed]
24. Mause, S.F.; Weber, C. Microparticles: Protagonists of a novel communication network for intercellular information exchange. *Circ. Res.* **2010**, *107*, 1047–1057. [CrossRef]
25. Vickers, K.C.; Palmisano, B.T.; Shoucri, B.M.; Shamburek, R.D.; Remaley, A.T. MicroRNAs are transported in plasma and delivered to recipient cells by high-density lipoproteins. *Nat. Cell Biol.* **2011**, *13*, 423–435. [CrossRef] [PubMed]
26. Niculescu, L.S.; Simionescu, N.; Sanda, G.M.; Carnuta, M.G.; Stancu, C.S.; Popescu, A.C.; Popescu, M.R.; Vlad, A.; Dimulescu, D.R.; Simionescu, M.; et al. MiR-486 and miR-92a Identified in Circulating HDL Discriminate between Stable and Vulnerable Coronary Artery Disease Patients. *PLoS ONE* **2015**, *10*, e0140958. [CrossRef] [PubMed]
27. Auber, M.; Fröhlich, D.; Drechsel, O.; Karaulanov, E.; Krämer-Albers, E.M. Serum-free media supplements carry miRNAs that co-purify with extracellular vesicles. *J. Extracell. Vesicles* **2019**, *8*, 1656042. [CrossRef] [PubMed]
28. Jeppesen, D.K.; Fenix, A.M.; Franklin, J.L.; Higginbotham, J.N.; Zhang, Q.; Zimmerman, L.J.; Liebler, D.C.; Ping, J.; Liu, Q.; Evans, R.; et al. Reassessment of Exosome Composition. *Cell* **2019**, *177*, 428–445. [CrossRef] [PubMed]
29. Albanese, M.; Chen, Y.-F.A.; Hüls, C.; Gärtner, K.; Tagawa, T.; Keppler, O.T.; Göbel, C.; Zeidler, R.; Hammerschmidt, W. Micro RNAs Are Minor Constituents of Extracellular Vesicles and Are Hardly Delivered to Target Cells. Available online: https://www.biorxiv.org/content/10.1101/2020.05.20.106393v1.abstract (accessed on 26 July 2020).
30. O'Brien, K.; Breyne, K.; Ughetto, S.; Laurent, L.C.; Breakefield, X.O. RNA delivery by extracellular vesicles in mammalian cells and its applications. *Nat. Rev. Mol. Cell Biol.* **2020**, *21*, 585–606. [CrossRef]
31. Park, C.Y.; Choi, Y.S.; McManus, M.T. Analysis of microRNA knockouts in mice. *Hum. Mol. Genet.* **2010**, *19*, 169–175. [CrossRef]
32. Bernstein, E.; Kim, S.Y.; Carmell, M.A.; Murchison, E.P.; Alcorn, H.; Li, M.Z.; Mills, A.A.; Elledge, S.J.; Anderson, K.V.; Hannon, G.J. Dicer is essential for mouse development. *Nat. Genet.* **2003**, *35*, 215–217. [CrossRef]
33. London, L. Motivator and Barriers to Latina's Participation in Clinical Trials. *Contemp. C* **2015**, *40*, 3–14. [CrossRef]
34. Van Rooij, E.; Quiat, D.; Johnson, B.A.; Sutherland, L.B.; Qi, X.; Richardson, J.A.; Kelm, R.J.; Olson, E.N. Expression and Muscle Performance. *Dev. Cell* **2009**, *17*, 662–673. [CrossRef] [PubMed]
35. Van Rooij, E.; Sutherland, L.B.; Qi, X.; Richardson, J.A.; Hill, J.; Olson, E.N. Control of stress-dependent cardiac growth and gene expression by a microRNA. *Science* **2007**, *316*, 575–579. [CrossRef] [PubMed]
36. Xin, M.; Small, E.M.; Sutherland, L.B.; Qi, X.; McAnally, J.; Plato, C.F.; Richardson, J.A.; Bassel-Duby, R.; Olson, E.N. MicroRNAs miR-143 and miR-145 modulate cytoskeletal dynamics and responsiveness of smooth muscle cells to injury. *Genes Dev.* **2009**, *23*, 2166–2178. [CrossRef]

37. Zhao, W.; Zhao, S.-P.; Zhao, Y.-H. MicroRNA-143/-145 in Cardiovascular Diseases. *Biomed. Res. Int.* **2015**, *2015*, 531740. [CrossRef]
38. Bang, C.; Batkai, S.; Dangwal, S.; Gupta, S.K.; Foinquinos, A.; Holzmann, A.; Just, A.; Remke, J.; Zimmer, K.; Zeug, A.; et al. Cardiac fibroblast-derived microRNA passenger strand-enriched exosomes mediate cardiomyocyte hypertrophy. *J. Clin. Invest.* **2014**, *124*, 2136–2146. [CrossRef]
39. Fu, F.; Jiang, W.; Zhou, L. Circulating Exosomal miR-17-5p and miR-92a-3p Predict Pathologic Stage and Grade of Colorectal Cancer. *Transl. Oncol.* **2018**, *11*, 221–232. [CrossRef]
40. Liu, T.; Zhang, Q.; Zhang, J.; Li, C.; Miao, Y.R.; Lei, Q.; Li, Q.; Guo, A.Y. EVmiRNA: A database of miRNA profiling in extracellular vesicles. *Nucleic Acids Res.* **2019**, *47*, 89–93. [CrossRef]
41. Yang, S.Y.; Wang, Y.Q.; Gao, H.M.; Wang, B.; He, Q. The clinical value of circulating MIR-99a in plasma of patients with acute myocardial infarction. *Eur. Rev. Med. Pharmacol. Sci.* **2016**, *20*, 5193–5197.
42. Schulte, C.; Barwari, T.; Joshi, A.; Theofilatos, K.; Zampetaki, A.; Barallobre-Barreiro, J.; Singh, B.; Sörensen, N.A.; Neumann, J.T.; Zeller, T.; et al. Comparative analysis of circulating noncoding rnas versus protein biomarkers in the detection of myocardial injury. *Circ. Res.* **2019**, *125*, 328–340. [CrossRef]
43. Mendell, J.T.; Olson, E.N. MicroRNAs in stress signaling and human disease. *Cell* **2012**, *148*, 1172–1187. [CrossRef] [PubMed]
44. Bonneau, E.; Neveu, B.; Kostantin, E.; Tsongalis, G.J.; De Guire, V. How close are miRNAs from clinical practice? A perspective on the diagnostic and therapeutic market. *Electron. J. Int. Fed. Clin. Chem. Lab. Med.* **2019**, *30*, 114–127.
45. Bajan, S.; Hutvagner, G. RNA-Based Therapeutics: From Antisense Oligonucleotides to miRNAs. *Cells* **2020**, *9*, 137. [CrossRef] [PubMed]
46. Mitra, S.; Deshmukh, A.; Sachdeva, R.; Lu, J.; Mehta, J.L. Oxidized Low-Density Lipoprotein and Atherosclerosis Implications in Antioxidant Therapy. *Am. J. Med. Sci.* **2011**, *342*, 135–142. [CrossRef] [PubMed]
47. Linton, M.F.; Yancey, P.G.; Davies, S.S.; Jerome, W.G.; Linton, E.F.; Vickers, K.C. *The Role of Lipids and Lipoproteins in Atherosclerosis*; MDText: South Dartmouth, MA, USA, 2000.
48. Bairey Merz, C.N.; Pepine, C.J.; Walsh, M.N.; Fleg, J.L.; Camici, P.G.; Chilian, W.M.; Clayton, J.A.; Cooper, L.S.; Crea, F.; Di Carli, M.; et al. Ischemia and No Obstructive Coronary Artery Disease (INOCA). *Circulation* **2017**, *135*, 1075–1092. [CrossRef] [PubMed]
49. Tse, K.; Tse, H.; Sidney, J.; Sette, A.; Ley, K. T cells in atherosclerosis. *Int. Immunol.* **2013**, *25*, 615–622. [CrossRef] [PubMed]
50. Golledge, J.; Norman, P.E. Atherosclerosis and abdominal aortic aneurysm: Cause, response, or common risk factors? *Arterioscler. Thromb. Vasc. Biol.* **2010**, *30*, 1075–1077. [CrossRef]
51. Koroleva, I.A.; Nazarenko, M.S.; Kucher, A.N. Role of microRNA in development of instability of atherosclerotic plaques. *Biochemistry* **2017**, *82*, 1380–1390. [CrossRef]
52. Sharma, S.; Jackson, P.G.; Makan, J. Cardiac troponins. *J. Clin. Pathol.* **2004**, *57*, 1025–1026. [CrossRef]
53. Omland, T.; de Lemos, J.A.; Sabatine, M.S.; Christophi, C.A.; Rice, M.M.; Jablonski, K.A.; Tjora, S.; Domanski, M.J.; Gersh, B.J.; Rouleau, J.L.; et al. A sensitive cardiac troponin T assay in stable coronary artery disease. *N. Engl. J. Med.* **2009**, *361*, 2538–2547. [CrossRef]
54. Speidl, W.S.; Graf, S.; Hornykewycz, S.; Nikfardjam, M.; Niessner, A.; Zorn, G.; Wojta, J.; Huber, K. High-sensitivity C-reactive protein in the prediction of coronary events in patients with premature coronary artery disease. *Am. Heart J.* **2002**, *144*, 449–455. [CrossRef]
55. Sara, J.D.S.; Prasad, M.; Zhang, M.; Lennon, R.J.; Herrmann, J.; Lerman, L.O.; Lerman, A. High-sensitivity C-reactive protein is an independent marker of abnormal coronary vasoreactivity in patients with non-obstructive coronary artery disease. *Am. Heart J.* **2017**, *190*, 1–11. [CrossRef] [PubMed]
56. Tahhan, A.S.; Sandesara, P.; Hayek, S.S.; Hammadah, M.; Alkhoder, A.; Kelli, H.M.; Topel, M.; O'Neal, W.T.; Ghasemzadeh, N.; Ko, Y.A.; et al. High-sensitivity troponin I levels and coronary artery disease severity, progression, and long-term outcomes. *J. Am. Heart Assoc.* **2018**, *7*, e007914. [CrossRef]
57. Zimmerli, L.U.; Schiffer, E.; Zürbig, P.; Good, D.M.; Kellmann, M.; Mouls, L.; Pitt, A.R.; Coon, J.J.; Schmieder, R.E.; Peter, K.H.; et al. Urinary proteomic biomarkers in coronary artery disease. *Mol. Cell. Proteomics* **2008**, *7*, 290–298. [CrossRef]

58. Ibrahim, N.E.; Januzzi, J.L.; Magaret, C.A.; Gaggin, H.K.; Rhyne, R.F.; Gandhi, P.U.; Kelly, N.; Simon, M.L.; Motiwala, S.R.; Belcher, A.M.; et al. A Clinical and Biomarker Scoring System to Predict the Presence of Obstructive Coronary Artery Disease. *J. Am. Coll. Cardiol.* **2017**, *69*, 1147–1156. [CrossRef] [PubMed]
59. D'Alessandra, Y.; Devanna, P.; Limana, F.; Straino, S.; Di Carlo, A.; Brambilla, P.G.; Rubino, M.; Carena, M.C.; Spazzafumo, L.; De Simone, M.; et al. Circulating microRNAs are new and sensitive biomarkers of myocardial infarction. *Eur. Heart J.* **2010**, *31*, 2765–2773. [CrossRef]
60. Condorelli, G.; Latronico, M.V.G.; Dorn, G.W. MicroRNAs in heart disease: Putative novel therapeutic targets? *Eur. Heart J.* **2010**, *31*, 649–658. [CrossRef] [PubMed]
61. Fichtlscherer, S.; De Rosa, S.; Fox, H.; Schwietz, T.; Fischer, A.; Liebetrau, C.; Weber, M.; Hamm, C.W.; Röxe, T.; Müller-Ardogan, M.; et al. Circulating microRNAs in patients with coronary artery disease. *Circ. Res.* **2010**, *107*, 677–684. [CrossRef] [PubMed]
62. Raitoharju, E.; Lyytikäinen, L.-P.; Levula, M.; Oksala, N.; Mennander, A.; Tarkka, M.; Klopp, N.; Illig, T.; Kähönen, M.; Karhunen, P.J.; et al. miR-21, miR-210, miR-34a, and miR-146a/b are up-regulated in human atherosclerotic plaques in the Tampere Vascular Study. *Atherosclerosis* **2011**, *219*, 211–217. [CrossRef]
63. Raitoharju, E.; Oksala, N.; Lehtimäki, T. MicroRNAs in the atherosclerotic plaque. *Clin. Chem.* **2013**, *59*, 1708–1721. [CrossRef]
64. Chan, M.C.; Hilyard, A.C.; Wu, C.; Davis, B.N.; Hill, N.S.; Lal, A.; Lieberman, J.; Lagna, G.; Hata, A. Molecular basis for antagonism between PDGF and the TGF b family of signalling pathways by control of miR-24 expression. *EMBO J.* **2009**, *29*, 559–573. [CrossRef] [PubMed]
65. Davis, B.N.; Hilyard, A.C.; Nguyen, P.H.; Lagna, G.; Hata, A. Induction of MicroRNA-221 by platelet-derived growth factor signaling is critical for modulation of vascular smooth muscle phenotype. *J. Biol. Chem.* **2009**, *284*, 3728–3738. [CrossRef]
66. Liu, X.; Cheng, Y.; Chen, X.; Yang, J.; Xu, L.; Zhang, C. MicroRNA-31 regulated by the extracellular regulated kinase is involved in vascular smooth muscle cell growth via large tumor suppressor homolog 2. *J. Biol. Chem.* **2011**, *286*, 42371–42380. [CrossRef] [PubMed]
67. Zhang, Y.; Wang, Y.; Wang, X.; Zhang, Y.; Eisner, G.M.; Asico, L.D.; Jose, P.A.; Zeng, C. Insulin promotes vascular smooth muscle cell proliferation via microRNA-208-mediated downregulation of p21. *J. Hypertens.* **2011**, *152*, 66. [CrossRef]
68. Leeper, N.J.; Raiesdana, A.; Kojima, Y.; Chun, H.J.; Azuma, J.; Maegdefessel, L.; Kundu, R.K.; Quertermous, T.; Tsao, P.S.; Spin, J.M. MicroRNA-26a is a novel regulator of vascular smooth muscle cell function. *J. Cell. Physiol.* **2011**, *226*, 1035–1043. [CrossRef]
69. Hutcheson, R.; Chaplin, J.; Hutcheson, B.; Borthwick, F.; Proctor, S.; Gebb, S.; Jadhav, R.; Smith, E.; Russell, J.C.; Rocic, P. miR-21 normalizes vascular smooth muscle proliferation and improves coronary collateral growth in metabolic syndrome. *FASEB J.* **2014**, *28*, 4088–4099. [CrossRef] [PubMed]
70. Zhou, J.; Shao, G.; Chen, X.; Yang, X.; Huang, X.; Peng, P.; Ba, Y. miRNA 206 and miRNA 574-5p are highly expression in coronary artery disease. *Biosci. Rep.* **2016**, *36*, e00295. [CrossRef] [PubMed]
71. Li, H.Y.; Zhao, X.; Liu, Y.Z.; Meng, Z.; Wang, D.; Yang, F.; Shi, Q.W. Plasma MicroRNA-126-5p is Associated with the Complexity and Severity of Coronary Artery Disease in Patients with Stable Angina Pectoris. *Cell. Physiol. Biochem.* **2016**, *39*, 837–846. [CrossRef]
72. Wang, H.W.; Lo, H.H.; Chiu, Y.L.; Chang, S.J.; Huang, P.H.; Liao, K.H.; Tasi, C.F.; Wu, C.H.; Tsai, T.N.; Cheng, C.C.; et al. Dysregulated miR-361-5p/VEGF axis in the plasma and endothelial progenitor cells of patients with coronary artery disease. *PLoS ONE* **2014**, *9*, e98070. [CrossRef]
73. Wang, M.; Ji, Y.; Cai, S.; Ding, W. MiR-206 suppresses the progression of coronary artery disease by modulating vascular endothelial growth factor (VEGF) expression. *Med. Sci. Monit.* **2016**, *22*, 5011–5020. [CrossRef]
74. Adachi, T.; Nakanishi, M.; Otsuka, Y.; Nishimura, K.; Hirokawa, G.; Goto, Y.; Nonogi, H.; Iwai, N. Plasma microRNA 499 as a biomarker of acute myocardial infarction. *Clin. Chem.* **2010**, *56*, 1183–1185. [CrossRef] [PubMed]
75. Corsten, M.F.; Dennert, R.; Jochems, S.; Kuznetsova, T.; Devaux, Y.; Hofstra, L.; Wagner, D.R.; Staessen, J.A.; Heymans, S.; Schroen, B. Circulating MicroRNA-208b and MicroRNA-499 reflect myocardial damage in cardiovascular disease. *Circ. Cardiovasc. Genet.* **2010**, *3*, 499–506. [CrossRef] [PubMed]
76. Ji, X.; Takahashi, R.; Hiura, Y.; Hirokawa, G.; Fukushima, Y.; Iwai, N. Plasma miR-208 as a biomarker of myocardial injury. *Clin. Chem.* **2009**, *55*, 1944–1949. [CrossRef] [PubMed]

77. Ai, J.; Zhang, R.; Li, Y.; Pu, J.; Lu, Y.; Jiao, J.; Li, K.; Yu, B.; Li, Z.; Wang, R.; et al. Circulating microRNA-1 as a potential novel biomarker for acute myocardial infarction. *Biochem. Biophys. Res. Commun.* **2010**, *391*, 73–77. [CrossRef] [PubMed]
78. Hoekstra, M.; van der Lans, C.A.C.; Halvorsen, B.; Gullestad, L.; Kuiper, J.; Aukrust, P.; van Berkel, T.J.C.; Biessen, E.A.L. The peripheral blood mononuclear cell microRNA signature of coronary artery disease. *Biochem. Biophys. Res. Commun.* **2010**, *394*, 792–797. [CrossRef]
79. Takahashi, Y.; Satoh, M.; Minami, Y.; Tabuchi, T.; Itoh, T.; Nakamura, M. Expression of miR-146a/b is associated with the Toll-like receptor 4 signal in coronary artery disease: Effect of renin-angiotensin system blockade and statins on miRNA-146a/b and Toll-like receptor 4 levels. *Clin. Sci.* **2010**, *119*, 395–405. [CrossRef]
80. Satoh, M.; Tabuchi, T.; Minami, Y.; Takahashi, Y.; Itoh, T.; Nakamura, M. Expression of let-7i is associated with Toll-like receptor 4 signal in coronary artery disease: Effect of statins on let-7i and Toll-like receptor 4 signal. *Immunobiology* **2012**, *217*, 533–539. [CrossRef]
81. Willeit, P.; Zampetaki, A.; Dudek, K.; Kaudewitz, D.; King, A.; Kirkby, N.S.; Crosby-Nwaobi, R.; Prokopi, M.; Drozdov, I.; Langley, S.R.; et al. Circulating MicroRNAs as novel biomarkers for platelet activation. *Circ. Res.* **2013**, *112*, 595–600. [CrossRef]
82. Das, A.; Samidurai, A.; Salloum, F.N. Deciphering Non-coding RNAs in Cardiovascular Health and Disease. *Front. Cardiovasc. Med.* **2018**, *5*, 73. [CrossRef]
83. Zhang, Y.; Zhang, L.; Wang, Y.; Ding, H.; Xue, S.; Qi, H.; Li, P. MicroRNAs or long noncoding RNAs in diagnosis and prognosis of coronary artery disease. *Aging Dis.* **2019**, *10*, 353–366. [CrossRef]
84. Elmén, J.; Lindow, M.; Silahtaroglu, A.; Bak, M.; Christensen, M.; Lind-Thomsen, A.; Hedtjärn, M.; Hansen, J.B.; Hansen, H.F.; Straarup, E.M.; et al. Antagonism of microRNA-122 in mice by systemically administered LNA-antimiR leads to up-regulation of a large set of predicted target mRNAs in the liver. *Nucleic Acids Res.* **2008**, *36*, 1153–1162. [CrossRef]
85. Dong, J.; Liang, Y.Z.; Zhang, J.; Wu, L.J.; Wang, S.; Hua, Q.; Yan, Y.X. Potential role of lipometabolism-related microRNAs in peripheral blood mononuclear cells as biomarkers for coronary artery disease. *J. Atheroscler. Thromb.* **2017**, *24*, 430–441. [CrossRef] [PubMed]
86. Moore, K.J.; Rayner, K.J.; Suárez, Y.; Fernández-Hernando, C. The role of microRNAs in cholesterol efflux and hepatic lipid metabolism. *Annu. Rev. Nutr.* **2011**, *31*, 49–63. [CrossRef]
87. Marquart, T.J.; Allen, R.M.; Ory, D.S.; Baldán, Á. miR-33 links SREBP-2 induction to repression of sterol transporters. *Proc. Natl. Acad. Sci. USA* **2010**, *107*, 12228–12232. [CrossRef] [PubMed]
88. Iliopoulos, D.; Drosatos, K.; Hiyama, Y.; Goldberg, I.J.; Zannis, V.I. MicroRNA-370 controls the expression of MicroRNA-122 and Cpt1α and affects lipid metabolism. *J. Lipid Res.* **2010**, *51*, 1513–1523. [CrossRef] [PubMed]
89. Faccini, J.; Ruidavets, J.B.; Cordelier, P.; Martins, F.; Maoret, J.J.; Bongard, V.; Ferrières, J.; Roncalli, J.; Elbaz, M.; Vindis, C. Circulating MIR-155, MIR-145 and let-7c as diagnostic biomarkers of the coronary artery disease. *Sci. Rep.* **2017**, *7*, 42916. [CrossRef] [PubMed]
90. Li, X.; Kong, D.; Chen, H.; Liu, S.; Hu, H.; Wu, T.; Wang, J.; Chen, W.; Ning, Y.; Li, Y.; et al. MiR-155 acts as an anti-inflammatory factor in atherosclerosis-Associated foam cell formation by repressing calcium-regulated heat stable protein 1. *Sci. Rep.* **2016**, *6*, 21789. [CrossRef] [PubMed]
91. Cheng, H.S.; Sivachandran, N.; Lau, A.; Boudreau, E.; Zhao, J.L.; Baltimore, D.; Delgado-Olguin, P.; Cybulsky, M.I.; Fish, J.E. MicroRNA-146 represses endothelial activation by inhibiting pro-inflammatory pathways. *EMBO Mol. Med.* **2013**, *5*, 949–966. [CrossRef]
92. Huang, R.S.; Gamazon, E.R.; Ziliak, D.; Wen, Y.; Im, H.K.; Zhang, W.; Wing, C.; Duan, S.; Bleibel, W.K.; Cox, N.J.; et al. Population differences in microRNA expression and biological implications. *RNA Biol.* **2011**, *8*, 692–701. [CrossRef]
93. Rawlings-Goss, R.A.; Campbell, M.C.; Tishkoff, S.A. Global population-specific variation in miRNA associated with cancer risk and clinical biomarkers. *BMC Med. Genomics* **2014**, *7*, 53. [CrossRef]
94. Meder, B.; Backes, C.; Haas, J.; Leidinger, P.; Stähler, C.; Großmann, T.; Vogel, B.; Frese, K.; Giannitsis, E.; Katus, H.A.; et al. Influence of the confounding factors age and sex on microRNA profiles from peripheral blood. *Clin. Chem.* **2014**, *60*, 1200–1208. [CrossRef] [PubMed]
95. Simon, L.M.; Edelstein, L.C.; Nagalla, S.; Woodley, A.B.; Chen, E.S.; Kong, X.; Ma, L.; Fortina, P.; Kunapuli, S.; Holinstat, M.; et al. Human platelet microRNA-mRNA networks associated with age and gender revealed by integrated plateletomics. *Blood* **2014**, *123*, 37–45. [CrossRef] [PubMed]

96. Sayed, A.S.M.; Xia, K.; Li, F.; Deng, X.; Salma, U.; Li, T.; Deng, H.; Yang, D.; Haoyang, Z.; Yang, T.L.; et al. The diagnostic value of circulating microRNAs for middle-aged (40–60-year-old) coronary artery disease patients. *Clinics* **2015**, *70*, 257–263. [CrossRef]
97. Olivieri, F.; Bonafè, M.; Spazzafumo, L.; Gobbi, M.; Prattichizzo, F.; Recchioni, R.; Marcheselli, F.; La Sala, L.; Galeazzi, R.; Rippo, M.R.; et al. Age- and glycemia-related miR-126-3p levels in plasma and endothelial cells. *Aging* **2014**, *6*, 771–786. [CrossRef] [PubMed]
98. Ultimo, S.; Zauli, G.; Martelli, A.M.; Vitale, M.; McCubrey, J.A.; Capitani, S.; Neri, L.M. Cardiovascular disease-related miRNAs expression: Potential role as biomarkers and effects of training exercise. *Oncotarget* **2018**, *9*, 17238–17254. [CrossRef] [PubMed]
99. Gupta, S.K.; Foinquinos, A.; Thum, S.; Remke, J.; Zimmer, K.; Bauters, C.; de Groote, P.; Boon, R.A.; de Windt, L.J.; Preissl, S.; et al. Preclinical Development of a MicroRNA-Based Therapy for Elderly Patients With Myocardial Infarction. *J. Am. Coll. Cardiol.* **2016**, *68*, 1557–1571. [CrossRef]
100. De Lucia, C.; Komici, K.; Borghetti, G.; Femminella, G.D.; Bencivenga, L.; Cannavo, A.; Corbi, G.; Ferrara, N.; Houser, S.R.; Koch, W.J.; et al. MicroRNA in cardiovascular aging and age-related cardiovascular diseases. *Front. Med. Lausanne* **2017**, *4*, 74. [CrossRef]
101. Van Almen, G.C.; Verhesen, W.; van Leeuwen, R.E.W.; van de Vrie, M.; Eurlings, C.; Schellings, M.W.M.; Swinnen, M.; Cleutjens, J.P.M.; van Zandvoort, M.A.M.J.; Heymans, S.; et al. MicroRNA-18 and microRNA-19 regulate CTGF and TSP-1 expression in age-related heart failure. *Aging Cell* **2011**, *10*, 769–779. [CrossRef]
102. Zhou, M.; Cai, J.; Tang, Y.; Zhao, Q. MiR-17-92 cluster is a novel regulatory gene of cardiac ischemic/reperfusion injury. *Med. Hypotheses* **2013**, *81*, 108–110. [CrossRef]
103. Zhong, Z.; Hou, J.; Zhang, Q.; Zhong, W.; Li, B.; Li, C.; Liu, Z.; Yang, M.; Zhao, P. Circulating microRNA expression profiling and bioinformatics analysis of dysregulated microRNAs of patients with coronary artery disease. *Medicine* **2018**, *97*, e11428. [CrossRef]
104. Wang, K.; Yuan, Y.; Cho, J.H.; McClarty, S.; Baxter, D.; Galas, D.J. Comparing the MicroRNA spectrum between serum and plasma. *PLoS ONE* **2012**, *7*, e41561. [CrossRef] [PubMed]
105. Blondal, T.; Jensby Nielsen, S.; Baker, A.; Andreasen, D.; Mouritzen, P.; Wrang Teilum, M.; Dahlsveen, I.K. Assessing sample and miRNA profile quality in serum and plasma or other biofluids. *Methods* **2013**, *59*, 1–6. [CrossRef] [PubMed]
106. Kroh, E.M.; Parkin, R.K.; Mitchell, P.S.; Tewari, M. Analysis of circulating microRNA biomarkers in plasma and serum using quantitative reverse transcription-PCR (qRT-PCR). *Methods* **2010**, *50*, 298–301. [CrossRef] [PubMed]
107. Sunderland, N.; Skroblin, P.; Barwari, T.; Huntley, R.P.; Lu, R.; Joshi, A.; Lovering, R.C.; Mayr, M. MicroRNA Biomarkers and Platelet Reactivity: The Clot Thickens. *Circ. Res.* **2017**, *120*, 418–435. [CrossRef] [PubMed]
108. Peirson, S.N.; Butler, J.N. RNA Extraction From Mammalian Tissues. In *Methods in Molecular Biology*; Rosato, E., Ed.; Humana Press: Totowa, NJ, USA, 2007; pp. 315–327. ISBN 978-1-59745-257-1.
109. Glinge, C.; Clauss, S.; Boddum, K.; Jabbari, R.; Jabbari, J.; Risgaard, B.; Tomsits, P.; Hildebrand, B.; Kääb, S.; Wakili, R.; et al. Stability of Circulating Blood-Based MicroRNAs—Pre-Analytic Methodological Considerations. *PLoS ONE* **2017**, *12*, e0167969. [CrossRef]
110. Mayeux, R. Biomarkers: Potential Uses and Limitations. *NeuroRx* **2004**, *1*, 182–188. [CrossRef]
111. Jansen, F.; Yang, X.; Proebsting, S.; Hoelscher, M.; Przybilla, D.; Baumann, K.; Schmitz, T.; Dolf, A.; Endl, E.; Franklin, B.S.; et al. MicroRNA expression in circulating microvesicles predicts cardiovascular events in patients with coronary artery disease. *J. Am. Heart Assoc.* **2014**, *3*, e001249. [CrossRef]
112. Calin, G.A.; Dumitru, C.D.; Shimizu, M.; Bichi, R.; Zupo, S.; Noch, E.; Aldler, H.; Rattan, S.; Keating, M.; Rai, K.; et al. Frequent deletions and down-regulation of micro-RNA genes miR15 and miR16 at 13q14 in chronic lymphocytic leukemia. *Proc. Natl. Acad. Sci. USA* **2002**, *99*, 15524–15529. [CrossRef]
113. Hayes, J.; Peruzzi, P.P.; Lawler, S. MicroRNAs in cancer: Biomarkers, functions and therapy. *Trends Mol. Med.* **2014**, *20*, 460–469. [CrossRef]
114. Hongyan, Z.; Guo-chang, F. Extracellular/circulating microRNAs and their potential role in cardiovascular disease. *Am. J. Cardiovasc. Dis.* **2011**, *1*, 138–149.
115. Trzybulska, D.; Vergadi, E.; Tsatsanis, C. MiRNA and other non-coding RNAs as promising diagnostic markers. *Electron. J. Int. Fed. Clin. Chem. Lab. Med.* **2018**, *29*, 221–226.
116. Pogribny, I.P. MicroRNAs as biomarkers for clinical studies. *Exp. Biol. Med.* **2018**, *243*, 283–290. [CrossRef] [PubMed]

117. Kreth, S.; Hübner, M.; Hinske, L.C. MicroRNAs as clinical biomarkers and therapeutic tools in perioperative medicine. *Anesth. Analg.* **2018**, *126*, 670–681. [CrossRef]
118. Wang, J.; Yan, Y.; Song, D.; Liu, B. Reduced Plasma miR-146a is a Predictor of Poor Coronary Collateral Circulation in Patients with Coronary Artery Disease. *Biomed Res. Int.* **2016**, *2016*, 4285942. [CrossRef] [PubMed]
119. Li, S.; Lee, C.; Song, J.; Lu, C.; Liu, J.; Cui, Y.; Liang, H.; Cao, C.; Zhang, F.; Chen, H. Circulating microRNAs as potential biomarkers for coronary plaque rupture. *Oncotarget* **2017**, *8*, 48145–48156. [CrossRef] [PubMed]
120. Li, X.D.; Yang, Y.J.; Wang, L.Y.; Qiao, S.B.; Lu, X.F.; Wu, Y.J.; Xu, B.; Li, H.F.; Gu, D.F. Elevated plasma miRNA-122, -140-3p, -720, -2861, and -3149 during early period of acute coronary syndrome are derived from peripheral blood mononuclear cells. *PLoS ONE* **2017**, *12*, e0184256. [CrossRef]
121. Jansen, F.; Schäfer, L.; Wang, H.; Schmitz, T.; Flender, A.; Schueler, R.; Hammerstingl, C.; Nickenig, G.; Sinning, J.; Werner, N. Kinetics of Circulating MicroRNAs in Response to Cardiac Stress in Patients With Coronary Artery Disease. *J. Am. Heart Assoc.* **2017**, *6*, e005270. [CrossRef]
122. Soeki, T.; Yamaguchi, K.; Niki, T.; Uematsu, E.; Bando, S.; Matsuura, T.; Ise, T.; Kusunose, K.; Hotchi, J.; Tobiume, T.; et al. Plasma microRNA-100 is associated with coronary plaque vulnerability. *Circ. J.* **2015**, *79*, 413–418. [CrossRef]
123. Liu, C.Z.; Zhong, Q.; Huang, Y.Q. Elevated plasma miR-29a levels are associated with increased carotid intima-media thickness in atherosclerosis patients. *Tohoku J. Exp. Med.* **2017**, *241*, 183–188. [CrossRef]
124. Wang, X.; Lian, Y.; Wen, X.; Guo, J.; Wang, Z.; Jiang, S.; Hu, Y. Expression of miR-126 and its potential function in coronary artery disease. *Afr. Health Sci.* **2017**, *17*, 474–480. [CrossRef]
125. Al-Kafaji, G.; Al-Mahroos, G.; Abdulla Al-Muhtaresh, H.; Sabry, M.A.; Abdul Razzak, R.; Salem, A.H. Circulating endothelium-enriched microRNA-126 as a potential biomarker for coronary artery disease in type 2 diabetes mellitus patients. *Biomarkers* **2017**, *22*, 268–278. [CrossRef] [PubMed]
126. Al-Muhtaresh, H.A.; Salem, A.H.; Al-Kafaji, G. Upregulation of Circulating Cardiomyocyte-Enriched miR-1 and miR-133 Associate with the Risk of Coronary Artery Disease in Type 2 Diabetes Patients and Serve as Potential Biomarkers. *J. Cardiovasc. Transl. Res.* **2019**, *12*, 347–357. [CrossRef]
127. Boon, R.A. Non-coding RNAs in cardiovascular health and disease. *Non Coding RNA Res.* **2018**, *3*, 99. [CrossRef]
128. Wang, H.W.; Huang, T.S.; Lo, H.H.; Huang, P.H.; Lin, C.C.; Chang, S.J.; Liao, K.H.; Tsai, C.H.; Chan, C.H.; Tsai, C.F.; et al. Deficiency of the MicroRNA-31-MicroRNA-720 pathway in the plasma and endothelial progenitor cells from patients with coronary artery disease. *Arterioscler. Thromb. Vasc. Biol.* **2014**, *34*, 857–869. [CrossRef] [PubMed]
129. Zhang, Y.; Li, H.-H.; Yang, R.; Yang, B.-J.; Gao, Z.-Y. Association between circulating microRNA-208a and severity of coronary heart disease. *Scand. J. Clin. Lab. Investig.* **2017**, *77*, 379–384. [CrossRef] [PubMed]
130. Han, H.; Qu, G.; Han, C.; Wang, Y.; Sun, T.; Li, F.; Wang, J.; Luo, S. MiR-34a, miR-21 and miR-23a as potential biomarkers for coronary artery disease: A pilot microarray study and confirmation in a 32 patient cohort. *Exp. Mol. Med.* **2015**, *47*, 138. [CrossRef] [PubMed]
131. Gao, H.; Guddeti, R.R.; Matsuzawa, Y.; Liu, L.P.; Su, L.X.; Guo, D.; Nie, S.P.; Du, J.; Zhang, M. Plasma levels of microRNA-145 are associated with severity of coronary artery disease. *PLoS ONE* **2015**, *10*, e0123477. [CrossRef] [PubMed]
132. Ren, J.; Zhang, J.; Xu, N.; Han, G.; Geng, Q.; Song, J.; Li, S.; Zhao, J.; Chen, H. Signature of circulating MicroRNAs As potential biomarkers in vulnerable coronary artery disease. *PLoS ONE* **2013**, *8*, e80738. [CrossRef] [PubMed]
133. Chen, J.; Xu, L.; Hu, Q.; Yang, S.; Zhang, B.; Jiang, H. MiR-17-5p as circulating biomarkers for the severity of coronary atherosclerosis in coronary artery disease. *Int. J. Cardiol.* **2015**, *197*, 123–124. [CrossRef] [PubMed]
134. Lin, B.; Feng, D.-G.; Wang, F.; Wang, J.-X.; Xu, C.-G.; Zhao, H.; Cheng, Z.-Y. MiR-365 participates in coronary atherosclerosis through regulating IL-6. *Eur. Rev. Med. Pharmacol. Sci.* **2016**, *20*, 5186–5192.
135. Cipollone, F.; Felicioni, L.; Sarzani, R.; Ucchino, S.; Spigonardo, F.; Mandolini, C.; Malatesta, S.; Bucci, M.; Mammarella, C.; Santovito, D.; et al. A unique MicroRNA signature associated with plaque instability in humans. *Stroke* **2011**, *42*, 2556–2563. [CrossRef] [PubMed]
136. Kumar, S.; Kim, C.W.; Simmons, R.D.; Jo, H. Role of flow-sensitive microRNAs in endothelial dysfunction and atherosclerosis—"Mechanosensitive Athero-miRs". *Arter. Thromb Vasc Biol.* **2014**, *22*, 313–333. [CrossRef]

137. Tian, F.J.; An, L.N.; Wang, G.K.; Zhu, J.Q.; Li, Q.; Zhang, Y.Y.; Zeng, A.; Zou, J.; Zhu, R.F.; Han, X.S.; et al. Elevated microRNA-155 promotes foam cell formation by targeting HBP1 in atherogenesis. *Cardiovasc. Res.* **2014**, *103*, 100–110.
138. Horie, T.; Baba, O.; Kuwabara, Y.; Chujo, Y.; Watanabe, S.; Kinoshita, M.; Horiguchi, M.; Nakamura, T.; Chonabayashi, K.; Hishizawa, M.; et al. MicroRNA-33 deficiency reduces the progression of atherosclerotic plaque in ApoE$^{-/-}$ mice. *J. Am. Heart Assoc.* **2012**, *1*, e003376.
139. Fang, Y.; Shi, C.; Manduchi, E.; Civelek, M.; Davies, P.F. MicroRNA-10a regulation of proinflammatory phenotype in athero-susceptible endothelium in vivo and in vitro. *Proc. Natl. Acad. Sci. USA* **2010**, *107*, 13450–13455.
140. Shan, Z.; Qin, S.; Li, W.; Wu, W.; Yang, J.; Chu, M.; Li, X.; Huo, Y.; Schaer, G.L.; Wang, S.; et al. An Endocrine Genetic Signal Between Blood Cells and Vascular Smooth Muscle Cells: Role of MicroRNA-223 in Smooth Muscle Function and Atherogenesis. *J. Am. Coll. Cardiol.* **2015**, *65*, 2526–2537.
141. Bidzhekov, K.; Gan, L.; Denecke, B.; Rostalsky, A.; Hristov, M.; Koeppel, T.A.; Zernecke, A.; Weber, C. microRNA expression signatures and parallels between monocyte subsets and atherosclerotic plaque in humans. *Thromb. Haemost.* **2012**, *107*, 619–625.
142. Jansen, F.; Yang, X.; Hoelscher, M.; Cattelan, A.; Schmitz, T.; Proebsting, S.; Wenzel, D.; Vosen, S.; Franklin, B.S.; Fleischmann, B.K.; et al. Endothelial microparticle-mediated transfer of microRNA-126 promotes vascular endothelial cell repair via spred1 and is abrogated in glucose-damaged endothelial microparticles. *Circulation* **2013**, *128*, 2026–2038.
143. Schulte, C.; Molz, S.; Appelbaum, S.; Karakas, M.; Ojeda, F.; Lau, D.M.; Hartmann, T.; Lackner, K.J.; Westermann, D.; Schnabel, R.B.; et al. MiRNA-197 and miRNA-223 predict cardiovascular death in a cohort of patients with symptomatic coronary artery disease. *PLoS ONE* **2015**, *10*, e0145930.
144. Hulsmans, M.; Sinnaeve, P.; Van Der Schueren, B.; Mathieu, C.; Janssens, S.; Holvoet, P. Decreased miR-181a expression in monocytes of obese patients is associated with the occurrence of metabolic syndrome and coronary artery disease. *J. Clin. Endocrinol. Metab.* **2012**, *97*, 1213–1218.

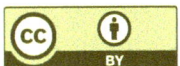 © 2020 by the authors. Licensee MDPI, Basel, Switzerland. This article is an open access article distributed under the terms and conditions of the Creative Commons Attribution (CC BY) license (http://creativecommons.org/licenses/by/4.0/).

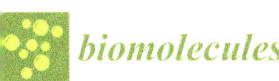 

*Article*

# Nourin-Dependent miR-137 and miR-106b: Novel Early Inflammatory Diagnostic Biomarkers for Unstable Angina Patients

Salwa A. Elgebaly [1,2,*], Robert H. Christenson [3], Hossam Kandil [4], Nashwa El-Khazragy [5], Laila Rashed [6], Beshoy Yacoub [4], Heba Eldeeb [4], Mahmoud Ali [4], Roshanak Sharafieh [2,7], Ulrike Klueh [7,8] and Donald L. Kreutzer [2,7]

1. Research & Development, Nour Heart, Inc., Vienna, VA, 22180, USA
2. Department of Surgery, School of Medicine, UConn Health, Farmington, CT, 06032, USA; rsharafieh@uchc.edu (R.S.); kreutzer@uchc.edu (D.L.K.)
3. Department of Pathology, University of Maryland School of Medicine, Baltimore, MD 21201, USA; rchristenson@som.umaryland.edu
4. Department of Cardiology, Kasr Alainy Faculty of Medicine, Cairo University, Cairo 11562, Egypt; Hossamkandil@kasralainy.edu.eg (H.K.); beshoy.ayuob@gmail.com (B.Y.); hebamostafakamel@gmail.com (H.E.); mahmoudbe1@hotmail.com (M.A.)
5. Department of Clinical Pathology-Hematology, Ain Shams Medical Research Institute (MASRI), Faculty of Medicine, Ain Shams University, Cairo 11566, Egypt; nashwaelkhazragy@med.asu.edu.eg
6. Department of Biochemistry and Molecular Biology, Kasr Alainy Faculty of Medicine, Cairo University, Cairo 11562, Egypt; lailarashed@kasralainy.edu.eg
7. Cell & Molecular Tissue Engineering, LLC Farmington, CT 06032, USA; klueh@wayne.edu
8. Integrative Biosciences Center (IBio), Department of Biomedical Engineering, Wayne State University, Detroit, MI 48202, USA
* Correspondence: selgebaly@nourheart.com; Tel.: +1-860-680-8860

**Abstract:** Background: Currently, no blood biomarkers exist that can diagnose unstable angina (UA) patients. Nourin is an early inflammatory mediator rapidly released within 5 min by reversible ischemic myocardium, and if ischemia persists, it is also released by necrosis. Nourin is elevated in acute coronary syndrome (ACS) patients but not in symptomatic noncardiac and healthy subjects. Recently, circulating microRNAs (miRNAs) have been established as markers of disease, including cardiac injury and inflammation. Objectives: To profile and validate the potential diagnostic value of Nourin-dependent *miR-137* (marker of cell damage) and *miR-106b-5p* (marker of inflammation) as early biomarkers in suspected UA patients and to investigate the association of their target and regulating genes. Methods: Using Nourin amino acid sequence, an integrated bioinformatics analysis was conducted. Analysis indicated that Nourin is a direct target for *miR-137* and *miR-106b-5p* in myocardial ischemic injury. Two linked molecular networks of lncRNA/miRNAs/mRNAs were also retrieved, including *CTB89H12.4/miR-137/FTHL-17* and *CTB89H12.4/miR-106b-5p/ANAPC11*. Gene expression profiling was assessed in serum samples collected at presentation to an emergency department (ED) from: (1) UA patients ($n = 30$) (confirmed by invasive coronary angiography with stenosis greater than 50% and troponin level below the clinical decision limit); (2) patients with acute ST elevation myocardial infarction (STEMI) ($n = 16$) (confirmed by persistent ST-segment changes and elevated troponin level); and (3) healthy subjects ($n = 16$). Results: Gene expression profiles showed that *miR-137* and *miR-106b-5p* were significantly upregulated by 1382-fold and 192-fold in UA compared to healthy, and by 2.5-fold and 4.6-fold in STEMI compared to UA, respectively. Healthy subjects showed minimal expression profile. Receiver operator characteristics (ROC) analysis revealed that the two miRNAs were sensitive and specific biomarkers for assessment of UA and STEMI patients. Additionally, Spearman's correlation analysis revealed a significant association of miRNAs with the associated mRNA targets and the regulating lncRNA. Conclusions: Nourin-dependent gene expression of *miR-137* and *miR-106b-5p* are novel blood-based biomarkers that can diagnose UA and STEMI patients at presentation and stratify severity of myocardial ischemia, with higher expression in STEMI compared to UA. Early diagnosis of suspected UA patients using

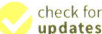

**Citation:** Elgebaly, S.A.; Christenson, R.H.; Kandil, H.; El-Khazragy, N.; Rashed, L.; Yacoub, B.; Eldeeb, H.; Ali, M.; Sharafieh, R.; Klueh, U.; et al. Nourin-Dependent miR-137 and miR-106b: Novel Early Inflammatory Diagnostic Biomarkers for Unstable Angina Patients. *Biomolecules* 2021, 11, 368. https://doi.org/10.3390/biom11030368

Academic Editors: Clara Crescioli and Pietro Scicchitano

Received: 19 December 2020
Accepted: 23 February 2021
Published: 28 February 2021

**Publisher's Note:** MDPI stays neutral with regard to jurisdictional claims in published maps and institutional affiliations.

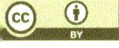

Copyright: © 2021 by the authors. Licensee MDPI, Basel, Switzerland. This article is an open access article distributed under the terms and conditions of the Creative Commons Attribution (CC BY) license (https://creativecommons.org/licenses/by/4.0/).

the novel Nourin biomarkers is key for initiating guideline-based therapy that improves patients' health outcomes.

**Keywords:** unstable angina; Nourin; miRNAs; inflammatory diagnostic biomarkers; reversible myocardial ischemia; acute coronary syndromes

## 1. Introduction

Acute coronary syndromes encompass a spectrum of ischemic conditions that include acute myocardial infarction (AMI) with ST-segment elevation (STEMI) or without (NSTEMI) and unstable angina [1,2]. Currently, patients with chest pain are assessed by risk score algorithms [3,4], electrocardiogram (ECG), cardiac enzymes, and occasionally coronary computed tomographic angiography [5,6]. However, the diagnosis still has major challenges especially for patients with atypical symptoms and completely normal or dynamic come-and-go ECG changes [7]. Although the introduction of high-sensitive cardiac troponins has improved the detection rate of NSTEMI, in the absence of myocardial necrosis, patients with unstable angina (UA) often undergo a lengthy assessment in a hospital emergency department (ED) or require hospital admissions [8]. Additionally, to date, no inflammatory blood-based biomarkers exist that can quickly diagnose reversible ischemic injury in UA patients [9]. Thus, there is a clear need to identify and validate new blood-based biomarkers to identify reversible ischemic injury as seen in UA patients before progressing to necrosis.

Elgebaly et al. [10–15] reported that Nourin is a 3 KDa formyl peptide that is released within five minutes by human and animal hearts in response to ischemic injury. Nourin is unique because of its rapid release by reversible ischemic myocardium when cells are initially injured, but still alive and not dead. If ischemia persists, Nourin is also released by necrotic cells. Nourin is a potent inflammatory mediator, and its release is associated with post-ischemic cardiac inflammation in early ischemia/reperfusion animal models of AMI, cardiopulmonary bypass surgery, as well as heart failure. A schematic diagram illustrating the release of the leukocyte chemotactic factor Nourin by ischemic myocardium, followed by leukocyte recruitment and cardiac inflammation, is presented in Figure 1. In our earlier publications, Nourin was referred to as cardiac-derived leukocyte chemotactic factor. Nourin was purified from cardioplegic solutions collected during cardiac arrest (reversible myocardial ischemia) from cardiopulmonary bypass patients when they underwent coronary revascularization [11], and its amino acid sequence was determined. As a formyl peptide, Nourin binds to formyl peptide receptor (FPR) on leukocytes and vascular endothelial cells (VECs). A number of competitive antagonists were identified, including cyclosporin H, spinorphin, t-Boc-Phe-D.Leu-Phe-D.Leu-Phe, and soluble FPR fragment 17 aa loop peptide, which inhibited Nourin activity and tissue inflammation. Additionally, the bioenergetic compound, Cyclocreatine Phosphate (CCrP) prevented ischemic injury by preserving elevated levels of cellular adenosine triphosphate (ATP) during ischemia, thus reducing Nourin intracellular formation and circulating levels, resulting in reduction of early reperfusion cardiac inflammation and restoration of contractile function in animal models of AMI, global cardiac arrest, cardiopulmonary bypass, heart transplantation, as well as heart failure [10,13]. As a potent inflammatory mediator, Nourin stimulates leukocyte chemotaxis and VEC migration and activates human monocytes, neutrophils, and VECs to express high levels of cytokine storm mediators, digestive enzymes, and free radicals, including tumor necrosis factor-$\alpha$ (TNF-$\alpha$, a key stimulant of apoptosis), interleukin 1$\beta$ (IL-1$\beta$), interleukin 8 (IL-8), leukocyte-endothelial cell adhesion molecule 1 (LECAM-1), intercellular adhesion molecule 1 (ICAM-1), and endothelial-leukocyte adhesion molecule 1 (ELAM-1), as well as collagenase type IV, N-acetyl-B-glucosaminidase, gelatinases, and superoxide anion [10]. Several of these mediators were reported by other investigators to play a crucial role in recruiting and activating neutrophils during post-ischemic early reperfusion, and thus may contribute to the no-reflow phenomenon. Furthermore, since the above-described Nourin inhibitors/antagonists are aimed at controlling the level and activity of Nourin, they will likely reduce early post-reperfusion leukocyte influx/activation and inflammation-induced damage without interfering with the crucial cardiac repair process that occurs a few days following myocardial infarction [ ]. Additionally, an independent study indicated that high levels of TNF-α, IL-1β, and IL-8 were detected in UA patients during the early disease phase [ ], suggesting a role of Nourin-induced proinflammatory cytokines in the pathogenesis of UA. Clinically, using Nourin ELISA and chemotaxis assay, we demonstrated that high levels of Nourin were detected in blood samples collected at presentation to hospital EDs from symptomatic acute coronary syndromes (ACS) patients and patients with documented AMI but not in symptomatic noncardiac patients and healthy subjects [ ]. These results suggest the potential use of the Nourin biomarker to rule out myocardial ischemia for symptomatic patients having noncardiac causes.

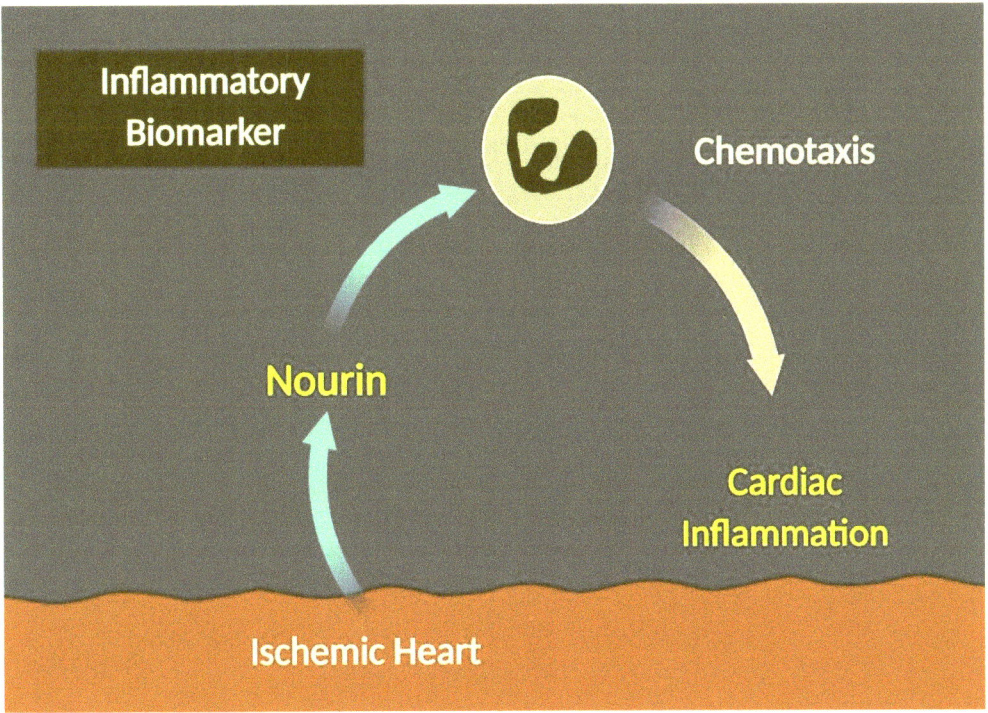

**Figure 1.** Schematic diagram illustrating the release of the leukocyte chemotactic factor Nourin by ischemic myocardium, followed by leukocyte recruitment and cardiac inflammation.

Non-coding RNA molecules are nonprotein coding genes that regulate 60% of protein coding genes. Non-coding RNAs are either: (1) short noncoding of approximately 22–24 nucleotides, named miRNAs post-transcriptional regulator, or (2) long noncoding (>200 nucleotides) [ ]. They are involved in numerous biological processes, including cell proliferation, differentiation, and apoptosis, thereby contributing to various pathological conditions [ ]. With the development of high-throughput next-generation sequencing (NGS), about 30 miRNAs have been reported as specific diagnostic and prognostic blood-based biomarkers in AMI patients, including *miR-155, miR-380, miR-208b,* and *miR-133a.* On the other hand, a cluster of the three miRNAs—(*miR-150/186/132*), miR-133a, and *miR-108b*—are linked to UA patients [ , ]. The role of miR-137 in ischemic stroke and their potential therapeutic targets have also been reported in recent studies [22,23]. Although the focus was restricted to cerebral [22] and retinal hypoxia [24], the signaling pathway was directly related to hypoxic conditions. Li et al. reported that *miR-137* is a hypoxia-responsive gene, and its overexpression aggravates hypoxia-induced cell apoptosis [24]. Additionally, recent bioinformatics analysis has suggested that *miR-106b-5p* serves as a robust inflammatory mediator for apoptosis and angiogenesis in AMI [25–27].

In the current study, we applied an integrative bioinformatics analysis using the Nourin amino acid sequence to retrieve the Nourin-associated miRNAs in UA and acute STEMI patients. The two miRNAs, *miR-137* and *miR-106b-5p*, which are linked to myocardial ischemia, were selected. Both miRNAs are found to be expressed in human hearts and they were identified as cardiac-enriched miRNAs that are found to be overexpressed at a much higher level during cardiac tissue injury and in AMI patients, but undetectable in healthy individuals. Furthermore, the lncRNA/miRNA/mRNA network for each miRNA was constructed and a quantitative real time PCR (qPCR) was performed to determine whether the Nourin-dependent miRNAs, *miR-137* and *miR-106b-5p*, can diagnose ischemia-induced injury in UA patients when troponin levels are below the clinical decision limit or in STEMI patients with elevated troponin level. A schematic diagram illustrating the signaling pathway of Nourin-dependent *miR-137* and *miR-106b-5p* in myocardial ischemic injury is presented in Figure 2. Specifically, downregulation of *lncR-CTB89H12.4* due to ischemia resulted in upregulation of both miR-137 (marker of cell damage) and miR-106b-5p (marker of inflammation), as well as activation of *mRNA-FTHL-17* and *mRNA-ANAPC11* with a likely increased translation and production of Nourin protein. Thus, the association of these miRNAs with their regulatory molecular networks outlines a novel underlying mechanistic signaling pathway in myocardial ischemic injury.

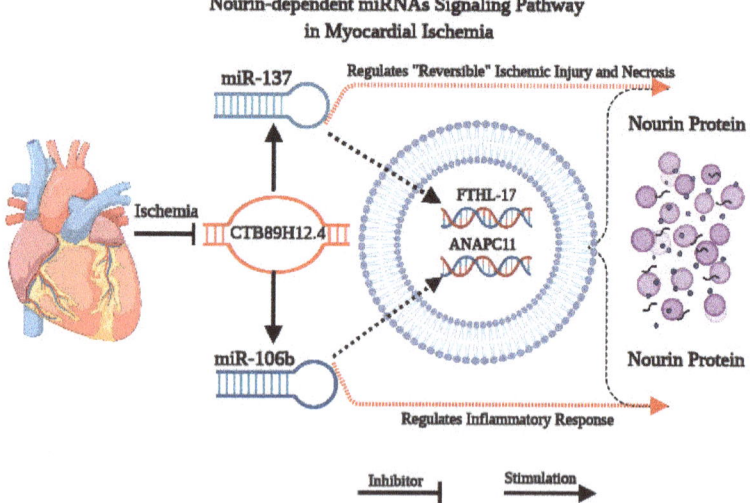

**Figure 2.** Schematic diagram illustrating the mechanism of Nourin-dependent miRNAs, *miR-137* and *miR-106b-5p*, in myocardial ischemic injury and their associated molecular network, based on integrative bioinformatics analysis. Downregulation of *CTB89H12.4* due to ischemia resulted in upregulation of both *miR-137* (marker of cell damage) and *miR-106b-5p* (marker of inflammation) and activation of *mRNA-FTHL-17* and *mRNA-ANAPC11*, with a likely increased translation and production of Nourin protein.

## 2. Subjects and Methods

### 2.1. Bioinformatics Analysis

A comprehensive bioinformatics analysis was conducted to analyze different expressed genes (DEGs) that are incorporated with myocardial ischemic injury and related to Nourin protein, then the Nourin protein interaction was mapped through functional gathering analysis using the incorporated gene ontology (GO) and Kyoto Encyclopedia of Genes and Genomes (KEGG) databases, and finally, a pathway enrichment analysis of the DEGs was performed using the online The Database for Annotation, Visualization and Integrated Discovery (DAVID) tools. A $p$-value < 0.05 indicates significance. To construct a protein–protein interaction (PPI) network, the Nourin-dependent DEGs were uploaded to an interacting genes/proteins database (STRING), which provides a systematic functional organization of the proteome. The data obtained revealed that ferritin heavy chain like 17 (*FTHL-17*) and anaphase promoting complex subunit 11 (*ANAPC11*) genes directly targeted Nourin protein, and they were significantly dysregulated in myocardial ischemic injury. In addition, they were minimally expressed in normal myocardial tissue. To construct lncRNA/miRNA/mRNA networks for the two selected genes, these target genes were further analyzed to predict specific miRNAs, using miRDB, TargetScan and miRTarBase databases. Analysis showed that *miR-137* and *miR-106b-5p* are candidate targets for *FTHL-17* and *ANAPC11*, respectively. Each mRNA was recognized by three different databases to ensure that data accuracy and selection were based on detection of high complementarity binding sites. Finally, the *lncRNA-CTB89H12.4* (*CTB89H12.4*) was selected to control the expression of both miRNAs using the DIANA-LncBasev3, Starbase and CHIP databases [ ]. The in silico prediction of each network was verified by Clustal 2 multiple sequence alignment software to validate the alignment between the candidate genes in each network.

### 2.2. Study Design/Participant's Selection

A prospective observational study was conducted on UA and acute STEMI patients presented with chest pain at Kasr-Alainy hospital during the period from October 2019 to March 2020. The study complied with the Declaration of Helsinki and was approved by the Ethics Community of Faculty of Medicine, Cairo University. A written consent was obtained from each patient and healthy subject before enrollment.

In the current pilot study, all 62 subjects met the inclusion/exclusion criteria before being enrolled, including UA ($n$ = 30) and STEMI ($n$ = 16) patients with acute chest pain within the first 10 h of symptoms, as well as healthy subjects ($n$ = 16). Unstable angina patients were defined as patients with prolonged angina pain at rest, new onset angina, or recent destabilization of previously stable angina. Diagnosis of UA patients was conducted using (1) high-sensitive cardiac troponin T (hs-cTnT) (Elecsys Troponin T hs, and some Troponin I, Roche Diagnostics) and (2) invasive coronary angiography. Acute STEMI patients were diagnosed using ECG ST-segment changes and troponin levels. Healthy participants ($n$ = 16) underwent standard clinical physical evaluation, measured troponin levels and exercised on an ECG/treadmill stress test for 10 min to confirm absence of myocardial ischemia. The following patients were excluded from the study: patients with recent attack of AMI, positive c-reactive protein (CRP), cardiomyopathy, congenital heart disease, heart failure, renal failure, hepatitis, hepatic failure, bleeding disorders, malignancy, and autoimmune diseases, including arthritis and inflammatory bowel disease.

### 2.3. Total and miRNA Extraction and Purification

Venous blood (3 mL) was collected at zero-time from patients at presentation to the hospital ED with acute chest pain; blood was centrifuged at 1300× $g$ at 4 °C for 20 min, and the serum was immediately stored at −80 °C until analyzed. In a limited study, venous blood was also collected, centrifuged at 1300× $g$ at 4 °C for 20 min, and the plasma (EDTA) was immediately stored at −80 °C until analyzed. Total RNA and miRNAs were extracted from sera samples using the RNeasy Mini Kit (Qiagen, Hilden, Germany) according to the manufacturer's protocol, and the concentration and purity of RNA were evaluated spectrophotometrically at 260 and 280 nm, respectively. RNA integrity was visually confirmed by agarose gel electrophoresis. Using miScript RT Kit (Qiagen, Hilden, Germany), cDNA was synthesized by reverse transcription reaction.

### 2.4. Gene Amplification Analysis by Quantitative Real Time PCR (qPCR)

cDNA was amplified for miRNA, mRNA, and lncRNA expression using miScript primer assay for miRNA amplification (Hs_miR-137_1 and Hs_miR-106b-5p_1 miScript primer assay) and Quantitect primer assays for mRNAs (Hs_FTHL17_1 and Hs_ANAPC11_1_SG QuantiTect primer assays) and lncRNA ($RT^2$_CTB89H12.4 primer assay). The Hs_RNU6-2_11 and Hs_GAPDH genes were used as reference housekeeper genes. The thermal cycling was adjusted according to manufacture instructions. The PCR analysis was conducted on Rotor-Gene Q 5plex HRM Platform (Qiagen, Hilden, Germany). The fluorescence data were collected at the extension step. Following amplification, gene expression was calculated using the $2^{\Delta\Delta Ct}$ method.

### 2.5. Statistical Analysis

Statistical analysis was performed using GraphPad Prism software, version no: 8.0.2. Calculation of median and range was used for skewed data, while calculation of mean $\pm$ SD was used for normally distributed numerical data. Calculation of number of cases and percentages used cross-tabulation. The nonparametric Mann–Whitney U test was used to compare the expression of genes between two groups, and ANOVA was used to evaluate the difference in gene expression for more than two groups. The diagnostic potential of miRNAs for UA and acute STEMI was evaluated by receiver operator characteristics (ROC) analysis, then the biomarker sensitivities and specificities were calculated according to the optimum cut-off value. Significance was set at $p \leq 0.05$.

## 3. Results

### 3.1. Demographic Characteristics of Participants

The clinical characteristics of patients with UA (n = 30), patients with acute STEMI (n = 16) and 16 healthy controls are presented in Table 1.

**Table 1.** Clinical Characteristics of Patient Populations.

| Variables | ACS (n = 46) | | Healthy (n = 16) | p-Value |
|---|---|---|---|---|
| | UA (n = 30) | STEMI (n = 16) | | |
| Age (years) mean $\pm$ SD | 60.1 $\pm$ 8.1 | 54.4 $\pm$ 12.7 | 32.9 $\pm$ 9.9 | 0.001 |
| Sex: Males: n (%) | 19 (63.3) | 12 (75) | 16 (100) | 0.014 |
| Risk factors | | | | |
| BMI (kg/m$^2$) mean $\pm$ SD | 29.3 $\pm$ 7.1 | 31.4 $\pm$ 4.8 | | 0.145 |
| Smoking: n (%) | 16 (53.3) | 10 (52.5) | 26.8 $\pm$ 4.7 | 0.09 |
| Diabetes Mellitus: n (%) | 16 (53.3) | 6 (37.5) | 8 (50) | 0.001 |
| Hypertension: n (%) | 19 (63.3) | 7 (43) | | 0.001 |
| Dyslipidemia: n (%) | 12 (40) | 5 (31.3) | | 0.001 |

ASC: Acute coronary syndrome, UA: Unstable angina, STEMI: ST-segment elevated myocardial infarction, BMI: Body mass index, n: Number of cases, %: Percentage of cases calculated as percentage in the group, SD: Standard deviation, p-value > 0.05 considered statistically insignificant, and p-value < 0.05 considered statistically significant.

### 3.2. Assessment of CTB89H12.4/miR-137/FTHL-17 Network

The expression of candidate genes was verified using qPCR. For *miR-137* expression (Figure 3a), there was significant upregulation by 1382-fold ($p$ = 0.001) in UA patients compared to healthy control, while *FTHL-17* expression (Figure 3b) had a 1.7-fold increase in UA patients compared to healthy. However, the *CTB89H12.4* gene was downregulated by 20-fold in UA compared to healthy ($p = 0.0001$) and by 3.4-fold in acute STEMI compared to UA ($p = 0.001$) (Figure c) (Table ). Interestingly, comparing gene expression of *miR-137* and *FTHL-17* in UA to acute STEMI patients revealed that *miR-137* (Figure a) showed a significant increase by 2.5-fold ($p < 0.01$) in patients with STEMI compared to UA and that *FTHL-17* (Figure b) also showed a significant increase by 7.5-fold ($p < 0.0001$) in patients with acute STEMI compared to UA. Additionally, the expression pattern for miR-137 in UA and acute STEMI patients was plotted in an XY graph to illustrate the marked elevated expression levels in UA and STEMI patients compared to the observed minimal expression in healthy controls (Figure f).

Table 2. Gene Expression Profiles in Patients with UA versus Healthy, as well as Patients with UA versus Acute STEMI.

| Genes | Median Expression Level ($\log_{10}$) | | | Statistics FC (*p*-Value) | |
|---|---|---|---|---|---|
| | Healthy | UA | STEMI | UA/Healthy | STEMI/UA |
| *miR-137* ($\log_{10}$) | 0.9 | 1244 | 3163 | 1382 (<0.0001) | 2.5 (<0.001) |
| *FTHL-17* ($\log_{10}$) | 3.76 | 6.6 | 50.4 | 1.7 (<0.0001) | 7.5 (<0.0001) |
| *miR-106b-5p* ($\log_{10}$) | 1.08 | 207 | 953 | 192 (<0.001) | 4.6 (<0.001) |
| *ANAPC11* ($\log_{10}$) | 0.86 | 7.36 | 8.39 | 8.5 (<0.0001) | 1.1 (>0.05) |
| *CTB89H12.4* ($\log_{10}$) | 65.3 | 3.27 | 0.94 | 20 (<0.0001) | 3.4 (<0.001) |

UA: Unstable angina, STEMI: ST-segment elevated myocardial infarction, FC: Fold change, *FTHL-17*, ferritin heavy chain like 17, *ANAPC11*: Anaphase promoting complex subunit, *p*-value > 0.05 considered statistically insignificant, and *p*-value < 0.05 considered statistically significant.

Furthermore, an ROC curve analysis was conducted to evaluate the reliability of miR-137 as a diagnostic biomarker for UA and STEMI patients. Comparing UA to healthy controls, the calculated cut-off value was 195.4 (Figure a). The *miR-137* biomarker sensitivity and specificity were 97% and 94%, respectively, to discriminate UA from healthy controls (area under the curve (AUC): 0.99, Youden's index: 0.91, *J* value = 195.4). Additionally, at an optimum cut-off value of 2488, miR-137 expression level could potentially discriminate UA from patients with acute STEMI (AUC: 0.84, Youden's index: 0.58, *J* value = 157) (Figure b) with sensitivity of 75% and specificity of 83%.

*3.3. Assessment of CTB89H12.4/miR-106b-5p/ANAPC11 Network*

Serum *miR-106b-5p* gene expression was associated with myocardial ischemia, where *miR-106b-5p* (Figure d) and ANAPC11 (Figure e) were significantly ($p = 0.001$) upregulated by 192-fold and 8.5-fold in UA patients compared to healthy subjects, respectively. Comparing gene expression in UA with STEMI patients, *miR-106b-5p* (Figure d) expression was significantly increased by 4.6-fold ($p < 0.001$) in patients with acute STEMI compared to UA, but there was no statistically significant difference in *ANAPC11* gene expression between UA and STEMI (Figure e). The *CTB89H12.4* gene was downregulated by 20-fold in UA compared to healthy ($p = 0.0001$) and by 3.4-fold in STEMI compared to UA ($p = 0.001$) (Figure c) (Table ). In addition, the expression pattern for *miR-106b-5p* in UA and STEMI patients was plotted in an XY graph to illustrate the sizable difference in expression level in UA and STEMI compared to the observed minimal expression in healthy controls (Figure g). The diagnostic potential of *miR-106b-5p* was assessed and the ROC analysis revealed that *miR-106b-5p* is a reliable biomarker for UA and STEMI. The calculated biomarker sensitivities and specificities were 87% and 88%, respectively, to discriminate UA from healthy controls; the optimum cut-off value was 90.4 (AUC: 0.9, Youden's index: 0.75, *J* value: 157) (Figure a). To discriminate UA from STEMI patients (Figure b), results indicated that at a cut-off value of 385.0 (AUC: 0.95, Youden's index: 0.76, *J* value: 175), the diagnostic sensitivity was 86% and specificity was 90%.

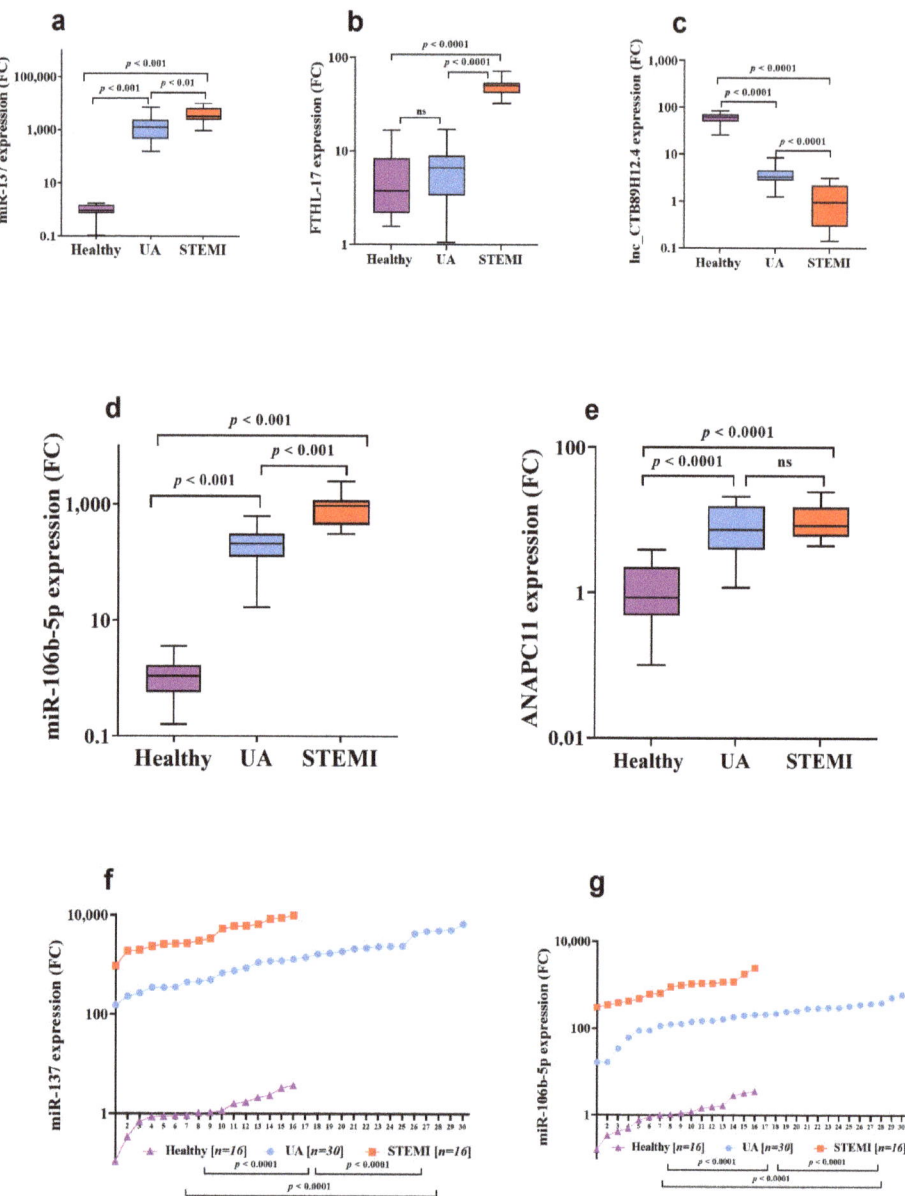

**Figure 3.** Expression profiles of candidate miRNAs in patients with UA and acute STEMI in comparison to healthy controls. The two candidate miRNAs, *miR-137* and *miR-106b-5p*, were measured with qRT-PCR using 62 serum samples, including 16 Healthy (non-ACS) as well as 30 UA and 16 STEMI patients (ACS samples). *miR-137* (**a**) and *miR-106b-5p* (**d**) were significantly upregulated in the UA and STEMI groups compared to Healthy (**a**,**d**). In addition, similar upregulation was observed for the associated mRNA targets *FTHL-17* (**b**) and *ANAPC11* (**e**), while the *lnc-CTB89H12.4* regulating gene was significantly decreased in UA and STEMI patients (**c**). (**f**,**g**) demonstrate the expression pattern of *miR-137* and *miR-106b-5p* in the three studied groups (UA, STEMI and Healthy). Abbreviation: ns: no significant difference.

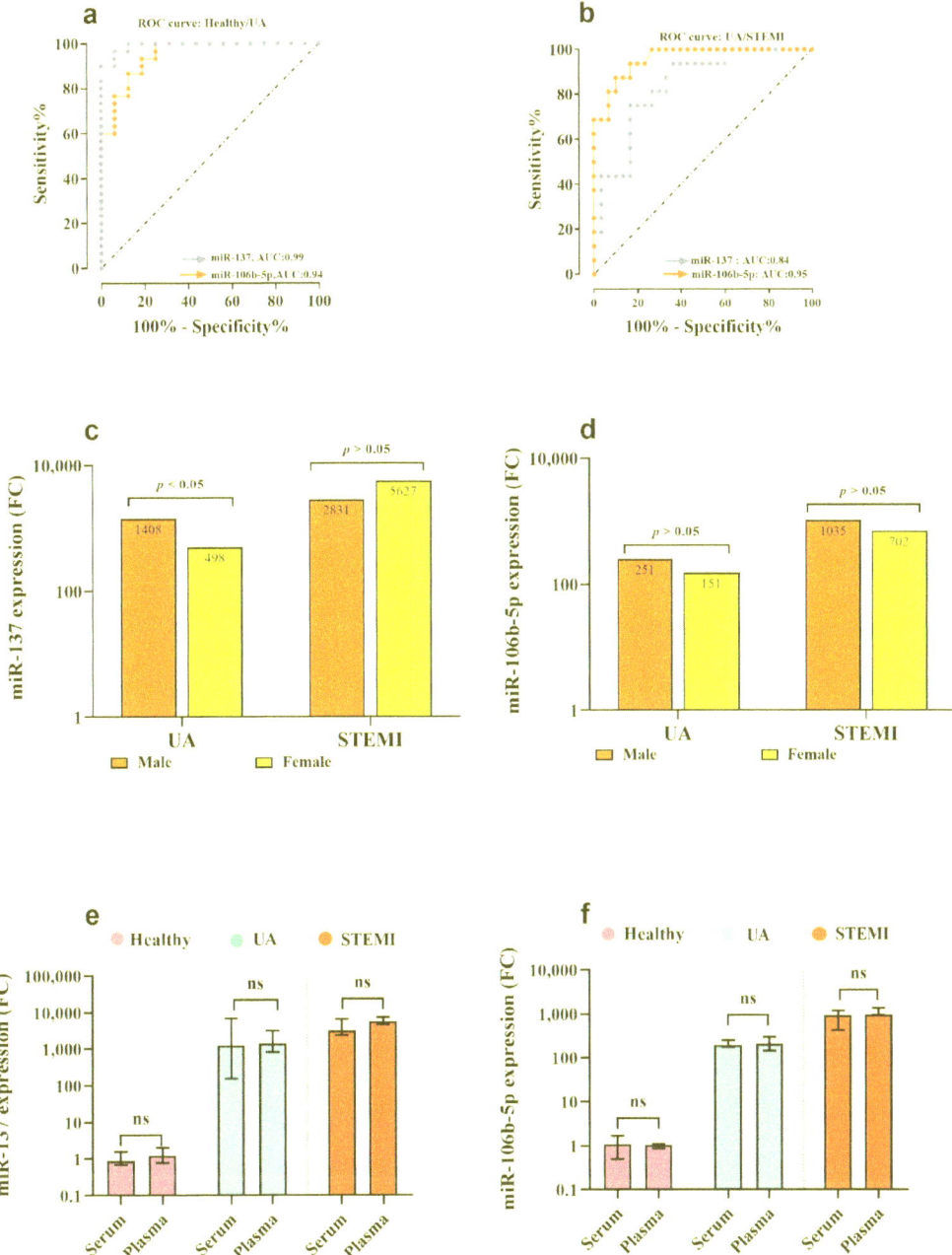

**Figure 4.** Receiver operator characteristics (ROC) curve illustrating the diagnostic value of the two miRNAs (*miR-137* and *miR-106b-5p*) in discriminating UA from Healthy (**a**) and UA from STEMI (**b**). (**c**,**d**) show the nonsignificant association of miR-106b-5p expression level between genders in UA and AMI patients, respectively. Finally, the serum and plasma expression levels for *miR-137* (**e**) and *miR-106b-5p* (**f**) were compared, and results indicate no significant difference was reached. Abbreviations: UA: unstable angina, STEMI: ST-elevation myocardial infarction, AUC: area under the curve, $p$-value > 0.05 considered statistically insignificant, and $p$-value < 0.05 considered statistically significant.

There was no gender difference in *miR-137* (Figure 4c) and *miR-106b-5p* (Figure 4d) gene expression level in STEMI patients ($p > 0.05$). However, there was higher expression of *miR-137* in males UA compared to females ($p < 0.05$) (Figure 4c) but no gender difference in *miR-106b-5p* gene expression in UA patients (Figure 4d). Additionally, in a limited study ($n = 4$ for each group), the gene expression levels of *miR-137* and *miR-106b-5p* were measured in plasma samples and compared to their levels in serum samples. There was no significant difference ($p > 0.05$) in *miR-137* (Figure 4e) and *miR-106b-5p* (Figure 4f) gene expression detected between serum and plasma samples collected from UA, STEMI, and healthy.

Troponin analysis indicated that during serial sampling at the 0/3 h, 67% of UA patients had hs-cTnT levels consistently below the 99th percentile value (14 ng/L), while only 33% of patients showed low-to-mild elevation of hs-cTnT levels above the 99th percentile values within the range of 15 ng/L to 51 ng/L but without significant delta change in serial samples. Unstable angina was further confirmed by invasive coronary angiography, where more than 50% of UA patients had coronary artery stenosis. Contrary to the limited elevation of hs-cTnT levels of <1 to 3-fold over the cutoff of 14 ng/L in only 33% of UA patients, Nourin miRNAs were markedly elevated in 100% of UA patients, with a significant increase of 1382-fold for *miR-137* and 192-fold for *miR-106b-5p* over baseline gene expression levels in healthy subjects. For acute STEMI patients, myocardial infarction was confirmed by persistent ST-segment changes and significant high elevation of hs-cTnT in all patients, similar to the marked elevation of Nourin miRNAs in the same 16 STEMI patients compared to healthy (1535-fold increase for *miR-137* and 177-fold for *miR-106b-5p*). Healthy participants represented the negative control group, and their troponin levels were below the clinical decision limit and showed negative ECG/treadmill stress tests, indicative of absence of myocardial ischemia. Healthy subjects also showed minimum gene expression of Nourin miRNAs.

### 3.4. Correlation between lncRNA/miRNA/mRNA Genes in Acute Coronary Syndrome (ACS) Patients

Since there was no significant association detected between the expression of *miR-137*, *FTHL-17*, and *CTB89H12.4*, as well as for *miR-106b-5p*, *ANAPC11*, and *CTB89H12.4* genes for UA or patients with STEMI, we combined the two groups (UA and acute STEMI) into one group called ACS group, and then a Spearman's analysis was conducted between the two paired genes in each network. Results revealed a positive significant correlation between *miR-137* and *FTHL-17* ($r$: 0.5, 95% CI: 0.2–0.7, $p = 0.001$) and between *miR-106b-5p* and *ANAPC11* ($r$: 0.4, 95% CI: 0.4–0.6, $p = 0.02$) genes in ACS patients. In contrary, *CTB89H12.4* showed a significant negative correlation with either *FTHL-17* or *ANAPC11*. Lower expression levels of *CTB89H12.4* were significantly associated with higher expression levels of *FTHL-17* and *ANAPC11* in ACS patients ($p < 0.01$).

In summary, Nourin *miR-137* (marker of cell damage) and *miR-106b-5p* (marker of inflammation) gene expression measured in serum samples collected from patients with acute chest pain at presentation to the hospital ED, could (1) detect unstable angina patients with chest pain secondary to reversible myocardial ischemia and confirmed by invasive coronary angiography to have greater than 50% coronary artery stenosis and troponin level below the clinical decision, and (2) detect acute STEMI patients with chest pain secondary to irreversible myocardial ischemia (necrosis) and confirmed by persistent ST-segment changes and elevated troponin level. Additionally, both biomarkers showed consistent elevation of Nourin *miR-137* and *miR-106b* gene expression in all 30 UA patients and 16 acute STEMI patients. Therefore, Figure 2 presents an underlying molecular mechanism associated with the Nourin protein and its RNA molecular network in UA and acute STEMI patients. The downregulation of *CTB89H12.4* after myocardial ischemia results in an increase in the expression of miR-137 and miR-106b-5p, which sequentially activates the *FTHL-17* and *ANAPC11*, respectively, with an increased translation and production of Nourin protein. Results also support the ontology bioinformatics evidence that *CTB89H12.4/miR-137/FTHL-17* and *CTB89H12.4/miR-106b-5p/ANAPC11* networks synergistically regulate the Nourin protein expression in myocardial ischemia, and thus provide a novel molecular mechanism in ischemic heart disease.

## 4. Discussion

Acute coronary syndrome is a life threatening condition owing to high morbidity and mortality worldwide, due partially to the lack of early blood-based biomarkers that can diagnose reversible myocardial ischemia before progressing to necrosis, and thus can guide treatment decisions [ ]. Although high sensitivity troponin represents the gold standard cardiac specific biomarker [ ], the major limitation is its inability to diagnose unstable angina patients [ ], and its low specificity in differentiating ACS patients from other nonischemic clinical emergency syndromes, such as acute myocarditis, heart failure without CAD, stress-induced cardiomyopathy, and pulmonary embolism [ ]. Accordingly, there is an ultimate need to identify novel early and sensitive biomarkers to specifically diagnose unstable angina patients and assist in their therapeutic approaches.

Nourin is a novel blood biomarker with a known mode of action as an early potent inflammatory mediator released within 5 min by ischemic myocardial tissue and it is associated with the initiation and amplification of post-ischemic cardiac inflammation [ – ]. Clinically high levels of Nourin were detected in ACS and AMI patients, but not in symptomatic noncardiac patients and healthy subjects [ ], suggesting a potential use of the Nourin biomarker to rule out myocardial ischemia for symptomatic patients having noncardiac causes. Recently, aberrant miRNAs have been reported to play a role in the pathogenesis of cardiovascular diseases, and they are involved in vascular dysfunction, apoptosis, autophagy, inflammation, and angiogenesis [ , , – ]. In the present study, we applied a bioinformatics analysis to elucidate the underlying molecular mechanism associated with Nourin protein, and accordingly, the topological characteristics between Nourin protein sequence and miRNAs-mediated interactions network associated with myocardial ischemia were retrieved. The two networks, *CTB89H12.4/miR-137/FTHL-17* and *CTB89H12.4/miR-106b-5p/ANAPC11*, were selected based on novelty, their direct interaction with Nourin protein, as well as association with myocardial ischemia. Both networks showed high tendency to interact with each other through sharing in the lncRNA *CTB89H12.4*. Standard qPCR was used in order to evaluate the diagnostic efficacy of Nourin-dependent miRNAs (*miR-137* as a marker of cell damage and *miR-106b-5p* as a marker of inflammation) for ruling in patients with UA when troponin level was below the clinical decision limit for diagnosis and patients had greater than 50% coronary artery stenosis by invasive coronary angiography. Gene expression profiles of circulating *miR-137* and *miR-106b-5p* and the association with their target genes *FTHL-17*, *ANAPC11*, and *CTB89H112.4* were investigated in patients with UA ($n = 30$), acute STEMI ($n = 16$) and healthy subjects ($n = 16$). Results indicate that *miR-137* and *miR-106b-5p* were significantly upregulated in UA and acute STEMI patients compared to healthy controls and that both miRNAs can diagnose symptomatic UA patients with high sensitivity and specificity, as well as stratify severity of myocardial ischemia with higher expression in acute STEMI compared to UA. Furthermore, the significant association of *miR-137* and *miR-106b-5p* with their regulatory target genes *FTHL-17*, *ANAPC11*, and *CTB89H12.4* supported the bioinformatics data and outlined a novel underlying mechanistic signaling pathway in myocardial ischemic injury. However, the small sample size reflects the limitation of the study and, thus, a large-scale sample size study is needed with focus on the Nourin underlying mechanistic pathways as novel cardiac biomarkers.

Recent evidence has demonstrated that *miR-137* is a hypoxia-responsive gene overexpressed in ischemic-cell injury [ ]. Moreover, recent studies have reported that downregulation of *miR-137* inhibits oxidative stress-induced cardiomyocytes apoptosis by targeting the *KLF15* gene [ ] and protects cells against ischemia-induced apoptosis through *CDC42* [ , ]. On the other hand, high expression levels of *miR-137* have been observed in dexamethasone-treated multiple myeloma cells by targeting *MCL-1* and *MITF* genes [ , ], thus inhibiting cancer cell proliferation and inducing apoptosis [ , ]. These findings suggest a regulatory mechanistic pathway of *miR-137* in ischemia-induced cell injury, which has been investigated in neural cells on wide scale [22]. Recently, the therapeutic value of *miR-137* has been reported in hypoxia-induced retinal diseases, through targeting the Notch1 signaling pathway [41].

In addition to the reported inflammatory mechanism of *miR-106b-5p* in myocardial tissue, it was described as a hypoxia-associated miRNA in myocardial infarction [27], as well as various human cancers [42,43]. MiR-106b-5p exerts cell degradation through a lysosomal-dependent mechanism. Upregulation of *miR-106b-5p* has been demonstrated in myocardial tissue with dilated cardiomyopathy in which the autophagy mechanism is mediated through the *miR-106b-5p/FYCO1*-dependent pathway [44]. Additionally, *miR-106b-5p* was found to be the most significant miRNA in 746 altered miRNAs in atherosclerotic vascular diseases; it targets multiple inflammatory signaling pathways including PI3K, Akt, mTOR, TGF-β, TNF, TLR, and HIF-1α [44]. In vitro experimental studies have reported its biological role in cholesterol homeostasis [45] and spermatogenesis [46]. The regulatory role of *miR-106b-5p* in cardiomyocytes apoptosis has been investigated to illustrate the underlying signaling pathway in myocardial infarction [27]. Recent evidence suggested that suppression of *miR-106b-5p* promotes hypoxia-induced cell apoptosis, an observation that explains the early increase in its serum level in response to ischemia-induced myocardial injury. As miRNAs are tissue specific, a previous study suggested that p21 is the direct target of *miR-106b-5p* in cardiomyocytes that mediate an anti-apoptotic effect under hypoxic conditions [27]. It has been established that *miR-137* and *miR-106b* are strongly linked to the pathogenesis of atherosclerosis [47]. Recently, *miR-137* was shown to directly suppress the insulin-like growth factor-binding protein 5 (IGFBP-5), which further suppresses cell proliferation and migration of vascular smooth muscle cells (VSMCs) [48]. Additionally, overexpression of *miR-137* in VSMCs suppresses the activity of mTOR/STAT3 signaling, and *miR-106b* modulates angiogenesis in vascular endothelial cells by targeting STAT3 [49].

As reported here, a significant positive correlation was detected in UA and acute STEMI patients between *miR-137* and *FTHL-17*, as well as between *miR-106b-5p* and *ANAPC11*. However, a significant negative correlation was detected between the two miRNAs (*miR-137* and *miR-106b-5p*) and *lnc-CTB89H12.4*. In the context of identifying new cardiac diagnostic biomarkers with high sensitivity and specificity, it is more beneficial to use a network of functionally linked biomarkers such as the Nourin RNA molecular network rather than depending on a single biomarker. Specifically, the Nourin-dependent *FTHL-17* gene is a novel type of ferritin gene, located on X chromosome. It encodes for ferritin-like protein but without ferroxidase activity. The partial nuclear localization of *FTHL-17* suggests its specific biological functions apart from iron storage regulation [50]. Similarly, the Nourin-dependent *ANAPC11* genes are a complex of subunits that promote cell cycle progression and induce G1 arrest through ubiquitination-mediated cell destruction and have two novel insights, including protein degradation and epigenetic regulation [51]. Based on gene database records, the two genes (*FTHL-17* and *ANAPC11*) and their miRNAs regulators (*miR-137* and *miR-106b-5p*) are highly expressed in cardiomyocytes and skeletal muscles, which strongly support their symbiotic interaction. Additionally, the role of *lnc-CTB89H12.4*, also called *lncRNA-RP11-175K6.1*, has been reported in atherosclerosis and angiogenesis, which highlights its strong association with angiogenesis and cardiomyocytes [52,53].

The study has points of strength and some limitations. The relatively small sample size of patients at zero time, as well as the limited baseline miRNA measurements, represent the first limiting point. The second point is that despite the increased quality of the study design by accurate diagnosis of patients through elective coronary angiography, the study population does not represent the general population, since all cardiac patients were enrolled from a single hospital, Kasr-Alainy Hospital. In addition, we used a combination of two Nourin-dependent miRNAs biomarkers measured with highly sensitive PCR technique, which enabled us to avoid bias created by a raised number of false positive results. Finally, the study showed restricted interpretation of results due to lack of long-term follow-up and correlation with severity of myocardial injury.

## 5. Conclusions

Despite availability of high-sensitivity cardiac troponin, there is a need for new biomarkers with high diagnostic sensitivity and specificity for the detection of myocardial ischemia in suspected ACS patients with troponin levels below the clinical decision limit. We showed that the Nourin-dependent *miR-137* and *miR-106b-5p* are a novel promising rule-in test that can (1) diagnose unstable angina among patients presenting to hospital EDs with acute chest pain, and (2) stratify severity of myocardial ischemia, with higher expression in acute STEMI compared to UA patients. The diagnostic potential of *miR-137* and *miR-106b-5p* indicated that both miRNAs are reliable biomarkers for UA and acute STEMI patients. Finally, early diagnosis of suspected unstable angina patients using the novel Nourin biomarkers is key for initiating guideline-based therapy that improves patients' health outcomes.

**Author Contributions:** Study design and plan was prepared by S.A.E. All authors contributed to material preparation, data collection, and analysis. The first draft of the manuscript was written by N.E.-K. and S.A.E., and all authors commented on previous versions of the manuscript. All authors have read and agreed to the published version of the manuscript.

**Funding:** This study was supported by Nour Heart, Inc., Vienna, Virginia and Cell and Molecular Tissue Engineering LLC, Avon, Connecticut.

**Institutional Review Board Statement:** The study was conducted according to the guidelines of the Declaration of Helsinki, and approved by the Research Ethics Committee, Faculty of Medicine, Cairo University, Egypt, dated 12/10/2019.

**Informed Consent Statement:** Informed consent was obtained from all subjects involved in the study.

**Data Availability Statement:** The data presented in this study are available on request from the corresponding author. The data presented in this study are available on request from the corresponding author. The data are not publicly due to privacy.

**Conflicts of Interest:** S.A.E. is the founder of Nour Heart, Inc. R.H.C. reports receiving a research grant from Spingotech Diagnostics, Roche Diagnostics, Siemens Diagnostics, Becton Dickinson. U.K. and D.L.K. are founders of Cell and Molecular Tissue Engineering, LLC. The other authors have no conflicts of interest to disclose.

## Abbreviations

| | |
|---|---|
| UA | unstable angina |
| STEMI | ST-elevation myocardial infarction |
| ACS | acute coronary syndrome |
| CAD | coronary artery disease |
| ED | emergency department |
| FTHL-17 | ferritin heavy chain like 17 |
| ANAPC11 | anaphase promoting complex subunit |
| CTB89H12.4 | lncRNA-CTB89H12.4 |
| PI3K | phosphatidylinositol-3 kinase |
| Akt | protein kinase B (PKB) |
| mTOR | mammalian target of rapamycin |
| Jak-STAT | janus kinase/signal transducer and activator of transcription |
| NGS | next-generation sequencing |
| TNF-$\alpha$ | tumor necrosis factor-$\alpha$ |
| IL-1$\beta$ | interleukin 1$\beta$ |
| IL-8 | interleukin 8 |
| LECAM-1 | leukocyte-endothelial cell adhesion molecule 1 |
| ICAM-1 | intercellular adhesion molecule 1 |

| | |
|---|---|
| ELAM-1 | endothelial-leukocyte adhesion molecule 1 |
| FPR | formyl peptide receptor |
| CRP | c-reactive protein |
| TLR | toll-like receptor |
| HIF-1α | hypoxia-inducible factor-1α |
| ROC | receiver operator characteristics |
| AUC | area under the curve |
| VECs | vascular endothelial cells |
| DEGs | different expressed genes |
| GO | gene ontology |
| KEGG | Kyoto Encyclopedia of Genes and Genomes |
| PPI | protein–protein Interaction |
| ATP | adenosine triphosphate |

## References

1. Kaski, J.C.; Crea, F.; Gersh, B.J.; Camic, P.G.i. Reappraisal of Ischemic Heart Disease: Fundamental Role of Coronary Microvascular Dysfunction in the Pathogenesis of Angina Pectoris. *Circulation* **2018**, *138*, 1463–1480. [CrossRef] [PubMed]
2. Collet, J.-P.; Thiele, H.; Barbato, E.; Barthélémy, O.; Bauersachs, J.; Bhatt, D.L.; Dendale, P.; Dorobantu, M.; Edvardsen, T.; Folliguet, T.; et al. 2020 ESC Guidelines for the management of acute coronary syndromes in patients presenting without persistent ST-segment elevationThe Task Force for the management of acute coronary syndromes in patients presenting without persistent ST-segment elevation of the European Society of Cardiology (ESC). *Eur. Heart J.* **2020**, 1–79. [CrossRef]
3. Jakimov, T.; Mrdović, I.; Filipović, B.; Zdravković, M.; Djoković, A.; Hinić, S.; Milić, N.; Filipović, B. Comparison of RISK-PCI, GRACE, TIMI risk scores for prediction of major adverse cardiac events in patients with acute coronary syndrome. *Croat. Med. J.* **2017**, *58*, 406–415. [CrossRef]
4. Yan, A.T.; Yan, R.T.; Tan, M.; Casanova, A.; Labinaz, M.; Sridhar, K.; Fitchett, D.H.; Langer, A.; Goodman, S.G. Risk scores for risk stratification in acute coronary syndromes: Useful but simpler is not necessarily better. *Eur. Heart J.* **2007**, *28*, 1072–1078. [CrossRef] [PubMed]
5. Singh, T.; Bing, R.; Dweck, M.R.; van Beek, E.J.R.; Mills, N.L.; Williams, M.C.; Villines, T.C.; Newby, D.E.; Adamson, P.D. Exercise Electrocardiography and Computed Tomography Coronary Angiography for Patients With Suspected Stable Angina Pectoris: A Post Hoc Analysis of the Randomized SCOT-HEART Trial. *JAMA Cardiol.* **2020**, *5*, 920–928. [CrossRef] [PubMed]
6. BreweR, L.C.; Svatikova, A.; Mulvagh, S.L. The Challenges of Prevention, Diagnosis and Treatment of Ischemic Heart Disease in Women. *Cardiovasc. Drugs Ther.* **2015**, *29*, 355–368. [CrossRef]
7. Parsonage, W.A.; Cullen, L.; Younger, J.F. The approach to patients with possible cardiac chest pain. *Med. J. Aust.* **2013**, *199*, 30–34. [CrossRef]
8. Aydin, S.; Ugur, K.; Aydin, S.; Sahin, I.; Yardim, M. Biomarkers in acute myocardial infarction: Current perspectives. *Vasc. Health Risk Manag.* **2019**, *15*, 1–10. [CrossRef]
9. Cavarretta, E.; Frati, G. MicroRNAs in Coronary Heart Disease: Ready to Enter the Clinical Arena? *Biomed Res. Int.* **2016**, *2016*, 2150763. [CrossRef]
10. Elgebaly, S.A.; Poston, R.; Todd, R.; Helmy, T.; Almaghraby, A.M.; Elbayoumi, T.; Kreutzer, D.L. Cyclocreatine protects against ischemic injury and enhances cardiac recovery during early reperfusion. *Expert Rev. Cardiovasc. Ther.* **2019**, *17*, 683–697. [CrossRef]
11. Elgebaly, S.A.; Hashmi, F.H.; Houser, S.L.; Allam, M.E.; Doyle, K. Cardiac-derived neutrophil chemotactic factors: Detection in coronary sinus effluents of patients undergoing myocardial revascularization. *J. Thorac. Cardiovasc. Surg.* **1992**, *103*, 952–959. [CrossRef]
12. Elgebaly, S.A.; Masetti, P.; Allam, M.; Forouhar, F. Cardiac derived neutrophil chemotactic factors; preliminary biochemical characterization. *J. Mol. Cell. Cardiol.* **1989**, *21*, 585–593. [CrossRef]
13. Elgebaly, S.A.; van Buren, C.; Todd, R.; Poston, R.; Rabie, M.A.; Mohamed, A.F.; Ahmed, L.A.; El Sayed, N.S. Cyclocreatine Phosphate: A Novel Mechanism for Preventing Development of Heart Failure. *Circulation* **2020**, *142* (Suppl. 3), A13311.
14. Elgebaly, S.A.; Christenson, R.H.; Kandil, H.; El-Khazragy, N.; Rashed, L.; Yacoub, B.; Sharafieh, R.; Klue, U.; Kreutzer, D.L. Nourin-dependent Mirna-137: A Novel Early Diagnostic Biomarker for Unstable Angina Patients. *Circulation* **2020**, *142* (Suppl. 3), A13051. [CrossRef]
15. Elgebaly, S.A.; Christenson, R.H.; Kandil, H.; Elkhazragy, N.; Rashed, L.; Yacou, B.; Sharafieh, R.; Klueh, U.; Kreutzer, D.L. Nourin-dependent Mirna-106b: A Novel Early Inflammatory Diagnostic Biomarker for Cardiac Injury. *Circulation* **2020**, *142* (Suppl. 3), A13103. [CrossRef]
16. Ozeren, A.; Aydin, M.; Tokac, M.; Demircan, N.; Unalacak, M.; Gurel, A.; Yazici, M. Levels of serum IL-1beta, IL-2, IL-8 and tumor necrosis factor-alpha in patients with unstable angina pectoris. *Mediat. Inflamm.* **2003**, *12*, 361–365. [CrossRef]
17. Elgebaly, S.; Christenson, R.; Schiffmann, E.; Yi, Q.; Kreutzer, D. Early identification of cardiac ischemia patients in the emergency department. *Catheter. Cardiovasc. Interv.* **2013**, *81* (Suppl. 1), S2–S3.
18. Cordeddu, L.; Pilbrow, A.P.; Cameron, V.A.; Troughton, R.W.; Richards, M.A.; Foo, R.S. Circulating miRNAs as Biomarkers in Acute Coronary Syndrome. *Circ. Res.* **2012**, *111*, A290. [CrossRef]

19. Elbaz, M.; Faccini, J.; Laperche, C.; Grousset, E.; Roncalli, J.; Ruidavets, J.B.; Vindis, C. Identification of a miRNA Based-Signature Associatetd with Acute Coronary Syndrome: Evidence from the FLORINF Study. *J. Clin. Med.* **2020**, *9*, 1674. [CrossRef]
20. Gacoń, J.; Kabłak-Ziembicka, A.; Stępień, E.; Enguita, F.J.; Karch, I.; Derlaga, B.; Żmudka, K.; Przewłocki, T. Decision-making microRNAs (miR-124,-133a/b,-34a and -134) in patients with occluded target vessel in acute coronary syndrome. *Kardiol. Pol.* **2016**, *74*, 280–288.
21. Wang, A.; Kwee, L.C.; Grass, E.; Neely, M.L.; Gregory, S.G.; Fox, K.A.A.; Armstrong, P.W.; White, H.D.; Ohman, E.M.; Roe, M.T.; et al. Whole blood sequencing reveals circulating microRNA associations with high-risk traits in non-ST-segment elevation acute coronary syndrome. *Atherosclerosis* **2017**, *261*, 19–25. [CrossRef]
22. Zhang, M.; Ge, D.J.; Su, Z.; Qi, B. miR-137 alleviates focal cerebral ischemic injury in rats by regulating JAK1/STAT1 signaling pathway. *Hum. Exp. Toxicol.* **2020**, *39*, 816–827. [CrossRef]
23. Suzuki, T.; Toba, K.; Kato, K.; Ozawa, T.; Higasimura, M.; Kitajima, T.; Oda, H.; Tsuchida, K.; Tomosugi, N.; Saitoh, H.; et al. Serum ferritin levels adversely affect cardiac function in patients with ST-elevation myocardial infarction who underwent successful percutaneous coronary intervention. *Int. J. Cardiol.* **2013**, *167*, 286–288. [CrossRef]
24. Li, H.; Zhu, Z.; Liu, J.; Wang, J.; Qu, C. MicroRNA-137 regulates hypoxia-induced retinal ganglion cell apoptosis through Notch1. *Int. J. Mol. Med.* **2018**, *41*, 1774–1782. [CrossRef]
25. Gorabi, A.M.; Kiaie, N.; Sathyapalan, T.; Al-Rasadi, K.; Jamialahmadi, T.; Sahebkar, A. The Role of MicroRNAs in Regulating Cytokines and Growth Factors in Coronary Artery Disease: The Ins and Outs. *J. Immunol. Res.* **2020**, *2020*, 5193036. [CrossRef]
26. Bostjancic EGlavac, D. miRNome in myocardial infarction: Future directions and perspective. *World J. Cardiol.* **2014**, *6*, 939–958. [CrossRef] [PubMed]
27. Liu, Z.; Yang, D.; Xie, P.; Ren, G.; Sun, G.; Zeng, X.; Sun, X. MiR-106b and MiR-15b modulate apoptosis and angiogenesis in myocardial infarction. *Cell. Physiol. Biochem.* **2012**, *29*, 851–862. [CrossRef]
28. Li, J.; Fan, G. Identification of key genes and pathways in obstructive coronary artery disease by integrated analysis. *J. Xiangya Med.* **2020**, *5*, 14. [CrossRef]
29. Park, K.C.; Gaze, D.C.; Collinson, P.O.; Marber, M.S. Cardiac troponins: From myocardial infarction to chronic disease. *Cardiovasc. Res.* **2017**, *113*, 1708–1718. [CrossRef] [PubMed]
30. Neumann, J.T.; Sörensen, N.A.; Ojeda, F.; Renné, T.; Schnabel, R.B.; Zeller, T.; Karakas, M.; Blankenberg, S.; Westermann, D. Early diagnosis of acute myocardial infarction using high-sensitivity troponin I. *PLoS ONE* **2017**, *12*, e0174288. [CrossRef]
31. Pleister, A.; Selemon, H.; Elton, S.M.; Elton, T.S. Circulating miRNAs: Novel biomarkers of acute coronary syndrome? *Biomark. Med.* **2013**, *7*, 287–305. [CrossRef]
32. Barraclough, J.Y.; Joglekar, M.V.; Januszewski, A.S.; Martínez, G.; Celermajer, D.S.; Keech, A.C.; Hardikar, A.A.; Patel, S. A MicroRNA Signature in Acute Coronary Syndrome Patients and Modulation by Colchicine. *J. Cardiovasc. Pharmacol. Ther.* **2020**, *25*, 444–455. [CrossRef]
33. Oerlemans, M.I.F.J.; Mosterd, A.; Dekker, M.S.; de Very, E.A.; van Mil, A.; Pasterkamp, G.; Doevendans, P.A.; Hoes, A.W.; Sluijter, J.P.G. Early assessment of acute coronary syndromes in the emergency department: The potential diagnostic value of circulating microRNAs. *EMBO Mol. Med.* **2012**, *4*, 1176–1185. [CrossRef]
34. Zhao, T.; Qiu, Z.; Gao, Y. MiR-137-3p exacerbates the ischemia-reperfusion injured cardiomyocyte apoptosis by targeting KLF15. *Naunyn-Schmiedeberg's Arch. Pharmacol.* **2020**, *393*, 1013–1024. [CrossRef]
35. Wang, J.; Xu, R.; Wu, J.; Li, Z. MicroRNA-137 Negatively Regulates H$_2$O$_2$-Induced Cardiomyocyte Apoptosis Through CDC42. *Med. Sci. Monit.* **2015**, *21*, 3498–3504. [CrossRef] [PubMed]
36. Li, J.; Li, J.; Wei, T.; Li, J. Down-Regulation of MicroRNA-137 Improves High Glucose-Induced Oxidative Stress Injury in Human Umbilical Vein Endothelial Cells by Up-Regulation of AMPKalpha1. *Cell. Physiol. Biochem.* **2016**, *39*, 847–859. [CrossRef]
37. Yang, Y.; Li, F.; Saha, M.N.; Abdi, J.; Qiu, L.; Chang, H. miR-137 and miR-197 Induce Apoptosis and Suppress Tumorigenicity by Targeting MCL-1 in Multiple Myeloma. *Clin. Cancer Res.* **2015**, *21*, 2399–2411. [CrossRef]
38. Zhang, B.; Ma, L.; Wei, J.; Hu, J.; Zhao, Z.; Wang, Y.; Chen, Y.; Zhao, F. miR-137 Suppresses the Phosphorylation of AKT and Improves the Dexamethasone Sensitivity in Multiple Myeloma Cells Via Targeting MITF. *Curr. Cancer Drug Targets* **2016**, *16*, 807–817. [CrossRef] [PubMed]
39. Hao, N.-B.; He, Y.-F.; Li, X.-Q.; Wang, K.; Wang, R.-L. The role of miRNA and lncRNA in gastric cancer. *Oncotarget* **2017**, *8*, 81572–81582. [CrossRef] [PubMed]
40. Wang, Y.; Chen, R.; Zhou, X.; Guo, R.; Yin, J.; Li, Y.; Ma, G. miR-137: A Novel Therapeutic Target for Human Glioma. *Mol. Ther. Nucleic Acids* **2020**, *21*, 614–622. [CrossRef] [PubMed]
41. Yu, B.; Song, B. Notch 1 signalling inhibits cardiomyocyte apoptosis in ischaemic postconditioning. *Heart Lung Circ.* **2014**, *23*, 152–158. [CrossRef]
42. Guarnieri, A.L.; Towers, C.G.; Drasin, D.J.; Oliphant, M.U.J.; Andrysik, Z.; Hotz, T.J.; Vartuli, R.L.; Linklater, E.S.; Pandey, A.; Khana, S.L.; et al. The miR-106b-25 cluster mediates breast tumor initiation through activation of NOTCH1 via direct repression of NEDD4L. *Oncogene* **2018**, *37*, 3879–3893. [CrossRef] [PubMed]
43. Wang, Y.-X.; Lang, F.; Liu, Y.-X.; Yang, C.-Q.; Gao, H.-J. In situ hybridization analysis of the expression of miR-106b in colonic cancer. *Int. J. Clin. Exp. Pathol.* **2015**, *8*, 786–792. [PubMed]
44. Zhang, J.; Li, S.F.; Chen, H.; Song, J.X. Role of miR-106b-5p in the regulation of gene profiles in endothelial cells. *Beijing Da Xue Xue Bao Yi Xue Ban* **2019**, *51*, 221–227. [PubMed]

45. Kim, J.; Yoon, H.; Ramírez, C.M.; Lee, S.M.; Hoe, H.S.; Fernández-Hernando, C.; Kim, J. MiR-106b impairs cholesterol efflux and increases Aβ levels by repressing ABCA1 expression. *Exp. Neurol.* **2012**, *235*, 476–483. [CrossRef] [PubMed]
46. Tong, M.H.; Mitchell, D.A.; McGowan, S.D.; Evanoff, R.; Griswold, M.D. Two miRNA clusters, Mir-17-92 (Mirc1) and Mir-106b-25 (Mirc3), are involved in the regulation of spermatogonial differentiation in mice. *Biol. Reprod.* **2012**, *86*, 72. [CrossRef]
47. Novák, J.; Olejníčková, V.; Tkáčová, N.; Santulli, G. Mechanistic Role of MicroRNAs in Coupling Lipid Metabolism and Atherosclerosis. *Adv. Exp. Med. Biol.* **2015**, *887*, 79–100.
48. Pan, J.; Li, K.; Huang, W.; Zhang, X. MiR-137 inhibited cell proliferation and migration of vascular smooth muscle cells via targeting IGFBP-5 and modulating the mTOR/STAT3 signaling. *PLoS ONE* **2017**, *12*, e0186245. [CrossRef]
49. Maimaiti, A.; Maimaiti, A.; Yang, Y.; Ma, Y. MiR-106b exhibits an anti-angiogenic function by inhibiting STAT3 expression in endothelial cells. *Lipids Health Dis.* **2016**, *15*, 51. [CrossRef]
50. Eid, R.; Boucher, E.; Gharib, N.; Khoury, C.; Arab, N.T.T.; Murray, A.; Young, P.G.; Mandato, C.A.; Greenwood, M.T. Identification of human ferritin, heavy polypeptide 1 (FTH1) and yeast RGI1 (YER067W) as pro-survival sequences that counteract the effects of Bax and copper in Saccharomyces cerevisiae. *Exp. Cell Res.* **2016**, *342*, 52–61. [CrossRef]
51. Zhong, S.; Xu, Y.; Yu, C.; Zhang, X.; Li, L.; Ge, H.; Ren, G.; Wang, Y.; Ma, J.; Zheng, Y.; et al. Anaphase-promoting complex/cyclosome regulates RdDM activity by degrading DMS3 in Arabidopsis. *Proc. Natl. Acad. Sci. USA* **2019**, *116*, 3899–3908. [CrossRef] [PubMed]
52. Zhang, X.; Zhuang, J.; Liu, L.; He, Z.; Liu, C.; Ma, X.; Li, J.; Ding, X.; Sun, C. Integrative transcriptome data mining for identification of core lncRNAs in breast cancer. *PeerJ* **2019**, *7*, e7821. [CrossRef] [PubMed]
53. Saddic, L.A.; Sigurdsson, M.I.; Chang, T.-W.; Mazaika, E.; Heydarpour, M.; Shernan, S.K.; Seidman, C.E.; Seidman, J.G.; Aranki, S.F.; Body, S.C.; et al. The Long Noncoding RNA Landscape of the Ischemic Human Left Ventricle. *Circ. Cardiovasc. Genet.* **2017**, *10*, e001534. [CrossRef] [PubMed]

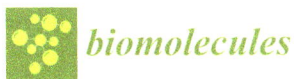 

Article

# The Ser290Asn and Thr715Pro Polymorphisms of the *SELP* Gene Are Associated with A Lower Risk of Developing Acute Coronary Syndrome and Low Soluble P-Selectin Levels in A Mexican Population [†]

Gabriel Herrera-Maya [1,‡], Gilberto Vargas-Alarcón [1,‡], Oscar Pérez-Méndez [1], Rosalinda Posadas-Sánchez [2], Felipe Masso [3], Teresa Juárez-Cedillo [4], Galileo Escobedo [5], Andros Vázquez-Montero [1] and José Manuel Fragoso [1,*]

1. Department of Molecular Biology, Instituto Nacional de Cardiología Ignacio Chávez, Mexico City 14080, Mexico; mayadermata@ciencias.unam.mx (G.H.-M.); gvargas63@yahoo.com (G.V.-A.); opmendez@yahoo.com (O.P.M.); koapa_93and@hotmail.com (A.V.-M.)
2. Department of Endocrinology, Instituto Nacional de Cardiología Ignacio Chávez, Mexico City 14080, Mexico; rossy_posadas_s@yahoo.it
3. Laboratory of Translational Medicine, UNAM-INC Research Unit, Instituto Nacional de Cardiología, Ignacio Chávez, Mexico City 14080, Mexico; f_masso@yahoo.com
4. Commissioned of the Research Unit in Clinical Epidemiology, Hospital Regional No. 1, Dr. Carlos McGregor Sánchez Navarro, Instituto Mexicano del Seguro Social, Mexico City 14080, Mexico; terezillo@exalumno.unam.mx
5. Unit of the Experimental Medicine, Hospital General de Mexico, Dr. Eduardo Liceaga, Mexico City 14080, Mexico; gescobedog@msn.com
* Correspondence: mfragoso1275@yahoo.com.mx; Tel.: (52-55)-5573-2911 (ext. 26302); Fax: (52-55)-5573-0926
† Running Head: SELP gene polymorphisms in acute coronary syndrome.
‡ The contributions by G. Herrera-Maya and G. Vargas-Alarcón are equal and the order of authorship is arbitrary.

Received: 14 January 2020; Accepted: 10 February 2020; Published: 11 February 2020

**Abstract:** Recent studies have shown that P-selectin promotes the early formation of atherosclerotic plaque. The aim of the present study was to evaluate whether the *SELP* gene single nucleotide polymorphisms (SNPs) are associated with presence of acute coronary syndrome (ACS) and with plasma P-selectin levels in a case-control association study. The sample size was estimated for a statistical power of 80%. We genotyped three *SELP* (*SELP* Ser290Asn, *SELP* Leu599Val, and *SELP* Thr715Pro) SNPs using 5′ exonuclease TaqMan assays in 625 patients with ACS and 700 healthy controls. The associations were evaluated with logistic regressions under the co-dominant, dominant, recessive, over-dominant and additive inheritance models. The genotype contribution to the plasma P-selectin levels was evaluated by a Student's t-test. Under different models, the *SELP* Ser290Asn (OR = 0.59, $pC_{Co\text{-}Dominant}$ = 0.047; OR = 0.59, $pC_{Dominant}$ = 0.014; OR = 0.58, $pC_{Over\text{-}Dominant}$ = 0.061, and OR = 0.62, $pC_{Additive}$ = 0.015) and *SELP* Thr715Pro (OR = 0.61, $pC_{Dominant}$ = 0.028; OR = 0.63, $pC_{Over\text{-}Dominant}$ = 0.044, and OR = 0.62, $pC_{Additive}$ = 0.023) SNPs were associated with a lower risk of ACS. In addition, these SNPs were associated with low plasma P-selectin levels. In summary, this study established that the *SELP* Ser290Asn and *SELP* Thr715Pro SNPs are associated with a lower risk of developing ACS and with decreased P-selectin levels in plasma in a Mexican population.

**Keywords:** acute coronary syndrome; P-selectin; genetics; polymorphisms; susceptibility

## 1. Introduction

Acute coronary syndrome (ACS) comprises a spectrum of obstructive coronary artery diseases that most commonly arise from plaque rupture and/or erosion, leaving the vulnerable lipid-rich core exposed to the circulation. As a result, platelets and the coagulation cascade are activated, leading to acute thrombotic occlusion [1,2]. This syndrome is a consequence of atherosclerosis associated with a strong inflammatory component, which is immune mediated by chemokines. These molecules have an important role in the development of atherosclerotic plaque [3–5]. P-selectin is a chemokine, which mediates lymphocyte and monocyte recruitment, rolling, and diapedesis to the areas of inflammation [4–6]. Experimental studies have shown that higher expression of SELP increases adhesion, monocytes rolling to the vascular wall, accumulation of oxidized low-density lipoproteins, and the early formation of atherosclerotic plaque and other inflammatory diseases [4–7].

P-selectin contains 17 exons and is encoded by the *SELP* gene located on chromosome 1q21-q24 spanning <50 kb [8]. Recently, three single nucleotide polymorphism (SNPs) in the *SELP* gene in the exons 7, 12, and 13 [positions *G1057A* Ser290Asn (rs6131), *G1980T* Leu599Val (rs6133), and *A2331C* Thr715Pro (rs6136)] have been associated with myocardial infarction, hypertension, coronary heart disease, lupus erythematosus, type 2 diabetes mellitus (T2DM), and atherosclerosis [8–13]. Nonetheless, the association between these SNPs and other inflammatory diseases, such as diabetic retinopathy and multiple sclerosis is controversial, with negative results [14,15].

Considering the prominent role of P-selectin as a key in the chain of events leading to atherosclerotic plaque formation, the aim of this study was to investigate the association of three *SELP* SNPs (Ser290Asn, Leu599Val and Thr715Pro) with the risk of developing ACS. Furthermore, we evaluated whether these SNPs were associated with plasma P-selectin levels in a Mexican population sample.

## 2. Subjects and Methods

### 2.1. Study Population

This case-control study was carried out at the Instituto Nacional de Cardiologia Ignacio Chavez. The sample size was calculated for unmatched cases and controls with OpenEpi software (http://www.openepi.com/SampleSize/SSCC.html) with a statistical power of 80% and an alpha error of 0.05. Using this criterion, we included 625 patients with ACS (82% men and 18% women with a mean age of 57.97 ± 10.5 years) who were diagnosed based on clinical characteristics, electrocardiographic changes and biochemical markers of cardiac necrosis, according to guidelines from the European Society of Cardiology (ESC) and American College of Cardiology (ACC) [16,17]. The exclusion criteria were (1) patients with clear inflammatory pathologies on admission, such as infection established by clinical, laboratory, or image investigations, and (2) patients with an autoimmune disease or cancer previously diagnosed or documented during their hospitalization. Moreover, we included 700 healthy controls (66% men and 34% women with a mean age of 54.37 ± 7.65 years) coming from the Genetics of Atherosclerosis Disease (GEA) Mexican study previously described by Rosalinda-Posadas et al [18]. All healthy controls were asymptomatic and apparently healthy individuals without a family history of CAD and with a negative calcium score, indicative of the absence of subclinical atherosclerosis [18]. The exclusion criteria included not only the use anti-dyslipidemic, anti-hypertensive, and anti-diabetic drugs at the time of the study, but also congestive heart failure, as well as liver, renal, thyroid or oncological disease. All GEA participants were unrelated and of self-reported Mexican ancestry (3 generations). A Mexican mestizo was defined as a person who (1) was born in Mexico and (2) is a descendant of the original autochthonous inhabitants and of individuals (Caucasian and/or African, mainly Spaniards) who migrated to America in or after the XVI century. This study was conducted according to the principles of the Declaration of Helsinki and was approved by the Ethics and Research committee of our institution (registration number: 17CI09012010). Written informed consent was obtained from all individuals enrolled in the study.

## 2.2. Laboratory Analyses

After a 12-h overnight fast, EDTA blood samples were drawn and centrifuged within 15 min after collection; the plasma was separated into aliquots and immediately analyzed or frozen at −80 °C until analysis. Cholesterol and triglyceride plasma concentrations were determined by enzymatic/colorimetric assays (Randox Laboratories, UK). The phosphotungstic acid-$Mg^{2+}$ method was used to determine HDL-C concentrations. LDL-C was estimated in samples with a triglyceride level lower than 400 mg/dl, using the modified Friedewald formula [ ]. Plasma lipid concentrations were determined within 24 h after blood sample collection. We followed the National Cholesterol Education Project (NCEP) Adult Treatment Panel (ATP III) guidelines and thus defined dyslipidemia with the following levels: cholesterol > 200 mg/dl, LDL-C > 130 mg/dl, HDL-C < 40 mg/dl, and triglyceride > 150 mg/dl (http://www.nhlbi.nih.gov/guidelines/cholesterol/atp3_rpt.htm). Type 2 diabetes mellitus (T2DM) was defined with a fasting glucose ≥ 126 mg/dL and was also considered when participants reported glucose-lowering treatment or a physician diagnosis of T2DM. Hypertension was defined by a systolic blood pressure ≥ 140 mmHg and/or diastolic blood pressure ≥ 90 mmHg, or the use of oral antihypertensive therapy [ ].

## 2.3. Genetic Analysis

DNA extraction was performed from peripheral blood in agreement with the method of Lahiri and Nurnberger [ ]. The *SELP G1057A* Ser290Asn, *SELP G1980T* Leu599Val, and *SELP A2331C* Thr715Pro SNPs were genotyped using 5′ exonuclease TaqMan assays on a 7900HT Fast Real-Time PCR system according to manufacturer's instructions (Applied Biosystems, foster City, CA, USA). In order to avoid genotyping errors, ten percent of the samples were determined twice; the results were concordant for all cases.

## 2.4. Determination of P-Selectin Levels

Samples were aliquoted and stored at −70 °C for further use. Plasma P-selectin levels were measured using a quantitative sandwich enzyme immunoassay technique (ELISA) kit in accordance with the manufacturer's instructions (Human P-Selectin/CD62P Quantikine ELISA Kit, R&D systems). The detection range was 0.8–50.00 ng/mL and the sensitivity was equal to the minimal detectable dose of this kit (≥ 0.121 ng/mL).

## 2.5. Functional Prediction Analysis

Two in silico programs, the ESEfinder (http://rulai.cshl.edu/cgi-bin/tools/ESE3/esefinder.cgi?process=home) and SNP Function Prediction (http://snpinfo.niehs.nih.gov/cgi-bin/snpinfo/snpfunc.cgi) were used to predict the possible functional effect of the *SELP* SNPs. Both programs (ESEfinder2.0 and SNPinfo) analyzed the localization of the SNPs (e.g., 5′-upstream, 3′-untranslated regions, intronic) and their possible functional effects, such as amino acid changes in protein structure, transcription factor binding sites in promoter or intronic enhancer regions, and alternative splicing regulation by disrupting exonic splicing enhancers (*ESE*) or silencers [ , ].

## 2.6. Statistical Analysis

All statistical analysis in this study was performed using SPSS version 18.0 (SPSS, Chicago, Il). Data of continuous variables were expressed as median and percentiles (25th–75th), while data of discrete variables [e.g., frequency (n, %)] were analyzed using Chi-squared or Fisher's exact tests. We used logistic regression tests to associate the SNPs with ACS under five inheritance models [ ]. The correction of the p-values (pC) was performed with the Bonferroni test. Using the HAPLOVIEW version 4.1 software (Cambridge, MA, USA), we performed the haplotypes construction and linkage disequilibrium analysis (LD, D″). We tested whether our study population was in Hardy–Weinberg equilibrium (HWE) with a Chi-square test. Furthermore, we used the QUANTO software [http://biostats.usc.edu/software] to calculate the statistical power of our study and found it was 0.80. Using the Student's t-test, we analyzed the contribution of the genotypes on the P-selectin plasma levels. The values were expressed as means ± SD. The level of significance was set at $p < 0.05$.

## 3. Results

### 3.1. Characteristics of the Study Population

Clinical and biochemical characteristics of the ACS patients and healthy controls are shown in Table 1. There were significant differences between the ACS patients and healthy controls. Compared to healthy controls, the ACS patients had a higher frequency of T2DM, hypertension, dyslipidemia, and smoking habit. Conversely, the total cholesterol, triglycerides, and LDL-C levels in ACS patients were lower than those in the control group; this effect may be due to their treatment with statins.

**Table 1.** Clinical characteristics and biochemical parameters of the study individuals.

|  |  | ACS (n = 625) | Healthy Controls (n = 700) | p-Value |
|---|---|---|---|---|
|  |  | Median (percentile 25–75) | Median (percentile 25–75) |  |
| Age (years) |  | 57.72 (51–65) | 54.39 (49–59) | <0.001 |
| BMI (kg/m$^2$) |  | 27.3 (25–29) | 28.3 (26–31) | 0.001 |
| Blood pressure (mmHg) | Systolic | 130.61 (114–144) | 117.32 (106–126) | <0.001 |
|  | Diastolic | 80.1 (70–90) | 72.47 (66–77) | <0.001 |
| Glucose (mg/dl) |  | 158.51 (102–188) | 98.73 (84–99) | <0.001 |
| Total cholesterol (mg/dl) |  | 164.22 (128–198) | 190.4 (164–210) | <0.001 |
| HDL-C (mg/dl) |  | 38.32 (32–44) | 44.6 (35–53) | <0.001 |
| LDL-C (mg/dl) |  | 106.4 (76–133) | 115.8 (94–134) | <0.001 |
| Triglycerides (mg/dl) |  | 169.2 (109–201) | 175.1 (112–208) | 0.218 |
| Gender n (%) | Male | 510 (82) | 463 (66) | <0.001 |
|  | Female | 115 (18) | 237 (34) |  |
| Smoking n (%) | Yes | 225 (35) | 155 (22) | <0.001 |
| Hypertension | Yes | 355 (57) | 206 (29) | <0.001 |
| Diabetes mellitus | Yes | 218 (35) | 68 (10) | <0.001 |
| Dyslipidemia n (%) | Yes | 534 (85) | 501 (71) | <0.001 |

Data are expressed as median and percentiles (25th–75th). p-values were estimated using Mann–Whitney U test for continuous variables and chi-square test for categorical values. ACS: acute coronary syndrome patients.

### 3.2. Allele and Genotype Frequencies

Genotype frequencies of the SNPs were in HWE. The frequencies of the *SELP Leu599Val* SNP was similar in ACS patients and healthy controls. Nonetheless, the SNPs [*SELP* Ser290Asn, and *SELP* Thr715Pro] were associated with a lower risk of ACS (Table 2). Under co-dominant, dominant, over-dominant, and additive models, the *A* (290Asn) allele of the *SELP* Ser290Asn SNP was associated with a lower risk of ACS (OR = 0.59, $pC_{Co\text{-}Dom}$ = 0.047; OR = 0.59, $pC_{Dom}$ = 0.014; OR = 0.58, $pC_{Over\text{-}Dom}$ = 0.061, and OR = 0.62, $pC_{Add}$ = 0.015, respectively). In the same way, under dominant, over-dominant, and additive models, the C (715Pro) allele of the *SELP* Thr715Pro SNP was associated with a lower risk of ACS (OR = 0.61, $pC_{Dom}$ = 0.028; OR = 0.63, $pC_{Over\text{-}Dom}$ = 0.044, and OR = 0.62, $pC_{Add}$ = 0.023, respectively). All models were adjusted for gender, age, blood pressure, BMI, glucose, total cholesterol, HDL-C, LDL-C, triglycerides, and smoking habit.

**Table 2.** Distribution of *SEL-P* polymorphisms in ACS patients and healthy controls.

| | | | | MAF | Model | OR (95%CI) | pC |
|---|---|---|---|---|---|---|---|
| | *SELP G1057A* Ser290Asn (rs6131) | | | | | | |
| | GG | GA | AA | | | | |
| Control (n = 691) | 569 (0.823) | 115 (0.166) | 7 (0.010) | 0.09 | Co-dominant | 0.59 (0.38–0.92) | 0.047 |
| | | | | | Dominant | 0.59 (0.39–0.90) | 0.014 |
| | | | | | Recessive | 0.58 (0.12–2.83) | 0.49 |
| ACS (n = 617) | 541 (0.877) | 73 (0.118) | 3 (0.005) | 0.06 | Over-dominant | 0.61 (0.39–0.92) | 0.019 |
| | | | | | Additive | 0.62 (0.42–0.92) | 0.015 |
| | *SELP G1980T* Leu599Val (rs6133) | | | | | | |
| | GG | GT | TT | | | | |
| Control (n = 682) | 563 (0.825) | 114 (0.167) | 5 (0.007) | 0.09 | Co-dominant | 0.28 (0.02–3.32) | 0.46 |
| | | | | | Dominant | 1.07 (0.73–1.58) | 0.73 |
| | | | | | Recessive | 0.27 (0.02–3.26) | 0.26 |
| ACS (n = 611) | 505 (0.827) | 105 (0.172) | 1 (0.002) | 0.09 | Over-dominant | 1.12 (0.75–1.66) | 0.57 |
| | | | | | Additive | 1.02 (0.71–1.49) | 0.90 |
| | *SELP A2331C* Thr715Pro (rs6136) | | | | | | |
| | AA | AC | CC | | | | |
| Control (n = 685) | 580 (0.847) | 97 (0.141) | 8 (0.012) | 0.08 | Co-dominant | 0.63 (0.40–0.99) | 0.075 |
| | | | | | Dominant | 0.61 (0.39–0.95) | 0.028 |
| | | | | | Recessive | 0.36 (0.04–2.95) | 0.32 |
| ACS (n = 607) | 537 (0.884) | 67 (0.110) | 3 (0.005) | 0.06 | Over-dominant | 0.63 (0.40–0.99) | 0.044 |
| | | | | | Additive | 0.62 (0.41–0.94) | 0.023 |

ACS, acute coronary syndrome, MAF, minor allele frequency, OR, odds ratio, CI, confidence interval, pC, p-value corrected. The p-values were calculated by the logistic regression analysis, and the ORs were adjusted for gender, age, blood pressure, BMI, glucose, total cholesterol, HDL-C, LDL-C, triglycerides, and smoking habit.

Considering that the prevalence of T2DM (35%) and hypertension (57%) are highest in ACS patients versus healthy controls (10% and 29%, respectively), we performed a sub-analysis of the polymorphisms associated with a low risk of ACS (*SELP* Ser290Asn and *SELP* Thr715Pro). This analysis was made comparing individuals with and without T2DM and the other hand, individuals with and without hypertension. The results show that both polymorphisms were not associated with T2DM or with hypertension (Supplementary Tables S1 and S2). Therefore, this analysis corroborates that the genetic variation of these polymorphisms of the *SELP* gene are associated to the ACS, and not comes of the T2DM or hypertension.

*3.3. Linkage Disequilibrium Analysis*

We used the Haploview version 4.1 program for the analysis of the linkage disequilibrium and construction of haplotypes. In this analysis, the *SELP* Thr715Pro and *SELP* Leu599Val SNPs showed a strong linkage disequilibrium (D' = 0.95). In addition, Haploview revealed strong evidence of recombination of the polymorphisms *SELP* Thr715Pro versus *SELP* Ser290Asn and *SELP* Leu599Val versus *SELP* Ser290Asn (D'= 0.17 and D' = 0.28, respectively; data not shown). This analysis marked three haplotypes with different distributions in ACS patients and healthy controls (Table ). The "Thr-Leu-Ser" haplotype was associated with a higher risk of developing ACS (OR = 1.28, 95% CI: 1.05–1.54, pC = 0.006), while the "Pro-Leu-Ser" and "Thr-Leu-Asn" haplotypes were associated with a lower risk of developing ACS (OR = 0.72, 95% CI: 0.52-0.99, pC = 0.022, and OR = 0.71, 95% CI: 0.51–1.00, pC = 0.027, respectively).

**Table 3.** Haplotype frequencies (Hf) of *SEL-P* haplotypes in ACS patients and healthy controls.

| Haplotypes | Thr715Pro | Leu599Val | Ser290Asn | ACS (n = 605) | Controls (n = 676) | OR | 95%CI | P |
|---|---|---|---|---|---|---|---|---|
| | | | | Hf | Hf | | | |
| H1 | Thr | Leu | Ser | 0.804 | 0.763 | 1.28 | 1.05–1.54 | **0.006** |
| H2 | Thr | Val | Ser | 0.073 | 0.067 | 1.08 | 0.80–1.47 | 0.32 |
| H3 | Pro | Leu | Ser | 0.057 | 0.077 | 0.72 | 0.52–0.99 | **0.022** |
| H4 | Thr | Leu | Asn | 0.049 | 0.066 | 0.71 | 0.51–1.00 | **0.027** |
| H5 | Pro | Val | Asn | 0.014 | 0.022 | 0.62 | 0.33–1.13 | 0.063 |

Abbreviations: Hf, Haplotype frequency; P, p-value; OR, odds ratio; 95% CI, confidential interval. The order of the polymorphisms in the haplotypes is according to the positions in the chromosome (*SELP A2331C* Thr715Pro (rs6136), *SELP G1980T* Leu599Val (rs6133), and *SELP G1057A* Ser290Asn (rs6131). Bold numbers indicate significant associations.

### 3.4. Association of Polymorphisms with Plasma P-Selectin Levels

In order to define the functional effect of the *SELP* Ser290Asn and *SELP* Thr715Pro SNPs associated with a lower risk of ACS, we determined the plasma levels of P-selectin in individuals with different genotypes of these two polymorphisms. For this analysis, we included a subgroup of 30 healthy controls for *SELP* Ser290Asn (7 *AA*, 11 *GA* and 12 *GG*) and a subgroup of 30 healthy controls for the *SELP* Thr715Pro SNP (8 *CC*, 11 *AC* and 11 *AA*). In this study, we did not include the analysis of plasma P-selectin levels in patients with ACS, due to the fact that in the setting of the coronary syndrome, the comorbidities, such as insulin resistance/T2DM, hypertension, and inflammatory processes, as well as the use of the anti-dyslipidemic and/or anti-hypertensive drugs, may have altered the inflammatory markers levels, such as inflammatory cytokines, adhesion molecules, and C-reactive protein, masking the real impact of *SELP* polymorphisms on plasma P-selectin levels [23–25]. In this context, subjects carrying the *AA* (Ans/Ans) genotype of the *SELP* Ser290Asn SNP had a lower P-selectin plasma concentration (33.93 ± 9.79 ng/mL) than carriers of the *GG* (Ser/Ser) (44.76 ± 6.54 ng/mL, $p = 0.032$) or *GA* (Ser/Ans) genotypes (48.04 ± 16.57 ng/mL, $p = 0.049$) (Figure 1A). On the other hand, the analysis of the *SELP* Thr715Pro polymorphism showed that individuals with the *CC* (Pro/Pro) genotype had a lower concentration of P-selectin (26.44 ± 10.77 ng/mL) than *AA* (Thr/Thr) carriers (55.35 ± 14.05 ng/dl, $p = 0.001$). In addition, the individuals with the *AC* (Thr/Pro) genotype had lower P-selectin levels than *AA* (Thr/Thr) carriers (34.91 ± 14.46 ng/dl, $p = 0.005$) (Figure 1B).

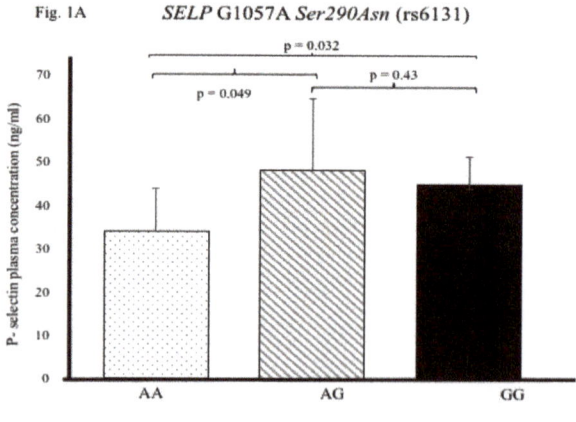

Fig. 1A    *SELP G1057A Ser290Asn* (rs6131)

**Figure 1.** *Cont.*

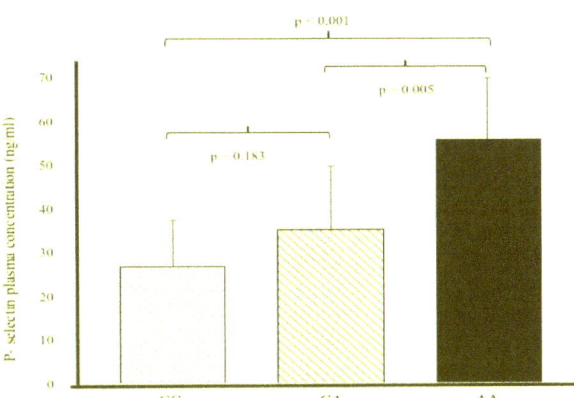

**Figure 1.** Genetic contribution of the *SELP G1057A* and *SELP A2331C* polymorphisms on P-selectin levels. (**A**) P-selectin plasma levels in individuals with different genotypes of the *SELP G1057A* polymorphism. (**B**) P-selectin plasma levels in individuals with different genotypes of the *SELP A2331C* polymorphism.

*3.5. Functional Prediction*

The functional prediction analysis showed that the presence of the *A* (Asn) allele of the *SELP* Ser290Asn polymorphism potentially produces a binding motif for Srp40 protein. In contrast, no evidence of potentially functional motifs was found for the *SELP* Thr715Pro polymorphism.

**4. Discussion**

In this study, we analyzed three relevant polymorphisms (Ser290Asn, Leu599Val, and Thr715Pro, respectively) of the *SELP* gene. The association of these SNPs with several inflammatory diseases in different populations is controversial, with positive and negative results [ – ]. In our study, the distribution of the *SELP* Leu599Val SNP was similar in both ACS patients and healthy controls. Nonetheless, the presence of the 290*Asn* and 715*Pro* alleles (*SELP* Ser290Asn and *SELP* Thr715Pro polymorphisms, respectively) was associated with a lower risk of developing ACS. In the same way, Reiner et al. reported in the CARDIA study that the *SELP* Ser290Asn and *SELP* Thr715Pro SNPs are associated with carotid intima-media thickness in young adults; however, these associations are different in European-American and African-American individuals [ ]. In line with these data, Nasibullin et al. reported that the 290*Ans* allele of the *SELP* Ser290Asn SNP is associated with a lower risk of MI in a Russian population [ ]. Similarly, the study of the risk of atherosclerosis in communities (ARIC), as well as the study of the Framingham heart (FHS) have shown that the genotype Pro715Pro is associated with a decreased risk of atherosclerosis in American and European populations [ , ]. In contrast with these data, in the ARIC study, Volcik et al. reported that the 290*Ans* and 715*Pro* alleles (*SELP* Ser290Asn and *SELP* Thr715Pro SNPs, respectively) were associated with the development of coronary heart disease in white but not in African Americans [ ]. Similarly, Timasheva et al. reported that the 290*Ans* allele of the *SELP* Ser290Asn SNP is associated with the development of hypertension in ethnic Tatars originating from the Republic of Bashkortostan (Russian Federation) [ ]. By the same token, Kou et al. reported that *Thr715Pro* or *Pro715Pro* genotypes of the *SELP* Thr715Pro polymorphism increased the risk of developing cardiovascular diseases (CVD) in a Chinese Han population [ ]. Additionally, we found that the H3 (Pro-Leu-Ser) and H4 (Thr-Leu-Asn) haplotypes were associated with a lower risk of developing ACS, whereas H1 (Thr-Leu-Ser) was associated with a higher risk. As can be seen, the haplotypic combinations between *SELP* Thr715Pro and *SELP* Ser290Asn polymorphisms were not in linkage disequilibrium. Nonetheless, the protection haplotypes carry *715Pro* and *290Ans* alleles, and both of them were associated independently with a lower risk of cardiovascular diseases and other inflammatory diseases. This finding corroborated the role of these two alleles with the presence of ACS, whether they were analyzed independently or as haplotypes.

It is important to note that ACS patients and the healthy donors have much greater variation in blood glucose (102-188 versus 84-99) and diabetes mellitus (35% versus 10%). Considering these data, it is important to establish whether the polymorphisms are associated with T2DM or hypertension. In a sub-analysis, we showed that both polymorphisms were not associated with T2DM or with hypertension.

As can be seen, the associations of the *SELP* Ser290Asn and *SELP* Thr715Pro polymorphisms with ACS are contradictory in different study populations. We suggest that these discrepancies could be due to the classical cardiovascular risk factors and the environmental factors, such as diet, exercise, and lifestyle, which have an important role in the development of inflammatory diseases [29,30]. Another reason may be the fact that the allelic distribution of these polymorphisms varies according to the ethnic origin of the study populations. According to data obtained from the National Center for Biotechnology Information, populations from European, Asian, and African ancestry in Southwest US present a higher frequency of the *A* allele of the *SELP G1057A* Ser290Asn (rs6131) polymorphism (21.7%, 20.2% and 32.9%, respectively) when compared to Mexican mestizos and white American populations with a lower frequency of the *A* allele (9% and 14%, respectively). Concerning the *SELP A2331C* Thr715Pro (rs6136) SNP, Mexican mestizos, Europeans, and white Americans present a higher frequency of the *C* allele (8%, 8.8%, and 8.2%, respectively) than populations with Asian and African ancestry (0.2% and 2.5%, respectively) (https://www.ncbi.nlm.nih.gov/variation/tools/1000genomes/), (https://www.ensembl.org/index.html).

We further determined the effect of the *SELP* gene polymorphisms on plasma P-selectin levels using genotype groups. We found that the *AA* (290 Asn/Asn) and *CC* (715 Pro/Pro) genotypes were associated with low P-selectin levels. As far as we know, this is the first study that showed the association of the *SELP* Ser290Asn and *SELP* Thr715Pro polymorphisms in P-selectin levels in individuals without the use of the anti-dyslipidemic or anti-hypertensive drugs. These drugs may modify the levels of the inflammatory markers, such as pro-inflammatory cytokines, adhesion molecules and C-reactive protein, masking the real impact of *SELP* gene polymorphisms on plasma P-selectin [23–25]. Nonetheless, the results concerning the association between P-selectin plasma levels and heart diseases are still contradictory. For example, Reiner et al. reported in the CARDIA study that the *A* (290Asn) and *C* (715Pro) alleles are associated with decreased plasma P-selectin levels and with the risk of developing atherosclerosis [9]. By the same token, Volcik et al. documented that the 715Pro allele is associated with lower P-selectin levels in the Atherosclerosis Risk in Communities (ARIC) study [27]. Similarly, Lee et al. determined that the lower serum levels of P-selectin decreased the risk of atherosclerosis [26]. At the same time, other reports have shown that the 715Pro (C) allele increased the expression of SELP mRNA, as well as the concentration of P-selectin levels in other inflammatory diseases, such as rheumatoid arthritis and T2DM [8,31]. As far as we know, the precise mechanism by which low and/or high P-selectin levels are associated with ACS remains to be elucidated. Nonetheless, recent data provide evidence that P-selectin upregulation on the endothelial cell surface mediates the effects of angiotensin II (Ang II), which has an important role in the development atherosclerosis [32]. In addition, Ang II stimulates not only the production of several molecules (adhesion molecules, chemokines, and cytokines) but also the oxidation and uptake of LDL, which promotes endothelial dysfunction [6,32]. On the other hand, Ang II triggers the synthesis of matrix metalloproteinases, the plasminogen activator inhibitor-1, and the proliferation of vascular smooth cells; this effect leads to the destabilization of atherosclerotic plaques [6]. Furthermore, using bioinformatics tools, we determined the potential effect of the *SELP* gene polymorphisms associated with ACS. The analysis of the *SELP* Thr715Pro polymorphism did not provide evidence of potential functional motifs. Nonetheless, the analysis of the *SELP* Ser290Asn polymorphism showed that the 290 Asn (*A*) allele generates a binding site for the Srp40 proteins. These proteins have multiple functions in the pre-mRNA splicing process, as well as in the regulation of alternative splicing, which leads to the production of protein isoforms [ , ]. In this context, we think that future investigations are warranted to understand the effect of these polymorphisms on P-selectin levels.

Some limitations should be considered. The P-selectin levels were only measured in a small sample of control individuals and experiments on RNA transcription or protein stability were not made. Considering these limitations, the effect of the SNPs on P-selectin plasma levels should be taken with care and studies in a large number of individuals are necessary to corroborate this association. In the same way, in our study it was not possible to determine the expression levels of P-selectin on the leukocyte's surface to confirm the data obtained in plasma.

In summary, this study demonstrated that the *SELP* Ser290Asn and *SELP* Thr715Pro polymorphisms are associated with a lower risk of developing ACS in a Mexican population. It was possible to distinguish two haplotypes (Pro-Leu-Ser and Thr-Leu-Asn) associated with a lower risk of developing ACS. On the other hand, both polymorphisms were associated with lower P-selectin levels in plasma. Lastly, due to the specific genetic characteristics of the Mexican population, we consider that additional studies will need to be undertaken in a larger number of individuals and in populations with different ethnic origins; these studies could help define the true role of these polymorphisms as markers of risk or protection from developing ACS and other cardiovascular events.

**Supplementary Materials:** The following are available online at http://www.mdpi.com/2218-273X/10/2/270/s1, Table **S1.** Distribution of Ser290Asn and Thr715Pro SEL-P polymorphisms in individuals with and without T2DM. **Table S2.** Distribution of Ser290Asn and Thr715Pro SEL-P polymorphisms in individuals with and without hypertension.

**Author Contributions:** Conceptualization, G.H.-M., G.V.-A., O.P.-M. and J.M.F.; Data curation, O.P.-M., T.J.-C. and A.V.-M.; Formal analysis, G.H.-M., R.P.-S., F.M., T.J.-C., G.E., A.V.-M. and J.M.F.; Investigation, G.V.-A., O.P.-M. and J.M.F.; Methodology, O.P.-M., R.P.-S., F.M., G.E. and A.V.-M.; Resources, G.H.-M., O.P.-M., T.J.-C. and G.E.; Software, G.H.-M., R.P.-S., F.M., T.J.-C., G.E. and A.V.-M.; Supervision, J.M.F.; Validation, A.V.-M.; Writing – original draft, J.M.F.; Writing – review & editing, G.V.-A. and J.M.F. All authors have read and agreed to the published version of the manuscript.

**Funding:** This research was funded by the Consejo Nacional de Ciencia y Tecnología (CONACyT), Mexico City, Mexico (Project number 233277).

**Acknowledgments:** This work was submitted in fulfilment of the requirements to obtaining the Doctoral degree of Gabriel Herrera-Maya in the PhD program of Biological Sciences of the Universidad Nacional Autónoma de Mexico (UNAM). Gabriel Herrera-Maya was supported by a fellowship from the *Consejo Nacional de Ciencia y Tecnología* (*CONACyT*) Mexico City, Mexico with **CVU number 545322**. The authors are grateful to the study participants. Institutional Review Board approval was obtained for all sample collections. The authors would like to thank the technicians Silvestre Ramirez-Fuentes and Marva Arellano-Gonzalez for their participation in sample collection and DNA extraction.

**Conflicts of Interest:** The authors declare no conflict of interest.

## Abbreviations

| | |
|---|---|
| HDL-C | High-density lipoprotein–cholesterol |
| LDL | Low-density lipoprotein–cholesterol |
| SELP | P-selectin gene |
| T2DM | Type 2 diabetes mellitus |
| SNP | Single nucleotide polymorphism |
| ACS | Acute coronary syndrome |

## References

1. Libby, P. Inflammation and Atherosclerosis. *Nature* **2002**, *420*, 868–874. [ ]
2. Virmani, R.; Kolodgie, F.D.; Burke, A.P.; Finn, A.V.; Gold, H.K.; Tulenko, T.N.; Wrenn, S.P.; Narula, J. Atherosclerotic plaque progression and vulnerability to rupture: angiogenesis as a source of intraplaque hemorrhage. *Arterioscler. Thromb. Vasc. Biol.* **2005**, *25*, 2054–2061. [ ] [ ]

3. Achar, S.A.; Kundu, S.; Norcross, W.A. Diagnosis of acute coronary syndrome. *Am. Fam. Physician.* **2005**, *72*, 119–126. [PubMed]
4. Braunersreuther, V.; Mach, F.; Steffens, S. The specific role of chemokines in atherosclerosis. *Thromb. Haemost* **2007**, *97*, 714–721. [CrossRef]
5. Aukrust, P.; Halvorsen, B.; Yndestad, A.; Ueland, T.; Oie, E.; Otterdal, K.; Gullestad, L.; Damås, J.K. Chemokines and cardiovascular risk. *Arterioscler. Thromb. Vasc. Biol.* **2008**, *28*, 1909–1919. [CrossRef]
6. Montezano, A.C.; Nguyen Dinh Cat, A.; Rios, F.J.; Touyz, R.M. Angiotensin II and Vascular Injury. *Curr. Hypertens Rep.* **2014**, *16*, 431. [CrossRef]
7. Bland, A.D.; Nadar, S.K.; Lip, G.Y.H. The adhesion molecule P-selectin and cardiovascular disease. *Eur. Heart J.* **2003**, *24*, 2166–2179. [CrossRef]
8. Kaur, R.; Singh, J.; Kapoor, R.; Kaur, M. Association of SELP polymorphisms with soluble P-selectin levels and vascular risk in patients with type 2 diabetes mellitus: a case-control study. *Biochem. Genet.* **2019**, *57*, 73–97. [CrossRef]
9. Reiner, A.P.; Carlson, C.S.; Thyagarajan, B.; Reider, M.J.; Polak, J.F.; Siscovick, D.S.; Nickerson, D.A.; Jacobs, D.R., Jr.; Gross, M.D. Soluble P-selectin, SELP polymorphisms, and atherosclerotic risk European-American and African-African young adults: the coronary artery risk development in young adults (CARDIA) study. *Arterioscler. Thromb. Vasc. Biol.* **2008**, *28*, 1549–1555. [CrossRef]
10. Morris, D.L.; Graham, R.R.; Erwig, L.P.; Gaffney, P.M.; Moser, K.L.; Behrens, T.W.; Vyse, T.J.; Graham, D.C. Variation in the upstream region of P-selectin (SELP) is a risk factor for SLE. *Genes Immun.* **2009**, *10*, 404–413. [CrossRef] [PubMed]
11. Volcik, K.A.; Ballantyne, C.M.; Coresh, J.; Folsom, A.R.; Boerwinkle, E. Specific P-selectin and P-selectin glycoprotein ligand-1 genotypes/haplotypes are associated with risk of incidence CHD and ischemic stroke: the atherosclerosis risk in communities (ARIC) study. *Atherosclerosis* **2007**, *195*, e76–e82. [CrossRef] [PubMed]
12. Timasheva, Y.R.; Nasibullin, T.R.; Imaeva, E.B.; Erdman, V.; Kruzliak, P.; Tuktarova, I.A.; Nikolaeva, I.E.; Mustafina, O.E. Polymorphisms of inflammatory markers and risk of essential hypertension in Tartars from Russia. *Clin. Exp. Hypertens.* **2015**, *37*, 398–403. [CrossRef] [PubMed]
13. Nasibullin, T.R.; Timasheva, Y.R.; Sadikova, R.I.; Tuktarova, I.A.; Erdman, V.V.; Nikolaeva, I.E.; Sabo, J.; Kruzliak, P.; Mustafina, O.E. Genotype/allelic combinations as potential predictors of myocardial infarction. *Mol. Bio. Rep.* **2016**, *43*, 11–16. [CrossRef] [PubMed]
14. Kolahdouz, P.; Yazd, E.F.; Tajamolian, M.; Manaviat, M.R.; Sheikhha, M.H. The rs3917779 polymorphism of P-selectin significant association with proliferative diabetic retinopathy in Yazd, Iran. *Graefes Arch. Clin. Exp. Ophthalmol.* **2015**, *253*, 1967–1972. [CrossRef] [PubMed]
15. Fenoglio, C.; Scalabrini, D.; Piccio, L.; de Ris, M.; Venturelli, E.; Cortini, F.; Villa, C.; Serpente, M.; Parks, B.; Rinker, J.; et al. Candidate gene analysis of selectin cluster in patients with multiple sclerosis. *J. Neurol.* **2009**, *256*, 832–833. [CrossRef] [PubMed]
16. Cannon, C.P.; Battler, A.; Brindis, R.G.; Cox, J.L.; Ellis, S.G.; Every, N.R.; Flaherty, J.T.; Harrington, R.A.; Krumholz, H.M.; Simoons, M.L.; et al. American College of Cardiology key data elements and definitions for measuring the clinical management and outcomes of patients with acute coronary syndromes. A report of the American College of Cardiology Task Force on Clinical Data Standards (Acute Coronary Syndromes Writing Committee). *J. Am. Coll. Cardiol.* **2001**, *38*, 2114–2130.
17. Hamm, C.W.; Bassand, J.P.; Agewall, S.; Bax, J.; Boersma, E.; Bueno, H.; Caso, P.; Dudek, D.; Gielen, S.; Huber, K. ESC Guidelines for the management of acute coronary syndromes in patients presenting without persistent ST-segment elevation: The Task Force for the management of acute coronary syndromes (ACS) in patients presenting without persistent ST-segment elevation of the European Society of Cardiology (ESC). *Eur. Heart J.* **2011**, *32*, 2999–3054.
18. Posadas-Sanchez, R.; Perez-Hernandez, N.; Angeles-Martinez, J.; Lopez-Bautista, F.; Villarreal-Molina, T.; Rodríguez-Perez, J.M.; Fragoso, J.M.; Posadas-Romero, C.; Vargas-Alarcón, G. Interleukin 35 Polymorphisms Are Associated with Decreased Risk of Premature Coronary Artery Disease, Metabolic Parameters, and IL-35 Levels: The Genetics of Atherosclerotic Disease (GEA) Study. *Mediators Inflamm.* **2017**, *2017*, 6012795. [CrossRef]
19. DeLong, D.M.; DeLong, E.R.; Wood, P.D.; Lippel, K.; Rifkind, B.M. A comparison of methods for the estimation of plasma low- and very low-density lipoprotein cholesterol. The Lipid Research Clinics Prevalence Study. *JAMA.* **1986**, *256*, 2372–2377. [CrossRef]

20. Lahiri, D.K.; Nurnberger, J.I., Jr. A rapid non-enzymatic method for the preparation HMW DNA from blood for RFLP studies. *Nucleic Acids Res.* **1991**, *19*, 5444. [CrossRef]
21. Smith, P.J.; Zhang, C.; Wang, J.; Chew, S.L.; Zhang, M.Q.; Krainer, A.R. An increased specificity score matrix for the prediction of SF2/ASF-specific exonic splicing enhancers. *Hum. Mol. Genet.* **2006**, *15*, 2490–2508. [CrossRef] [PubMed]
22. Xu, Z.; Taylor, J.A. SNPinfo: integrating GWAS and candidate gene information into functional SNP selection for genetic association studies. *Nucleic Acids Res.* **2009**, *37*, W600–W605. [CrossRef] [PubMed]
23. Agabiti Rosei, E.; Morelli, P.; Rizzoni, D. Effects of nifedipine GITS 20 mg or enalapril 20 mg on blood pressure and inflammatory markers in patients with mild-moderate hypertension. *Blood Press Suppl.* **2005**, *1*, 14–22. [CrossRef] [PubMed]
24. Golia, E.; Limongelli, G.; Natale, F.; Fimiani, F.; Maddaloni, V.; Pariggiano, I.; Bianchi, R.; Crisci, M.; Giordano, R.; Di Palma, G.; et al. Inflamation and cardiuovascular disease: From pathogenesis and therapeutic target. *Curr. Atheroscler. Rep.* **2014**, *16*, 435. [CrossRef]
25. Ruszkowski, P.; Masajtis-Zagajewska, A.; Nowicki, M. Effects of combined statin and ACE inhibitor therapy on endothelial function and blood pressure in essential hypertension-a radomised double-blind, placebo controlled crossover study. *J. Renin. Angiotensin Aldosterone Syst.* **2019**, *20*, 1–9. [CrossRef]
26. Lee, D.S.; Larson, M.G.; Lunetta, K.L.; Dupuis, J.; Rong, J.; Keaney, J.F., Jr.; Lipinska, I.; Baldwin, C.T.; Vasan, R.S.; Benjamin, E.J. Clinical and genetic correlates of soluble P-selectin in the community. *J. Thromb. Haemost.* **2008**, *6*, 20–31. [CrossRef]
27. Volcik, K.A.; Catellier, D.; Folson, A.R.; Matijevic, N.; Wasserman, B.; Boerwinkle, E. SELP and SELPG genetic variation is associated with cell surface measures of SELp and SELPG: the atherosclerosis risk in communities (ARIC) study. *Clin. Chem.* **2009**, *55*, 1076–1082. [CrossRef]
28. Kuo, L.; Yang, N.; Dong, B.; Li, Y.; Tang, J.; Qin, Q. Interaction between SELP genetic polymorphisms with inflammatory cytokine interleukin-6 (IL_6) gene variants on cardiovascular disease in Chinese Han population. *Mamm. Genome* **2017**, *28*, 436–442.
29. Bielinski, S.J.; Berardi, C.; Decker, P.A.; Kirsch, P.S.; Larson, N.B.; Pankow, J.S.; Sale, M.; De Andrade, M.; Sicotte, H.; Tang, W.; et al. P-selectin and subclinical and clinical atherosclerosis: the multi-ethnic study of atherosclerosis (MESA). *Atherosclerosis* **2015**, *240*, 3–9. [CrossRef]
30. Nettleton, J.A.; Matijevic, N.; Follis, J.L.; Folsom, A.R.; Boerwinkle, E. Associations between dietary patterns and flow cytometry-measured biomarkers of inflammation and cellular activation in the Atherosclerosis Risk in Communities (ARIC) Carotid Artery MRI Study. *Atherosclerosis* **2010**, *212*, 260–267. [CrossRef]
31. Burkhardt, J.; Blume, M.; Petit-Teixeira, E.; Hugo Teixeira, V.; Steiner, A.; Quente, E.; Wolfram, G.; Scholz, M.; Pierlot, C.; Migliorini, P.; et al. Cellular Adhesion Gene SELP Is Associated with Rheumatoid Arthritis and Displays Differential Allelic Expression. *PLoS ONE* **2014**, *9*, e103872. [CrossRef] [PubMed]
32. Piqueras, L.; Kubes, P.; Alvarez, A.; O'Connor, E.; Issekutz, A.C.; Esplugues, J.V.; Sanz, M.J. Angiotensin II Induces leukocyte–endothelial cell interactions in vivo via AT1 and AT2 receptor-mediated P-selectin upregulation. *Circulation* **2000**, *102*, 2118–2123. [CrossRef] [PubMed]
33. Tardos, J.G.; Eisenreich, A.; Deikus, G.; Bechhofer, D.H.; Chandradas, S.; Zafar, U.; Rauch, U.; Bogdanov, V.Y. SR proteins ASF/SF2 and SRp55 participoate in tissue factor biosynthesis in human monocyte cells. *J. Thromb. Haemost.* **2008**, *6*, 877–884. [CrossRef] [PubMed]
34. Graveley, B.R. Sorting out the complexity of SR protein functions. *RNA* **2000**, *6*, 1197–1211. [CrossRef] [PubMed]

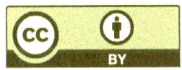

© 2020 by the authors. Licensee MDPI, Basel, Switzerland. This article is an open access article distributed under the terms and conditions of the Creative Commons Attribution (CC BY) license (http://creativecommons.org/licenses/by/4.0/).

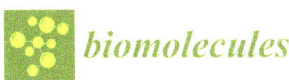 

*Review*

# Sarcomeric Gene Variants and Their Role with Left Ventricular Dysfunction in Background of Coronary Artery Disease

**Surendra Kumar [1],[†], Vijay Kumar [2],[\*],[†] and Jong-Joo Kim [2],[\*]**

[1] Department of Anatomy, All India Institute of Medical Sciences, New Delhi 110029, India; surendrakhedarcbt@gmail.com
[2] Department of Biotechnology, Yeungnam University, Gyeongsan, Gyeongbuk 38541, Korea
\* Correspondence: vijaykumarcbt@gmail.com (V.K.); kimjj@ynu.ac.kr (J.-J.K.); Tel.: +82-53-810-3027 or +82-10-9668-3464 (J.-J.K.); Fax: +82-53-801-3464 (J.-J.K.)
[†] These authors contributed equally to this work.

Received: 1 March 2020; Accepted: 11 March 2020; Published: 12 March 2020

**Abstract:** Cardiovascular diseases are one of the leading causes of death in developing countries, generally originating as coronary artery disease (CAD) or hypertension. In later stages, many CAD patients develop left ventricle dysfunction (LVD). Left ventricular ejection fraction (LVEF) is the most prevalent prognostic factor in CAD patients. LVD is a complex multifactorial condition in which the left ventricle of the heart becomes functionally impaired. Various genetic studies have correlated LVD with dilated cardiomyopathy (DCM). In recent years, enormous progress has been made in identifying the genetic causes of cardiac diseases, which has further led to a greater understanding of molecular mechanisms underlying each disease. This progress has increased the probability of establishing a specific genetic diagnosis, and thus providing new opportunities for practitioners, patients, and families to utilize this genetic information. A large number of mutations in sarcomeric genes have been discovered in cardiomyopathies. In this review, we will explore the role of the sarcomeric genes in LVD in CAD patients, which is a major cause of cardiac failure and results in heart failure.

**Keywords:** sarcomere; dilated cardiomyopathy; left ventricle dysfunction; actin; myosin; troponin; tropomyosin

---

## 1. Introduction:

Cardiac diseases are one of the main causes of death these days, generally originating as coronary artery disease (CAD) or hypertension. In later stages, many patients may develop left ventricle dysfunction (LVD). Left ventricular ejection fraction (LVEF) is the most determining factor for the prognosis of CAD patients [1–3].

LVD is a complex multifactorial condition in which the left ventricle becomes functionally compromised. In the cardiovascular system, the left ventricle plays a central role in the maintenance of circulation because of its role as the major pump in the heart. In the case of LVD, the pumping function of the heart is reduced, leading to symptoms of congestive heart failure (CHF). CAD patients with severe LVD have a higher mortality than those with preserved LV function, and this mortality rate is proportional to the severity of LVD. The rising number of patients with ischemic LVD contributes significantly to the increased morbidity and mortality of cardiac arrests. Impaired pumping by the heart leads to other cardiovascular complications, such as heart failure, myocardial infarction, cardiomyopathies, etc. [4–6].

LVD includes two distinctive morphologies: hypertrophy and dilation. In LV hypertrophy, ventricular chamber volume remains the same, but the wall of the chamber is thickened. In LV dilation, the chamber volume of the left ventricle gets enlarged when the walls are either normal or thinned. These two conditions are associated with specific hemodynamic variations. In hypertrophic conditions, only diastolic relaxation is impaired, while in the dilated condition, systolic functions are diminished. This results in a change of heart shape from an elliptical to a more spherical form, which causes considerable mechanical inefficiency and deterioration, resulting in CHF [3,6]. Sarcomeric proteins are basic contractile units of the myocyte/myocardium. Several sarcomeric genes have been identified and associated with the pathogenesis of CHF.

This review will highlight the genetic basis of LVD in the background of CAD. We review the role of common sarcomeric genes (MYBPC3, TNNT2, TTN, Myospryn) and their genetic variants with LVD in CAD patients.

## 2. Common Sarcomeric Protein and Associated Gene Polymorphism

In recent years, remarkable developments have been made in identifying the genetic association of cardiac diseases, resulting in a better understanding of the underlying molecular mechanisms. Several genetic studies have found an association between LVD and dilated cardiomyopathy (DCM). Various sarcomeric protein-encoding genes such as cardiac myosin-binding protein C (MYBPC3), myosin heavy polypeptide, and cardiac troponin I gene mutations, as well as other gene mutations have been identified in DCM [7–13]. The common sarcomeric gene polymorphisms with their locations and functional roles are given in Table 1.

Table 1. Common sarcomeric gene polymorphism.

| Genes | Location | Type of Polymorphism | Functional Role | Ref. |
|---|---|---|---|---|
| MYBPC3 | 11p11.2 | 25 bp Ins/del | MYBPC3 gene mutation is associated with inherited cardiomyopathies and an increased heart failure risk | [14–18] |
| TNNT2 | 1q32 | 5 bp Ins/del | The 5 bp (CTTCT) deletion in intron 3 of the TNNT2 gene at the polypyrimidine tract was found to affect the gene splicing and branch site selection | [10,19,20] |
| TTN | 2q31 | 18 bp Ins/del | This deletion is present within the PEVK region of titin gene that regulates the extensibility of the protein | [21,22] |
| Myospryn | 5q14.1 | K2906N | This polymorphism is associated with cardiac adaptation in response to pressure overload, left ventricular hypertrophy, and left ventricular diastolic dysfunction in hypertensive patients | [23] |

## 3. Sarcomeric Proteins

A sarcomere is the functional unit of striated muscle tissue. Skeletal muscles are composed of myocytes formed during myogenesis. Muscle fibers are composed of numerous tubular myofibrils. These myofibrils are a bundle of sarcomeres with repeating units, which appear as alternating dark and light bands under a microscope. Sarcomeric proteins drive muscle contraction and relaxation as these protein filaments slide past each other during these processes. The main components of sarcomere myofilament are actin, myosin, tropomyosin (Tm), and troponin complex (TnT, TnC, and TnI). Myosin protein present in the center of the sarcomere in the form of a thick filament, while actin is thin myofilament and overlaps with myosin. Titin protein's C-terminus attaches to M-line, while N-terminus attaches to Z-disc. Titin is anchored to Z-disc by attaching both actin and myosin proteins [24–27]. During muscle contraction, a conformational rearrangement in the troponin complex is generated by binding calcium ions to TnC, resulting in the movement of Tm, which provides a space for myosin binding on actin, leading to a cross-bridge creation with the help of energy provided by ATP. The contractility of muscles is regulated by calcium ion, which acts on the thin filament's receptor molecule troponin. Calcium ion is bounded to TnC that successively binds to TnI, releasing it from its inhibitory site on actin [ – ]. The details are shown in Figure 1.

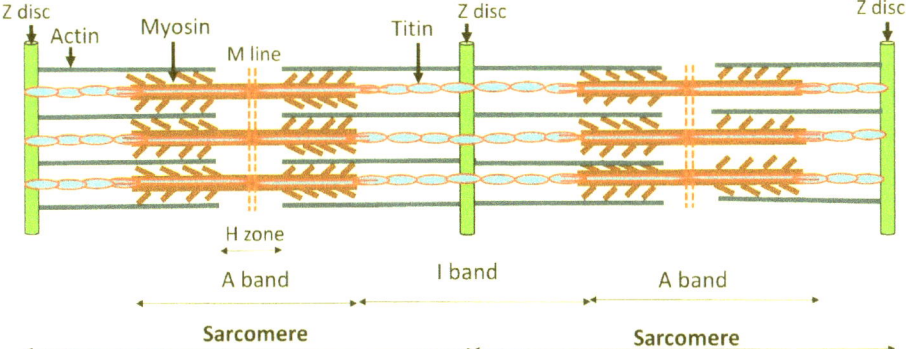

**Figure 1.** The location and arrangement of the thick and thin myofilament in the sarcomere.

*3.1. Myofilament Proteins*

Sarcomeres are in the form of thick and thin myofilament proteins. The thick filament is made up of C protein and myosin, while the thin filament is formed from actin, Tm, and troponin complex.

3.1.1. Myosin

Myosin is a motor molecule with actin myofilament, and generates force and motion. Myosin consists of two light chains (MLCs) and two heavy chains (MHCs) [ ]. Cardiac MHCs have two isoforms in mammals (α and β-isoform) [ ]. The α-isoform is related to better actomyosin ATPase activity than β-isoform. Thus, α-isoform has a fast-contractile velocity than β-isoform [ ].

MHCs' isoform expression is sensitive to hormonal changes and cardiovascular stress [ , ]. Isoform shift was observed in human failing myocardium [ , ]. An increase in β-isoform was observed in cardiomyopathy, thyroid depletion, aging, and pressure overload condition [ ]. In addition, mammalian myocardium normally primarily expresses α-isoform, but during experimental stimulation of heart failure, it shows upregulation of β-isoform and downregulation of α-isoform [ ]. A localized shift of α and β isoforms is noticed in tissues of human ventricles. There is a higher expression of α-isoform in the sub-epicardial than in the sub-endocardial layer [ ]. This localized shift of α and β isoforms is consistent with contraction duration and the shorter action potential in the sub-epicardium compared with sub-endocardium [ ]. About 80% of atria tissues, present in human ventricular tissues, consist of α-isoform [ ]. In atrial fibrillation, the β-isoform expression is approximately doubled [ ], and in failing ventricles, α-isoform expression is decreased [ ]. In sum, the MHC isoforms' transition may occur in human atrial and ventricular myocardial disease.

The β-myosin heavy chain (*MYH7*) gene is located on Chr. 14q11.2 and encodes the β isoform in the cardiac myosin heavy chain. Gene mutation in the *MYH7* gene leads to abnormal sarcomeric protein function. The deficiency or altered function of these proteins results in impaired muscle contraction, which results in heart failure [ , ].

3.1.2. Actin

Actin is essential for various cell functions. Actin isoforms in mammals are highly conserved. It consists of six isoforms encoded by six different genes. α-skeletal actin, α-cardiac actin, α-smooth actin, and γ-smooth actin are specific in their location and present in skeletal, cardiac, and smooth muscle, respectively. The other two isoforms, β-cyto actin and γ-cyto actin, are universally expressed in tissues [ ]. The delicate variations in ratios of actin isoform may lead to alterations in contractility [ ].

Additionally, evidence indicates that a reduction in cardiac contractility is associated with decreased expressions of α-cardiac isoform and aberrant expressions of γ-smooth isoform [47]. Humans generally have higher levels of α-skeletal isoform in the heart, compared to rats and mice [48].

### 3.1.3. Myospryn

In humans, myospryn protein is a large protein with 4069 amino acid residues (mol. wt. 449 kDa). The C-terminal portion of the protein is made up of approximately 570 amino acids and has tripartite motif (TRIM) proteins-like structure, while the rest of the protein consists of multiple glutamate-rich sequences. Based on this structure, myospryn has also been known as TRIM76 (HGNC Database 2008). Myospryn protein expression is restricted to cardiac and skeletal muscle only [49]. Myospryn protein is localized primarily in a Z-disc of sarcomere below the sarcolemma [50,51].

*Myospryn* gene is situated on Chr 5q14.1 and is related to Z-disc. The *Myospryn* gene is expressed in striated muscle cells, co-localized with the α-actinin sarcomeric protein. In the past, studies have reported an association of *Myospryn* K2906N (rs6859595) polymorphism with left ventricular hypertrophy, cardiac adaptation due to pressure overload [52], and LV diastolic dysfunction in hypertensive patients [23].

### 3.2. Regulatory Proteins

#### 3.2.1. Tropomyosin (Tm)

Tropomyosin is a major regulatory protein, present in a supercoiled form by wrapping around each other—a dimer of two α-helical coil chains. In cells, Tm-isoforms collectively regulate the functional role of actin filaments. Tm-isoforms have two types—(a) muscle Tm-isoforms and (b) non-muscle Tm-isoforms [53]. The interactions between actin and myosin are controlled by these Tm-isoforms and play a pivotal role in controlling $Ca^{++}$ sensitive regulation of contraction [54–56]. In humans, Tm-isoforms are encoded by four different genes (TPM1, TPM2, TPM3, and TPM4) [57]. α-Tm and κ-Tm from the *TPM1* gene, β-Tm from the *TPM2* gene, and γ-Tm transcribed from the *TPM3* gene are major Tm-isoforms present in human striated muscles. The ratio of β to α-Tm isomer varies from one species to another [58].

The Tm-isoform transition leads to cardiovascular disease. Purcell et al. reported that α-Tm isoform is exclusively expressed by failing heart ventricular muscles [59]. In the heart of chronic DCM patients was found increased expression of κ-Tm-isoform [60,61]. Tm-isoforms regulate cardiac contraction/relaxation, calcium sensitivity, and sarcomeric tension. Tm-isoform shifting potentially affects the overall cardiovascular system.

#### 3.2.2. Troponins

The troponin complex controls the interaction of actin and myosin in striated muscle in response to calcium. This complex contains three regulatory subunits: Troponin-C (TnC; calcium-binding protein), Troponin-I (TnI; inhibitory protein), and Troponin-T (TnT; tropomyosin binding protein).

Troponin-C (TnC): Troponin-C is expressed in cardiac and skeletal muscle and has two isoforms, encoded by genes (*TNNC1* and *TNNC2*). The two isoforms are slow skeleton TnC isoform (ssTnC), encoded by the *TNNC1* gene and expressed in slow muscles and heart muscles; and the fast-skeletal isoform (fsTnC), encoded by the *TNNC2* gene. ssTnC is referred to as cTnC in the heart. The ssTnC/cTnC isoform has been expressed in both developing and adult hearts [55,62].

Troponin-I (TnI): Troponin-I has three isoforms: (a) ssTnI (slow skeletal muscle), (b) fsTnI (fast skeletal muscle), and (c) cTnI isoform (cardiac muscle), encoded by *TNNI1*, *TNNI2*, and *TNNI3* genes, respectively. During development, the ssTnI:cTnI ratio is continuously decreased, and the adult heart has mostly cTnI isoform [63,64]. As the developed heart only expresses cTnI, it does not go through isoform switching under pathological conditions such as DCM, ischemic, and heart failure [65]. In adult transgenic mice, due to increased calcium sensitivity, slow TnI overexpression may impair relaxation and diastolic cardiac function [ ]. The cTnI knockout mice show developmental downregulation of ssTnI. TnI depletion changes the mechanical properties of the myocardium. Under relaxed conditions, the myocytes in ventricles show reduced sarcomeres, raised resting tension, and a decreased calcium sensitivity under activating conditions [ ].

Troponin-T (TnT): The Tn-t protein is present in three isoforms: slow skeletal isoform (ssTnT), fast skeletal isoform (fsTnT), and cardiac isoform (cTnT), encoded by these genes: TNNT1, TNNT3, and TNNT2, respectively [ , ]. The human heart possesses four common isoforms of cardiac Tn-T (cTnT) i.e., (cTnT1, cTnT2, cTnT3, and cTnT4). A normal adult heart expresses only cTnT3 isoform, while the failing adult heart, as well as the fetal heart, expresses the cTnT4 isoform [ ]. Unusual cTnT isoform expressions have been associated with heart ailments. An exon 4 skipped isoform was found highly expressed in failing human hearts [ ], and familial HCM human hearts [ ]. An over-expression of exon7-excluded cTnT isoform was observed by Craig et al. in a transgenic mouse heart leading to impaired systolic function [ ]. The heterogeneous group of TnT isoforms or co-presence of multiple TnT isoforms desynchronize the calcium activation of thin filaments, resulting in cardiac performance reduction [ ]. In comparison to wild–type controls, overexpression of one or more functionally different cardiac TnT isoforms in mice resulted in lower left ventricular pressure, declined stroke volume, and slower contractile and relaxation velocities. The author also suggests that co-expression of functionally distinct cTnT isoforms may impair cardiac function in adult ventricular muscle [ ].

Troponin T (TNNT2) Gene: TNNT2 gene is located on Chr. 1q32. and encodes a tropomyosin-binding subunit of the troponin complex. This protein is situated on the thin filament of striated muscles and controls muscle contractility in response to $Ca^{++}$ signals. Mutations in the TNNT2 gene have been positively associated with DCM and familial HCM [ , , ]. It has been reported that a 5-bp (CTTCT) I/ D polymorphism present in intron 3 of the TNNT2 gene may impair the skipping of exon 4 and lead to LVD [ , , ].

### 3.3. Sarcomeric Cytoskeletal Proteins

Cytoskeletal proteins provide mechanical resistance, morphological integrity, and play a major role in maintaining the cell shape of cardiomyocytes. Titin, α-actinin, myomesin, myosin-binding protein C (MyBP-C), and M-protein are the main constituent proteins of this group [ ].

#### 3.3.1. Titin Protein and Associated Gene Polymorphism

Titin is also known as connectin and encoded by the TTN gene, which is located on Chr. 2q31. It is a giant muscle protein of striated muscles that act as a molecular spring and are responsible for passive elasticity. Like a spring, it provides the force to control sarcomere contraction and signaling [ , – ]. Titin is the third most abundant protein in cardiac muscle, after myosin and actin. It spans half of the sarcomere and connects M-line to Z-line. It is the key determinant of myocardial passive tension and plays an important role in the elasticity of cardiac myocytes. These proteins also contribute to the diastolic function of LV filling. Titin consists of two types of protein domains: 1) fibronectin type III domain and 2) immunoglobulin domain. The N-terminal of titin is located in the I-band and connected to Z-disc, and have elastic property. This I-band elastic region has a spring-like PEVK segment, rich in proline, glutamate, valine, and lysine [ – , , ].

A single gene encodes three major isoforms of titin through alternative splicing [ , ]. Change in ratios of cardiac titin isoforms has been associated with cardiovascular disease. Itoh-Satoh et al. found four possible DCM-associated mutations. The mutated gene expresses a non-functional titin protein that is unable to rotate half sarcomere and decreases binding affinities to Z-line proteins [ ]. A familial DCM locus maps to Chr. 2q31 and causes early-onset congestive heart failure (CHF) [ ]. RNA binding motif 20 (Rbm20) is a muscle-specific splicing factor, regulating alternative splicing of titin [ ]. The Rbm20 knockout rats express a most compliant titin isoform that causes DCM [ , ]. This mutation is associated with the expression of a larger, compliant fetal cardiac titin isoform in severe DCM patients [ ].

An 18 bp (TTTTCCTCTTCAGGAGCAA/T) I/D polymorphism falls within the PEVK region that controls the contractile nature of titin. It was previously reported that mutations in the *TTN* gene have been related to different forms of cardiomyopathy, including HCM, DCM, and arrhythmogenic right ventricular cardiomyopathy (ARVC) [9,21,22].

3.3.2. Myosin-Binding Protein C (Mybp-C) and Associated Gene Polymorphism

MyBP-C is a thick filament-associated striated muscle protein situated in the C zones cross-bridge of A-bands and binds to titin and myosin. MyBP-C and titin collectively form a firm ternary complex, where titin act as a molecular ruler and MyBP-C as a regulatory protein [85–87]. In the adult heart, MyBP-C is present in three isoforms in striated muscles, while skeletal muscle expresses only two isoforms. The fsMyBP-C is the fast-skeletal isoform encoded by the gene *MYBPC2* in humans. In humans, MYBPC1 encodes for ssMyBP-C, the slow form of skeletal muscle [88] while *MYBPC3* encodes for human cardiac MyBP-C (cMyBP-C) [89]. In the same sarcomere, fsMyBP-C and ssMyBP-C isoforms can be expressed simultaneously [90] and the diverse arrangements of the specific sarcomere bands are due to the co-existence of fsMyBP-C and ssMyBP-C in variable proportions [91]. The cMyBP-C isoform is found only in cardiac muscle and cannot be trans-complemented by skeletal MyBP-Cs [92].

The *MYBPC3* gene located on Chr. 11p11.2 and mutations in this gene were reported in HCM and DCM patients [17,93–95]. In 2–6% of Southeast Asian populations, *MYBPC3* 25 bp deletion, located in intron 32 at 3′ region of the gene is noted and associated with a high risk of LVD (left ventricular ejection fraction < 45). This 25-bp intronic deletion results in exon 33 skipping and incorporated missense amino acids at the C-terminal of the protein [14,18]. Incorporation of this mutated protein in myofibrils [14] may cause sarcomere breakdown. Moreover, authors have reported through a protein model that this deletion disrupts the α-helical stretch in the cMyBP-C and an additional α-helix and β-pleated sheets are incorporated in the mutated protein. As the cMyBP-C protein directly binds a subset of Ig domains with titin and myosin through its C8, C9, and C10 domains, any conformational changes in the mutated protein may cause alterations in conformation or direction of the C10 domain. Thus, the inability of myosin binding may have severe effects on sarcomeric organization, suggesting its involvement in the morphological and functional changes of cardiac muscle.

The pathophysiology of cardiac muscles due to truncated and missense MyBP-C has been explained by other mechanisms as well. Due to these mutations, MyBP-C3 mRNA may undergo nonsense-mediated mRNA decay (NMD), which disrupts its proteins through the UPS and may result in cardiac dysfunction [96]. UPS functions also decline with high oxidative stress and the age of an individual. Further, mutated protein may accumulate and disturb cellular homeostasis, and can initiate LVD [97,98]. This deletion polymorphism is also associated with other parameters of LV remodeling, i.e., LV dimensions (LV end-systolic and diastole dimension). This deletion may play an important role in conferring LVD risk in Southeast Asian populations and can be used as an early risk predictor [15].

The *MYBPC3* 25-bp deletion polymorphism is quite common with varied frequency in South Asian inhabitants. Studies have suggested that this deletion might have not been present in initial settlers who arrived 50000 to 20000 years ago from Africa, but might have surfaced later in India. The high frequency of this deleterious mutation is somewhat surprising. It has been suggested that with carrier frequency of 2–8% gradation from North to South India, this variation may contribute significantly to the burden of cardiac diseases in the subcontinent [14,99,100].

4. Common Sarcomeric Variants Reported with LVD

Studies have reported numerous genetic variants that play a vital role in the pathophysiology of left ventricular dysfunction [15,16,101]. Previously, the *TTN* and *TNNT2* gene variants were studied with various cardiac remodeling phenotypes. Mutation in the *TTN* and *TNNT2* genes were associated with different phenotypes of cardiac remodeling. In intron 3 of the *TNNT2* gene, a 5bp I/D polymorphism is associated with cardiac hypertrophy [20]. The DD genotype is associated with wall thickening of the ventricles and a greater LV mass in the hypertrophy population. Farza et al., however, observed no clinical importance of this variant in cardiac hypertrophy [ ]. Rani et al. observed that 5bp deletion in this polymorphism leads to exon 4 skipping at the time of splicing, and is present in a significantly high concentration in HCM patients [ ]. Nakagami et al. observed an association between cardiac hypertrophy and myospryn polymorphisms. Authors have reported that in the *Myospryn* gene, AA genotype of K2906N polymorphism plays a risk allele for left ventricular diastolic dysfunction in hypertensive patients [ ]. Kumar et al. conducted a case-control study to explore the association of MYBPC3, titin, troponin T2, and myosporin gene deletion polymorphisms. A total of 988 angiographically proved CAD patients and 300 healthy controls were enrolled in this study. Of the 988 CAD patients, 253 were categorized as LVD with reduced left ventricular ejection fraction (LVEF $\leq$ 45%). The study concluded that there is a significant association of MYBPC3 25-bp deletion polymorphism with elevated risk of LVD (LVEF < 45) (healthy controls v/s LVD: OR = 3.85, $p$ value < 0.001; and non-LVD v/s LVD: OR = 1.65, $p$ value = 0.035), while the other three studied polymorphisms (Myosporin, TNNT2, TTN) do not seem to play a direct role in LVD as well as CAD risk in north Indians [ , , , ].

Several truncated and missense mutations were reported in MyBP-C, which generates poison peptides and haplo-insufficiency. Due to these mutations, MyBP-C3 mRNA may undergo nonsense-mediated mRNA decay (NMD), which disrupts its proteins through the UPS and may result in cardiac dysfunction [ ]. UPS function also declines with high oxidative stress and age. Further, the mutated protein may accumulate and disturb cellular homeostasis and initiate LVD [ , ]. During adrenergic stimulation, cardiac contractility is regulated by MyBP-C. With the help of cyclic AMP-dependent protein kinase and calcium/calmodulin-dependent protein kinase II, MyBP-C goes through reversible phosphorylation [ , ]. A 25-bp deletion in the MyBP-C3 gene causes severe ischemic damage to the cardiac muscle and can develop severe LVD in CAD patients who carry this deletion [ ]. In the South Asian population, this 25 bp deletion is relatively common. Analysis of this deletion in different subgroups based on LV ejection fraction (LVEF) shows a significant association of this polymorphism with severe LVD. Patients with LVEF (30–40%) and below 30% have a higher percentage of this deletion genotype. Additionally, this deletion polymorphism is also associated with echocardiogram results such as LV systolic and end-diastolic dimension. To rule out the possibilities of the development of LVD in CAD patients due to confounding factors such as diabetes, smoking, hypertension, and ST-elevation myocardial infarction, the authors performed a multivariate analysis, which shows that the above-stated association was only due to this 25 bp deletion only. This deletion may be responsible, for the development of LVD in CAD patients [ ], alone or in combination with hypertension. Based on the above discussion, we proposed a model for left ventricular dysfunction (LVD)/heart failure (Figure ).

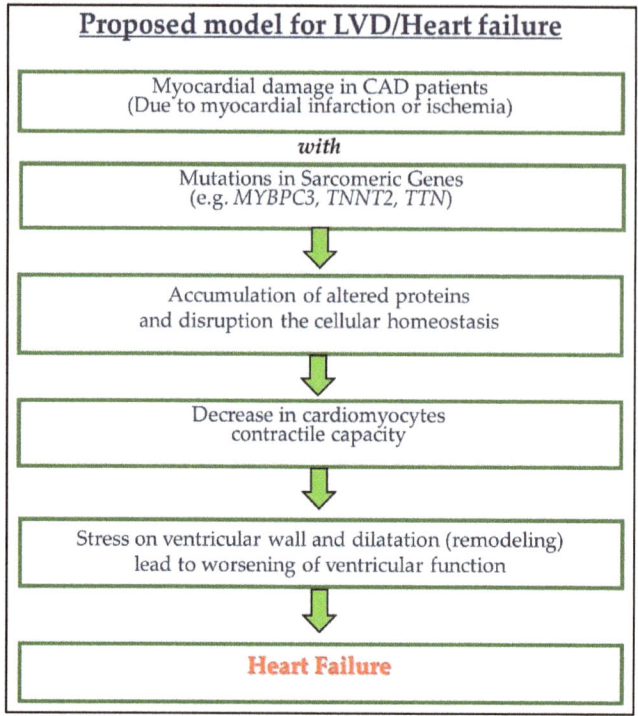

**Figure 2.** A model for left ventricular dysfunction (LVD)/heart failure. Coronary artery disease (CAD).

## 5. Conclusions

It is well established that left ventricular dysfunction is a complex condition, caused by numerous factors—mechanical, neurohormonal, and genetic. Some potential modifiers are shown in Table 2. Sarcomeric genes [15,16], matrix metalloproteinases (MMPs) [106], renin-angiotensin-aldosterone system (RAAS) [101], and inflammatory pathway genes [107] was previously associated with left ventricular dysfunction. In complex diseases, most genetic variants are known to exert minor, but significant effects on disease phenotype. It may be worthy to perform genome-wide association studies to identify novel loci, which may have a vital impact on the development of LVD. Moreover, it is suggested that large, well-designed association studies with functional studies for validation are conducted to establish the combined roles of SNPs in the predisposition and severity of the disease. Moreover, it is important to identify and validate novel mutations in sarcomeric genes using next-generation sequencing and microarrays methods for a complete analysis of genes involved in LVD.

**Table 2.** Potential modifier of Left Ventricular Dysfunction (LVD).

| Common Factors | Effect | Ref. |
|---|---|---|
| **Environmental Risk Factors** | | |
| Age | Higher in older patients | [ ] |
| Gender | More in men | [ ] |
| Ethnicity | High in African Athletes | [ ] |
| Smoking status | Higher in smoker patients | [ ] |
| Obesity | Higher in obese patients | [ ] |
| Hypertension | Higher in hypertensive patients | [ ] |
| Coronary artery disease | Higher in CAD patients | [ ] |
| Renal disease | Higher in CKD patients | [ ] |
| **Genetic Risk Factors** | | |
| Sarcomeric gene mutations–*MYBPC3, TNNT2, TTN, MYH7, Myospryn*, etc. | ↑ ventricular remodeling and LVD | [ , ] |
| Renin–Angiotensin–Aldosterone System (RAAS) pathway–*ACE* and *AT1* Gene | ↑ ventricular remodeling and LVD | [ , ] |
| Matrix Metalloproteinase (MMPs)–*MMP2, MMP7* and *MMP9* | ↑ LVD | [ , ] |
| Adrenergic pathway–*ADRB1, ADRA2A, ADRB3* | ↑ ventricular remodeling and LVD | [ ] |
| Inflammatory pathway–*NFKB1, IL6*, and *TNF-α* | ↑ ventricular remodeling and LVD | [ , ] |

Coronary artery disease (CAD); Chronic kidney disease (CKD); Left ventricle dysfunction (LVD).

**Author Contributions:** Conceptualization, S.K., V.K.; methodology, S.K., V.K.; writing—original draft preparation, S.K., V.K.; writing—review and editing J.-J.K., S.K., V.K. All authors have read and agreed to the published version of the manuscript.

**Funding:** This research did not receive any specific grants from funding agencies in the public, commercial, or not-for-profit sectors.

**Conflicts of Interest:** The authors declare no conflict of interest.

# References

1. Ghai, A.; Silversides, C.; Harris, L.; Webb, G.D.; Siu, S.C.; Therrien, J. Left ventricular dysfunction is a risk factor for sudden cardiac death in adults late after repair of tetralogy of Fallot. *J. Am. Coll. Cardiol.* **2002**, *40*, 1675–1680. [ ]
2. McMurray, J.J.; Ezekowitz, J.A.; Lewis, B.S.; Gersh, B.J.; van Diepen, S.; Amerena, J.; Bartunek, J.; Commerford, P.; Oh, B.H.; Harjola, V.P.; et al. Left ventricular systolic dysfunction, heart failure, and the risk of stroke and systemic embolism in patients with atrial fibrillation: Insights from the ARISTOTLE trial. *Circ. Heart Fail.* **2013**, *6*, 451–460. [ ] [ ]
3. Al-Khatib, S.M.; Stevenson, W.G.; Ackerman, M.J.; Bryant, W.J.; Callans, D.J.; Curtis, A.B.; Deal, B.J.; Dickfeld, T.; Field, M.E.; Fonarow, G.C.; et al. 2017 AHA/ACC/HRS Guideline for Management of Patients With Ventricular Arrhythmias and the Prevention of Sudden Cardiac Death. *Circulation* **2018**, *138*, e272–e391.
4. Stevens, S.M.; Reinier, K.; Chugh, S.S. Increased left ventricular mass as a predictor of sudden cardiac death: Is it time to put it to the test? *Circ. Arrhythm. Electrophysiol.* **2013**, *6*, 212–217. [ ] [ ]
5. Chonchol, M.; Goldenberg, I.; Moss, A.J.; McNitt, S.; Cheung, A.K. Risk factors for sudden cardiac death in patients with chronic renal insufficiency and left ventricular dysfunction. *Am. J. Nephrol.* **2007**, *27*, 7–14. [ ]
6. Benito, B.; Josephson, M.E. Ventricular tachycardia in coronary artery disease. *Rev. Esp. Cardiol.* **2012**, *65*, 939–955. [ ] [ ]
7. Mestroni, L.; Brun, F.; Spezzacatene, A.; Sinagra, G.; Taylor, M.R. Genetic Causes of Dilated Cardiomyopathy. *Prog. Pediatr. Cardiol.* **2014**, *37*, 13–18. [ ]

8. Favalli, V.; Serio, A.; Grasso, M.; Arbustini, E. Genetic causes of dilated cardiomyopathy. *Heart* **2016**, *102*, 2004–2014. [CrossRef]
9. McNally, E.M.; Mestroni, L. Dilated Cardiomyopathy: Genetic Determinants and Mechanisms. *Circ. Res.* **2017**, *121*, 731–748. [CrossRef]
10. Mattos, B.P.; Scolari, F.L.; Torres, M.A.; Simon, L.; Freitas, V.C.; Giugliani, R.; Matte, U. Prevalence and Phenotypic Expression of Mutations in the MYH7, MYBPC3 and TNNT2 Genes in Families with Hypertrophic Cardiomyopathy in the South of Brazil: A Cross-Sectional Study. *Arq. Bras. Cardiol.* **2016**, *107*, 257–265. [CrossRef]
11. Rafael, J.F.; Cruz, F.F.; Carvalho, A.C.C.; Gottlieb, I.; Cazelli, J.G.; Siciliano, A.P.; Dias, G.M. Myosin-binding Protein C Compound Heterozygous Variant Effect on the Phenotypic Expression of Hypertrophic Cardiomyopathy. *Arq. Bras. Cardiol.* **2017**, *108*, 354–360. [CrossRef] [PubMed]
12. Bienengraeber, M.; Olson, T.M.; Selivanov, V.A.; Kathmann, E.C.; O'Cochlain, F.; Gao, F.; Karger, A.B.; Ballew, J.D.; Hodgson, D.M.; Zingman, L.V.; et al. ABCC9 mutations identified in human dilated cardiomyopathy disrupt catalytic KATP channel gating. *Nat. Genet.* **2004**, *36*, 382–387. [CrossRef] [PubMed]
13. Kimura, A. Molecular basis of hereditary cardiomyopathy: Abnormalities in calcium sensitivity, stretch response, stress response and beyond. *J. Hum. Genet.* **2010**, *55*, 81–90. [CrossRef]
14. Dhandapany, P.S.; Sadayappan, S.; Xue, Y.; Powell, G.T.; Rani, D.S.; Nallari, P.; Rai, T.S.; Khullar, M.; Soares, P.; Bahl, A.; et al. A common MYBPC3 (cardiac myosin binding protein C) variant associated with cardiomyopathies in South Asia. *Nat. Genet.* **2009**, *41*, 187–191. [CrossRef] [PubMed]
15. Kumar, S.; Mishra, A.; Srivastava, A.; Bhatt, M.; Garg, N.; Agarwal, S.K.; Pande, S.; Mittal, B. Role of common sarcomeric gene polymorphisms in genetic susceptibility to left ventricular dysfunction. *J. Genet.* **2016**, *95*, 263–272. [CrossRef]
16. Srivastava, A.; Garg, N.; Mittal, T.; Khanna, R.; Gupta, S.; Seth, P.K.; Mittal, B. Association of 25 bp deletion in MYBPC3 gene with left ventricle dysfunction in coronary artery disease patients. *PLoS ONE* **2011**, *6*, e24123. [CrossRef]
17. Tanjore, R.R.; Rangaraju, A.; Kerkar, P.G.; Calambur, N.; Nallari, P. MYBPC3 gene variations in hypertrophic cardiomyopathy patients in India. *Can. J. Cardiol.* **2008**, *24*, 127–130. [CrossRef]
18. Waldmuller, S.; Sakthivel, S.; Saadi, A.V.; Selignow, C.; Rakesh, P.G.; Golubenko, M.; Joseph, P.K.; Padmakumar, R.; Richard, P.; Schwartz, K.; et al. Novel deletions in MYH7 and MYBPC3 identified in Indian families with familial hypertrophic cardiomyopathy. *J. Mol. Cell Cardiol.* **2003**, *35*, 623–636. [CrossRef]
19. Rani, D.S.; Nallari, P.; Dhandapany, P.S.; Tamilarasi, S.; Shah, A.; Archana, V.; AshokKumar, M.; Narasimhan, C.; Singh, L.; Thangaraj, K. Cardiac Troponin T (TNNT2) mutations are less prevalent in Indian hypertrophic cardiomyopathy patients. *DNA Cell Biol.* **2012**, *31*, 616–624. [CrossRef]
20. Komamura, K.; Iwai, N.; Kokame, K.; Yasumura, Y.; Kim, J.; Yamagishi, M.; Morisaki, T.; Kimura, A.; Tomoike, H.; Kitakaze, M.; et al. The role of a common TNNT2 polymorphism in cardiac hypertrophy. *J. Hum. Genet.* **2004**, *49*, 129–133. [CrossRef]
21. Bang, M.L.; Centner, T.; Fornoff, F.; Geach, A.J.; Gotthardt, M.; McNabb, M.; Witt, C.C.; Labeit, D.; Gregorio, C.C.; Granzier, H.; et al. The complete gene sequence of titin, expression of an unusual approximately 700-kDa titin isoform, and its interaction with obscurin identify a novel Z-line to I-band linking system. *Circ. Res.* **2001**, *89*, 1065–1072. [CrossRef]
22. Granzier, H.L.; Radke, M.H.; Peng, J.; Westermann, D.; Nelson, O.L.; Rost, K.; King, N.M.; Yu, Q.; Tschope, C.; McNabb, M.; et al. Truncation of titin's elastic PEVK region leads to cardiomyopathy with diastolic dysfunction. *Circ. Res.* **2009**, *105*, 557–564. [CrossRef] [PubMed]
23. Nakagami, H.; Kikuchi, Y.; Katsuya, T.; Morishita, R.; Akasaka, H.; Saitoh, S.; Rakugi, H.; Kaneda, Y.; Shimamoto, K.; Ogihara, T. Gene polymorphism of myospryn (cardiomyopathy-associated 5) is associated with left ventricular wall thickness in patients with hypertension. *Hypertens. Res.* **2007**, *30*, 1239–1246. [CrossRef] [PubMed]
24. Gregorio, C.C.; Trombitas, K.; Centner, T.; Kolmerer, B.; Stier, G.; Kunke, K.; Suzuki, K.; Obermayr, F.; Herrmann, B.; Granzier, H.; et al. The NH2 terminus of titin spans the Z-disc: Its interaction with a novel 19-kD ligand (T-cap) is required for sarcomeric integrity. *J. Cell Biol.* **1998**, *143*, 1013–1027. [CrossRef] [PubMed]

25. Guo, W.; Bharmal, S.J.; Esbona, K.; Greaser, M.L. Titin diversity–alternative splicing gone wild. *J. Biomed. Biotechnol.* **2010**, *2010*, 753675. [CrossRef]
26. Dos Remedios, C.; Gilmour, D. An historical perspective of the discovery of titin filaments. *Biophys. Rev.* **2017**, *9*, 179–188. [CrossRef]
27. Gonzalez-Morales, N.; Holenka, T.K.; Schock, F. Filamin actin-binding and titin-binding fulfill distinct functions in Z-disc cohesion. *PLoS Genet.* **2017**, *13*, e1006880. [CrossRef]
28. Gordon, A.M.; Homsher, E.; Regnier, M. Regulation of contraction in striated muscle. *Physiol. Rev.* **2000**, *80*, 853–924. [CrossRef]
29. Hamdani, N.; Kooij, V.; van Dijk, S.; Merkus, D.; Paulus, W.J.; Remedios, C.D.; Duncker, D.J.; Stienen, G.J.; van der Velden, J. Sarcomeric dysfunction in heart failure. *Cardiovasc. Res.* **2008**, *77*, 649–658. [CrossRef]
30. Tskhovrebova, L.; Trinick, J. Roles of titin in the structure and elasticity of the sarcomere. *J. Biomed. Biotechnol.* **2010**, *2010*, 612482. [CrossRef]
31. Rall, J.A. What makes skeletal muscle striated? Discoveries in the endosarcomeric and exosarcomeric cytoskeleton. *Adv. Physiol. Educ.* **2018**, *42*, 672–684. [CrossRef] [PubMed]
32. Rayment, I.; Holden, H.M.; Whittaker, M.; Yohn, C.B.; Lorenz, M.; Holmes, K.C.; Milligan, R.A. Structure of the actin-myosin complex and its implications for muscle contraction. *Science* **1993**, *261*, 58–65. [CrossRef] [PubMed]
33. Yamauchi-Takihara, K.; Sole, M.J.; Liew, J.; Ing, D.; Liew, C.C. Characterization of human cardiac myosin heavy chain genes. *Proc. Natl. Acad. Sci. USA* **1989**, *86*, 3504–3508. [CrossRef]
34. Holubarsch, C.; Goulette, R.P.; Litten, R.Z.; Martin, B.J.; Mulieri, L.A.; Alpert, N.R. The economy of isometric force development, myosin isoenzyme pattern and myofibrillar ATPase activity in normal and hypothyroid rat myocardium. *Circ. Res.* **1985**, *56*, 78–86. [CrossRef] [PubMed]
35. Allen, D.L.; Leinwand, L.A. Postnatal myosin heavy chain isoform expression in normal mice and mice null for IIb or IId myosin heavy chains. *Dev. Biol.* **2001**, *229*, 383–395. [CrossRef]
36. Lowes, B.D.; Minobe, W.; Abraham, W.T.; Rizeq, M.N.; Bohlmeyer, T.J.; Quaife, R.A.; Roden, R.L.; Dutcher, D.L.; Robertson, A.D.; Voelkel, N.F.; et al. Changes in gene expression in the intact human heart. Downregulation of alpha-myosin heavy chain in hypertrophied, failing ventricular myocardium. *J. Clin. Invest.* **1997**, *100*, 2315–2324. [CrossRef]
37. Miyata, S.; Minobe, W.; Bristow, M.R.; Leinwand, L.A. Myosin heavy chain isoform expression in the failing and nonfailing human heart. *Circ. Res.* **2000**, *86*, 386–390. [CrossRef]
38. Lompre, A.M.; Schwartz, K.; d'Albis, A.; Lacombe, G.; Van Thiem, N.; Swynghedauw, B. Myosin isoenzyme redistribution in chronic heart overload. *Nature* **1979**, *282*, 105–107. [CrossRef]
39. Swynghedauw, B. Developmental and functional adaptation of contractile proteins in cardiac and skeletal muscles. *Physiol. Rev.* **1986**, *66*, 710–771. [CrossRef]
40. Takahashi, T.; Schunkert, H.; Isoyama, S.; Wei, J.Y.; Nadal-Ginard, B.; Grossman, W.; Izumo, S. Age-related differences in the expression of proto-oncogene and contractile protein genes in response to pressure overload in the rat myocardium. *J. Clin. Invest.* **1992**, *89*, 939–946. [CrossRef]
41. Herron, T.J.; McDonald, K.S. Small amounts of alpha-myosin heavy chain isoform expression significantly increase power output of rat cardiac myocyte fragments. *Circ. Res.* **2002**, *90*, 1150–1152. [CrossRef]
42. Reiser, P.J.; Portman, M.A.; Ning, X.H.; Schomisch Moravec, C. Human cardiac myosin heavy chain isoforms in fetal and failing adult atria and ventricles. *Am. J. Physiol. Heart Circ. Physiol.* **2001**, *280*, H1814–H1820. [CrossRef]
43. Eiras, S.; Narolska, N.A.; van Loon, R.B.; Boontje, N.M.; Zaremba, R.; Jimenez, C.R.; Visser, F.C.; Stooker, W.; van der Velden, J.; Stienen, G.J. Alterations in contractile protein composition and function in human atrial dilatation and atrial fibrillation. *J. Mol. Cell Cardiol.* **2006**, *41*, 467–477. [CrossRef]
44. Meredith, C.; Herrmann, R.; Parry, C.; Liyanage, K.; Dye, D.E.; Durling, H.J.; Duff, R.M.; Beckman, K.; de Visser, M.; van der Graaff, M.M.; et al. Mutations in the slow skeletal muscle fiber myosin heavy chain gene (MYH7) cause laing early-onset distal myopathy (MPD1). *Am. J. Hum. Genet.* **2004**, *75*, 703–708. [CrossRef]
45. Darin, N.; Tajsharghi, H.; Ostman-Smith, I.; Gilljam, T.; Oldfors, A. New skeletal myopathy and cardiomyopathy associated with a missense mutation in MYH7. *Neurology* **2007**, *68*, 2041–2042. [CrossRef]
46. Suurmeijer, A.J.; Clement, S.; Francesconi, A.; Bocchi, L.; Angelini, A.; Van Veldhuisen, D.J.; Spagnoli, L.G.; Gabbiani, G.; Orlandi, A. Alpha-actin isoform distribution in normal and failing human heart: A morphological, morphometric, and biochemical study. *J. Pathol.* **2003**, *199*, 387–397. [CrossRef]

47. Kumar, A.; Crawford, K.; Flick, R.; Klevitsky, R.; Lorenz, J.N.; Bove, K.E.; Robbins, J.; Lessard, J.L. Transgenic overexpression of cardiac actin in the mouse heart suggests coregulation of cardiac, skeletal and vascular actin expression. *Transgenic Res.* **2004**, *13*, 531–540. [CrossRef]
48. Boheler, K.R.; Carrier, L.; de la Bastie, D.; Allen, P.D.; Komajda, M.; Mercadier, J.J.; Schwartz, K. Skeletal actin mRNA increases in the human heart during ontogenic development and is the major isoform of control and failing adult hearts. *J. Clin. Invest.* **1991**, *88*, 323–330. [CrossRef]
49. Benson, M.A.; Tinsley, C.L.; Blake, D.J. Myospryn is a novel binding partner for dysbindin in muscle. *J. Biol. Chem.* **2004**, *279*, 10450–10458. [CrossRef]
50. Durham, J.T.; Brand, O.M.; Arnold, M.; Reynolds, J.G.; Muthukumar, L.; Weiler, H.; Richardson, J.A.; Naya, F.J. Myospryn is a direct transcriptional target for MEF2A that encodes a striated muscle, alpha-actinin-interacting, costamere-localized protein. *J. Biol. Chem.* **2006**, *281*, 6841–6849. [CrossRef]
51. Kouloumenta, A.; Mavroidis, M.; Capetanaki, Y. Proper perinuclear localization of the TRIM-like protein myospryn requires its binding partner desmin. *J. Biol. Chem.* **2007**, *282*, 35211–35221. [CrossRef]
52. Kielbasa, O.M.; Reynolds, J.G.; Wu, C.L.; Snyder, C.M.; Cho, M.Y.; Weiler, H.; Kandarian, S.; Naya, F.J. Myospryn is a calcineurin-interacting protein that negatively modulates slow-fiber-type transformation and skeletal muscle regeneration. *FASEB J.* **2011**, *25*, 2276–2286. [CrossRef]
53. Pittenger, M.F.; Kazzaz, J.A.; Helfman, D.M. Functional properties of non-muscle tropomyosin isoforms. *Curr. Opin. Cell Biol.* **1994**, *6*, 96–104. [CrossRef]
54. Janco, M.; Suphamungmee, W.; Li, X.; Lehman, W.; Lehrer, S.S.; Geeves, M.A. Polymorphism in tropomyosin structure and function. *J. Muscle Res. Cell Motil.* **2013**, *34*, 177–187. [CrossRef]
55. Murakami, K.; Yumoto, F.; Ohki, S.Y.; Yasunaga, T.; Tanokura, M.; Wakabayashi, T. Structural basis for Ca2+-regulated muscle relaxation at interaction sites of troponin with actin and tropomyosin. *J. Mol. Biol.* **2005**, *352*, 178–201. [CrossRef]
56. Pathan-Chhatbar, S.; Taft, M.H.; Reindl, T.; Hundt, N.; Latham, S.L.; Manstein, D.J. Three mammalian tropomyosin isoforms have different regulatory effects on nonmuscle myosin-2B and filamentous beta-actin in vitro. *J. Biol. Chem.* **2018**, *293*, 863–875. [CrossRef]
57. Perry, S.V. Vertebrate tropomyosin: Distribution, properties and function. *J. Muscle Res. Cell Motil.* **2001**, *22*, 5–49. [CrossRef]
58. Denz, C.R.; Narshi, A.; Zajdel, R.W.; Dube, D.K. Expression of a novel cardiac-specific tropomyosin isoform in humans. *Biochem. Biophys. Res. Commun.* **2004**, *320*, 1291–1297. [CrossRef]
59. Purcell, I.F.; Bing, W.; Marston, S.B. Functional analysis of human cardiac troponin by the in vitro motility assay: Comparison of adult, foetal and failing hearts. *Cardiovasc. Res.* **1999**, *43*, 884–891. [CrossRef]
60. Karam, C.N.; Warren, C.M.; Rajan, S.; de Tombe, P.P.; Wieczorek, D.F.; Solaro, R.J. Expression of tropomyosin-kappa induces dilated cardiomyopathy and depresses cardiac myofilament tension by mechanisms involving cross-bridge dependent activation and altered tropomyosin phosphorylation. *J. Muscle Res. Cell Motil.* **2011**, *31*, 315–322. [CrossRef]
61. Rajan, S.; Jagatheesan, G.; Karam, C.N.; Alves, M.L.; Bodi, I.; Schwartz, A.; Bulcao, C.F.; D'Souza, K.M.; Akhter, S.A.; Boivin, G.P.; et al. Molecular and functional characterization of a novel cardiac-specific human tropomyosin isoform. *Circulation* **2010**, *121*, 410–418. [CrossRef]
62. Filatov, V.L.; Katrukha, A.G.; Bulargina, T.V.; Gusev, N.B. Troponin: Structure, properties, and mechanism of functioning. *Biochemistry* **1999**, *64*, 969–985. [PubMed]
63. Wilkinson, J.M.; Grand, R.J. Comparison of amino acid sequence of troponin I from different striated muscles. *Nature* **1978**, *271*, 31–35. [CrossRef]
64. Wade, R.; Eddy, R.; Shows, T.B.; Kedes, L. cDNA sequence, tissue-specific expression, and chromosomal mapping of the human slow-twitch skeletal muscle isoform of troponin I. *Genomics* **1990**, *7*, 346–357. [CrossRef]
65. Sasse, S.; Brand, N.J.; Kyprianou, P.; Dhoot, G.K.; Wade, R.; Arai, M.; Periasamy, M.; Yacoub, M.H.; Barton, P.J. Troponin I gene expression during human cardiac development and in end-stage heart failure. *Circ. Res.* **1993**, *72*, 932–938. [CrossRef]
66. Fentzke, R.C.; Buck, S.H.; Patel, J.R.; Lin, H.; Wolska, B.M.; Stojanovic, M.O.; Martin, A.F.; Solaro, R.J.; Moss, R.L.; Leiden, J.M. Impaired cardiomyocyte relaxation and diastolic function in transgenic mice expressing slow skeletal troponin I in the heart. *J. Physiol.* **1999**, *517*((Pt. 1)), 143–157. [CrossRef]

67. Huang, X.; Pi, Y.; Lee, K.J.; Henkel, A.S.; Gregg, R.G.; Powers, P.A.; Walker, J.W. Cardiac troponin I gene knockout: A mouse model of myocardial troponin I deficiency. *Circ. Res.* **1999**, *84*, 1–8. [CrossRef]
68. Sheng, J.J.; Jin, J.P. Gene regulation, alternative splicing, and posttranslational modification of troponin subunits in cardiac development and adaptation: A focused review. *Front. Physiol.* **2014**, *5*, 165. [CrossRef]
69. Samson, F.; Mesnard, L.; Mihovilovic, M.; Potter, T.G.; Mercadier, J.J.; Roses, A.D.; Gilbert, J.R. A new human slow skeletal troponin T (TnTs) mRNA isoform derived from alternative splicing of a single gene. *Biochem. Biophys. Res. Commun.* **1994**, *199*, 841–847. [CrossRef]
70. Anderson, P.A.; Malouf, N.N.; Oakeley, A.E.; Pagani, E.D.; Allen, P.D. Troponin T isoform expression in humans. A comparison among normal and failing adult heart, fetal heart, and adult and fetal skeletal muscle. *Circ. Res.* **1991**, *69*, 1226–1233. [CrossRef]
71. Thierfelder, L.; Watkins, H.; MacRae, C.; Lamas, R.; McKenna, W.; Vosberg, H.P.; Seidman, J.G.; Seidman, C.E. Alpha-tropomyosin and cardiac troponin T mutations cause familial hypertrophic cardiomyopathy: A disease of the sarcomere. *Cell* **1994**, *77*, 701–712. [CrossRef]
72. Craig, R.; Offer, G. The location of C-protein in rabbit skeletal muscle. *Proc. R Soc. Lond. B. Biol. Sci.* **1976**, *192*, 451–461. [PubMed]
73. Wakabayashi, T. Mechanism of the calcium-regulation of muscle contraction–in pursuit of its structural basis. *Proc. Jpn. Acad. Ser. B Phys. Biol. Sci.* **2015**, *91*, 321–350. [CrossRef] [PubMed]
74. Li, Y.D.; Ji, Y.T.; Zhou, X.H.; Li, H.L.; Zhang, H.T.; Xing, Q.; Hong, Y.F.; Tang, B.P. TNNT2 Gene Polymorphisms are Associated with Susceptibility to Idiopathic Dilated Cardiomyopathy in Kazak and Han Chinese. *Med. Sci. Monit.* **2015**, *21*, 3343–3347. [CrossRef]
75. Ripoll-Vera, T.; Gamez, J.M.; Govea, N.; Gomez, Y.; Nunez, J.; Socias, L.; Escandell, A.; Rosell, J. Clinical and Prognostic Profiles of Cardiomyopathies Caused by Mutations in the Troponin T Gene. *Rev. Esp. Cardiol.* **2016**, *69*, 149–158. [CrossRef]
76. Hein, S.; Kostin, S.; Heling, A.; Maeno, Y.; Schaper, J. The role of the cytoskeleton in heart failure. *Cardiovasc. Res.* **2000**, *45*, 273–278. [CrossRef]
77. Whiting, A.; Wardale, J.; Trinick, J. Does titin regulate the length of muscle thick filaments? *J. Mol. Biol.* **1989**, *205*, 263–268. [CrossRef]
78. Miller, M.K.; Granzier, H.; Ehler, E.; Gregorio, C.C. The sensitive giant: The role of titin-based stretch sensing complexes in the heart. *Trends Cell Biol.* **2004**, *14*, 119–126. [CrossRef]
79. LeWinter, M.M.; Granzier, H.L. Cardiac titin and heart disease. *J. Cardiovasc. Pharmacol.* **2014**, *63*, 207–212. [CrossRef]
80. Itoh-Satoh, M.; Hayashi, T.; Nishi, H.; Koga, Y.; Arimura, T.; Koyanagi, T.; Takahashi, M.; Hohda, S.; Ueda, K.; Nouchi, T.; et al. Titin mutations as the molecular basis for dilated cardiomyopathy. *Biochem. Biophys. Res. Commun.* **2002**, *291*, 385–393. [CrossRef]
81. Siu, B.L.; Niimura, H.; Osborne, J.A.; Fatkin, D.; MacRae, C.; Solomon, S.; Benson, D.W.; Seidman, J.G.; Seidman, C.E. Familial dilated cardiomyopathy locus maps to chromosome 2q31. *Circulation* **1999**, *99*, 1022–1026. [CrossRef] [PubMed]
82. Guo, W.; Schafer, S.; Greaser, M.L.; Radke, M.H.; Liss, M.; Govindarajan, T.; Maatz, H.; Schulz, H.; Li, S.; Parrish, A.M.; et al. RBM20, a gene for hereditary cardiomyopathy, regulates titin splicing. *Nat. Med.* **2012**, *18*, 766–773. [CrossRef] [PubMed]
83. Guo, W.; Pleitner, J.M.; Saupe, K.W.; Greaser, M.L. Pathophysiological defects and transcriptional profiling in the RBM20-/- rat model. *PLoS ONE* **2013**, *8*, e84281. [CrossRef]
84. Li, S.; Guo, W.; Dewey, C.N.; Greaser, M.L. Rbm20 regulates titin alternative splicing as a splicing repressor. *Nucleic Acids Res.* **2013**, *41*, 2659–2672. [CrossRef]
85. Flashman, E.; Redwood, C.; Moolman-Smook, J.; Watkins, H. Cardiac myosin binding protein C: Its role in physiology and disease. *Circ. Res.* **2004**, *94*, 1279–1289. [CrossRef] [PubMed]
86. Kensler, R.W.; Craig, R.; Moss, R.L. Phosphorylation of cardiac myosin binding protein C releases myosin heads from the surface of cardiac thick filaments. *Proc. Natl. Acad. Sci. USA* **2017**, *114*, E1355–E1364. [CrossRef]
87. Mamidi, R.; Gresham, K.S.; Verma, S.; Stelzer, J.E. Cardiac Myosin Binding Protein-C Phosphorylation Modulates Myofilament Length-Dependent Activation. *Front. Physiol.* **2016**, *7*, 38. [CrossRef]

88. Weber, F.E.; Vaughan, K.T.; Reinach, F.C.; Fischman, D.A. Complete sequence of human fast-type and slow-type muscle myosin-binding-protein C (MyBP-C). Differential expression, conserved domain structure and chromosome assignment. *Eur. J. Biochem.* **1993**, *216*, 661–669. [CrossRef]
89. Gautel, M.; Zuffardi, O.; Freiburg, A.; Labeit, S. Phosphorylation switches specific for the cardiac isoform of myosin binding protein-C: A modulator of cardiac contraction? *EMBO J.* **1995**, *14*, 1952–1960. [CrossRef]
90. Dhoot, G.K.; Hales, M.C.; Grail, B.M.; Perry, S.V. The isoforms of C protein and their distribution in mammalian skeletal muscle. *J. Muscle Res. Cell Motil.* **1985**, *6*, 487–505. [CrossRef]
91. Reinach, F.C.; Masaki, T.; Fischman, D.A. Characterization of the C-protein from posterior latissimus dorsi muscle of the adult chicken: Heterogeneity within a single sarcomere. *J. Cell Biol.* **1983**, *96*, 297–300. [CrossRef] [PubMed]
92. Gautel, M.; Furst, D.O.; Cocco, A.; Schiaffino, S. Isoform transitions of the myosin binding protein C family in developing human and mouse muscles: Lack of isoform transcomplementation in cardiac muscle. *Circ. Res.* **1998**, *82*, 124–129. [CrossRef] [PubMed]
93. James, J.; Robbins, J. Signaling and myosin-binding protein C. *J. Biol. Chem* **2011**, *286*, 9913–9919. [CrossRef] [PubMed]
94. Sadayappan, S.; de Tombe, P.P. Cardiac myosin binding protein-C as a central target of cardiac sarcomere signaling: A special mini review series. *Pflugers Arch.* **2014**, *466*, 195–200. [CrossRef] [PubMed]
95. Seidman, C.E.; Seidman, J.G. Identifying sarcomere gene mutations in hypertrophic cardiomyopathy: A personal history. *Circ. Res.* **2011**, *108*, 743–750. [CrossRef]
96. Sarikas, A.; Carrier, L.; Schenke, C.; Doll, D.; Flavigny, J.; Lindenberg, K.S.; Eschenhagen, T.; Zolk, O. Impairment of the ubiquitin-proteasome system by truncated cardiac myosin binding protein C mutants. *Cardiovasc. Res.* **2005**, *66*, 33–44. [CrossRef]
97. Bulteau, A.L.; Szweda, L.I.; Friguet, B. Age-dependent declines in proteasome activity in the heart. *Arch. Biochem. Biophys.* **2002**, *397*, 298–304. [CrossRef]
98. Okada, K.; Wangpoengtrakul, C.; Osawa, T.; Toyokuni, S.; Tanaka, K.; Uchida, K. 4-Hydroxy-2-nonenal-mediated impairment of intracellular proteolysis during oxidative stress. Identification of proteasomes as target molecules. *J. Biol. Chem.* **1999**, *274*, 23787–23793. [CrossRef]
99. Simonson, T.S.; Zhang, Y.; Huff, C.D.; Xing, J.; Watkins, W.S.; Witherspoon, D.J.; Woodward, S.R.; Jorde, L.B. Limited distribution of a cardiomyopathy-associated variant in India. *Ann. Hum. Genet.* **2010**, *74*, 184–188. [CrossRef]
100. Anand, A.; Chin, C.; Shah, A.S.V.; Kwiecinski, J.; Vesey, A.; Cowell, J.; Weber, E.; Kaier, T.; Newby, D.E.; Dweck, M.; et al. Cardiac myosin-binding protein C is a novel marker of myocardial injury and fibrosis in aortic stenosis. *Heart* **2018**, *104*, 1101–1108. [CrossRef]
101. Mishra, A.; Srivastava, A.; Mittal, T.; Garg, N.; Mittal, B. Impact of renin-angiotensin-aldosterone system gene polymorphisms on left ventricular dysfunction in coronary artery disease patients. *Dis. Markers* **2012**, *32*, 33–41. [CrossRef] [PubMed]
102. Farza, H.; Townsend, P.J.; Carrier, L.; Barton, P.J.; Mesnard, L.; Bahrend, E.; Forissier, J.F.; Fiszman, M.; Yacoub, M.H.; Schwartz, K. Genomic organisation, alternative splicing and polymorphisms of the human cardiac troponin T gene. *J. Mol. Cell Cardiol.* **1998**, *30*, 1247–1253. [CrossRef] [PubMed]
103. Kumar, S.; Mishra, A.; Srivastava, A.; Mittal, T.; Garg, N.; Mittal, B. Significant role of ADRB3 rs4994 towards the development of coronary artery disease. *Coron. Artery Dis.* **2014**, *25*, 29–34. [CrossRef]
104. Mishra, A.; Srivastava, A.; Mittal, T.; Garg, N.; Mittal, B. Genetic predisposition to left ventricular dysfunction: A multigenic and multi-analytical approach. *Gene* **2014**, *546*, 309–317. [CrossRef] [PubMed]
105. Sadayappan, S.; Osinska, H.; Klevitsky, R.; Lorenz, J.N.; Sargent, M.; Molkentin, J.D.; Seidman, C.E.; Seidman, J.G.; Robbins, J. Cardiac myosin binding protein C phosphorylation is cardioprotective. *Proc. Natl. Acad. Sci. USA* **2006**, *103*, 16918–16923. [CrossRef] [PubMed]
106. Mishra, A.; Srivastava, A.; Mittal, T.; Garg, N.; Mittal, B. Association of matrix metalloproteinases (MMP2, MMP7 and MMP9) genetic variants with left ventricular dysfunction in coronary artery disease patients. *Clin. Chim. Acta* **2012**, *413*, 1668–1674. [CrossRef] [PubMed]
107. Mishra, A.; Srivastava, A.; Mittal, T.; Garg, N.; Mittal, B. Role of inflammatory gene polymorphisms in left ventricular dysfunction (LVD) susceptibility in coronary artery disease (CAD) patients. *Cytokine* **2013**, *61*, 856–861. [CrossRef]

108. Akasheva, D.U.; Plokhova, E.V.; Tkacheva, O.N.; Strazhesko, I.D.; Dudinskaya, E.N.; Kruglikova, A.S.; Pykhtina, V.S.; Brailova, N.V.; Pokshubina, I.A.; Sharashkina, N.V.; et al. Age-Related Left Ventricular Changes and Their Association with Leukocyte Telomere Length in Healthy People. *PLoS ONE* **2015**, *10*, e0135883. [CrossRef]
109. Hayward, C.S.; Kalnins, W.V.; Kelly, R.P. Gender-related differences in left ventricular chamber function. *Cardiovasc. Res.* **2001**, *49*, 340–350. [CrossRef]
110. Kishi, S.; Reis, J.P.; Venkatesh, B.A.; Gidding, S.S.; Armstrong, A.C.; Jacobs, D.R., Jr.; Sidney, S.; Wu, C.O.; Cook, N.L.; Lewis, C.E.; et al. Race-ethnic and sex differences in left ventricular structure and function: The Coronary Artery Risk Development in Young Adults (CARDIA) Study. *J. Am. Heart Assoc.* **2015**, *4*, e001264. [CrossRef]
111. Alshehri, A.M.; Azoz, A.M.; Shaheen, H.A.; Farrag, Y.A.; Khalifa, M.A.; Youssef, A. Acute effects of cigarette smoking on the cardiac diastolic functions. *J. Saudi Heart Assoc.* **2013**, *25*, 173–179. [CrossRef] [PubMed]
112. Triposkiadis, F.; Giamouzis, G.; Parissis, J.; Starling, R.C.; Boudoulas, H.; Skoularigis, J.; Butler, J.; Filippatos, G. Reframing the association and significance of co-morbidities in heart failure. *Eur J. Heart Fail.* **2016**, *18*, 744–758. [CrossRef] [PubMed]
113. Mishra, A.; Srivastava, A.; Kumar, S.; Mittal, T.; Garg, N.; Agarwal, S.K.; Pande, S.; Mittal, B. Role of angiotensin II type I (AT1 A1166C) receptor polymorphism in susceptibility of left ventricular dysfunction. *Indian Heart J.* **2015**, *67*, 214–221. [CrossRef] [PubMed]

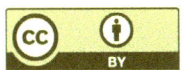

© 2020 by the authors. Licensee MDPI, Basel, Switzerland. This article is an open access article distributed under the terms and conditions of the Creative Commons Attribution (CC BY) license (http://creativecommons.org/licenses/by/4.0/).

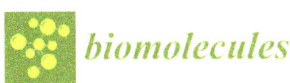 

Article

# Biophysical and Lipidomic Biomarkers of Cardiac Remodeling Post-Myocardial Infarction in Humans

Valerie Samouillan [1], Ignacio Miguel Martinez de Lejarza Samper [2,3], Aleyda Benitez Amaro [4,5], David Vilades [2,3], Jany Dandurand [1], Josefina Casas [6,7], Esther Jorge [2,3], David de Gonzalo Calvo [4,5], Alberto Gallardo [8], Enrique Lerma [8], Jose Maria Guerra [2,3], Francesc Carreras [2,3], Ruben Leta [2,3] and Vicenta Llorente Cortes [3,4,5,*]

[1] CIRIMAT, Université de Toulouse, Université Paul Sabatier, Equipe PHYPOL, 31062 Toulouse, France; valerie.samouillan@univ-tlse3.fr (V.S.); jany.lods@univ-tlse3.fr (J.D.)
[2] Department of Cardiology, Hospital de la Santa Creu i Sant Pau, Biomedical Research Institute Sant Pau (IIB Sant Pau), Universitat Autonoma de Barcelona, 08193 Barcelona, Spain; IMartinezL@santpau.cat (I.M.M.d.L.S.); DVilades@santpau.cat (D.V.); EJorge@santpau.cat (E.J.); JGuerra@santpau.cat (J.M.G.); FCarreras@santpau.cat (F.C.); RLeta@santpau.cat (R.L.)
[3] CIBERCV, Institute of Health Carlos III, 28029 Madrid, Spain
[4] Institute of Biomedical Research of Barcelona (IIBB), Spanish National Research Council (CSIC), 08036 Barcelona, Spain; ABenitez@santpau.cat (A.B.A.); david.degonzalo@gmail.com (D.d.G.C.)
[5] Group of Lipids and Cardiovascular Pathology, Biomedical Research Institute Sant Pau (IIB Sant Pau), Hospital de la Santa Creu i Sant Pau, 08041 Barcelona, Spain
[6] Research Unit on BioActive Molecules (RUBAM), Department of Biological Chemistry, Institute for Advanced Chemistry of Catalonia (IQAC-CSIC), 08034 Barcelona, Spain; fina.casas@iqac.csic.es
[7] CIBEREHD Institute of Health Carlos III, 28029 Madrid, Spain
[8] Department of Pathology, Hospital de la Santa Creu i Sant Pau, 08041 Barcelona, Spain; AGallardo@santpau.cat (A.G.); ELerma@santpau.cat (E.L.)
* Correspondence: cllorente@santpau.cat or vicenta.llorente@iibb.csic.es; Tel.: +34-935565888

Received: 16 September 2020; Accepted: 21 October 2020; Published: 22 October 2020

**Abstract:** Few studies have analyzed the potential of biophysical parameters as markers of cardiac remodeling post-myocardial infarction (MI), particularly in human hearts. Fourier transform infrared spectroscopy (FTIR) illustrates the overall changes in proteins, nucleic acids and lipids in a single signature. The aim of this work was to define the FTIR and lipidomic pattern for human left ventricular remodeling post-MI. A total of nine explanted hearts from ischemic cardiomyopathy patients were collected. Samples from the right ventricle (RV), left ventricle (LV) and infarcted left ventricle (LV INF) were subjected to biophysical (FTIR and differential scanning calorimetry, DSC) and lipidomic (liquid chromatography–high-resolution mass spectrometry, LC–HRMS) studies. FTIR evidenced deep alterations in the myofibers, extracellular matrix proteins, and the hydric response of the LV INF compared to the RV or LV from the same subject. The lipid and esterified lipid FTIR bands were enhanced in LV INF, and both lipid indicators were tightly and positively correlated with remodeling markers such as collagen, lactate, polysaccharides, and glycogen in these samples. Lipidomic analysis revealed an increase in several species of sphingomyelin (SM), hexosylceramide (HexCer), and cholesteryl esters combined with a decrease in glycerophospholipids in the infarcted tissue. Our results validate FTIR indicators and several species of lipids as useful markers of left ventricular remodeling post-MI in humans.

**Keywords:** biophysical markers; cardiac remodeling post-MI; lipidomics; Fourier transform infrared spectroscopy; heart failure

## 1. Introduction

Ischemic heart disease is the primary cause of death in Western countries, and myocardial infarction occupies about 50% of deaths in this group. Despite the important improvements in the management of myocardial infarction, adverse left ventricular remodeling, which occurs in up to 30% of cases following ST-segment elevation myocardial infarction (STEMI), is strongly associated with poor patient outcomes. Chronic left ventricular remodeling (LVR) is, apart from infarct size and infarct wound healing, the primary determinant of heart failure post-myocardial infarction (MI) [1,2]. Adverse LVR after MI involves crucial changes in the composition and organization of the extracellular matrix (ECM) [3].

The location, size and shape of MI is commonly determined by imaging techniques at the clinical level or by histopathology at the experimental level. Detailed information about the chemical composition and physical structure of infarct zones post-MI remains limited. Previous studies from our group have shown that Fourier transform infrared (FTIR) spectroscopy has the potential to highlight the main alterations that occur in cardiac remodeling in a post-MI mice model [4], as well as in a pig model of tachycardia-induced dilated cardiomyopathy [5]. The FTIR spectra of freeze-dried mice's left ventricles showed amides I and II to be the major absorptions bands. Collagen possesses a specific band at 1338 $cm^{-1}$ [6] that can be used to compile a collagen/protein indicator. Finally, the sub-resolution of the FTIR spectra determined by Fourier self-deconvolution (FSD) and the second derivative method in the amide I/II zone is useful for determining the secondary structures of proteins [7]. In a mice model, we showed that an increase in the collagen indicator in the infarcted tissue is associated with the predominance of the triple helical conformation of proteins, evidencing a deep remodeling of this zone.

In addition to structural remodeling, infarcted tissue undergoes what is called "metabolic remodeling", which includes a set of metabolic changes that occur in the cardiac tissue exposed to ischemia. These metabolic changes include partial insulin resistance, associated with reduced fatty acid oxidation and impaired mitochondrial biogenesis [8,9], downregulation of metabolic genes [10], and upregulation of lipoprotein receptors that contribute to increasing the intracellular lipids in cardiomyocytes [11–14]. A high prevalence of myocardial lipids has been found in areas of chronic MI in humans [15]. Patients with cardiac lipid deposition had larger infarctions, as well as decreased wall thickening and impaired endocardial wall motion. The hydrolysis of lipid species such as phospholipids in the membrane of cardiomyocytes during ischemic processes is intimately linked to the pathogenesis of myocardial infarction [16,17]. Clinical studies have identified new circulating metabolites that are derived from phospholipidic metabolism in serum and are useful as potential new biomarkers in cardiac remodeling post-MI [18–22]. To the best of our knowledge, only one lipidomic study has been performed in cardiac infarcted tissues, and was developed using pigs [13].

The objective of the current investigation was to identify conformational, biophysical, and lipidomic alterations that are useful as biomarkers of cardiac adverse remodeling in human infarcted hearts.

## 2. Materials and Methods

### 2.1. Collection of Human Samples

A total of 9 explanted human hearts from ischemic cardiomyopathy patients were collected and immediately processed. These hearts were from patients undergoing cardiac transplantation in the Department of Cardiology. The myocardial samples from the explanted hearts were collected in the Department of Pathology (both departments from Santa Creu I Sant Pau Hospital, Barcelona). Clinical data, electrocardiograms, Doppler echocardiography, hemodynamic studies, and coronary angiography were available for all patients. All patients were functionally classified according to the New York Heart Association (NYHA) criteria and received medical treatment according to the guidelines of the European Society of Cardiology [23] using diuretics 89%, angiotensin-converting enzyme inhibitors 86%, β-blockers 48%, aldosterone antagonists 71%, digoxin 49% and statins 82% (Table 1).

**Table 1.** Clinical and echocardiographic characteristics from whom explanted ischemic hearts were obtained.

|  | ICM ($n = 9$) |
|---|---|
| Age (years) | 57.67 ± 12.02 |
| Gender male (%) | 78 |
| Prior Hypertension (%) | 44 |
| Diabetes mellitus (%) | 11 |
| Dislipemia (%) | 75 |
| Perfusion abnormalities * (%) | 72 |
| Echo-Doppler study | |
| Ejection fraction (%) | 29.88 ± 8.90 |
| Intraventricular septum in diastole (mm) | 11.63 ± 4.63 |
| Left ventricular posterior wall in diastole (mm) | 9.53 ± 0.75 |
| Left ventricular end-diastolic diameter (mm) | 60.38 ± 14.15 |
| Left ventricular end-systolic diameter (mm) | 56.25 ± 2.79 |
| Treatment (%) | |
| Diuretics | 89 |
| Angiotensin-converting enzyme inhibitors | 86 |
| β-blockers | 48 |
| Aldosteron antagonists | 71 |
| Digoxin | 49 |
| Statins | 82 |

ICM, ischemic cardiomyopathy; * the patients with perfusion abnormalities were considered those subjected to coronary interventions (i.e. by-pass, angioplasty, stents and others).

Hearts were weighed and measured, and samples from the right ventricle (RV) ($n = 9$), left ventricle (LV) ($n = 9$), and infarcted left ventricle (LV INF) ($n = 9$) were excised and frozen at −80 °C for immunohistochemical, biophysical and lipidomic studies. The project was approved by the local Ethics Committee of Hospital de la Santa Creu i Sant Pau, Barcelona, Spain, and was conducted in accordance with the guidelines of the Declaration of Helsinki. All patients gave written informed consent that was obtained according to our institutional guidelines.

*2.2. Tissue Homogenization and Preparation of the Samples for the Different Studies*

One portion of collected tissue was embedded in optimal cutting temperature compound (OCT) and used for immunohistochemical studies. Other portion was frozen under $N_2$, pulverized using a mortar and a pestle in liquid nitrogen and used for the biophysical studies. A 5 mg aliquot was freeze dried and used for vibrational characterization and a 25 mg aliquot was used for differential scanning calorimetry (DSC). Another aliquot of pulverized tissue (500 µg) was dissolved in a lysis buffer (Tris-HCl 1 M, KCl 1 M, and protease inhibitors 1 µg/mL) and used for the lipidomic studies.

*2.3. Immunohistochemical Analysis*

Myocardial collagen was immunohistochemically assessed by Sirius Red Staining as previously described [ ].

## 2.4. Vibrational Characterization

The Fourier transform infrared spectroscopy/attenuated total reflectance (FTIR/ATR) spectra of the freeze-dried tissues were acquired using a Nicolet 5700 FTIR instrument (Thermo Fisher Scientific, Waltham, MA, USA) equipped with an ATR device with a KBr beam splitter and an MCT/B detector. The ATR accessory used was a Smart Orbit with a type IIA diamond crystal (refractive index 2.4, Thermo Fisher Scientific, Waltham, MA, USA). Samples were directly deposited on the entire active surface of the crystal and gently compressed using a Teflon tip to ensure good contact. For each sample, 80 interferograms were recorded in the 4000–450 $cm^{-1}$ region, co-added and Fourier-transformed to generate an average spectrum of the segmented heart part with a nominal resolution of 1 $cm^{-1}$ using Omnic 8.0 (Thermo Fisher Scientific, Waltham, MA, USA). The single-beam background spectrum was collected from the clean diamond crystal before each experiment, and this background was subtracted from the spectra.

To circumvent the attenuation of penetration depth in the samples at large wave numbers in the ATR mode, spectra were subjected to advanced ATR correction. Then, the spectra were baseline corrected and normalized using the maximum of the amide II peak. These spectra were subsequently used to calculate the integrated band intensities and their ratios. For semi-quantitative comparison between groups, the areas of the different absorption bands were computed from the individual spectrum of each tissue, and the appropriate ratio of areas was used according to the literature data in trans-reflectance or ATR mode [25,26]. Second derivatives were used to enhance the chemical information present in the overlapping infrared absorption bands of the spectra. All spectra processing was performed using Omnic 8.0. The spectra presented for each group were calculated by averaging the spectra of all samples within each group.

## 2.5. Differential Scanning Calorimetry

Calorimetric analyses were performed using a DSC Pyris calorimeter (Perkin Elmer, Waltham, MA). The calorimeter was calibrated using Hg and In resulting in a temperature accuracy of 0.1 °C and an enthalpy accuracy of 0.2 J/g. Fresh samples, 5–10 mg in weight, were set into hermetic aluminum pans and equilibrated at the initial temperature for 5 min before cooling to −100 °C at 10 °C/min. Then, the thermograms were recorded during heating at 10 °C/min until reaching 90 °C. After the DSC measurements were performed, the pans were reweighed to check that they had been correctly sealed.

## 2.6. Lipidomic Analysis of the Heart

Phospholipids (PLs) and sphingolipids (SLs extracts) were prepared and analyzed using the following protocols previously described [27,28], with minor modifications.

### 2.6.1. Phospholipids and Neutral Lipids

A 750 µL methanol–chloroform (1:2, v/v) solution containing standards was transferred to borosilicate glass test tubes with Teflon caps, and 0.25 mL methanol and 0.5 mL chloroform were subsequently added. This mixture was fortified with the internal standards of lipids (200 pmol each). The following standards were added to myocardial samples: 16:0 D31_18:1 phosphocholine, 16:0 D31_18:1 phosphoethanolamine, 16:0 D31-18:1 phosphoserine, 17:0 lyso-phosphocholine, 17:1 lyso-phosphoethanolamine, 17:1 lyso-phosphoserine, 17:0/17:0/17:0 triacylglycerol, and C17:0 cholesteryl ester; 0.2 nmol of each standard (from Avanti Polar Lipids). The samples were vortexed and sonicated until they appeared dispersed and were then incubated at 48 °C overnight. The solvent was removed using a Speed Vac Savant SPD131DDA (Thermo Scientific). Lipids were solubilized in 0.5 mL of methanol and transferred to 1.5 mL Eppendorf tubes and evaporated again. The samples were resuspended in 150 µL of methanol. The tubes were centrifuged at 13,000× g for 3 min, and 130 µL of the supernatants was transferred to ultra-performance liquid chromatography (UPLC) vials for injection and analysis.

## 2.6.2. Sphingolipids

A 750 µL methanol–chloroform (2:1, *v/v*) solution containing internal standards (N-dodecanoylsphingosine, N-dodecanoylglucosylsphingosine, N-dodecanoylsphingosylphosphorylcholine, and C17-sphinganine, 0.2 nmol each, from Avanti Polar Lipids) was added to the myocardial samples. The samples were extracted at 48 °C overnight and cooled. Then, 75 µL of 1 M KOH in methanol was added to saponify phospholipids and prevent their possible interference in the detection of sphingolipids, and the mixture was incubated for 2 h at 37 °C. Following the addition of 75 µL of 1 M acetic acid, the samples were evaporated to dryness, and stored at −20 °C until analysis. Before analysis, 150 µL of methanol was added to the samples. Then, the samples were centrifuged at 13,000× $g$ for 5 min, and 130 µL of the supernatant was transferred to a new vial and injected.

## 2.6.3. UPLC Coupled to HRMS Analysis

Ultra Performance Liquid chromatography (UPLC) coupled to high-resolution mass spectrometry (HRMS) analysis was performed using an Acquity ultra-high-performance liquid chromatography (UHPLC) system (Waters, USA) connected to a Time of Flight (LCT Premier XE) Detector. The full-scan spectra from 50 to 1800 Da were acquired, and individual spectra were summed to produce data points each being 0.2 s. Mass accuracy at a resolving power of 10,000 and reproducibility were maintained using an independent reference spray via LockSpray interference.

Lipid extracts were injected onto an Acquity UPLC BEH C8 column (1.7 µm particle size, 100 mm × 2.1 mm, Waters Ireland) at a flow rate of 0.3 mL/min and a column temperature of 30 °C. The mobile phases were water with 2 mM of ammonium formate and 0.2% of formic acid (A) and methanol with 2 mM of ammonium formate and 0.2% of formic acid (B).The UPLC conditions were programmed as follows: 0.0 min_80% B; 3 min_90% B (linear gradient); 6 min_90% B (isocratic); 15 min_99% B (linear gradient); 18 min_99% B (isocratic); 20 min_80% B (linear gradient); 22 min_80% B (isocratic).

Positive identification of compounds was based on the accurate mass measurement and its LC retention time, compared with that of a standard (<2%). Selected ions for SLs and glycerophospholipids correspond to $[M + H]^+$, whereas ammonia adduct were used for neutral lipids (Table S1). The ceramide (Cer) standards used were N-palmitoyl-sphingosine, N-stearoyl-sphingosine, N-lignoceroyl-sphingosine and N-nervonoyl-sphingosine. The sphingomyelin (SM) standards used were N-palmitoylsphingosyl phosphorylcholine, egg SMs (predominant C16:0SM) and brain SMs (C18:0SM, C24:0SM and C24:1SM in known percentages). The glucosylceramide standard used was N-palmitoylglucosylsphingosine. The lactosylceramide standard used was N-palmitoyl-lactosylsphingosine. The diacylphospholipid standards used were 1,2-dipalmitoyl-snglycero-3-phosphocholine, 1-palmitoyl-2-oleoyl-sn-glycero-3-phosphocholine, 1-palmitoyl-2-oleoyl-sn-glycero-3-phosphoethanolamine and 1-palmitoyl-2-oleoyl-sn-glycero-3-phospho-L-serine. The lysophospholipid standards used were 1-stearoyl-2-hydroxy-sn-glycero-3-phosphocholine, 1-oleoyl-2-hydroxy-sn-glycero-3-phosphoethanolamine and 1-oleoyl-2-hydroxy-sn-glycero-3-phospho-L-serine. The triacylglycerol standard used was 1,2,3-tri-(9Z-octadecenoyl)-glycerol. The cholesteryl ester standard used was cholesteryl cis-9-octadecenoate. When authentic standards were not available, identification was achieved based on their accurate mass measurement, elemental composition, calculated mass, error, double-bond equivalents and retention times. Quantification was carried out using the extracted ion chromatogram of each compound, obtained with a mass chromatogram absolute window value of 0.05 Da. As an example, representative ion chromatograms for sphingolipids (Figure S1), glycerophospholipids (Figures S2 and S3) and neutral lipids (Figure S4) of the right, left and infarcted left ventricle from the same patient are shown. The linear dynamic range was determined by injecting mixtures of internal and natural standards indicated above. If values were above the linear dynamic range, samples were diluted and analyzed again. Since standards for all identified lipids were not available, the amounts of lipids are given as pmol equivalents relative to each specific standard (Table S1).

Sphingolipids (Cer: ceramide; SM: sphingomyelin; CDH: Ceramide dihexoside; HexCer: hexosylceramides), glycerophospholipids (PC: phosphatidylcholine; LPC: lysophosphatidylcholine; PE: phosphatidylethanolamine; LPE: lysophosphatidylethanolamine; PS: phosphatidylserine; LPS: lysophosphatidylserine, PG: phosphatidylglycerol), and neutral lipids (TAG: triacylglycerol; CE: cholesteryl esters; free cholesterol: FC) were detected. All glycerophospholipid and neutral lipid species were annotated using the "lipid subclass" and "C followed by the total fatty acid (FA) chain length:total number of unsaturated bonds" (e.g., PC (32:2)).

### 2.7. Statistical Analysis

Variables were compared two by two among the 3 groups (RV, LV and LV INF) using Student's *t*-test or a Mann–Whitney U test for paired samples (myocardial samples were from the same patient), respectively, depending on whether the variables were normal. Normality was tested with a Shapiro–Wilk and Lilliefors test. *p* values were adjusted with Bonferroni's correction, we performed 3 comparisons for each variable.

The correlations between variables were studied in each group using Pearson's correlation. *p* values were adjusted with Bonferroni's correction because we tested the correlation among all lipidomic and biophysical variables. $p < 0.05$ was considered statistically significant.

Lipidomic variables whose differences were significant in some of the study groups were represented in a heatmap. Each variable was represented as a logarithm of the quotient of the group mean and the mean value in all groups.

Statistical power was calculated afterwards as few lipidomic studies in human hearts have been performed until now and it was difficult to estimate the effect size in some lipidomic variables. Assuming the differences obtained in the significant variables as the real effect size, we obtained a range of values of statistical power between 0.64 and 0.98 in differential analysis and a range between 0.79 and 1 in correlation analysis.

All data analyses were performed using R 4.0.2 software [29].

## 3. Results

### 3.1. Identification of the Main FTIR Bands in the Human Heart

To compare the spectral signature of the human heart with previous data collected from animal hearts [4,5], the average FTIR spectra of mice, pig, and human right ventricles were superimposed (Figure 1). Table S2 summarizes the different FTIR absorption bands detected in human compared to pig and mice right ventricles, as well as their assignments, according to previously published data in transmission or ATR mode [5,6,30–37]. The major absorption bands in these spectra were the amide A, the amide I, and the amide II, which are mainly associated with proteins in freeze-dried tissues. Since Amide A is located in the large wave number zone where FTIR-ATR is not the more appropriate mode, the intensity of this mode has not been used for further semi-quantitative analysis. The primary ventricular proteins are cardiomyocyte myofibrillar (myosin, α-actin) and sarcoplasmic proteins and the structural proteins of the extracellular matrix (ECM), i.e., fibrillar collagens I and III. Among these different vibrations, the 1338 $cm^{-1}$ band (wagging of the proline side chain) [6,25,36] corresponds to a specific signature of the structural proteins of the ECM since it is the only one that does not overlap with absorption or other components, e.g., DNA, lipids, or proteoglycans. As shown in Figure 1, the spectral signatures of the structural proteins of the ECM and the myofibers from mice, pigs and humans are very similar.

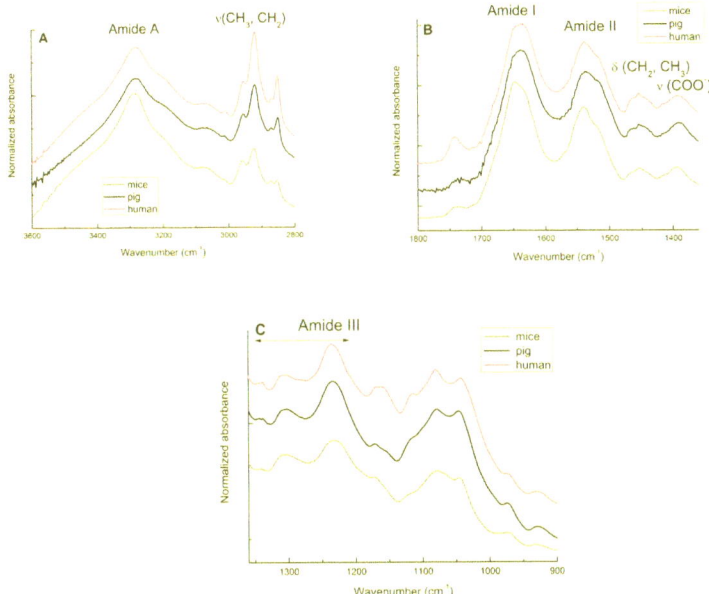

**Figure 1.** Averaged Fourier transform infrared spectroscopy (FTIR) spectra of the right ventricles from the mice, pig, and human samples. Line graphs showing the 3600–2800 cm$^{-1}$ (**A**), 1800–1350 cm$^{-1}$ (**B**), and 1350–900 cm$^{-1}$ (**C**) spectral regions of mice, pig, and human right ventricles.

The complex FTIR spectra of the ventricles also include lipids with their classic markers at 2800–3000 cm$^{-1}$ (especially the CH$_2$ stretching of long hydrocarbon chains) (Figure 1A) and at 1475–1450 cm$^{-1}$ (CH$_2$ scissoring and CH3 bending) (Figure 1B). These lipids are mainly phospholipids of the plasmatic membranes, confirmed by the presence of the C=O stretching of ester groups, the CO-O-C and PO$_2^-$ stretching bands, triglycerides, cholesteryl esters, free cholesterol and free fatty acids (C=O stretching at 1712 cm$^{-1}$ and COO$^-$ stretching at 1392 cm$^{-1}$). Unsaturated lipids are specifically marked by the 3013 cm$^{-1}$ band.

Where the band position of the lipids is quasi-identical among the three species, the lipid vibrational response is more intense in human ventricles (for both the ν(CH2) and ν(C=O) bands) than in pig and mice ventricles.

Finally, as shown in Figure 1C, other ventricular components contributed to this complex vibrational response including DNA, specifically at 974 cm$^{-1}$ [ ]; proteoglycans (contributing to the 1079 cm$^{-1}$ band and the overlapping 1226 cm$^{-1}$ band); glycogen; and other polysaccharides (1200–1000 cm$^{-1}$). The composite (1240–1100 cm$^{-1}$) zone is subjected to fine differences due to disparities in the nature or proportion of these components among the three compared species.

*3.2. Characterization of the Human Heart Lipidome*

UPLC–HRMS analysis electrospray ionization mass spectrometry revealed 44 species of sphingolipids, 60 species of glycerophospholipids, and 60 species of neutral lipids in the human heart. The relative amount of each lipid in the whole family was expressed as the percentage of each lipid area compared to the total number of lipids of the same family in the right and left ventricles (Figures S5–S7).

The relative abundance of the species present for each particular lipid among the family of sphingolipids in the human heart is also shown (Figure S5A–E). The most abundant sphingolipid in the human heart is sphingomyelin d18:1 (SM, 88.53%), particularly the species with long fatty acid chains (from 14 to 18 C) (Figure S5A). Minor species include ceramide d18:1 (Cer, 6.94%) (Figure S5B), followed by dihydrosphingomyelin d18:0 (dhSM, 3.56%) (Figure S5C), hexosylceramide (d18:1) (HexCer, 0.58%) (Figure S5D) and ceramide dihexoside (18:1) (CDH, 0.39%) (Figure S5E). CDH (d18:14:0) was significantly higher in LV than in RV ($p = 0.045$) (Figure S5E).

The most abundant glycerophospholipids in human cardiac tissue are phosphatidylcholine (PC, 75.24%), mainly species with long fatty acid (FA) chains (from 32 to 38 C) (Figure S6A); followed by phosphatidylserine (PS, 8.43%) (Figure S6B); lyso-phosphatidylcholine (LPC, 6.62%) (Figure S6C), phosphatidylethanolamine (PE, 4.96%) (Figure S6D), lyso-phosphatidylethanolamine (LPE, 2.88%) (Figure S6E), lyso- phosphatidylserine (LPS, 1.12%) (Figure S6F) and phosphatidylglycerol (PG, 0.76%) (Figure S6G).

Finally, as shown in Figure S7, the neutral lipids in the human hearts contain a high percentage of triglycerides (TAG, 97.06%) (Figure S7A). Several TAG species with longer unsaturated chains of fatty acids (FAs), decreased in the LV compared to the RV. These TAG species were C53:2 ($p = 0.041$), C54:1 ($p = 0.036$), and C54:2 ($p = 0.033$). The decrease in TAG in human LV compared to RV was previously reported in a porcine model [5] and likely reflects a higher effort and more energetic consumption of LV. Most of the cholesterol was found in the form of free cholesterol (FC, 2.03%) (Figure S7B), with a minor proportion found as cholesteryl esters (CE, 0.90%) (Figure S7C). There were no statistically significant differences in FC or CE between RV and LV.

*3.3. Identification of the Alterations of the FTIR Bands Related to Myofibers and Structural Extracellular Matrix Proteins in Human LV INF compared to LV and RV*

Table S3 shows a comparison of the IR bands between RVs, LVs and LV INFs of the human hearts compiled from IR spectra. Specific assignments of these bands were performed according to the literature [5,6,30–37]. Most of the IR bands previously described in murine and porcine cardiac control tissues are also present in the RV, LV, and LV INF of human hearts.

In agreement with the deep remodeling of infarcted tissue assessed by immunohistochemistry (Figure 2A), FTIR analyses revealed the profound alteration of the IR band pattern at 1300–860 cm$^{-1}$ in the LV INF compared to the LV or RV samples (Figure 2B). A distinct feature of the collagen-specific absorption band at 1338 cm$^{-1}$ was found in the human LV INF sample but not in the RV or LV samples. The indicator collagen/amide II (1338 cm$^{-1}$/1540 cm$^{-1}$), which reflects the content of structural proteins related to the total proteins, was significantly increased in LV INF compared to LV ($p = 0.023$) and RV ($p = 0.023$) (Figure 2C). The second derivative FTIR spectra (which allows increased resolution) showed the exclusive presence of certain IR bands in LV INF at 1140 and 1095 cm$^{-1}$ (Figure 2D, asterisks) in the $\nu$(C-O-C)/$\nu$(C-OH) absorption zone, indicating deep alterations in oligosaccharides and also in glycolipids, phospholipids, and nucleic acids in the infarcted area. In addition, intense absorptions at 1120 cm$^{-1}$ (characteristic of $\nu$(C-O) in lactate, polysaccharides, and glycogen), 1236 cm$^{-1}$ (amide III), and 1160 cm$^{-1}$ (hydroxyproline residues, collagen specific) were detected in human LV INF compared to LV and RV (Figure 2B,D, arrows). The increase of 1236 and 1160 cm$^{-1}$ band absorptions could be due to augmented collagen deposition in the infarcted zone, while that of 1120 cm$^{-1}$ is associated with elevated levels of lactate and/or polysaccharides in this zone ($p = 0.047$) (Figure 2E).

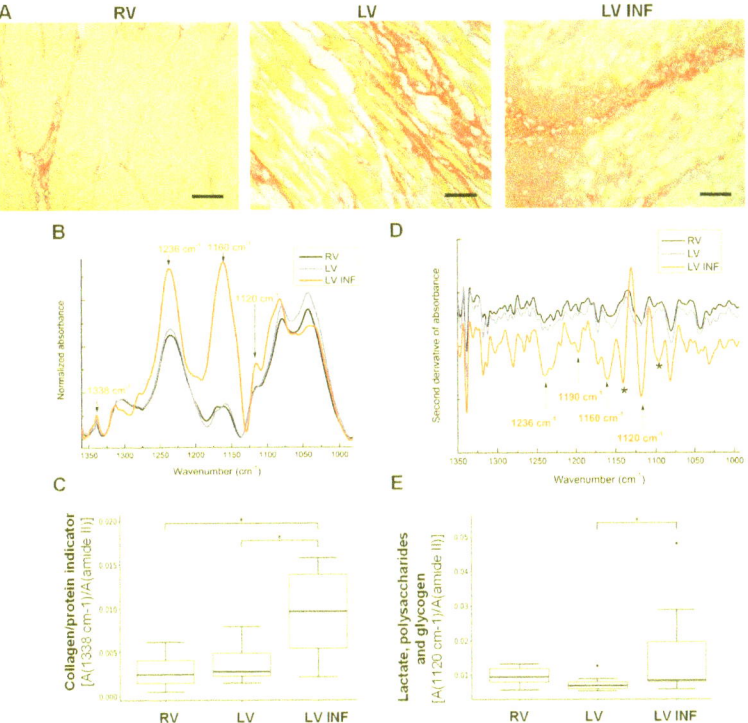

**Figure 2.** Immunohistochemical and FTIR analyses of fibrosis in human ventricle samples. Sirius Red Staining was used to distinguish the collagen (in red) in the right ventricle (RV), left ventricle (LV) and infarcted left ventricle (LV INF) samples. Scale Bar: 20 μm (**A**). Line graphs showing the 1350–1000 cm$^{-1}$ averaged FTIR spectra of RV, LV, and LV INF (**B**). Boxplot analysis of the FTIR collagen/protein indicator (1338 cm$^{-1}$/amide II) in the three groups (**C**). Line graphs showing the average second derivative spectra in the 1370–1000 cm$^{-1}$ region (**D**). Arrows indicate the bands altered in the LV INF samples. Asterisks indicate the occurrence of new absorption bands in the LV INF samples. Boxplots showing lactate, polysaccharide, and glycogen/protein indicator (1220 cm$^{-1}$/amide II) in the three groups ($n = 9$/group) (**E**). * $p < 0.05$. RV: right ventricle, LV: left ventricle, LV INF: infarcted left ventricle.

### 3.4. Identification of the Alterations in the FTIR Bands Corresponding to DNA Response in Human LV INF Compared to LV and RV

As reported in Figure A, FTIR spectra corresponding to 1000–850 cm$^{-1}$ where the DNA/RNA response prevails, showed differences between the three myocardial samples, which were quantified by the nucleic acid/protein indicator (band area ratio 974 cm$^{-1}$/1540 cm$^{-1}$, Figure B). There was a significant decrease in the DNA/protein ratio from the right to left ischemic ventricles, reaching significance in LV INF vs. LV ($p = 0.0056$) and RV ($p = 0.0061$) (Figure B).

This evolution is consistent with previous FTIR imaging results on infarcted myocardium, indicating that nucleic acids are widespread in a normal myocardium but destroyed in an infarcted myocardium [ ]. All changes revealed the profound remodeling of the ECM in human infarcted tissue.

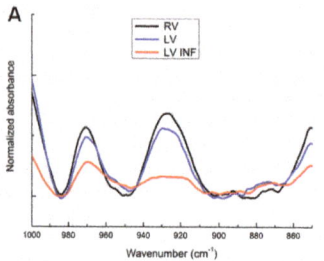 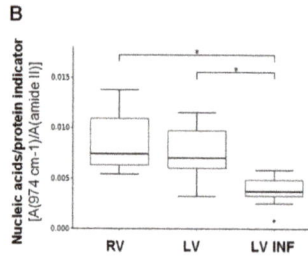

**Figure 3.** FTIR analysis of the nucleic acids in the human ventricle samples. Line graphs showing the 1000–850 cm$^{-1}$ average FTIR spectra corresponding to the signal of nucleic acids in the RV, LV, and LV INF samples (**A**). Boxplot analysis of nucleic acid/protein FITR indicator (974 cm$^{-1}$/amide II) (**B**) in the three groups (*n* = 9/group). * *p* < 0.05. RV: right ventricle, LV: left ventricle, LV INF: infarcted left ventricle.

### 3.5. Study of the Hydric Response of Human RV, LV and LV INF

Representative DSC thermograms (normalized to the initial mass) of fresh human ventricles corresponding to cooling from 20 to −100 °C and successive heating from −100 to 25 °C are reported in Figure S8A. The cooling thermograms are characterized by an intense exothermic peak corresponding to the crystallization of free water (namely, water not bound to hydrophilic components and able to form ice). The onset temperature of the peak (Ton) is attributed to the transition temperature of this thermal event. The heating thermograms are characterized by an endothermic peak corresponding to the melting of previously frozen water. Weak and multiple thermal events are detectable in the (50–85 °C) zone and attributed to the denaturation of cardiac muscle proteins, including myosin, sarcoplasmic proteins, collagen and actin as already observed in a previous study [4]. There is a significant decrease in the temperature of water crystallization Tc for LV INF compared to LV (*p* = 0.044) (Figure S8B). A similar trend is observed for the ice melting recorded in the heating scans. The increase in aqueous salt concentrations could explain such a depression of the melting/crystallization temperature. However, the typical signature of aqueous salts, namely the eutectic phase transition at lower temperature, was not detected in the DSC thermograms of myocardial samples. Since water crystallization and ice melting are related to the pore size in porous [39] and biological materials [40], the differences between the infarcted and non-infarcted zones can be interpreted as changes in the architecture associated with a decrease of the pore's nominal radius. Cardiac remodeling, including the replacement of myofibers by collagen fibers marking a difference in the tissue architecture (pore size), could explain this peculiar thermal behavior.

### 3.6. Study of the Associations between FITR Variables in Human RV, LV and LV INF

The FTIR spectra show that the CH$_2$ bands (2921 cm$^{-1}$ and 2850 cm$^{-1}$) in the (CH$_2$, CH$_3$) stretching zone (3000–2800 cm$^{-1}$) are mainly associated with the lipid signature (Figure 4A) and the C=O stretching zones of the ester carbonyl groups of phospholipids, triglycerides, and cholesteryl esters (Figure 4B). There was an intensification of the lipid bands in the left infarcted ventricles, and a close correlation (R = 1, *p* = 8.7 × 10$^{-8}$) between the total lipid (2921–2850 cm$^{-1}$/1540 cm$^{-1}$) and the esterified lipid (1745 cm$^{-1}$/1540 cm$^{-1}$) indicators (Figure 4C) in this zone. There were no correlations statistically significant between total and esterified lipids in RV or LV (R = 0.93, *p* = 1; R = 0.89, *p* = 1, respectively), suggesting that most of the lipids are esterified in the infarcted LV, but not in the RV or LV.

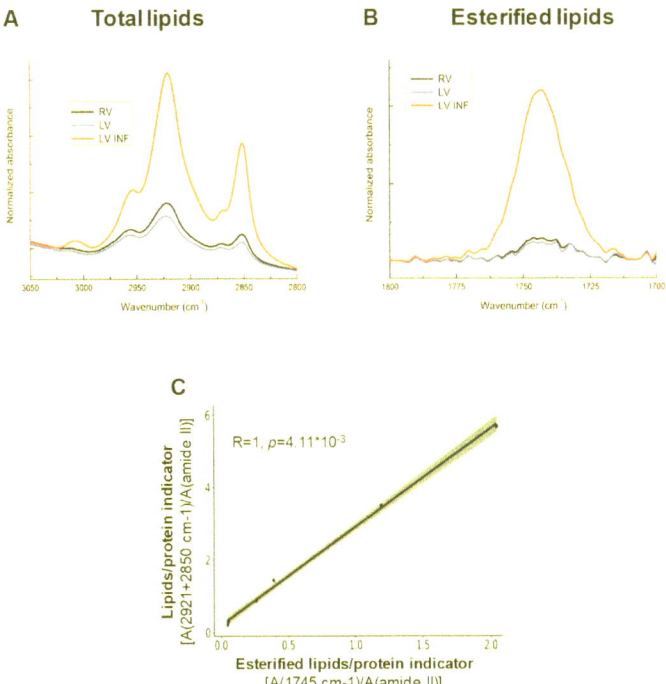

**Figure 4.** FTIR analysis of the total and esterified lipids in the human ventricle samples. Line graphs showing the 3050–2800 cm$^{-1}$ (**A**) and 1800–1700 cm$^{-1}$ (**B**) average FTIR spectra corresponding to the signals of the total and esterified lipids, respectively, in right ventricle (RV), left ventricle (LV), and infarcted left ventricle (LV INF). (**C**) Correlation analysis between the FTIR indicators of the total and esterified lipids in LV INF. The correlation was studied with Pearson's correlation, and the *p*-values were adjusted with Bonferroni's correction. RV: right ventricle, LV: left ventricle, LV INF: infarcted left ventricle.

*3.7. Identification of the Alterations in Sphingolipids, Glycerophospholipids and Neutral Lipids in Human LV INF Compared to LV and RV*

Lipidomic studies reflected deep lipid remodeling in the infarcted tissue. As visualized in the heatmap of Figure 5, cholesteryl ester and several sphingolipid species were significantly increased in LV INF compared to RV or LV, while most of the glycerophospholipid species were significantly decreased in the infarcted cardiac tissue. As shown in Table 2, SM 18:1 (14:0 and 14:1) and 16:1, dhSM 18:0 (16:0 and 18:0), and HexCer 18:1 species (16:0, 22:0, 24:0, 24:1) were significantly increased, while Cer 18:1 (18:0, 20:0, 20:1, 22:1 and 24:1) species were significantly decreased in the LV infarcted tissue (Table 2). There were no significant differences in CDH or the rest of the sphingolipid species between LV INF and LV or RV (Table S4). Like Cer, the main glycerophospholipids, including PE (34:2, 36:4), LPE (18:2), PC (32:2, 34:1, 34:2, 34:3, 34:4, 36:2, 36:3, 36:5), and PG (34:1, 34:2), were significantly decreased in human infarcted tissue (Table 3). There were no significant differences in the PS, LPS, or LPC and the rest of glycerophospholipid species between LV INF and LV or RV (Table S5). Finally, among the neutral lipids, only cholesteryl esters were found to be significantly increased in the infarcted tissue (18:3) (Table 3). There were no differences in the highly abundant TAG species or minor FC species between LV INF and LV or RV (Table S6).

## Differential lipid species in human ventricles from ischemic cardiomyopathy patients

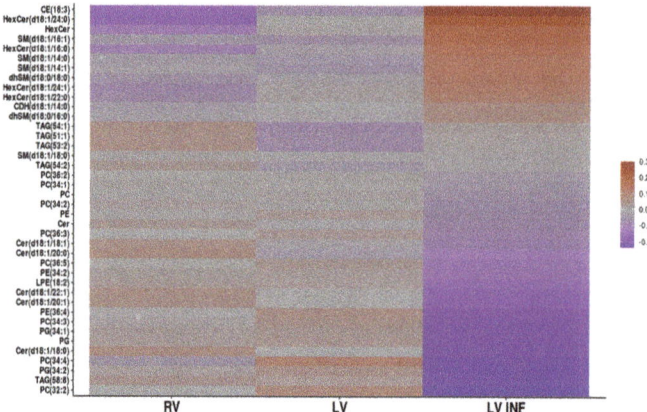

**Figure 5.** Lipidomic analysis of the human right ventricle, left ventricle and infarcted left ventricle. Heatmap of the nine human heart samples (in columns) based in the quantification of 40 differential lipid species (in rows) that exhibited statistically significant differences among right ventricle (RV), left ventricle (LV), and infarcted left ventricle (LV INF) samples. The heatmap colors represent a decimal logarithm of the quotient of the group mean and the mean value in all groups for each variable. Blue cells indicate values below the mean value of the variables in all groups, while red cells indicate values above the mean value of the variables in all groups. CE: cholesteryl esters, HexCer: hexosylceramide, SM: sphingomyelin, dhSM: dihydrosphingomyelin, CDH: ceramide dihexoside, TAG: triacylglycerols, PC: phosphatidylcholine, PE: phosphatidylethanolamine, LPE: lysophosphatidylethanolamine, Cer: ceramide, PG: phosphatidylglycerol. RV: right ventricle, LV: left ventricle, LV INF: infarcted left ventricle.

**Table 2.** Sphingolipid species with differential concentrations in the infarcted left ventricle compared to left ventricle or right ventricle from human explanted ischemic hearts.

| Variable | RV | LV | LV INF | $p$ vs. LV | $p$ vs. RV |
|---|---|---|---|---|---|
| SM(d18:1/14:0) | 308.5 ± 77.4 | 309.5 ± 95.9 | 430.5 ± 95.3 | 0.024 | 0.055 |
| SM(d18:1/14:1) | 3 ± 1.2 | 2.8 ± 1 | 3.9 ± 1.4 | 0.029 | 0.096 |
| SM(d18:1/16:1) | 164 ± 39.5 | 160.1 ± 56.8 | 258.8 ± 105.8 | 0.029 | 0.041 |
| SM(d18:1/18:0) | 1199.2 ± 156.3 | 1138.7 ± 128.5 | 1086.2 ± 142.7 | 0.485 | 0.038 |
| Total Cer | 753 ± 261.6 | 592.7 ± 240.1 | 549.5 ± 179.1 | 0.932 | 0.044 |
| Cer(d18:1/18:0) | 30.4 ± 13.5 | 22.9 ± 14.5 | 15 ± 4.9 | 0.115 | 0.029 |
| Cer(d18:1/18:1) | 7.2 ± 2.3 | 5.2 ± 2 | 4.6 ± 1.1 | 0.456 | 0.006 |
| Cer(d18:1/20:0) | 14.5 ± 3.6 | 11.1 ± 4 | 9.6 ± 2.8 | 0.457 | 0.01 |
| Cer(d18:1/20:1) | 4.4 ± 0.8 | 3.4 ± 1.3 | 2.6 ± 0.6 | 0.13 | 0.006 |
| Cer(d18:1/22:1) | 28.7 ± 22.9 | 20.2 ± 16.1 | 17.5 ± 20.1 | 0.804 | 0.018 |
| dhSM(d18:0/16:0) | 179.4 ± 41.3 | 207.5 ± 91.7 | 226.4 ± 65 | 0.931 | 0.029 |
| dhSM(d18:1/18:0) | 46.3 ± 13.4 | 49.5 ± 23.3 | 64.5 ± 16.3 | 0.174 | 0.041 |
| Total HexCer | 48.1 ± 26.6 | 63.9 ± 31.2 | 91.3 ± 36.6 | 0.114 | 0.006 |
| HexCer(d18:1/16:0) | 2.3 ± 1.5 | 3.2 ± 1.7 | 4.4 ± 3.1 | 0.474 | 0.023 |
| HexCer(d18:1/22:0) | 10.9 ± 5.8 | 16.1 ± 13.2 | 16 ± 5.6 | 1 | 0.012 |
| HexCer(d18:1/24:0) | 19.6 ± 10.4 | 25.3 ± 13.6 | 44.3 ± 25.1 | 0.127 | 0.018 |
| HexCer(d18:1/24:1) | 15.5 ± 10.5 | 20 ± 5.6 | 26.7 ± 13.5 | 0.102 | 0.006 |

Data are expressed as mean ± SD, $n = 9$ (RV, LV and LV INF). SM: sphingomyelin, Cer: Ceramide, dhSM: dihydrosphingomyelin, HexCer: Hexosylceramide, SD: standard deviation, RV: right ventricle, LV: left ventricle, LV INF: infarcted left ventricle.

**Table 3.** Glycerophospholipid species with differential concentrations in the infarcted left ventricle compared to left ventricle or right ventricle from human explanted ischemic hearts.

| Variable | RV | LV | LV INF | $p$ vs. LV | $p$ vs. RV |
| --- | --- | --- | --- | --- | --- |
| Total PC | 54,624.9 ± 11408.6 | 56,737 ± 5670.8 | 48,392.9 ± 4893.7 | 0.012 | 0.335 |
| PC(32:2) | 342.5 ± 146.2 | 389.6 ± 115.9 | 221.1 ± 103.4 | 0.029 | 0.102 |
| PC(34:1) | 14,602.8 ± 2506.6 | 15,143.9 ± 1769.8 | 13,505.1 ± 1492.7 | 0.029 | 0.556 |
| PC(34:2) | 13,397 ± 2572.8 | 13,827.1 ± 1685 | 11,574.9 ± 1501.8 | 0.006 | 0.232 |
| PC(34:3) | 120.7 ± 54.3 | 133.2 ± 46.3 | 71.9 ± 21.8 | 0.012 | 0.049 |
| PC(34:4) | 100.7 ± 52.6 | 133.8 ± 67.5 | 64.7 ± 34.1 | 0.041 | 0.077 |
| PC(36:2) | 4753.8 ± 1047.4 | 4902.2 ± 444.3 | 4439.5 ± 328.1 | 0.025 | 0.698 |
| PC(36:3) | 3650 ± 1035 | 3884.2 ± 936.2 | 2866.5 ± 856.6 | 0.003 | 0.122 |
| PC(36:5) | 391.6 ± 437.5 | 376.8 ± 327.3 | 236.4 ± 269.4 | 0.041 | 0.069 |
| Total PE | 3502.5 ± 1052.4 | 3840.7 ± 914.1 | 2986.4 ± 769 | 0.004 | 0.285 |
| PE(34:2) | 203.1 ± 65.5 | 205.2 ± 47 | 144.1 ± 37.9 | 0.008 | 0.028 |
| PE(36:4) | 1014.5 ± 300.8 | 1309.3 ± 502.6 | 629.4 ± 269.1 | 0.011 | 0.036 |
| LPE(18:2) | 144.7 ± 60.3 | 142.7 ± 43.4 | 95 ± 30.3 | 0.006 | 0.052 |
| Total PG | 538.9 ± 135.4 | 581.8 ± 188.7 | 329.2 ± 152.5 | 0.045 | 0.041 |
| PG(34:1) | 483 ± 121.9 | 523 ± 176.8 | 300.9 ± 139.4 | 0.052 | 0.042 |
| PG(34:2) | 55.9 ± 20.6 | 58.8 ± 19.1 | 28.3 ± 14.9 | 0.028 | 0.047 |

Data are expressed as mean ± SD, $n$ = 9 (RV, LV and LV INF). PC: phosphatidylcholine, PE: phosphatidylethanolamine, LPE: lysophosphatidylethanolamine, PG: phosphatidylglycerol, SD: standard deviation, RV: right ventricle, LV: left ventricle, LV INF: infarcted left ventricle.

**Table 4.** Neutral lipid species with differential concentrations in the infarcted left ventricle compared to left ventricle or right ventricle from human explanted ischemic hearts.

| Variable | RV | LV | LV INF | $p$ vs. LV | $p$ vs. RV |
| --- | --- | --- | --- | --- | --- |
| TAG(58:8) | 2856 ± 1534.1 | 3364.8 ± 3160.3 | 1978.9 ± 1520.3 | 0.018 | 0.075 |
| CE(18:3) | 269.5 ± 248.3 | 352.3 ± 319.7 | 575.9 ± 583.5 | 0.239 | 0.018 |

Data are expressed as mean ± SD, $n$ = 9 (RV, LV and LV INF). TAG: triacylglycerols, CE: cholesteryl esters, SD: standard deviation, RV: right ventricle, LV: left ventricle, LV INF: infarcted left ventricle.

### 3.8. Study of the Association between FTIR and Lipidomic Variables in RV, LV and LV INF

As shown in Figure , biophysical studies revealed that ECM remodeling was closely associated with lipid indicators, such as total lipids (2921–2850 cm$^{-1}$) (R = 1, $p$ = 1.6 × 10$^{-8}$) (Figure A) and esterified lipids (1745 cm$^{-1}$/amide II) (R = 0.99, $p$ = 9.3 × 10$^{-7}$) (Figure B) specifically in LV INF. In addition, other extracellular matrix markers such as lactate, polysaccharides, and glycogen, were also closely associated with total lipids (R = 1, $p$ = 3.6 × 10$^{-11}$) (Figure C) and esterified lipids (R = 0.99, $p$ = 9.1 × 10$^{-7}$) (Figure D) in the cardiac infarcted tissue. There was no significant correlation between lipid and ECM remodeling FITR indicators in human RV (R = 0.54, $p$ = 1) or LV (R = 0.68, $p$ = 1).

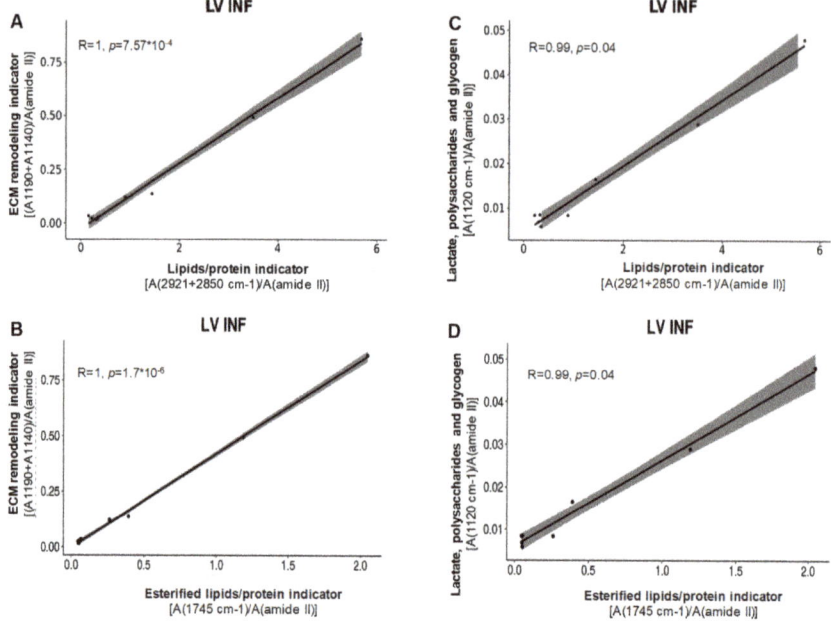

**Figure 6.** Correlation analysis of FTIR indicators of cardiac remodeling and lipids in the human heart. Correlation between the extracellular matrix (ECM) remodeling indicator and both total lipids (**A**) and esterified lipids (**B**), as well as between lactate, polysaccharide, and glycogen and both total lipids (**C**) and esterified lipids (**D**), in human infarcted left ventricle. The correlation was studied with Pearson's correlation, and *p* values were adjusted with Bonferroni's correction. LV INF: infarcted left ventricle.

## 4. Discussion

In this work, we used the FTIR spectrum to illustrate the overall variety of changes in proteins, nucleic acids, and lipids that occur in human cardiac infarcted tissue. FTIR spectroscopy is very sensitive to variations in cell metabolism, making it highly suitable for defining the structure in the infarcted areas where the tissue has undergone strong cardiometabolic alterations primarily associated with the process of ischemia [41].

The spectral signatures of the structural proteins of ECM and the myofibers in the human heart are similar to those previously reported in murine [4] and porcine hearts [5]. One of the most significant alterations observed in the FTIR spectra of human LV INF vs. LV or RV was a strong increase in the 1338 cm$^{-1}$ band, which has been shown to be specific to collagen [6,25,36]. The utility of this particular FTIR band to monitor the evolution of cardiac pathology and therapeutics was previously validated in a rat MI model [6]. Another FTIR band that is deeply altered in the context of MI is the 974 cm$^{-1}$ band assigned to nucleic acids that, as expected, suffered a strong decline in LV INF compared to LV and RV. These changes reflected a profound remodeling of the LV INF accompanying cardiomyocyte death in the context of myocardial infarction and highlighted the potential of infrared markers to trace the incidence of ischemia in cardiac remodeling.

The spectral signatures of lipids are also quasi-identical in the human heart to those in previous murine [4] and pig [5] hearts. The vibrational response of the lipids is much more intense (for both the ν(CH2) and ν(C=O) bands, corresponding to the total lipids and ester carbonyl groups of PL and neutral lipids) in human than in murine or porcine ventricles. Lipidomic analysis of the human heart revealed that the main lipids present are SM (d18:1) (88% of the total sphingolipids), PC (75% of the total glycerophospholipids) and TAGs (97% of the total neutral lipids). There are few detailed lipidomic studies of ventricles and almost none on humans, likely due to the difficulty of obtaining human heart samples. We found several species belonging to the sphingolipid, glycerophospholipid, and neutral lipid families that were altered in LV INF but not in RV and LV. Most of the glycerophospholipids decreased, while most of the sphingolipids and, specific species of cholesteryl esters increased in the infarcted human cardiac tissue.

Between sphingolipids, the levels of several species of SM, dhSM, and HexCer were increased in LV INF compared to LV or RV. The increase in the SM content of infarcted tissue found in the present work seems to be coherent with the decreased sphingomyelinase (SMase) activity previously described [ ]. The increase in SM that we found in humans differs from the results showing lower SM levels in the infarcted brains of in vivo models of ischemic stroke [ ]. The cleavage of SM by acid or neutral SMase results in the liberation of ceramide, a sphingolipid that acts as an intracellular messenger regulating the activity of kinases, phosphatases, and transcription factors. Ceramides were reported to be upregulated in the ischemic zones of the heart in several in vivo models of ischemia/reperfusion [ , , ]. This increase in ceramides after ischemia reperfusion appears to be transient and linked with reperfusion injury, as shown in a model of ischemic-reperfused myocardium in rats [ ]. It has also been shown that the post-MI increase in cardiac ceramide is not caused by increased SMase activity but instead by decreased ceramidase activity. In addition, it has been recently demonstrated that a transient increase in acid ceramidase is sufficient to induce cardioprotection post-MI [ ]. Ceramide is utilized for the synthesis of other bioactive sphingolipids, including sphingosine-1-phosphate, sphingosine, and the glycosphingolipids lactosylceramide and hexosylceramide (HexCer). Here, several species of HexCer were found accumulated in human infarcted hearts. Previous studies have reported the accumulation of HexCer in several organs from in vivo models of aging [ , ]. Clinically, increased circulating levels of both SM and Cer have been correlated with an increased risk of coronary artery disease [ , ].

Between glycerophospholipids, we found that the levels of the main PL, phosphatidylcholine (PC), and other less abundant PLs, such as phosphatidylethanolamine (PE) and phosphatidylglycerol (PG), were significantly decreased in LV INF compared to LV. These results are in agreement with previous studies performed in in vivo MI models [ , ] showing a strong PL decay caused by ischemia-induced phospholipolysis of the cardiomyocyte membranes. Increased phospholipolysis can be caused, among other factors, by the upregulatory effect of hypoxia on phospholipase activity [ , ]. Unbalanced levels of anionic phospholipids such as PG seem to have harmful consequences for mitochondrial morphology and function. PG plays a pivotal role in the formation of cardiolipin, which is essential in the control of mitochondrial inflammation and oxidative stress [ , ], and respiratory activity [ ]. In this study, we found a significant loss of PG that could, indeed, contribute to a serious decrease in mitochondrial oxidative metabolism in infarcted tissue. The strong decrease in mitochondrial respiratory activity combined with acute phospholipolysis, which actively generates fatty acids [ , ], could be a determinant for increased FA esterification. An additional source of esterified lipids in the infarcted tissue is circulating lipoproteins. Several groups, including ours, have reported the upregulatory effect of hypoxia/ischemia on lipoprotein receptors such as Very low-density lipoprotein receptor VLDLR and Low-density lipoprotein receptor related-protein 1 LRP1, which bind and internalize lipoproteins such as Very low-density lipoprotein (VLDL) and Low-density lipoprotein (LDL) (lipoproteins highly enriched in cholesteryl esters) [ – , , ]. Here, the close correlation between esterified lipids and remodeling in the human infarcted tissue pointed to FTIR lipid indicators as potential biomarkers of remodeling, at least in the context of ischemia. Previous studies from our group demonstrated that the levels of intracellular esterified lipids in cardiomyocytes determine the structural and physical characteristics of secreted tropoelastin through an increase in cathepsin S mature protein levels [ ]. The intracellular esterified lipids stored in lipid droplets are the subject of an intense debate over their potential beneficial/harmful effects on cell functionality [ ]. The differential implications of triglyceride and cholesteryl ester proportions in these lipid droplets are also under discussion [ ].

## 5. Conclusions

As a general conclusion, FTIR studies showed that human cardiac infarcted tissue suffers deep alterations in proteins, nucleic acids, and—especially—lipids. Liquid chromatography coupled to high-resolution mass spectrometry (LC–HRMS) revealed the strong lipid remodeling that results in reduced levels of PC, PE, LPE and PG and increased levels of SM, HexCer and cholesteryl esters in human cardiac infarcted tissue. We found a strong and positive association between esterified lipids and adverse cardiac remodeling in the context of human cardiac remodeling post-MI. The specific conclusions are that (i) there are deep alterations of the FTIR bands related to myofibers and structural extracellular matrix proteins in human LV INF compared to LV and RV, (ii) there are strong differences in the FTIR spectra corresponding to DNA responses in human LV INF compared to RV and LV, (iii) there is a differential hydric response of human LV INF compared to RV and LV, (iv) FTIR combined with lipidomic studies showed a strong intensification of lipids, particularly esterified lipids concomitantly with deep phospholipid remodeling in human infarcted hearts, and (v) esterified lipids are closely related with adverse cardiac remodeling in human infarcted heart. Thus, we have shown that FTIR lipid indicators are potential biomarkers of cardiac remodeling and validated certain lipid species as crucial in human pathological ventricular remodeling post-MI.

**Limitations of This Study:** The main limitation of this study is the low number of patients included due to the difficulty of (i) obtaining samples from ischemic cardiomyopathy patients and (ii) performing biophysical and lipidomic studies on an elevated number of series. However, great differences in some variables were found between ventricle samples, as well as strong correlations between variables. There was also a high correlation between ECM remodeling indicators and the total and esterified lipids in LV INF. Furthermore, we have obtained relatively high values of statistical power (between 0.64–0.98), despite the low number of samples, due to the big differences in some variables between the ventricles. Regardless, more studies are needed to confirm our results and provide higher statistical power. We also consider, as limitation of this study, the impossibility to characterize the infarcted right ventricle due to the low prevalence and diagnose of this entity. Finally, we could not assess the levels of cardiolipin, a crucial lipid in cardiovascular disease, due to the technical unavailability to perform this analysis.

**Supplementary Materials:** The following are available online at http://www.mdpi.com/2218-273X/10/11/1471/s1, Figure S1: Representative ion chromatograms of ceramides and sphingomyelins detected in the right, left and infarcted left ventricle of the same patient; Figure S2: Representative ion chromatograms of phosphatidylcholines (PCs) and phosphatidylethanolamines (PEs) detected in the right, left and infarcted left ventricle of the same patient; Figure S3: Representative ion chromatograms of phosphatidylserines (PSs) and lysophospholipids (PEs) detected in the right, left and infarcted left ventricle of the same patient; Figure S4: Representative ion chromatograms of neutral lipids detected in the right, left and infarcted left ventricle of the same patient; Figure S5: Levels of sphingolipids species in right and left ventricles from human explanted ischemic hearts; Figure S6: Levels of glycerolipids species in right and left ventricles from human explanted ischemic hearts; Figure S7: Levels of neutral lipid species in right and left ventricles from human explanted ischemic hearts; Figure S8: Hydric response of the right, left and left infarcted ventricles from human explanted ischemic hearts; Table S1: Lipids identified in the myocardial samples; Table S2: FTIR band position and assignment in human, pig and mice right ventricle samples; Table S3: FTIR band position and assignment in right, left and left infarcted ventricles from human explanted ischemic hearts; Table S4: Levels of sphingolipids species (pmol equiv/mg prot) in right, left and left infarcted ventricles from human ischemic hearts; Table S5: Levels of glycerophospholipid species (pmol equiv/mg prot) in right, left and left infarcted ventricles from human ischemic hearts; Table S6: Levels of neutral lipid species (pmol equiv/mg prot) in right, left and left infarcted ventricles from human ischemic hearts.

**Author Contributions:** Conceptualization, D.V., J.D., J.C., D.d.G.C., E.L., J.M.G., F.C., R.L., V.L.C.; Data curation, I.M.M.d.L.S., A.B.A.; Formal analysis, V.S., I.M.M.d.L.S., J.D., J.C., E.J., V.L.C.; Funding acquisition, V.L.C. and J.M.G.; Investigation, V.S., A.B.A., D.V., J.D., J.C., E.J., A.G., J.M.G., F.C., R.L.,V.L.C.; Methodology, V.S., I.M.M.d.L.S., A.B.A., J.D., J.C., D.d.G.C., A.G., E.L., V.L.C.; Project administration, V.S., A.B.A., F.C., V.L.C.; Resources, A.G., E.L., J.M.G., R.L., V.L.C.; Software, I.M.M.d.L.S.; Supervision, V.S., J.D., F.C., R.L., V.L.C.; Validation, I.M.M.d.L.S., D.V., D.d.G.C.; Writing—original draft, V.S., V.L.C. All authors have read and agreed to the published version of the manuscript.

**Funding:** This work was supported by grants from the Fundació La MARATÓ de TV3 (201516_10) and Fondo de Investigación Sanitaria, Instituto de Salud Carlos III (FIS PI18/01584 (to V.L.C.) and PI20/01702 (to J.M.G.) cofunded by ISCIII-Subdirección General de Evaluación y el Fondo Europeo de Desarrollo Regional (FEDER). CIBER Cardiovascular (CV) and CIBER Enfermedades Hepáticas y digestivas (EHD) are Instituto de Salud Carlos III Projects.

**Conflicts of Interest:** The authors declare no conflict of interest.

## References

1. Pfeffer, M.A.; Braunwald, E. Ventricular remodeling after myocardial infarction. Experimental observations and clinical implications. *Circulation* **1990**, *81*, 1161–1172.
2. Opie, L.H.; Commerford, P.J.; Gersh, B.J.; Pfeffer, M.A. Controversies in ventricular remodelling. *Lancet* **2006**, *367*, 356–367.
3. Jugdutt, B.I. Ventricular remodeling after infarction and the extracellular collagen matrix: When is enough enough? *Circulation* **2003**, *108*, 1395–1403.
4. Samouillan, V.; Revuelta-López, E.; Soler-Botija, C.; Dandurand, J.; Benitez-Amaro, A.; Nasarre, L.; de Gonzalo-Calvo, D.; Bayes-Genis, A.; Lacabanne, C.; Llorente-Cortés, V. Conformational and thermal characterization of left ventricle remodeling post-myocardial infarction. *Biochim. Biophys. Acta-Mol. Basis Dis.* **2017**, *1863*, 1500–1509.
5. Benitez-Amaro, A.; Samouillan, V.; Jorge, E.; Dandurand, J.; Nasarre, L.; de Gonzalo-Calvo, D.; Bornachea, O.; Amoros-Figueras, G.; Lacabanne, C.; Vilades, D.; et al. Identification of new biophysical markers for pathological ventricular remodelling in tachycardia-induced dilated cardiomyopathy. *J. Cell. Mol. Med.* **2018**, *22*, 4197–4208.
6. Cheheltani, R.; Rosano, J.M.; Wang, B.; Sabri, A.K.; Pleshko, N.; Kiani, M.F. Fourier transform infrared spectroscopic imaging of cardiac tissue to detect collagen deposition after myocardial infarction. *J. Biomed. Opt.* **2012**, *17*, 56014.
7. Kong, J.; Yu, S. Fourier Transform Infrared Spectroscopic Analysis of Protein Secondary Structures Protein FTIR Data Analysis and Band Assign- ment. *Acta Biochim. Biophys. Sin.* **2007**, *39*, 549–559.
8. Amorim, P.A.; Nguyen, T.D.; Shingu, Y.; Schwarzer, M.; Mohr, F.W.; Schrepper, A.; Doenst, T. Myocardial infarction in rats causes partial impairment in insulin response associated with reduced fatty acid oxidation and mitochondrial gene expression. *J. Thorac. Cardiovasc. Surg.* **2010**, *140*, 1160–1167.
9. Heather, L.C.; Clarke, K. Metabolism, hypoxia and the diabetic heart. *J. Mol. Cell. Cardiol.* **2011**, *50*, 598–605.
10. Rosenblatt-Velin, N.; Montessuit, C.; Papageorgiou, I.; Terrand, J.; Lerch, R. Postinfarction heart failure in rats is associated with upregulation of GLUT-1 and downregulation of genes of fatty acid metabolism. *Cardiovasc. Res.* **2001**, *52*, 407–416.
11. Cal, R.; Castellano, J.; Revuelta-López, E.; Aledo, R.; Barriga, M.; Farré, J.; Vilahur, G.; Nasarre, L.; Hove-Madsen, L.; Badimon, L.; et al. Low-density lipoprotein receptor-related protein 1 mediates hypoxia-induced very low density lipoprotein-cholesteryl ester uptake and accumulation in cardiomyocytes. *Cardiovasc. Res.* **2012**, *94*, 469–479.
12. Cal, R.; Juan-Babot, O.; Brossa, V.; Roura, S.; Gálvez-Montón, C.; Portoles, M.; Rivera, M.; Cinca, J.; Badimon, L.; Llorente-Cortés, V. Low density lipoprotein receptor-related protein 1 expression correlates with cholesteryl ester accumulation in the myocardium of ischemic cardiomyopathy patients. *J. Transl. Med.* **2012**, *10*, 160.
13. Drevinge, C.; Karlsson, L.O.; Ståhlman, M.; Larsson, T.; Perman Sundelin, J.; Grip, L.; Andersson, L.; Borén, J.; Levin, M.C. Cholesteryl Esters Accumulate in the Heart in a Porcine Model of Ischemia and Reperfusion. *PLoS ONE* **2013**, *8*, e61942.
14. De Lima, A.D.; Guido, M.C.; Tavares, E.R.; Carvalho, P.O.; Marques, A.F.; de Melo, M.D.T.; Salemi, V.M.C.; Kalil-Filho, R.; Maranhão, R.C. The Expression of Lipoprotein Receptors Is Increased in the Infarcted Area After Myocardial Infarction Induced in Rats With Cardiac Dysfunction. *Lipids* **2018**, *53*, 177–187.
15. Goldfarb, J.W.; Roth, M.; Han, J. Myocardial fat deposition after left ventricular myocardial infarction: Assessment by using MR water-fat separation imaging. *Radiology* **2009**, *253*, 65–73.
16. Turer, A.T. Using metabolomics to assess myocardial metabolism and energetics in heart failure. *J. Mol. Cell. Cardiol.* **2013**, *55*, 12–18.
17. Nam, M.; Jung, Y.; Ryu, D.H.; Hwang, G.S. A metabolomics-driven approach reveals metabolic responses and mechanisms in the rat heart following myocardial infarction. *Int. J. Cardiol.* **2017**, *227*, 239–246.
18. Feng, L.; Yang, J.; Liu, W.; Wang, Q.; Wang, H.; Shi, L.; Fu, L.; Xu, Q.; Wang, B.; Li, T. Lipid biomarkers in acute myocardial infarction before and after percutaneous coronary intervention by lipidomics analysis. *Med. Sci. Monit.* **2018**, *24*, 4175–4182.

19. Mundra, P.A.; Barlow, C.K.; Nestel, P.J.; Barnes, E.H.; Kirby, A.; Thompson, P.; Sullivan, D.R.; Alshehry, Z.H.; Mellett, N.A.; Huynh, K.; et al. Large-scale plasma lipidomic profiling identifies lipids that predict cardiovascular events in secondary prevention. *JCI Insight* **2018**, *3*. [CrossRef]
20. Floegel, A.; Kühn, T.; Sookthai, D.; Johnson, T.; Prehn, C.; Rolle-Kampczyk, U.; Otto, W.; Weikert, C.; Illig, T.; von Bergen, M.; et al. Serum metabolites and risk of myocardial infarction and ischemic stroke: A targeted metabolomic approach in two German prospective cohorts. *Eur. J. Epidemiol.* **2018**, *33*, 55–66. [CrossRef]
21. Lewis, G.D.; Asnani, A.; Gerszten, R.E. Application of Metabolomics to Cardiovascular Biomarker and Pathway Discovery. *J. Am. Coll. Cardiol.* **2008**, *52*, 117–123. [CrossRef] [PubMed]
22. Dang, V.T.; Huang, A.; Werstuck, G.H. Untargeted Metabolomics in the Discovery of Novel Biomarkers and Therapeutic Targets for Atherosclerotic Cardiovascular Diseases. *Cardiovasc. Hematol. Disord. Targets* **2018**, *18*, 166–175. [CrossRef] [PubMed]
23. Swedberg, K.; Cleland, J.; Dargie, H.; Drexler, H.; Follath, F.; Komajda, M.; Tavazzi, L.; Smiseth, O.A.; Gavazzi, A.; Haverich, A.; et al. Guidelines for the diagnosis and treatment of chronic heart failure: Executive summary (update 2005). *Eur. Heart J.* **2005**, *26*, 1115–1140. [CrossRef]
24. Kiernan, J.A. *Histological and Histochemical Methods: Theory and Practice*, 3rd ed.; Butterworth Heinemann: Oxford, UK, 1999; Volume 12, p. 679.
25. Staniszewska, E.; Malek, K.; Baranska, M. Rapid approach to analyze biochemical variation in rat organs by ATR FTIR spectroscopy. *Spectrochim. Acta. A Mol. Biomol. Spectrosc.* **2014**, *118*, 981–986. [CrossRef]
26. Wang, Q.; Sanad, W.; Miller, L.M.; Voigt, A.; Klingel, K.; Kandolf, R.; Stangl, K.; Baumann, G. Infrared imaging of compositional changes in inflammatory cardiomyopathy. *Vib. Spectrosc.* **2005**, *38*, 217–222. [CrossRef]
27. Simbari, F.; McCaskill, J.; Coakley, G.; Millar, M.; Maizels, R.M.; Fabriás, G.; Casas, J.; Buck, A.H. Plasmalogen enrichment in exosomes secreted by a nematode parasite versus those derived from its mouse host: Implications for exosome stability and biology. *J. Extracell. Vesicles* **2016**, *5*, 30741. [CrossRef]
28. Weber, M.; Mera, P.; Casas, J.; Salvador, J.; Rodríguez, A.; Alonso, S.; Sebastián, D.; Soler-Vázquez, M.C.; Montironi, C.; Recalde, S.; et al. Liver CPT1A gene therapy reduces diet-induced hepatic steatosis in mice and highlights potential lipid biomarkers for human NAFLD. *FASEB J.* **2020**, *34*, 11816–11837. [CrossRef]
29. R Core Team. R: A Language and Environment for Statistical Computing 2020. R Foundation for Statistical Computing: Vienna, Austria. Available online: https://www.R-project.org/ (accessed on 21 October 2020).
30. Bozkurt, O.; Severcan, M.; Severcan, F. Diabetes induces compositional, structural and functional alterations on rat skeletal soleus muscle revealed by FTIR spectroscopy: A comparative study with EDL muscle. *Analyst* **2010**, *135*, 3110. [CrossRef]
31. Gough, K.M.; Zelinski, D.; Wiens, R.; Rak, M.; Dixon, I.M.C. Fourier transform infrared evaluation of microscopic scarring in the cardiomyopathic heart: Effect of chronic AT1 suppression. *Anal. Biochem.* **2003**, *316*, 232–242. [CrossRef]
32. Jerônimo, D.P.; de Souza, R.A.; da Silva, F.F.; Camargo, G.L.; Miranda, H.L.; Xavier, M.; Sakane, K.K.; Ribeiro, W. Detection of creatine in rat muscle by FTIR spectroscopy. *Ann. Biomed. Eng.* **2012**, *40*, 2069–2077. [CrossRef]
33. Kirschner, C.; Ofstad, R.; Skarpeid, H.-J.; Høst, V.; Kohler, A. Monitoring of denaturation processes in aged beef loin by Fourier transform infrared microspectroscopy. *J. Agric. Food Chem.* **2004**, *52*, 3920–3929. [CrossRef]
34. Petibois, C.; Gouspillou, G.; Wehbe, K.; Delage, J.-P.; Déléris, G. Analysis of type I and IV collagens by FT-IR spectroscopy and imaging for a molecular investigation of skeletal muscle connective tissue. *Anal. Bioanal. Chem.* **2006**, *386*, 1961–1966. [CrossRef]
35. Zohdi, V.; Wood, B.R.; Pearson, J.T.; Bambery, K.R.; Black, M.J. Evidence of altered biochemical composition in the hearts of adult intrauterine growth-restricted rats. *Eur. J. Nutr.* **2013**, *52*, 749–758. [CrossRef]
36. Belbachir, K.; Noreen, R.; Gouspillou, G.; Petibois, C. Collagen types analysis and differentiation by FTIR spectroscopy. *Anal. Bioanal. Chem.* **2009**, *395*, 829–837. [CrossRef]
37. Wood, B.R. The importance of hydration and DNA conformation in interpreting infrared spectra of cells and tissues. *Chem. Soc. Rev.* **2016**, *45*, 1980–1998. [CrossRef]
38. Yang, T.T.; Weng, S.F.; Zheng, N.; Pan, Q.H.; Cao, H.L.; Liu, L.; Zhang, H.D.; Mu, D.W. Histopathology mapping of biochemical changes in myocardial infarction by Fourier transform infrared spectral imaging. *Forensic Sci. Int.* **2011**, *207*, e34–e39. [CrossRef] [PubMed]

39. Landry, M.R. Thermoporometry by differential scanning calorimetry: Experimental considerations and applications. *Thermochim. Acta* **2005**, *433*, 27–50. [CrossRef]
40. Fathima, N.N.; Kumar, M.P.; Rao, J.R.; Nair, B.U. A DSC investigation on the changes in pore structure of skin during leather processing. *Thermochim. Acta* **2010**, *501*, 98–102. [CrossRef]
41. Mignolet, A.; Derenne, A.; Smolina, M.; Wood, B.R.; Goormaghtigh, E. FTIR spectral signature of anticancer drugs. Can drug mode of action be identified? *Biochim. Biophys. Acta-Proteins Proteom.* **2016**, *1864*, 85–101. [CrossRef] [PubMed]
42. Zhang, D.X.; Fryer, R.M.; Hsu, A.K.; Zou, A.P.; Gross, G.J.; Campbell, W.B.; Li, P.L. Production and metabolism of ceramide in normal and ischemic-reperfused myocardium of rats. *Basic Res. Cardiol.* **2001**, *96*, 267–274. [CrossRef]
43. Wang, H.-Y.J.; Liu, C.B.; Wu, H.-W.; Kuo, S., Jr. Direct profiling of phospholipids and lysophospholipids in rat brain sections after ischemic stroke. *Rapid Commun. Mass Spectrom.* **2010**, *24*, 2057–2064. [CrossRef]
44. Beresewicz, A.; Dobrzyn, A.; Gorski, J. Accumulation of specific ceramides in ischemic/reperfused rat heart; effect of ischemic preconditioning. *J. Physiol. Pharmacol.* **2002**, *53*, 371–382.
45. Bielawska, A.E.; Shapiro, J.P.; Jiang, L.; Melkonyan, H.S.; Piot, C.; Wolfe, C.L.; Tomei, L.D.; Hannun, Y.A.; Umansky, S.R. Ceramide is involved in triggering of cardiomyocyte apoptosis induced by ischemia and reperfusion. *Am. J. Pathol.* **1997**, *151*, 1257–1263. [PubMed]
46. Hadas, Y.; Vincek, A.S.; Youssef, E.; Żak, M.M.; Chepurko, E.; Sultana, N.; Sharkar, M.T.K.; Guo, N.; Komargodski, R.; Kurian, A.A.; et al. Altering sphingolipid metabolism attenuates cell death and inflammatory response after myocardial infarction. *Circulation* **2020**, *141*, 916–930. [CrossRef] [PubMed]
47. Hernández-Corbacho, M.J.; Jenkins, R.W.; Clarke, C.J.; Hannun, Y.A.; Obeid, L.M.; Snider, A.J.; Siskind, L.J. Accumulation of long-chain glycosphingolipids during aging is prevented by caloric restriction. *PLoS ONE* **2011**, *6*, e20411. [CrossRef]
48. Trayssac, M.; Hannun, Y.A.; Obeid, L.M. Role of sphingolipids in senescence: Implication in aging and age-related diseases. *J. Clin. Investig.* **2018**, *128*, 2702–2712. [CrossRef]
49. Laaksonen, R.; Ekroos, K.; Sysi-Aho, M.; Hilvo, M.; Vihervaara, T.; Kauhanen, D.; Suoniemi, M.; Hurme, R.; März, W.; Scharnagl, H.; et al. Plasma ceramides predict cardiovascular death in patients with stable coronary artery disease and acute coronary syndromes beyond LDL-cholesterol. *Eur. Heart J.* **2016**, *37*, 1967–1976. [CrossRef]
50. Wang, D.D.; Toledo, E.; Hruby, A.; Rosner, B.A.; Willett, W.C.; Sun, Q.; Razquin, C.; Zheng, Y.; Ruiz-Canela, M.; Guasch-Ferré, M.; et al. Plasma ceramides, mediterranean diet, and incident cardiovascular disease in the PREDIMED trial (prevención con dieta mediterránea). *Circulation* **2017**, *135*, 2028–2040. [CrossRef]
51. Hazen, S.L.; Ford, D.A.; Gross, R.W. Activation of a membrane-associated phospholipase A2 during rabbit myocardial ischemia which is highly selective for plasmalogen substrate. *J. Biol. Chem.* **1991**, *266*, 5629–5633.
52. Ford, D.A.; Hazen, S.L.; Saffitz, J.E.; Gross, R.W. The rapid and reversible activation of a calcium-independent plasmalogen-selective phospholipase A2 during myocardial ischemia. *J. Clin. Investig.* **1991**, *88*, 331–335. [CrossRef]
53. Chen, W.W.; Chao, Y.J.; Chang, W.H.; Chan, J.F.; Hsu, Y.H.H. Phosphatidylglycerol Incorporates into Cardiolipin to Improve Mitochondrial Activity and Inhibits Inflammation. *Sci. Rep.* **2018**, *8*. [CrossRef]
54. Pokorná, L.; Čermáková, P.; Horváth, A.; Baile, M.G.; Claypool, S.M.; Griač, P.; Malínský, J.; Balážová, M. Specific degradation of phosphatidylglycerol is necessary for proper mitochondrial morphology and function. *Biochim. Biophys. Acta* **2016**, *1857*, 34–45. [CrossRef]
55. Castellano, J.; Aledo, R.; Sendra, J.; Costales, P.; Juan-Babot, O.; Badimon, L.; Llorente-Cortés, V. Hypoxia stimulates low-density lipoprotein receptor-related protein-1 expression through hypoxia-inducible factor-1α in human vascular smooth muscle cells. *Arterioscler. Thromb. Vasc. Biol.* **2011**, *31*, 1411–1420. [CrossRef]
56. Castellano, J.; Farré, J.; Fernandes, J.; Bayes-Genis, A.; Cinca, J.; Badimon, L.; Hove-Madsen, L.; Llorente-Cortés, V. Hypoxia exacerbates Ca(2+)-handling disturbances induced by very low density lipoproteins (VLDL) in neonatal rat cardiomyocytes. *J. Mol. Cell. Cardiol.* **2011**, *50*, 894–902. [CrossRef]
57. Samouillan, V.; Revuelta-López, E.; Dandurand, J.; Nasarre, L.; Badimon, L.; Lacabanne, C.; Llorente-Cortés, V. Cardiomyocyte intracellular cholesteryl ester accumulation promotes tropoelastin physical alteration and degradation: Role of LRP1 and cathepsin S. *Int. J. Biochem. Cell Biol.* **2014**, *55*, 209–219. [CrossRef]

58. Goldberg, I.J.; Reue, K.; Abumrad, N.A.; Bickel, P.E.; Cohen, S.; Fisher, E.A.; Galis, Z.S.; Granneman, J.G.; Lewandowski, E.D.; Murphy, R.; et al. Deciphering the role of lipid droplets in cardiovascular disease. *Circulation* **2018**, *138*, 305–315. [CrossRef]
59. Thiam, A.R.; Beller, M. The why, when and how of lipid droplet diversity. *J. Cell Sci.* **2017**, *130*, 315–324. [CrossRef]

**Publisher's Note:** MDPI stays neutral with regard to jurisdictional claims in published maps and institutional affiliations.

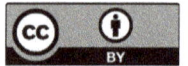

© 2020 by the authors. Licensee MDPI, Basel, Switzerland. This article is an open access article distributed under the terms and conditions of the Creative Commons Attribution (CC BY) license (http://creativecommons.org/licenses/by/4.0/).

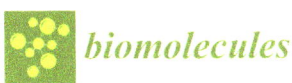 

*Article*

# The c.*52 *A/G* and c.*773 *A/G* Genetic Variants in the UTR'3 of the *LDLR* Gene Are Associated with the Risk of Acute Coronary Syndrome and Lower Plasma HDL-Cholesterol Concentration

Gilberto Vargas-Alarcon [1], Oscar Perez-Mendez [1,2], Julian Ramirez-Bello [3], Rosalinda Posadas-Sanchez [4], Hector Gonzalez-Pacheco [5], Galileo Escobedo [6], Betzabe Nieto-Lima [1], Elizabeth Carreon-Torres [1] and Jose Manuel Fragoso [1,*]

1. Department of Molecular Biology, Instituto Nacional de Cardiología Ignacio Chavez, Mexico City 14080, Mexico; gvargas63@yahoo.com (G.V.-A.); opmendez@yahoo.com (O.P.-M.); betsy@ciencias.unam.mx (B.N.-L.); qfbelizabethcm@yahoo.es (E.C.-T.)
2. School of Engineering and Scienses, Tecnologico de Monterrey, Campus Ciudad de Mexico, Mexico City 14380, Mexico
3. Research Unit on Endocrine and Metabolic Diseases, Hospital Juarez de México, Mexico City 01460, Mexico; dr.julian.ramirez.hjm@gmail.com
4. Department of Endocrinology, Instituto Nacional de Cardiología Ignacio Chavez, Mexico City 14080, Mexico; rossy_posadas_s@yahoo.it
5. Unit Coronary, Instituto Nacional de Cardiología Ignacio Chavez, Mexico City 14080, Mexico; hectorglezp@hotmail.com
6. Unit of the Experimental Medicine, Hospital General de Mexico, Dr. Eduardo Liceaga, Mexico City 06726, Mexico; gescobedog@msn.com
* Correspondence: mfragoso1275@yahoo.com.mx; Tel.: +52-5573-2911 (ext. 26302); Fax: +52-5573-0926

Received: 19 August 2020; Accepted: 24 September 2020; Published: 29 September 2020

**Abstract:** Dyslipidemia has a substantial role in the development of acute coronary syndrome (ACS). Low-density lipoprotein receptor (LDLR) plays a critical role in plasma lipoprotein hemostasis, which is involved in the formation of atherosclerotic plaque. This study aimed to evaluate whether *LDLR* gene polymorphisms are significantly associated with ACS and the plasma lipids profile. Three *LDLR* gene polymorphisms located in the *UTR'3* region (c.*52 *A/G*, c.*504 *A/G*, and c.* 773 *A/G*) were determined using TaqMan genotyping assays in a group of 618 ACS patients and 666 healthy controls. Plasma lipids profile concentrations were determined by enzymatic/colorimetric assays. Under co-dominant and recessive models, the *c.*52 A* allele of the *c.*52 A/G* polymorphism was associated with a higher risk of ACS (OR = 2.02, $pC_{Co\text{-}dom}$ = 0.033, and OR = 2.00, $pC_{Res}$ = 0.009, respectively). In the same way, under co-dominant and recessive models, the *c.*773 G* allele of the *c.*773 A/G* polymorphism was associated with a high risk of ACS (OR = 2.04, $pC_{Co\text{-}dom}$ = 0.027, and OR = 2.01, $pC_{Res}$ = 0.007, respectively). The "*AAG*" haplotype was associated with a high risk of ACS (OR = 1.22, $pC$ = 0.016). The *c.*52 AA* genotype showed a lower HDL-C concentration than individuals with the *GG* genotype. In addition, carriers of *c.*773 GG* genotype carriers had a lower concentration of the high-density lipoprotein-cholesterol (HDL-C) than subjects with the *AA* genotype. Our data suggest the association of the *LDLR c.*773 A/G* and *LDLR c.*52 A/G* polymorphisms with both the risk of developing ACS and with a lower concentration of HDL-C in the study population.

**Keywords:** genetics; single nucleotide polymorphism; acute coronary syndrome

## 1. Introduction

Acute coronary syndrome (ACS) constitutes a worldwide public health problem. It is a complex disease resulting from the interaction of genetic and environmental factors, as well as traditional cardiovascular risk factors [1,2]. This syndrome is a consequence of atherosclerosis by the excessive accumulation of cholesterol, which results in the formation of the atherosclerotic plaque associated with a strong inflammatory component [1–3]. The low-density lipoprotein receptor (LDLR) is a cell membrane glycoprotein that functions in the binding and internalization of circulating cholesterol-containing lipoprotein particles. The LDL receptor is ubiquitously expressed and is a key receptor for maintaining cholesterol homeostasis in humans [3–5]. This receptor mediates endocytosis of plasma lipoproteins containing apolipoprotein B, as well as remnants of triglyceride-rich lipoprotein metabolism, which are the precursors of plasma low-density lipoprotein cholesterol (LDL-C), which plays an important role in the atherosclerotic plaque [4–6].

Previous reports have shown a large number of the genetic variants in the *LDLR* gene that play an important role in the development of hypercholesterolemia and cardiovascular diseases in different populations; however, less than 15% have functional evidence [7,8]. Nonetheless, in recent years, three novel single nucleotide polymorphisms [*LDLR* UTR'3 c.*52 A/G (rs14158), *LDLR* UTR'3 c.*504 A/G (rs2738465), and *LDLR* UTR'3 c.* 773 A/G (rs2738466)] in the 3' untranslated region (UTR'3) of the *LDLR* gene (located in p13.1-13.3 of the chromosome 19) have been associated with higher levels of LDL-C and a greater risk of the developing hypercholesterolemia, the principal cardiovascular risk factor in atherosclerosis [9–11].

In this context, considering the important role of the LDL receptor in the uptake of low-density lipoprotein cholesterol (LDL-C) associated with the atherosclerotic plaque formation, the present study aimed to establish the role of the *LDLR* c.*52 A/G, *LDLR* c.*504 A/G, and *LDLR* c.* 773 A/G polymorphisms in the susceptibility to develop ACS. Furthermore, we evaluated whether these polymorphisms are associated with lipid profile plasma concentrations in a Mexican population sample.

## 2. Materials and Methods

### 2.1. Characteristics of the Study Population

We used the sample size calculation for unmatched cases and controls study with a power of 80% and an alpha error of 0.05 [12]. The study included 618 patients with ACS and 666 healthy controls unmatched by age or gender. From July 2010 to July 2015, 618 patients with ACS (82% men and 18% women, with a mean age of $58 \pm 10.5$ years) were referred to the Instituto Nacional de Cardiologia Ignacio Chavez. The patient inclusion criterion was the diagnosis of ACS; this disease was identified and classified by either an ST-elevation myocardial infarction (STEMI) or a non-ST-elevation ACS (NSTE-ACS) based on clinical characteristics, electrocardiographic changes, and biochemical markers of cardiac necrosis (creatinine kinase isoenzymes, creatinine phosphokinase, or troponin I above the upper limit of normal). The European Society of Cardiology (ESC) and American College of Cardiology (ACC) definitions were followed [13,14]. The diagnosis of NSTE-ACS included non-STEMI and unstable angina. The diagnosis of non-STEMI was angina or discomfort at rest with ST-segment changes on ECG indicating ischemia [ST-segment depression or transient elevation ($\geq 1$ mm) in at least two contiguous leads and/or prominent T-wave inversion] with a positive biomarker indicating myocardial necrosis. Patients with clinical features and/or electrocardiographic expression of non-STEMI (albeit with normal cardiac biomarker levels) were diagnosed with unstable angina [13,14]. Moreover, 666 healthy controls were included (68% men and 32% women with a mean age of $54 \pm 7.65$ years) from the cohort of the Genetics of Atherosclerotic Disease (GEA) Mexican study. The GEA study investigates the genetic factors associated with premature coronary artery disease (CAD), atherosclerosis, and other coronary risk factors in the Mexican population [15]. All subjects were asymptomatic and healthy individuals without a family history of premature CAD or atherosclerosis; they were recruited from June 2009 to June 2013 from blood bank donors and with the assistance of brochures posted in social service centers.

The exclusion criteria included the use of anti-dyslipidemic and anti-hypertensive drugs at the time of the study, congestive heart failure, and liver, renal, thyroid, or oncological disease. Additionally, the control subjects had a zero coronary calcium score determined by computed tomography, indicating the absence of subclinical atherosclerosis [ ]. To assess the contributions of the *LDLR* UTR'3 c.*52 *A/G*, *LDLR* UTR'3 c.*504 *A/G*, and *LDLR* UTR'3 c.* 773 *A/G* SNPs genotypes on the plasma lipids levels, we selected only the healthy controls group. All the included subjects were ethnically matched and considered Mexican mestizos only if they and their ancestors (at last three generations) had been born in the country. The study complies with the Declaration of Helsinki and was approved by the Ethics and Research commission of Instituto Nacional de Cardiologia Ignacio Chavez. Written informed consent was obtained from all individuals enrolled in the study.

*2.2. Laboratory Analyses*

Cholesterol and triglycerides plasma concentrations were determined by enzymatic/colorimetric assays (Randox Laboratories, Crumlin, Country Antrim, UK). HDL-cholesterol (C) concentrations were determined after precipitation of the apo B-containing lipoproteins by the method of the phosphotungstic acid-$Mg^{2+}$. The LDL-C concentration was determined in samples with a triglyceride level lower than 400 mg/dL with the Friedewald formula [ ]. Dyslipidemia was defined as the presence of one or more of the following conditions: cholesterol > 200 mg/dL, LDL-C > 130 mg/dL, HDL-C < 40 mg/dL, or triglycerides > 150 mg/dL, according to the guidelines of the National Cholesterol Education Project (NCEP) Adult Treatment Panel (ATP III) [ ]. Type 2 diabetes mellitus (T2DM) was defined with a fasting glucose ≥ 126 mg/dL; it was also considered when participants reported glucose-lowering treatment or a physician diagnosis of T2DM. Hypertension was defined by a systolic blood pressure ≥ 140 mmHg, diastolic blood pressure ≥ 90 mmHg, or the use of oral antihypertensive therapy [ ].

*2.3. Genetic Analysis*

DNA extraction was performed from peripheral blood in agreement with the method described by Lahiri and Nurnberger [ ]. The *LDLR* UTR'3 c.*52 *A/G* (rs14158), *LDLR* UTR'3 c.*504 *A/G* (rs2738465), and *LDLR* UTR'3 c.* 773 *A/G* (rs2738466) SNPs were genotyped using 5' exonuclease TaqMan genotyping assays on a 7900HT Fast Real-Time PCR System according to manufacturer's instructions (Applied Biosystems, Foster City, CA, USA). To avoid genotyping errors, 10% of the samples were assayed in duplicate; the results were concordant for all cases.

*2.4. Inheritance Models Analysis*

The association of the c.*52 *A/G*, c.*504 *A/G*, and c.* 773 *A/G* SNPs with ACS patients was perform under the following inheritance model: additive (major allele homozygotes versus heterozygotes versus minor allele homozygotes), codominant (major allele homozygotes versus minor allele homozygotes), dominant (major allele homozygotes versus heterozygotes + minor allele homozygotes), over-dominant (heterozygotes versus major allele homozygotes + minor allele homozygotes), and recessive (major allele homozygotes + heterozygotes versus minor allele homozygotes) using logistic regression, adjusting for cardiovascular risk factors.

*2.5. Analysis of the Haplotypes*

The linkage disequilibrium analysis (LD, D") and haplotypes construction were performed using Haploview version 4.1 (Broad Institute of Massachusetts Institute of Technology and Harvard University, Cambridge, MA, USA).

## 2.6. Functional Prediction Analysis

Two in silico programs, the ESEfinder 3.0 and SNP Function Prediction, were used to predict the possible functional effect of the LDLR SNPs. Both web-based tools (ESEfinder2.0 and SNPinfo) analyze the localization of the SNPs (e.g., 5′-upstream, 3′-untranslated regions, intronic) and their possible functional effects, such as amino acid changes in protein structure, transcription factor binding sites in the promoter or intronic enhancer regions, and alternative splicing regulation by disrupting exonic splicing enhancers (ESE) or silencers [19,20].

## 2.7. Statistical Analysis

All statistical analyses in this study were performed using SPSS version 18.0 (SPSS, Chicago, IL, USA). The Mann-Whitney $U$ test was used to compare the continuous variables (e.g., age, body mass index (BMI), blood pressure, glucose, total cholesterol, HDL-C, LDL-C, and triglycerides) between control and ACS groups. For the categorical variables (e.g., gender, hypertension, T2DM, dyslipidemia, and smoking habit), chi-squared or Fisher's exact tests were performed. All $p$-values were corrected (pC) by the Bonferroni test. The values of $pC < 0.05$ were considered statistically significant, and all odds ratios (OR) were presented with 95% confidence intervals. The occurrence of the ACS in our study was based in the OR values: (a) OR = 1 does not affect the odds of developing ACS, (b) OR > 1 is associated with higher odds of developing ACS, and (c) OR < 1 is associated with lower odds of developing ACS. To evaluate Hardy-Weinberg equilibrium (HWE), we used the chi-squared test. The Mann-Whitney U test was used for establishing the contributions of the genotypes on the lipid plasma levels. Values were expressed as means ± SD, and statistical significance was set at $p < 0.05$. The statistical power to detect an association with ACS was 0.80 according to the QUANTO software [21].

## 3. Results

### 3.1. Characteristics of the Study Population

Anthropometrics and biochemical parameters of the ACS patients and healthy controls are presented in Table 1. Patients with ACS have higher levels of blood pressure, glucose, and higher prevalence of hypertension, diabetes, and dyslipidemias than control subjects. On the other hand, ACS patients presented lower levels of total cholesterol, LDL-C, and triglycerides than healthy controls. This phenomenon could be due to the treatment with statins received by the group of patients.

### 3.2. Allele and Genotype Frequencies

Genotype frequencies in the polymorphic sites were in HWE. The allele and genotype frequencies of the *LDLR* SNPs in ACS patients and healthy controls are shown in Table 2. The frequencies allelic of the c.*52 A/G, c.*504 A/G, and c.*773 A/G SNPs located in the *LDLR* gene showed that the c.*52 A, c.*504 A, and c.*773 G alleles were associated with the risk of developing ACS (OR = 1.20, pC = 0.02, OR = 1.18, pC = 0.02, and OR = 1.22, pC = 0.01 respectively) (Table 2). In addition, we corroborated the association according to the inheritance models. In this context, the association of the c.*504 A/G polymorphism loses significance statistically (pC > 0.05). Nonetheless, the c.*52 A/G and c.*773 A/G polymorphisms were associated with the presence of ACS (Table 2). Under co-dominant and recessive models, the c.*52 AA genotype of the c.*52 A/G polymorphism was associated with a greater risk of ACS (OR = 2.02, $pC_{Co\text{-}dom}$ = 0.033, and OR = 2.00, $pC_{Res}$ = 0.009, respectively). In the same way, under co-dominant and recessive models, the c.*773 G genotype of the c.*773 A/G polymorphism was associated with a high risk of ACS (OR = 2.04, $pC_{Co\text{-}dom}$ = 0.027, and OR = 2.01, $pC_{Res}$ = 0.007, respectively). All models were adjusted for gender, age, blood pressure, BMI, glucose, total cholesterol, HDL-C, LDL-C, triglycerides, and smoking habits.

**Table 1.** Anthropometrics and biochemical parameters of the study individuals.

| Characteristic | | ACS Patients (n = 618) | Healthy Controls (n = 666) | p-Value |
|---|---|---|---|---|
| | | Median (percentile 25–75) | Median (percentile 25–75) | |
| Age (years) | | 58 (51–65) | 54 (49–59) | 0.001 |
| Gender n (%) | Male | 505 (82) | 453 (68) | <0.001 |
| | Female | 113 (18) | 213 (32) | |
| BMI (kg/m2) | | 27 (25–29) | 28 (26–31) | 0.521 |
| Blood pressure (mmHg) | Systolic | 132 (114–144) | 117 (106–126) | <0.001 |
| | Diastolic | 80 (70–90) | 73 (67–78) | <0.001 |
| Glucose (mg/dL) | | 159 (102–188) | 98 (84–99) | <0.001 |
| Total cholesterol (mg/dL) | | 164 (128–199) | 191 (165–210) | <0.001 |
| HDL-C (mg/dL) | | 39 (34–45) | 44 (35–53) | 0.017 |
| LDL-C (mg/dL) | | 106 (75–132) | 116 (94–134) | <0.001 |
| Triglycerides (mg/dL) | | 169 (109–201) | 176 (113–208) | 0.301 |
| Hypertension n (%) | Yes | 350 (57) | 201 (30) | <0.001 |
| Type II diabetes mellitus n (%) | Yes | 216 (35) | 63 (9) | <0.001 |
| Dyslipidemia n (%) | Yes | 528 (85) | 479 (72) | <0.001 |
| Smoking n (%) | Yes | 222 (36) | 147 (22) | <0.001 |

Data are expressed as median and percentiles (25th–75th). $p$ values were estimated using the Mann-Whitney $U$ test for continuous variables and the chi-squared test for categorical values. ACS: Acute coronary syndrome.

Table 2. Distribution of *LDLR* polymorphisms in ACS patients and healthy controls.

| Polymorphic Site | | n (Genotype Frequency) | | | Model | OR (95%CI) | pC | n (Allele Frequency) | | | OR | 95%CI | pC |
|---|---|---|---|---|---|---|---|---|---|---|---|---|---|
| *LDLR UTR'3* | c.*52 A/G (rs14158) | | | | | | | | | *Risk allele | | | |
| | | GG | AG | AA | | | | G | | *A | A vs. G | | |
| Control (n = 666) | | 385 (0.578) | 252 (0.378) | 29 (0.043) | | | | 1022 (0.766) | | 310 (0.232) | | | |
| ACS (n = 618) | | 337 (0.545) | 231 (0.374) | 50 (0.081) | Co-dominant | 2.02 (1.18–3.46) | 0.033 | 905 (0.732) | | 331 (0.267) | 1.20 | 1.00–1.44 | 0.02 |
| | | | | | Dominant | 1.13 (0.88–1.45) | 0.35 | | | | | | |
| | | | | | Recessive | 2.00 (1.18–3.39) | 0.009 | | | | | | |
| | | | | | Over-dominant | 0.96 (0.74–1.24) | 0.73 | | | | | | |
| | | | | | Additive | 1.20 (0.98–1.45) | 0.075 | | | | | | |
| *LDLR UTR'3* | c.*504 A/G (rs2738465) | | | | | | | | | | | | |
| | | GG | AG | AA | | | | G | | *A | A vs. G | | |
| Control (n = 666) | | 323 (0.485) | 283 (0.425) | 60 (0.090) | | | | 929 (0.696) | | 403 (0.302) | | | |
| ACS (n = 618) | | 280 (0.453) | 256 (0.414) | 82 (0.133) | Co-dominant | 1.50 (0.99–2.26) | 0.16 | 816 (0.660) | | 420 (0.339) | 1.18 | 1.00–1.40 | 0.02 |
| | | | | | Dominant | 1.15 (0.90–1.47) | 0.27 | | | | | | |
| | | | | | Recessive | 1.45 (0.98–2.16) | 0.06 | | | | | | |
| | | | | | Over-dominant | 0.99 (0.77–1.27) | 0.94 | | | | | | |
| | | | | | Additive | 1.17 (0.97–1.41) | 0.09 | | | | | | |
| *LDLR UTR'3* | c.*773 A/G (rs2738466) | | | | | | | | | | | | |
| | | AA | AG | GG | | | | A | | *G | G vs. A | | |
| Control (n = 666) | | 386 (0.580) | 250 (0.375) | 30 (0.045) | | | | 1022 (0.766) | | 310 (0.232) | | | |
| ACS (n = 618) | | 335 (0.542) | 231 (0.374) | 52 (0.084) | Co-dominant | 2.04 (1.35–3.45) | 0.027 | 901 (0.728) | | 335 (0.271) | 1.22 | 1.02–1.146 | 0.01 |
| | | | | | Dominant | 1.14 (0.88–1.46) | 0.32 | | | | | | |
| | | | | | Recessive | 2.01 (1.20–3.38) | 0.007 | | | | | | |
| | | | | | Over-dominant | 0.96 (0.74–1.24) | 0.73 | | | | | | |
| | | | | | Additive | 1.21 (0.99–1.48) | 0.062 | | | | | | |

ACS, Acute coronary syndrome; OR, odds ratio; CI, confidence interval; pC, p-value. The p-values were calculated with the logistic regression analysis, and ORs were adjusted for gender, age, blood pressure, BMI, glucose, total cholesterol, HDL-C, LDL-C, triglycerides, and smoking habit.

## 3.3. Linkage Disequilibrium Analysis

The linkage disequilibrium analysis between the c.*52 A/G, c.*504 A/G, and c.* 773 A/G SNPs located in the *LDLR* gene showed three common haplotypes (Table ). Two of them showed significant differences between patients with ACS and healthy controls. The "GGA" haplotype was associated with a low risk of developing ACS (OR = 0.84, 95% CI: 0.71–0.99, pC = 0.023), whereas the "AAG" haplotype was associated with high risk of developing the same syndrome (OR = 1.22, 95% CI: 1.02–1.46, pC = 0.016). In this study, we did not find any other haplotype because these SNPs are in almost complete linkage disequilibrium (D' ≈ 1), which results in the joint co-segregation of these polymorphisms in the cases and controls (data not shown).

**Table 3.** Frequencies of *LDLR* haplotypes in patients with ACS and healthy controls.

| c.*52 A/G Haplotype | c.*504 A/G | c.*773 A/G | ACS (n = 618) Hf | Controls (n = 666) Hf | OR | 95%CI | pC |
|---|---|---|---|---|---|---|---|
| G | G | A | 0.658 | 0.695 | 0.84 | 0.71–0.99 | 0.023 |
| A | A | G | 0.267 | 0.230 | 1.22 | 1.02–1.46 | 0.016 |
| A | G | A | 0.070 | 0.069 | 1.03 | 0.76–1.39 | 0.446 |

Abbreviations: ACS: acute coronary syndrome; Hf = Haplotype frequency, pC = p corrected. The order of the polymorphisms in the haplotypes is according to the positions in the chromosome (rs14158, rs2738465, rs2738466).

## 3.4. Functional Prediction

According, with the in silico programs ESEfinder 3.0 and SNP Function Prediction [ , ], the functional prediction analysis showed that the presence of the *A* allele of the c.*504 A/G polymorphism potentially produced a binding motif for the miR-200a microRNA. Moreover, a binding motif for miR-638 is predicted for the *G* allele of the c.* 773 A/G SNP. This analysis suggest that these polymorphisms located in the UTR'3 of the LDLR gene could be influence splicing or mRNA stability altering expression levels.

## 3.5. Association of Polymorphisms and Haplotypes with Plasma Lipids Levels

To define the possible functional effect of c.*52 A/G, c.*504 A/G, and c.*773 A/G SNPs, we determined the plasma lipids levels (total cholesterol, LDL-C, HDL-C, and triglycerides), as well as the risk cardiovascular factors (BMI, blood pressure, glucose) in individuals with different genotypes of these three polymorphisms. For this analysis, we selected only the healthy controls group. We did not include the plasma-lipid level analysis in patients with ACS because, in the setting of the coronary syndrome, these levels may be altered using anti-dyslipidemic or anti-hypertensive drugs [ – ]. The analysis showed that the c.*52 A/G, c.*504 A/G, and c.* 773 A/G SNPs were not associated with the following parameters: total cholesterol, LDL-C, triglycerides, BMI, blood pressure, and glucose (Supplementary Table S1). However, we observed significant differences in HDL-C plasma levels when subjects were grouped by these SNPs. As for the c.*52 A/G SNP, individuals with the *AA* genotype showed a lower concentration of HDL-C in plasma (38 ± 10.4 mg/dL) than individuals with either *AG* (45.5 ± 13.7 mg/dL, p = 0.002) or *GG* genotypes (44.3 ± 13.2 mg/dL, p = 0.007) (Figure A). Alternatively, subjects carrying c.*773 *GG* genotype had a lower HDL-C plasma concentration (38 ± 10.3 mg/dL) than carriers of either the *AA* (44.4 ± 13.1 mg/dL, p = 0.007) or *AG* genotype (45.4 ± 14.9 mg/dL, p = 0.003) (Figure C). Although the c.*504 A/G polymorphism was not associated with ACS development, individuals with the c.*504 *AA* genotype had a lower HDL-C plasma concentration than individuals with the *AG* genotype (41.7 ± 13.8 mg/dL, p = 0.039) (Figure B). In addition, the analysis of the haplotypes (GGA and AAG) showed significant differences when compared with HDL-C plasma concentrations. The "AAG" haplotype risk showed a lower concentration of HDL-C in plasma (39.9 ± 12.3 mg/dL) when compared to "GGA" haplotype of low risk (44.5 ± 13.24, p = 0.004) (Figure ).

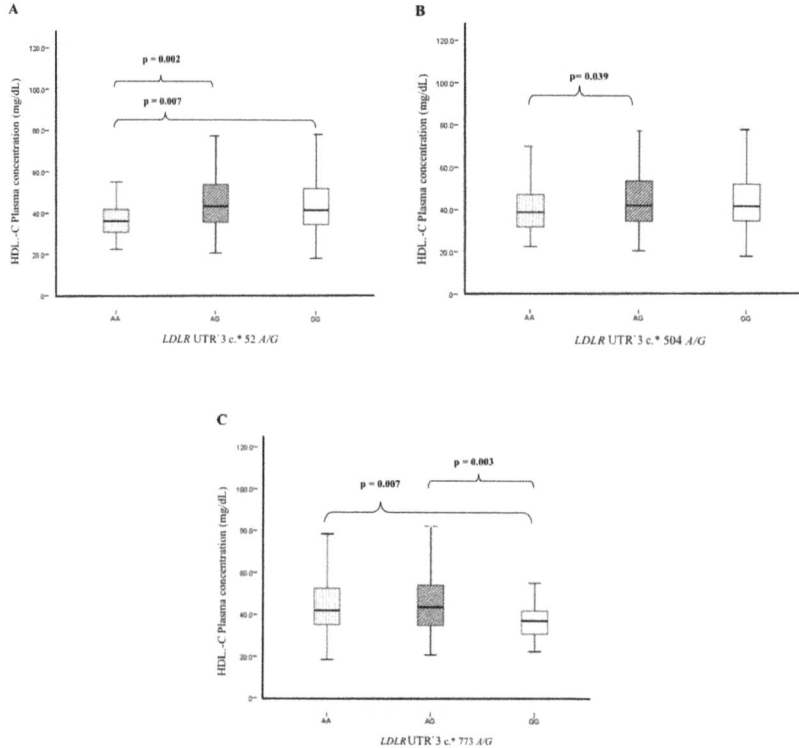

**Figure 1.** Genetic contribution of the *LDLR* UTR'3 c.*52 A/G, *LDLR* UTR'3 c.*504 A/G, and *LDLR* UTR'3 c.* 773 A/G polymorphisms on HDL-C levels. (**A**) The *AA* genotype of the *LDLR* UTR'3 c.*52 A/G SNP showed low HDL-C levels in plasma when compared to *AG/GG* genotypes. (**B**) The *AA* genotype of the *LDLR* UTR'3 c.*504 A/G polymorphism showed lower HDL-C levels in plasma than the *AG* genotype. (**C**) The *GG* genotype of the *LDLR* UTR'3 c.* 773 A/G showed low HDL-C levels in plasma when compared to *AA/AG* genotypes.

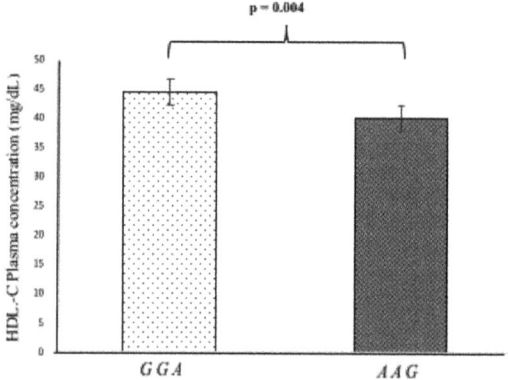

Comparison of HDL-C plasma concentrations between haplotypes associated.

**Figure 2.** Contribution of the "*GGA*" and "*AAG*" on HDL-C levels. The "*AAG*" haplotype risk showed a lower concentration of HDL-C in plasma when compared to "*GGA*" haplotype of low risk ($p = 0.004$).

## 4. Discussion

ACS is a multifactorial and polygenic disorder consequence of atherosclerosis, in which the excessive accumulation of cholesterol plays an important role. In the present study, we focused on the LDL receptor, which is a cell membrane glycoprotein that functions in the binding and internalization of circulating cholesterol-containing lipoprotein particles. The LDL receptor is ubiquitously expressed and is a key receptor for maintaining cholesterol homeostasis in humans [ – ]. We studied three polymorphisms (c.*52 A/G, c.*504 A/G, and c.*773 A/G) located in the 3′ untranslated region of the *LDLR* gene in ACS patients and healthy controls. According to our analysis, the c.*52 A/G and c.*773 A/G SNPs were associated with the risk of developing ACS, as well as with lower plasma HDL-C concentrations. To the best of our knowledge, this study is the first to describe the association between these polymorphisms and the presence of ACS. In this context, the association of these SNPs with several diseases in different populations is scarce and controversial. For example, in agreement with our data, van Zyl et al. reported that the *A* allele of the c.*52 A/G SNP increased the risk of developing familial hypercholesterolemia in the African population [ ]. In the same way, De Castro-Oros et al. reported that the hypercholesterolemic subjects with the c.*52 A, c.*504 A, and c.*773 G alleles have a lower response to the anti-dyslipidemic drug Armolipid Plus; in their study, the authors suggested that these SNPs increased the risk of developing hypercholesterolemia in a Spanish population [ ]. In contrast, Zambrano et al. reported that the *A* allele of the c.*52 A/G SNP decreased the risk of the developing hypercholesterolemia in a Brazilian population [ ]. By the same token, Chen et al. reported that c.*52 A/G, c.*504 A/G, and c.*773 A/G polymorphisms were not associated with the risk of developing coronary heart diseases in a Chinese population [ ]. Although in our study the c.*504 A/G polymorphism showed a moderate association with the risk of developing ACS ($pC = 0.06$), van Zyl et al. reported that this polymorphism increased the risk of developing familial hypercholesterolemia in an African population ($p = 0.051$) [ ]. In addition, we found that the "AAG" haplotype was associated with a high risk of developing ACS and with lower plasma HDL-C levels, whereas the "GGA" haplotype was associated with a low risk and higher plasma HDL-C levels.

According to data in the literature, the impact of the *LDLR* gene polymorphisms on lipid plasma concentration has been proposed as the mechanism that explains the relationship between these SNPs and the higher risk of developing familial hypercholesterolemia [ , ]. In this context, recent studies have associated the *LDLR* polymorphisms (c.*52 A/G, c.*504 A/G, and c.*773 A/G) with low levels of plasma lipids and the risk of developing familial hypercholesterolemia [ – , ]. For example, Li et al. reported that c.*773 G/G genotype is associated with decreased plasma levels of HDL-C in healthy individuals of China [ ]. In the same way, van Zyl et al. documented that c.*52 A/A and c.*504 A/A genotypes are associated with increased levels of LDL-C in the healthy black South African population [ ]. Our results showed that c.*52 A/A, c.*504 A/A, and c.*773 G/G genotypes were associated with low HDL-C levels. In contrast, Chen et al., studying a Chinese population, reported that these polymorphisms were not associated with altered plasma lipid levels in patients with coronary heart diseases and healthy controls [ ]. As far as we know, the precise mechanism by which low HDL-C levels are associated with hypercholesterolemia and adverse events, such as ACS, remains to be elucidated. Nonetheless, data in the literature provide evidence that the reduction of plasma HDL-C is due to the defective assembly of nascent HDL by hepatocyte Abca1 (ATP binding cassette transport A1) and increased plasma clearance of HDL protein and cholesteryl ester [ , ]. Moreover, experimental studies in mice have shown that (i) the hepatic LDL receptor stimulated plasma HDL selective cholesteryl ester uptake, and (ii) sterol trafficking into reverse cholesterol transport decreased HDL-C levels, when hepatocyte Abca1 was deficient [ – ]. Additionally, using bioinformatics tools, we determined the potential effect of the *LDLR* gene polymorphisms; no evidence of a functional motif was found for the c.*52 A/G polymorphism. Nonetheless, the analysis of the c.*504 A/G polymorphism showed that *A* allele produced a binding motif for miR-200a; this microRNA regulates the kelch-like EHC-associated protein 1 (Keap1)/nuclear factor erythroid 2-related factor (Nrf2) signaling axis, which plays an important role in regulating ischemic myocardial oxidative stress. Furthermore, the overexpression of miR-200a was found to protect cardiomyocytes from hypoxia-induced cell damage and the excessive production of reactive oxygen species [27]. On the other hand, the G allele of the *c.\*773 A/G* polymorphism produced a binding site for miR-638; this microRNA plays an important role in the vascular smooth muscle cell (VSMC) proliferation and migration in atherosclerotic plaque vulnerability through the regulation of the cyclin D and NOR1. Alternatively, miR-638 is a regulator of the platelet-derived growth factor-BB (PDGF-BB), which is released primarily by vascular endothelial cells and platelets at the sites of vascular injury. Of note, this miRNA has been identified as one of the most potent stimulants for the VSMC proliferation and migration, through the modulation of several transcription factors and key molecular signaling pathways [28,29]. However, the effects of miR-200a or miR-638 on plasma lipid levels has not been previously reported. Mechanistically, using bioinformatics tools, miRNAs predicted to recognize the polymorphic site were expected to decrease the LDL-R-mRNA half-life in the cytoplasm [19,20]. Consequently, LDL-cholesterol should have been higher in the risk allele carriers, but such difference was not observed. Speculative explanations to these observations include a mRNA stabilizing role of the micro RNAs or a limited or null association of the miRNA to the 3'UTR region. Based in the LDL-cholesterol plasma levels it is likely that the second result is more acceptable; the miR-200a and miR-638 seem to have a little impact on regulating LDL-R gene expression. Nevertheless, it cannot be discarded a contribution of these miRNAS to increasing LDL-cholesterol plasma levels. To our knowledge, there are no data describing the possible pathways altered specifically in ACS and/or other cardiovascular events by the miR-200a and miR-638, and binding sites harboring to the alleles c. * 52 A and c. * 773 G. Nonetheless, recent data have identified several SNPs that generates binding sites with microRNAs such as miR-33, miR-148a, and miR.128-1 that play an important role in the LDLR expression [30]. Future investigations are needed to understand the effect of these polymorphisms on LDL-R and HDL-C plasma levels and its potential relationship with miRNAs.

Finally, in our study, the *c.\*52 A/G* and *c.\*773 A/G* polymorphisms were associated with the presence of ACS; however, the participation of these polymorphisms is controversial in other populations. We think that the association of the *LDLR* polymorphisms with ACS could be due to the role of this receptor in the regulation of the circulating cholesterol-containing lipoprotein particles, which is, in turn, an important cardiovascular risk factor [11,23]. It is important to notice that the allele distribution of these polymorphisms varies according to the ethnic origin of the study populations. In this context, data obtained from the National Center for Biotechnology Information revealed that the individuals from Los Angeles with Mexican ancestry, Mexican mestizos, Caucasian, and Africans had a lower frequency of the c.*52 A allele (26, 23, 23, and 15%, respectively) than Asians (41%). Moreover, Mexican mestizos, Europeans, Africans, as well as individuals from Los Angeles with Mexican ancestry, have a lower frequency of the c.*773 G allele (23, 22, 16, and 26%, respectively) than the Asian population (41%) [31]. Of note, the Mexican population has a characteristic genetic background with important ethnic differences compared to other populations [32–34]. Therefore, we consider that studies with a greater sample in populations with different ethnic origins may explain the true role of *LDLR* SNPs in the risk of developing ACS.

In summary, this study demonstrated that the *c.\*52 A/G* and *c.\*773 A/G* polymorphisms of the *LDLR* gene are associated with the risk of developing ACS in a Mexican population. In addition, it was possible to distinguish one haplotype (*AAG*) associated with a higher risk of developing ACS. There was a statistically significant association of both c.*52 A/G and c.*773 A/G polymorphisms with lower HDL-C levels in plasma. Lastly, because of the specific genetic characteristics of the Mexican population, we consider that additional studies need to be undertaken in a larger number of individuals and in populations with different ethnic origins. This future research could help define the true role of these polymorphisms as markers of risk or protection from developing ACS and other cardiovascular events.

**Supplementary Materials:** The following are available online at https://www.mdpi.com/2218-273X/10/10/1381/s1, Table S1: Association of the LDLR gene SNPs with plasma lipids levels and anthropometric characteristics in the healthy control group (n = 666).

**Author Contributions:** Conceptualization, G.V.-A., O.P.-M., and J.M.F.; Data curation, O.P.-M., J.R.-B., H.G.-P., and E.C.-T.; Formal analysis, R.P.-S., G.E., B.N.-L., E.C.-T., and J.M.F.; Investigation, G.V.-A., O.P.-M., and J.M.F.; Methodology, O.P.-M., R.P.-S., G.E., and B.N.-L.; Resources, O.P.-M., J.R.-B., R.P.-S., H.G.-P., B.N.-L., and J.M.F.; Software, J.R.-B., R.P.-S., and G.E.; Supervision, J.M.F.; Validation, G.V.-A., O.P.-M., and J.M.F.; Writing—original draft, J.M.F.; Writing—review and editing, G.V.-A. and J.M.F. All authors have read and agreed to the published version of the manuscript.

**Funding:** This research was funded by the *Consejo Nacional de Ciencia y Tecnología (CONACyT)*, Mexico City, Mexico (Project Fronteras de la Ciencia-1958).

**Acknowledgments:** The authors are grateful to the study participants. Institutional Review Board approval was obtained for all sample collections. The authors are grateful to the technicians Silvestre Ramirez-Fuentes and Marva Arellano-Gonzalez for their participation in the collection of samples and extraction of DNA.

**Conflicts of Interest:** The authors declare that there is no conflict of interests regarding the publication of this article.

## Abbreviations

| | |
|---|---|
| LDLR | Low-density lipoprotein receptor |
| UTR'3 | Untranslated region-'3 |
| HDL-C | High-density lipoprotein-cholesterol |
| LDL-C | Low-density lipoprotein-cholesterol |
| T2DM | Type 2 diabetes mellitus |
| SNP | Single nucleotide polymorphism |
| ACS | Acute coronary syndrome |

## References

1. Libby, P.; Ridker, P.M.; Maseri, A. Inflammation and Atherosclerosis. *Circulation* **2002**, *105*, 1135–1143. [CrossRef] [PubMed]
2. Virmani, R.; Kolodgie, F.D.; Burke, A.; Finn, A.V.; Gold, H.K.; Tulenko, T.N.; Wrenn, S.P.; Narula, J. Atherosclerotic Plaque Progression and Vulnerability to Rupture. *Arter. Thromb. Vasc. Biol.* **2005**, *25*, 2054–2061. [CrossRef] [PubMed]
3. Zhang, Y.; Ma, K.; Ruan, X.Z.; Liu, B.C. Dysregulation of the Low-Density Lipoprotein Receptor Pathway Is Involved in Lipid Disorder-Mediated Organ Injury. *Int. J. Biol. Sci.* **2016**, *12*, 569–579. [CrossRef]
4. Litvinov, D.Y.; Savushkin, E.V.; Dergunov, A.D. Intracellular and Plasma Membrane Events in Cholesterol Transport and Homeostasis. *J. Lipids* **2018**, *2018*, 1–22. [CrossRef]
5. Abisambra, J.F.; Fiorelli, T.; Padmanabhan, J.; Neame, P.; Wefes, I.; Potter, H. LDLR Expression and Localization Are Altered in Mouse and Human Cell Culture Models of Alzheimer's Disease. *PLoS ONE* **2010**, *5*, e8556. [CrossRef] [PubMed]
6. Nikolic, J.; Belot, L.; Raux, H.; Legrand, P.; Gaudin, Y.; Albertini, A.A. Structural basis for the recognition of LDL-receptor family members by VSV glycoprotein. *Nat. Commun.* **2018**, *9*, 1029. [CrossRef] [PubMed]
7. Bourbon, M.; Alves, A.C.; Sijbrands, E.J.G. Low-density lipoprotein receptor mutational analysis in diagnosis of familial hypercholesterolemia. *Curr. Opin. Lipidol.* **2017**, *28*, 120–129. [CrossRef]
8. Defesche, J.C.; Gidding, S.S.; Harada-Shiba, M.; Hegele, R.A.; Santos, R.D.; Wierzbicki, A.S. Familial hypercholesterolaemia. *Nat. Rev. Dis. Primers* **2017**, *3*, 17093. [CrossRef]
9. Zambrano, T.; Hirata, M.H.; Cerda, Á.; Dorea, E.L.; Pinto, G.A.; Gusukuma, M.C.; Bertolami, M.C.; Salazar, L.A.; Hirata, R.D.C. Impact of 3′UTR genetic variants in PCSK9 and LDLR genes on plasma lipid traits and response to atorvastatin in Brazilian subjects: A pilot study. *Int. J. Clin. Exp. Med.* **2015**, *8*, 5978–5988.
10. De Castro-Orós, I.; Solà, R.; Valls, R.-M.; Brea, Á.; Mozas, P.; Puzo, J.; Pocovi, M. Genetic Variants of LDLR and PCSK9 Associated with Variations in Response to Antihypercholesterolemic Effects of Armolipid Plus with Berberine. *PLoS ONE* **2016**, *11*, e0150785. [CrossRef]

11. Van Zyl, T.; Jerling, J.C.; Conradie, K.R.; Feskens, E.J. Common and rare single nucleotide polymorphisms in the LDLR gene are present in a black South African population and associate with low-density lipoprotein cholesterol levels. *J. Hum. Genet.* **2013**, *59*, 88–94. [CrossRef] [PubMed]
12. Openepi.com. Available online: http://www.openepi.com/SampleSize/SSCC.html (accessed on 1 April 2020).
13. Cannon, C.P.; Battler, A.; Brindis, R.G.; Cox, J.L.; Ellis, S.G.; Every, N.R.; Flaherty, J.T.; Harrington, R.A.; Krumholz, H.M.; Simoons, M.L.; et al. American College of Cardiology key data elements and definitions for measuring the clinical management and outcomes of patients with acute coronary syndromes: A report of the American College of Cardiology Task Force on Clinical Data Standards (Acute Coronary Syndromes Writing Committee) Endorsed by the American Association of Cardiovascular and Pulmonary Rehabilitation, American College of Emergency Physicians, American Heart Association, Cardiac Society of Australia & New Zealand, National Heart Foundation of Australia, Society for Cardiac Angiography and Interventions, and the Taiwan Society of Cardiology. *J. Am. Coll. Cardiol.* **2001**, *38*, 2114–2130. [CrossRef]
14. Hamm, C.W.; Bassand, J.-P.; Agewall, S.; Bax, J.; Boersma, E.; Bueno, H.; Caso, P.; Dudek, D.; Gielen, S.; Huber, K.; et al. ESC Guidelines for the management of acute coronary syndromes in patients presenting without persistent ST-segment elevation: The Task Force for the management of acute coronary syndromes (ACS) in patients presenting without persistent ST-segment elevation of the European Society of Cardiology (ESC). *Eur. Heart J.* **2011**, *32*, 2999–3054. [CrossRef]
15. Posadas-Sánchez, R.; Pérez-Hernández, N.; Angeles-Martinez, J.; López-Bautista, F.; Villarreal-Molina, T.; Rodriguez-Perez, J.M.; Fragoso, J.M.; Posadas-Romero, C.; Vargas-Alarcón, G. Interleukin 35 Polymorphisms Are Associated with Decreased Risk of Premature Coronary Artery Disease, Metabolic Parameters, and IL-35 Levels: The Genetics of Atherosclerotic Disease (GEA) Study. *Mediat. Inflamm.* **2017**, *2017*, 1–10. [CrossRef] [PubMed]
16. Delong, D.M.; Delong, E.R.; Wood, P.D.; Lippel, K.; Rifkind, B.M. A Comparison of Methods for the Estimation of Plasma Low- and Very Low-Density Lipoprotein Cholesterol. *JAMA* **1986**, *256*, 2372–2377. [CrossRef] [PubMed]
17. ATP III Guidelines At-A-Glance Quick Desk Reference. Available online: https://www.nhlbi.nih.gov/files/docs/guidelines/atglance.pdf (accessed on 29 April 2020).
18. Lahiri, D.K.; Numberger, J.I. A rapid non-enzymatic method for the preparation of HMW DNA from blood for RFLP studies. *Nucleic Acids Res.* **1991**, *19*, 5444. [CrossRef]
19. Smith, P.J.; Zhang, C.; Wang, J.; Chew, S.L.; Zhang, M.Q.; Krainer, A. An increased specificity score matrix for the prediction of SF2/ASF-specific exonic splicing enhancers. *Hum. Mol. Genet.* **2006**, *15*, 2490–2508. [CrossRef]
20. Xu, Z.; Taylor, J.A. SNPinfo: Integrating GWAS and candidate gene information into functional SNP selection for genetic association studies. *Nucleic Acids Res.* **2009**, *37*, W600–W605. [CrossRef]
21. QUANTO. Available online: https://preventivemedicine.usc.edu/download-quanto/ (accessed on 3 April 2020).
22. Chen, W.; Wang, S.; Ma, Y.; Zhou, Y.; Liu, H.; Strnad, P.; Kraemer, F.B.; Krauss, R.M.; Liu, J. Analysis of polymorphisms in the 3′ untranslated region of the LDL receptor gene and their effect on plasma cholesterol levels and drug response. *Int. J. Mol. Med.* **2008**, *21*, 345–353. [CrossRef]
23. Li, Z.; Zhao, T.-Y.; Tan, X.-H.; Lei, S.; Huang, L.; Yang, L. Polymorphisms in PCSK9, LDLR, BCMO1, SLC12A3, and KCNJ1 are Associated with Serum Lipid Profile in Chinese Han Population. *Int. J. Environ. Res. Public Health* **2019**, *16*, 3207. [CrossRef]
24. Bashore, A.C.; Liu, M.; Key, C.-C.C.; Boudyguina, E.; Wang, X.; Carroll, C.M.; Sawyer, J.K.; Mullick, A.E.; Lee, R.G.; Macauley, S.L.; et al. Targeted Deletion of Hepatocyte Abca1 Increases Plasma HDL (High-Density Lipoprotein) Reverse Cholesterol Transport via the LDL (Low-Density Lipoprotein) Receptor. *Arter. Thromb. Vasc. Biol.* **2019**, *39*, 1747–1761. [CrossRef]
25. Joyce, C.; Wagner, E.M.; Basso, F.; Amar, M.J.; Freeman, L.A.; Shamburek, R.D.; Knapper, C.L.; Syed, J.; Wu, J.; Vaisman, B.L.; et al. ABCA1 Overexpression in the Liver of LDLr-KO Mice Leads to Accumulation of Pro-atherogenic Lipoproteins and Enhanced Atherosclerosis. *J. Biol. Chem.* **2006**, *281*, 33053–33065. [CrossRef] [PubMed]
26. Rinninger, F.; Heine, M.; Singaraja, R.; Hayden, M.; Brundert, M.; Ramakrishnan, R.; Heeren, J. High density lipoprotein metabolism in low density lipoprotein receptor-deficient mice. *J. Lipid Res.* **2014**, *55*, 1914–1924. [CrossRef] [PubMed]

27. Sun, X.; Zuo, H.; Liu, C.; Yang, Y. Overexpression of miR-200a protects cardiomyocytes against hypoxia-induced apoptosis by modulating the kelch-like ECH-associated protein 1-nuclear factor erythroid 2-related factor 2 signaling axis. *Int. J. Mol. Med.* **2016**, *38*, 1303–1311. [CrossRef]
28. Li, P.; Liu, Y.; Yi, B.; Wang, G.; You, X.; Zhao, X.; Summer, R.; Qin, Y.; Sun, J. MicroRNA-638 is highly expressed in human vascular smooth muscle cells and inhibits PDGF-BB-induced cell proliferation and migration through targeting orphan nuclear receptor NOR1. *Cardiovasc. Res.* **2013**, *99*, 185–193. [CrossRef]
29. Luque, A.; Farwati, A.; Krupinski, J.; Aran, J.M. Association between low levels of serum miR-638 and atherosclerotic plaque vulnerability in patients with high-grade carotid stenosis. *J. Neurosurg.* **2019**, *131*, 72–79. [CrossRef]
30. Aryal, B.; Singh, A.K.; Rotllan, N.; Price, N.D.; Fernández-Hernando, C. MicroRNAs and lipid metabolism. *Curr. Opin. Lipidol.* **2017**, *28*, 273–280. [CrossRef]
31. Ensembl.org. Available online: https://www.ensembl.org/Multi/Search/Results (accessed on 3 April 2020).
32. Lisker, R.; Granados, J.; Babinsky, V.; De Rubens, J.; Armendares, S.; Buentello, L.; Perez-Briceño, R. Gene frequencies and admixture estimates in a Mexico City population. *Am. J. Phys. Anthr.* **1986**, *71*, 203–207. [CrossRef]
33. Lisker, R.; Ramirez, E.; Briceño, R.P.; Granados, J.; Babinsky, V. Gene frequencies and admixture estimates in four Mexican urban centers. *Hum. Biol.* **1990**, *62*, 791–801. [PubMed]
34. Juárez-Cedillo, T.; Zúñiga, J.; Acuña-Alonzo, V.; Pérez-Hernández, N.; Rodriguez-Perez, J.M.; Barquera, R.; Gallardo, G.J.; Arenas, R.S.; García-Peña, M.D.C.; Granados, J.; et al. Genetic admixture and diversity estimations in the Mexican Mestizo population from Mexico City using 15 STR polymorphic markers. *Forensic Sci. Int. Genet.* **2008**, *2*, e37–e39. [CrossRef] [PubMed]

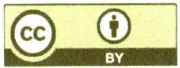

© 2020 by the authors. Licensee MDPI, Basel, Switzerland. This article is an open access article distributed under the terms and conditions of the Creative Commons Attribution (CC BY) license (http://creativecommons.org/licenses/by/4.0/).

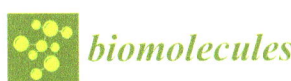 

*Review*

# The Role of Secretory Activity Molecules of Visceral Adipocytes in Abdominal Obesity in the Development of Cardiovascular Disease: A Review

Yuliya I. Ragino, Ekaterina M. Stakhneva *, Yana V. Polonskaya and Elena V. Kashtanova

Research Institute of Internal and Preventive Medicine - Branch of the Institute of Cytology and Genetics, Siberian Branch of Russian Academy of Sciences, Novosibirsk 630089, Russia; ragino@mail.ru (Y.I.R.); yana-polonskaya@yandex.ru (Y.V.P.); elekastanova@yandex.ru (E.V.K.)
* Correspondence: stahneva@yandex.ru; Tel.: +7-(383)-264-2516

Received: 4 December 2019; Accepted: 26 February 2020; Published: 28 February 2020

**Abstract:** Adipose tissue is considered one of the endocrine organs in the body because of its ability to synthesize and release a large number of hormones, cytokines, and growth and vasoactive factors that influence a variety of physiological and pathophysiological processes, such as vascular tone, inflammation, vascular smooth muscle cell migration, endothelial function, and vascular redox state. Moreover, genetic factors substantially contribute to the risk of obesity. Research into the biochemical effects of molecules secreted by visceral adipocytes as well as their molecular genetic characteristics is actively conducted around the world mostly in relation to pathologies of the cardiovascular system, metabolic syndrome, and diabetes mellitus. Adipokines could be developed into biomarkers for diagnosis, prognosis, and therapeutic targets in different diseases. This review describes the relevance of secretory activity molecules of visceral adipocytes in cardiovascular disease associated abdominal obesity.

**Keywords:** obesity; adipokines; biomolecules; biomarkers; leptin; resistin; visfatin

## 1. Introduction

At present, obesity is a relevant and important problem because of its rapidly increasing prevalence and severity of complications, which sometimes cause death at a young age [ , ].

According to the World Health Organization (WHO) in 2016, more than 1.9 billion adults over the age of 18 were overweight, and more than 650 million of them were obese. The worldwide prevalence of obesity nearly tripled between 1975 and 2016 [ ].

Visceral fat constitutes up to 10–20% of all adipose tissue in males and up to 5–8% in females. With age, in people of both sexes, there is an increase in the mass of visceral fat in the human body. Visceral adipose tissue contains a lot of large adipocytes. Visceral adipocytes are metabolically active and possess a higher lipolytic activity [ , ].

In recent years, there have been a number of biochemical and clinical–biochemical studies on the molecules generated by the secretory activity of visceral adipocytes, mostly in relation to the pathologies of the cardiovascular and endocrine systems.

The present review focuses on describing the current state of research in the field of cardiovascular diseases (CVDs) associated with abdominal obesity, discussion of the role of molecules of secretory activity of visceral adipocytes in the development of CVD, and their potential as biomarkers for diagnosis and prognosis.

## 2. Genetic Factors of Obesity

Genetic factors substantially contribute to the risk of obesity [6,7]. In recent years, there have been quite a few molecular genetic studies addressing the obesity problem in the world. It is thought that environmental risk factors related to changes in nutrition and physical activity can materialize only in the presence of genetic factors [8]. Accordingly, identification of candidate genes of obesity has aroused a lot of interest. Through medical examination of children and adults in various populations, investigators have uncovered more than 100 genetic polymorphisms associated with this disease [9,10].

Studies on the genetic polymorphisms in the Alaskan population have shown that the frequency of risk alleles of foodborne diseases in the ethnic groups of these regions is different from that in European and Asian populations [11,12]. A statistically significant association with excess body weight and obesity has been identified for two sequence variants (rs35682 and rs35683) of the adiponectin gene (*ADIPOQ*) in Americans of European origin in contrast to the residents of Alaska, who lack such associations [13]. In the population of Iceland, researchers have discovered a statistically significant association of obesity with polymorphic variant rs7566605 (of gene *INSIG2* regulating the synthesis of cholesterol, phospholipids, triglycerides (TG), and unsaturated fatty acids). This association is absent among the residents of Scandinavian countries, Americans of British origin, Russians living in Siberia, Koreans, and Chinese children and adolescents [14,15].

It is known that during visceral obesity, the increase in adipocyte size is related to the expression of genes FABP4, S100A9, and p53. The expression of p53, but not S100A9, in epicardial stromal cells is associated with adipocyte enlargement in obese patients with CVD [16]. In visceral adipose tissue from patients with IHD (ischemic heart disease), researchers have detected higher gene expression of such cytokines as interleukin-1β (IL-1β), monocytic chemotactic protein-1 (MCP-1), and natriuretic peptide receptor-C (NPR-C) [17]. In a study by Sacks et al., they investigated mRNA expression of 70 genes in visceral adipose tissue from patients with IHD. The authors found that 39 of the 70 analyzed genes were upregulated. Among the most actively expressed mRNAs was *IL8* mRNA, which manifested a threefold increase in expression [18]. It has been reported that circulating tumor necrosis factor-alpha (TNF-α) concentration and its mRNA expression are higher in patients with obesity and IHD (37 subjects) in comparison with patients without cardiovascular disorders (20 subjects). These data confirm the relation between changes in the secretome and transcriptome of adipose tissue in CVDs [19].

According to the above review, a small number of adipokines have been thoroughly studied (adiponectin is among the best-studied adipokines), as is the case for genes involved in the processes of adipogenesis and secretion of a protein product by adipocytes. Nonetheless, in the literature, there are data on some other factors. For instance, in adipocytes of epicardial adipose tissue and subcutaneous adipose tissue, researchers compared the expression of 307 genes participating in the regulation of angiogenesis, formation of vessel morphology, inflammation, and blood clotting. Among the 156 upregulated genes expressed in epicardial adipose tissue, 59 were found to be associated with angiogenesis and inflammation (e.g., *TNFRSF11B*, *PLAT*, *TGFB1*, *THBS2*, *HIF1A*, *GATA6*, and *SERPINE1*), whereas among the 166 downregulated genes, only 21 showed such associations (including *ANGPT1*, *ANGPTL1*, and *VEGFC*). These results indicate that epicardial adipocytes can participate in significant modulation of vascular inflammation [20].

## 3. Specific Molecules of Visceral Adipocytes

Recent studies suggest that visceral adipose tissue not only serves for the accumulation of energy-rich substrates but also acts as an endocrine gland of sorts, which produces various compounds exerting their effects both locally and at the systemic level. Products of secretion by the cells of visceral adipose tissue (adipocytes) are hormones (leptin, adiponectin, and resistin), proinflammatory cytokines (TNF-α, IL-6, IL-8, and others), and rennin–angiotensin system proteins; some of them take part in the functioning of the complement system and in vascular hemostasis (PAI1 and others) [21–26]. Research into biochemical effects of the molecules secreted by visceral adipocytes as well as their molecular genetic characteristics is actively conducted worldwide mostly in relation to pathologies of the cardiovascular system, metabolic syndrome, and diabetes mellitus.

## 4. Leptin

Many authors have lately addressed the contribution of leptin to cardiac remodeling in heart failure and the possible explanation of the obesity paradox by the influence of leptin on the metabolism, apoptosis, and remodeling of the extracellular matrix and on hypertrophy. Besides, obesity and hyperleptinemia are often linked with hypertension. We should not rule out the direct action of leptin on such phenomena as atherosclerosis, endothelial dysfunction, and thrombosis [ – ]. Unfortunately, extrapolation of the results of basic in vitro research (or research on animal models) to human physiology has turned out to be rather complicated. It is thought that leptin may be an important mediator between obesity and the development of CVDs. This mechanism is possibly driven by such leptin effects as the influence on arterial pressure, aggregation of platelets, formation of arterial thrombosis, and an inflammatory vascular response. Investigators believe that a high level of leptin is related to low arterial extensibility and participates in the pathogenesis of atherosclerosis via mechanisms different from vascular relaxation. Some authors have noted a connection between serum concentrations of leptin and various cardiovascular risks, including stroke, chronic heart failure, acute myocardial infarction, coronary artery disease, and left ventricle hypertrophy [ – ]. It seems worthwhile to study leptin/adiponectin ratios. As demonstrated by Kappelle et al. [ ] in a cohort case–control study of males with adjustment for age, the incidence of CVDs correlates with blood plasma levels of leptin, adiponectin, and the leptin/adiponectin ratio. After adjustment of the results for smoking status, waist circumference, hypertension, microalbuminuria, the TG/high-density lipoprotein (HDL) ratio, C-reactive protein (CRP), and the homeostasis model assessment of insulin resistance (HOMA-IR) index, the statistical significance of the link between CVD incidence and leptin and adiponectin levels disappeared. Thus, the authors concluded that the leptin/adiponectin ratio may be the most sensitive marker of CVD in males in comparison with leptin and adiponectin.

## 5. Adiponectin

In contrast to most other adipokines, the blood plasma level of adiponectin is lower during obesity and during the related pathologies, including CVDs, T2DM, and nonalcoholic fatty liver disease (NAFLD) [ – ]. Adiponectin levels were shown to be significantly lower in patients with NAFLD and NAFLD + T2DM than in the group of healthy subjects. Lower level of adiponectin was associated with the presence of T2DM and NAFLD independent of insulin resistance and obesity indices [ ]. The number of studies on the relationship between NAFLD and CVD is increasing year by year. These studies suggest that NAFLD can be actively involved in the pathogenesis of CVD [ , ].

Both mRNA expression of adiponectin and secretion of oligomeric adiponectin of high molecular weight are dysregulated in the adipose tissue of obese people. Epidemiological studies in various ethnic groups indicate that a low level of adiponectin in blood serum, and especially of its high-molecular-weight oligomer, is an independent risk factor of CVDs. There is a strong correlation between hypoadiponectinemia and CHD. Conversely, high blood plasma levels of adiponectin are related to a lower CHD risk, independently of other risk factors [ ]. Hypoadiponectinemia is independently associated with endothelial dysfunction in patients with diabetes. The inverse correlation between intima/media thickness and serum adiponectin has been detected in several clinical cohorts, which included both healthy subjects and patients with diabetes mellitus of both sexes. Moreover, the ratio of leptin to adiponectin is inversely related to the intima/media thickness of the vascular wall [ ] and has been suggested as an atherosclerotic indicator in patients with T2DM. Hyperadiponectinemia is an independent risk factor of diabetic cardiomyopathy. In healthy people, the levels of total adiponectin and high-molecular-weight adiponectin in the blood are linked with left ventricle hypertrophy, regardless of age and metabolic factors [ ]. A similar association has been noted in obese people [43]. These paradoxical findings can be explained by the development of adiponectin resistance [44] with age and with CVD progression.

## 6. Resistin

In 2001, researchers isolated a polypeptide named resistin, which is secreted mostly by preadipocytes and, to a lesser extent, by mature adipocytes located mostly in the abdomen [44,45]. There is evidence that CVDs are accompanied by changes in serum levels of resistin [46–48]. For instance, one study included 220 patients with chest pain and revealed that in patients with acute coronary syndrome (ACS), serum levels of resistin were significantly higher than those in the patients with stable angina pectoris. In the ACS group, an elevated serum level of resistin significantly correlated with high-sensitivity serum C-reactive protein (CRP) test results and with the leukocyte count; resistin also correlated with the number of coronary vessels with stenosis >50%. Overall, serum resistin was found to be a strong risk factor of ACS [49]. Moreover, resistin is a prognostic factor for death in type 2 diabetes [50].

There is a report of a substantial increase in the blood plasma level of resistin in patients with unstable angina pectoris in comparison to patients with stable angina pectoris or a control group; again, plasma resistin positively correlated with indicators of inflammation and of endothelium activation, e.g., the leukocyte count, CRP, and blood level of endothelin 1. Furthermore, resistin was found to be an independent predictor of the main adverse cardiovascular events, including cardiovascular death, myocardial infarction, and restenosis in patients after transcutaneous transluminal coronary angioplasty [51,52]. In a European cohort study on cancer and nutrition (the Potsdam study on 26,490 middle-aged patients without a history of acute myocardial infarction (AMI) or stroke; showing a relative risk of 2.09), the authors proposed to investigate the blood plasma level of resistin (adjusted for CRP) to predict the development of AMI. They noted elevated levels of resistin in patients with ACS and its correlation with severe myocardial injury and poor prognosis. A high level of resistin apparently is related to an adverse outcome after atherothrombotic ischemic stroke, regardless of other predictors of adverse outcomes [53]. Nevertheless, in some studies, researchers did not find a link between an elevated level of resistin circulating in the blood and the prevalence or outcome of IHD. Such discrepancies may have to do with differences in the demographics of the studied groups, differences in study design and in eligibility criteria for participants, as well as dissimilar methods of analysis. All these observations suggest that resistin plays an important part in the pathogenesis of CVDs, and currently, studies are underway to determine its involvement in atherogenesis and ACS.

## 7. Tumor Necrosis Factor Alpha (TNF-α)

Tumor necrosis factor-α is expressed by lymphocytes and adipocytes and has auto- and paracrine effects. The level of TNF-α in adipose tissue correlates with fat mass and hyperinsulinemia. The TNF-α stimulates leptin secretion, and this action is mediated by IL-1. In animal experiments, TNF-α administration reduces food intake, delays gastric emptying, inhibits insulin effects, modulates the levels of glucagon and glucocorticoids, and stimulates thermogenesis. Because of elevated secretion of TNF-α and IL-6, visceral fat exerts a proinflammatory action. These proinflammatory cytokines activate a transcription factor of the response to oxidative stress, NF-κB. The vascular endothelium is a specific target of TNF-α: the latter upregulates many proinflammatory, procoagulant, pro-proliferative, and proapoptotic genes [54,55]. The common initial stage for these changes is a decrease in the bioavailability of nitric oxide (NO), which is secondary to increased elimination of NO by reactive oxygen species (ROS) and/or decreased synthesis of NO. Vascular damage related to the main risk factors of CVDs [56] is characterized by endothelial dysfunction, formation and liberation of inflammatory cytokines such as TNF-α, prolonged activation of the systems producing ROS, and eventually, a decrease in endothelial bioavailability of NO. In isolated coronary arteries of type 2 diabetic mice, it was demonstrated that activated superoxide-generating systems reduced vasodilatation, and the concentration of circulating TNF-α increased. Inhibition of superoxide production [57] or lowering of superoxide content restores vasodilatation. In aged rats, there is an increase in the blood level of TNF-α, which is associated with endothelial dysfunction of coronary arteries, whereas chronic inhibition of TNF-α improves the slowing of blood flow in mesenteric arteries of the aged rats. Thus, TNF-α attenuates vasodilatation, mostly by lowering NO bioavailability and also because of ROS upregulation.

## 8. Interleukin-1 (IL-1)

Interleukin-1 is an apical proinflammatory mediator during acute and chronic inflammation and is a powerful inducer of an innate immune response [ ]. It triggers the synthesis and expression of several hundred mediators of the secondary alteration and upregulates its own production and processing: this stage is a key event in the pathogenesis of many autoinflammatory diseases [ – ]. Interleukin-1α and IL-1β, together with their negative regulator IL-1 receptor antagonist, play the most important role in the development of various CVDs, including atherosclerosis, AMI, myocarditis, dilated cardiomyopathy, infectious endocarditis, and cardiomyopathy. All other variants of the IL1 gene also correlate with a higher risk of CVDs. Two related genes encode two different proteins (IL-1α and IL-1β), which bind to the same receptor (type I). Interleukin-1α is synthesized as a fully active peptide, which remains bound to the membrane or may be liberated from the cytoplasm during cell death. Consequently, IL-1α participates more prominently in a local response to injury, and less frequently in a systemic inflammatory response [ , , ]. Interleukin-1β, the main form of circulating IL-1, is initially synthesized as a precursor (pro-IL-1β) and becomes active via cleavage of pro-IL-1β by caspase 1 under the conditions of a macromolecular structure known as a focus of inflammation [ ]. Caspase 1 also participates in the secretion of active IL-1, which can then bind to a membrane receptor of IL-1 on the same cell, on a neighboring cell, or on target cells [ ]. Inflammation activation after tissue injury causes a local increase in the IL-1β amount, thereby substantially enhancing the inflammatory response, attracting a large number of inflammatory cells, stimulating metalloproteinases, and eventually inducing the death (pyroptosis) of such inflammatory cells as leukocytes and resident cells [ , ]. In other words, the active form of IL-1 is a consequence of transformation of an inactive precursor through the NLRP3/caspase pathway after an infectious or inflammatory stimulus. Interleukin-1β possesses various biological properties and correlates with atherosclerosis, IHD, and tissue remodeling after AMI. IL-1α is constitutively active toward various cell types by binding to the same receptor as IL-1β binds, thereby exerting similar actions. Physiologically, IL-1α acts as a danger signal in response to sterile irritants, mostly owing to cell death as a consequence of necrosis taking place in AMI or stroke.

## 9. Interleukin-6 (IL-6)

Interleukin-6 is produced by activated monocytes or macrophages, by a vascular endothelium, fibroblasts, activated T cells, and by several nonimmune cell types [ ]. Interleukin-6 performs its biological functions via two signaling pathways: classical signaling through membrane-bound receptor of IL-6 (IL-6-R), which is responsible for anti-inflammatory processes, and signal transduction via a soluble receptor of IL-6 (sIL-6-R), which takes part in proinflammatory processes. Some effects caused by IL-6 are similar to those seen during the actions of IL-1 and TNF. Nonetheless, the main effect of IL-6 is related to its participation as a cofactor in the differentiation of B lymphocytes, their maturation, and conversion to plasma cells secreting immunoglobulins. In addition, IL-6 promotes IL-2 receptor expression on activated immune cells and induces IL-2 production by T cells. This cytokine stimulates T-lymphocyte proliferation and hematopoietic reactions. Furthermore, IL-6 mediates acute and chronic inflammatory reactions and regulates the acute phase reaction in hepatocytes, including the synthesis of CRP [ ]. Vascular effects of IL-6 depend on experimental conditions. In C57Bl/6 mice and in apoE-deficient mice, injection of recombinant IL-6 at supraphysiological doses enhances atherosclerosis. By contrast, at an early stage, deletion of the IL6 gene in apoE-deficient mice did not affect the disease relative to control mice, whereas at later stages, this knockout promoted atherosclerosis. Atherosclerotic plaques of humans contain IL-6, and a high plasma level of IL-6 is associated with a poor prognosis in people without a well-pronounced CVD and in patients with ACS. A large-scale analysis of 34 genetic studies, including 25,458 cases of IHD and 100,740 control cases of polymorphisms of the IL-6-R gene with cardiac events, revealed that polymorphism rs7529229 in IL6R, which is associated with elevated blood plasma levels of soluble IL-6-R, and lower levels of CRP correlate with lesser frequency of coronary artery diseases [67]. The similar findings of the two independent genetic studies indicate a causal link between IL-6 signaling and atherosclerosis in humans. Therefore, IL-6-R is a promising therapeutic target in IHD.

## 10. Interleukin-8 (IL-8)

Interleukin-8 bears the main responsibility for chemotaxis (recruiting) of monocytes and neutrophils: the characteristic cells of an acute inflammatory response. In vivo, a chemotactic gradient can be created by the binding of IL-8 to proteins of the basal membrane. This gradient helps to lead cells to an inflammation site and retains them as soon as they enter the site. Aside from recruitment of cells, IL-8 promotes activation of monocytes and neutrophils. Interleukin-8 emerges at an early stage of an inflammatory response but stays active for a long period: several days or even weeks. This feature distinguishes it from other inflammatory cytokines, which are usually produced and metabolized in vivo within several hours. IL-8 is very sensitive to oxidative agents, whereas antioxidants substantially downregulate the IL8 gene. The role of oxidative agents in the regulation of IL-8 and other chemokines is important in the pathogenesis of CVDs, where ischemia-induced oxidative stress is simultaneously a marker of the disease and a potential therapeutic target [68]. In the literature, there are plenty of data on the involvement of IL-8 in the pathogenesis of atherosclerosis. A popular field of research is elucidating whether IL-8 is a predictor of short-term and long-term outcomes in patients with IHD. Inoue et al. has found serum levels of 10 cytokines to be prognostically significant in an analysis of long-term outcomes of patients with stable IHD confirmed by angiography. The authors concluded that IL-8 is the only cytokine that predicts cardiovascular complications and does so regardless of nine other cytokines and high-sensitivity CRP test results [69].

It has been proven that IL-8 is a strong independent prognostic factor of cardiovascular and general mortality among patients with end-stage kidney failure. Investigators have found that the initial concentrations of IL-8 are substantially higher in IHD than in patients without IHD. Nonetheless, adjustment for additional cardiovascular and immunological risk factors weakened the observed relation, and the authors concluded that elevated blood levels of IL-8 precede the development of IHD but cannot serve as an independent risk factor. It is reported that lower levels of IL-8 after cardiovascular interventions are a prognostic indicator of more favorable short-term and long-term outcomes of the disease [70].

## 11. Interleukin-10 (IL-10)

Interleukin-10 controls the level of active forms of cyclooxygenase (COX). Sikka et al. has revealed that IL-10 deficiency causes COX activation and, therefore, activation of thromboxane receptor, which induces endothelial and cardiac dysfunction of blood vessels in mice. In mice with a low level of IL-10, cardiac and vascular dysfunctions develop with age [71]. On the other hand, Didion et al. has demonstrated that endogenous IL-10 reduces angiotensin II-mediated oxidative stress and vascular dysfunction both in vitro and in vivo, thereby confirming that at least some protective functions of IL-10 can be performed in the vessel wall [72]. Elevated initial levels of IL-10 are an independent predictor of a higher risk of subsequent death and AMI within one year. This finding is confirmed by the study by Cavusoglu and coauthors, who discovered that elevated levels of IL-10 in plasma are independently associated with a higher risk of death and of nonlethal myocardial infarction during 5-year follow-up in a group of males with ACS who were referred to coronary angiography. Additionally, the prognostic value of IL-10 in this regard did not depend on other biomarkers, including high-sensitivity CRP test results, and was comparable with their prognostic utility [73]. Elevated levels of IL-10 have also been found in patients with acute myocarditis, after which IL-10 was suggested as a pathogenic marker that can help to discriminate acute myocarditis and AMI [74]. Elevated levels of

IL-10 in blood serum have also been associated with a higher incidence of subsequent adverse events in patients with cardiomyopathy [ ]. Thus, IL-10, originally known as an anti-inflammatory cytokine with pleiotropic effects on the human body, probably plays an ambiguous role in CVDs.

## 12. Tissue Factor (TF)

As a strong initiator of coagulation, tissue factor (TF) is a crucial player in hemostasis and thrombogenesis. In general, TF is absent in the cells of a vascular endothelium, or if it is present, its conformation does not allow it to interact with factor VII. Nonetheless, after tissue and vascular endothelium are damaged, and the physical barrier separating intravessel factor VII from TF is disrupted, the factor VII–TF complex is formed. Furthermore, during stimulation of monocytes, macrophages, and endothelial cells by endotoxins, cytokines, and lectins, the expression of TF increases in these cells in parallel with an increase in procoagulant activity [ ]. In ACS, concentrations of inflammatory cytokines, such as TNF-$\alpha$ and interleukins, increase at the site of coronary artery occlusion to such an extent that TF is produced in vascular cells. There are several polymorphisms of the TF gene, and existing evidence suggests that certain mutations in gene TF and in the promoter of this gene may be related to a worse outcome of patients with ACS, possibly because of elevated production of TF by monocytes [ ]. In patients with tension-related unstable angina pectoris or myocardial infarction without elevation of the ST segment and a high index of intima/media thickness (TIMI $\geq$ 4), an elevated level of TF is detectable in blood plasma in comparison to patients with a low TIMI index (<3). Elevated levels of TF are present in people with cardiovascular risk factors and in patients with IHD. Tissue factor expression is higher in atherosclerotic plaques, and cellular and extracellular TF (contained in microparticles) come into contact with blood during endothelium erosion or plaque rupture. Consequently, TF plays a decisive part in the development of acute vascular events, such as AMI or stroke. On the other hand, TF can promote atherosclerosis progression by enhancing migration and proliferation of smooth muscle cells in the vessels.

## 13. Lipoportein Lipase (LPL)

In a large cross-sectional study by Khera et al., they found that the presence of rare damaging mutations in the lipoprotein lipase gene (LPL) was substantially associated with higher levels of TGs and a diagnosis of IHD [ ]. Similar results have been obtained by Lotta et al., who uncovered a relation between a polymorphism of the LPL gene and a lower risk of IHD among people carrying alleles corresponding to low TG levels in the blood, irrespective of genetic mechanisms lowering the level of low-density lipoprotein (LDL) cholesterol [ ]. In international literature, rather frequently, there are descriptions of both isolated cases and of meta-analyses suggesting that low levels of LPL in serum are linked with early atherosclerosis (before 55 years of age), whereas a higher LPL activity has a protective effect against the development of IHD. Xie and Li in a meta-analysis show that the risk of IHD varies depending on the polymorphism of LPL. For example, the HindIII polymorphism of LPL is substantially associated with a risk of IHD. For polymorphism Ser447X, investigators have discovered that only the XX genotype significantly correlates with IHD risk. Polymorphism PvuII did not manifest a significant link with the risk of IHD. Thus, LPL polymorphism HindIII may serve as a possible risk biomarker of IHD [ ].

## 14. Apolipoprotein E (ApoE)

Defects in ApoE lead to familial dysbetalipoproteinemia, also known as type III hyperlipoproteinemia, where elevated levels of cholesterol and TGs in blood plasma are caused by disrupted clearance of chylomicrons, very LDL, and LDL. Later, ApoE was studied regarding its participation in several biological processes not directly related to the transport of lipoproteins, e.g., Alzheimer's disease, immunoregulation, and cognitive functions. Isoform 4 of ApoE, encoded by an allele of APOE, has been implicated in the elevated level of calcium ions and apoptosis after mechanical damage [ ]. Data on the role of ApoE in the development of IHD are rather inconsistent. For instance, a large (~92,000 subjects) populational study on the link between ApoE and IHD clearly indicated that circulating ApoE raised the risk of IHD [82]. Sofat et al. made similar findings in their meta-analysis. It is reported that there is no evidence of a relation between ApoE blood concentration and CVD events. The validated link of an APOE genotype with CVD events may be explained by functions that are specific for isoforms and by other mechanisms rather than the concentrations of ApoE circulating with the blood [83]. By contrast, in their study, Corsetti et al. concluded that the levels of ApoE predicted CVD in females with high levels of HDL cholesterol and CRP [51]. In the elderly, high levels of ApoE in the blood precede upregulation of circulating CRP and strongly correlate with cardiovascular mortality, regardless of the APOE genotype and blood lipids.

## 15. Complement System

The complement system performs an important function in the pathogenesis of IHD and of heart failure [84,85]. The lectin pathway has a more prominent role in the induction of complement activation than do the classic and alternative pathways during ischemia-reperfusion injury [86]. Trendelenburg et al. has found that a serum level of mannose-binding lectin (MBL) is associated with lower mortality in patients with AMI who underwent transcutaneous transluminal coronary angioplasty [87]. Conversely, a low concentration of serine proteases associated with MBL is apparently a bad sign. For instance, Zhang et al. reported that the concentration of MBL-bound serine protease 2 was lower in the peripheral blood of patients after AMI, in comparison with a control group [88]. Taken together, these observations suggest that lower levels of MBL are a good sign because of a lower probability of lectin pathway activation. Several research papers have shown that an elevated level of C3 in serum and/or a higher C3/C4 ratio correlate with a higher risk of IHD. An elevated level of C4 in plasma is reported to be associated with a higher incidence of coronary events. Gombos et al. has demonstrated that higher levels of anaphylatoxin C3a in the plasma of patients with a left ventricular ejection fraction below 45% predict repeated hospitalization, cardiovascular events, and mortality [89].

## 16. Plasminogen Activator Inhibitor 1 (PAI-1)

It is reported that elevated levels of PAI1 are typically related to repeated myocardial infarction and IHD. Nonetheless, at present, the links among PAI1, early atherosclerosis, and IHD remain unclear. In several studies, it has been shown that PAI1 correlates with many traditional risk factors of IHD, such as obesity, hyperglycemia, T2DM [90], metabolic syndrome [91], and vessel wall thickness. Besides, higher expression of PAI1 is observed in coronary artery tissues in the presence of atherogenic lesions. Association of elevated levels of PAI1 in blood plasma with the incidence of IHD is noted in several prospective studies [92,93]. Nevertheless, this link has not always persisted after adjustment for cardiovascular risk factors. These discrepancies may have something to do with small sample sizes and/or limitations of the studies (e.g., only patients with T2DM, only obese people, or patients with HIV infection) [94].

## 17. Visfatin

There is evidence that the effects of visfatin on the accumulation of lipid depots are implemented by insulin receptors. By binding to these receptors, visfatin activates them. Administration of recombinant visfatin to mice acts on insulin receptor just as insulin does. The level of visfatin in circulating blood cells directly correlates with the body mass index, waist circumference, and the insulin resistance index. It is thought that visfatin participates in atherogenesis and in the pathogenesis of arterial hypertension in the presence of obesity and vascular complications of T2DM. Although further research will clarify the mechanisms behind the many well-studied physiological changes, it is already obvious that visfatin is a crucial immunoregulator with well-pronounced anti-inflammatory properties. A meta-analysis by Yu et al. [95], including 15 papers with 1053 cases of IHD and 714 control patients, suggests that, overall, visfatin concentration in peripheral blood is much higher in IHD cases than in controls. Group and meta-regression analyses revealed that the possible reasons for the heterogeneity are age, body mass index, race, diabetes mellitus, systolic arterial pressure, TGs, HDL cholesterol, and LDL cholesterol. These findings clearly show that an increase in the visfatin concentration in peripheral blood may be a risk marker of IHD. A study by Auguet et al. has revealed that the levels of visfatin are substantially higher in the secretome of the unstable atherosclerotic plaque from a carotid artery than in the secretome of a nonatherosclerotic thoracic artery. There were no differences in other analyzed adipo-/cytokines [ ]. Of note, in a study by Zheng et al. on the level of visfatin in patients with T2DM, the patients were subdivided into two groups by the presence of atherosclerotic plaques. Serum levels of visfatin were higher in the group with atherosclerotic plaques. In people with atherosclerotic plaques in the carotid artery, the level of visfatin was higher than that in patients with/without plaques in the femoral artery. Pearson's correlation analyses suggested that the serum levels of visfatin positively correlated with waist circumference, waist hip index, TGs, and the number of plaques. Logistic regression analysis revealed that a higher level of visfatin in serum is an independent predictor of the presence of atherosclerotic plaques [ ].

## 18. Angiotensin II

Numerous components of the renin–angiotensin system directly affect the physiology of adipocytes, and genetic animal models have provided a wealth of information about the mechanisms underlying these effects. In general, these studies indicate that angiotensin II in visceral adipose tissue promotes accumulation of energy. For example, transgenic activation of angiotensin in the adipose tissue of mice increases obesity [ ], whereas its conditional knockout in adipocytes does not affect either body weight or obesity but reduces inflammation in adipose tissue, raises metabolic activity, improves glucose tolerance, and lowers the predisposition to hypertension associated with obesity [ , ]. It is assumed that elevated levels of angiotensin in adipose tissue are sufficient for an increase in the adipose tissue volume, and that they are necessary for the inflammation associated with obesity as well as for the development of glucose tolerance impairment and hypertension. As for subtype 1 receptor of angiotensin II (AT1R), which may be involved in these phenomena, the following has been reported. Mice lacking AT1R in the whole body are resistant to diet-induced obesity, show smaller adipocytes, and do not show changes in adipocyte differentiation, indicating a possible role of AT1R in the growth of adipocytes, which manifests itself during diet-induced obesity.

## 19. Apelin

Apelin is considered a cardioprotective factor because it has effects opposite to those of the renin–angiotensin system. Apelin is expressed in several organs, including the hypothalamus, vascular endothelium, heart, lungs, and kidneys, as well as adipose tissue and the gastrointestinal tract. Its receptor APJ is widely expressed in endothelia, smooth muscles, and myocytes. In the systemic circulation, apelin causes NO-dependent vasodilatation, prevents vasoconstriction caused by angiotensin II, and exerts positive ionotropic and cardioprotective effects. Plasma levels of apelin are substantially lower in patients with atrial fibrillation than in healthy subjects. There are data on a higher risk of repeated atrial fibrillation in subjects with a lower level of apelin [ , ]. The level of apelin starts to decline early after AMI. Several days later, its level starts to grow but remains lowered until 24 weeks after AMI. This downregulation does not depend on the degree of ventricular dysfunction and prognosis [ , ]. As a rule, levels of apelin are lower in patients with IHD. In patients with unstable angina pectoris and AMI, levels of apelin are lower than those in patients with stable types of IHD. These levels also inversely correlate with the severity of coronary stenoses [ ]. There is a report of a beneficial influence of apelin on reperfusion damage after AMI. There is increased expression and production of apelin in the left ventricle, whereas mRNA levels of apelin in atria are unchanged, while in blood serum, the levels of apelin are lowered, as is the expression of apelin receptor AJP.

## 20. Omentin

Expression of the omentin gene and the omentin serum levels are lower in obese people and inversely correlate with the body mass index, waist circumference, insulin resistance, and IHD. Conversely, there is a positive correlation of omentin with serum adiponectin and HDL cholesterol. Furthermore, omentin increases insulin-induced glucose reuptake and participates in the regulation of insulin sensitivity and, therefore, may exert a protective action against the worsening of insulin resistance. Regarding the influence of omentin on the cardiovascular system, as mentioned above, lower levels of omentin are seen in patients with IHD [106,107]. In case of heart failure, the levels of omentin are significantly lower in people who experienced a greater number of cardiac events in the long term (death, repeated hospitalization) and in patients with more severe symptoms (with New York Heart Association (NYHA) class IV in comparison with NYHA II and III) [108].

## 21. Monocytic Chemoattractant Protein-1 (MCP-1)

Induction of chemokines is a characteristic feature of the inflammatory response associated with ischemia-reperfusion injury in many tissues. Analysis of biopsies from patients and animal models by hybridization and immunostaining in situ have revealed mRNA and protein expression of MCP1 in an ischemic myocardium. Elevated levels of MCP1 in blood serum have been detected in patients with IHD and were implicated in the risk of myocardial infarction and left ventricle dysfunction [109,110]. Quantitation of MCP1 in the coronary blood of patients with tension-related unstable angina pectoris has shown a link between the levels of MCP1 and the degree of coronary atherosclerosis as evidenced by coronary angiography. In the OPUS-TIMI 16 study, levels of MCP1 above the 75th percentile were associated with a higher risk of death or AMI after 10 months, even after adjustment for the traditional risk factors. Furthermore, according to Lee et al., the levels of circulating MCP1 positively correlate with a greater amount of visceral adipose tissue and IHD with multiple vascular damage [109]. Even though MCP1 is a promising biomarker, further research is needed to determine its clinical value.

## 22. Retinol-Binding Protein 4 (RBP4)

Upregulation of retinol-binding protein 4 (RBP4) in human blood serum is linked with insulin resistance, the development of T2DM, and such clinical manifestations of metabolic syndrome as obesity, glucose intolerance, dyslipidemia, and hypertension [111,112]. It has been demonstrated that patients with atherosclerosis of carotid arteries in combination with IHD have higher levels of RBP4 [113]. Liu et al. has noted that higher levels of RBP4 and adiponectin are related to higher rates of death from CVDs among males with T2DM [114]. Similar results have been obtained by Ingelsson et al. In the elderly, RBP4 concentrations correlate with metabolic syndrome and its components both in males and females as well as with a history of cerebrovascular disease in males [115]. In a study on a female population, Alkharfy et al. found that serum RBP4 concentration correlated with various well-established risk factors of CVDs; accordingly, they proposed that RBP4 may serve as an independent predictor of CVDs in females [116]. All the above data are consistent with the hypothesis that circulating RBP4 is a marker of metabolic complications, and possibly of atherosclerosis too.

## 23. Molecular and Genetic Studies

Recent years have witnessed a number of molecular genetic studies on the molecules of the secretory activity of visceral adipocytes, again, mostly in relation to pathologies of the cardiovascular and endocrine systems.

There has been research into the expression of adiponectin genes in patients with various types of cardiovascular pathologies [117,118]. One research group studied the mRNA expression of adiponectin in adipose tissue samples from 11 males after coronary artery bypass grafting and 10 males with a replaced heart valve. It was found that the mRNA expression was high in abdominal adipose tissue [119]. There is a report of a lower level of adiponectin with a concurrent increase in the expression of CD48 and MCP1 in the adipose tissue of patients with T2DM [120]. Underexpression of the adiponectin gene (*ADIPOQ*) and simultaneous upregulation of leptin (*LEP*) were detected in the analysis of the transcriptome from the adipocytes of patients with metabolic syndrome after coronary artery bypass grafting [121]. Other researchers have revealed that adiponectin expression is lower in patients with hypertension [122] or with IHD [123,124]. Another study has uncovered an insignificant increase in the expression of this gene in patients with IHD [12]. During induction of adipogenesis in the samples of visceral adipocytes from patients with IHD after a surgical intervention, investigators noted upregulation of *ADIPOQ* in response to various concentrations of glucose [125].

## 24. Conclusions and Future Perspectives

Thus, there is large number of biomarkers secreted by visceral adipocytes. All of them can substantially affect the development of atherosclerosis, vascular inflammation, and, as a consequence, stroke, myocardial infarction, and other cardiovascular events [126]. Nonetheless, the effects of most biomarkers discovered to date are usually either weak, poorly studied, or inconsistent and require further research.

It should be noted that the evidence accumulated so far regarding the secretory function of adipose tissue and its involvement in the pathogenesis of some socially significant diseases (such as obesity, T2DM, and atherosclerosis) suggests that it is important to continue studying the molecular basis of this secretory function. Today, there are virtually no data on the secretory function of adipose tissue and its role in the pathogenesis of various socially significant diseases and pathologies (not only cardiovascular and endocrine) in young adults at employable and reproductive age. These future studies seem to be especially relevant because they include medical examination of young adults living in strongly continental and subarctic climatic geographic conditions.

Overall, studies on the molecular genetic factors underlying adipose tissue function in the context of the above conditions may lead to a deeper understanding of the etiopathogenesis of not only cardiovascular but also other common socially significant diseases and pathologies in young adults as well as help to develop an effective strategy for their prophylaxis and management.

**Author Contributions:** Conceptualization, Y.I.R. and E.V.K.; methodology, Y.I.R.; data curation, Y.V.P.; writing—original draft preparation, Y.I.R., E.V.K. and Y.V.P.; writing—review and editing, E.M.S.; supervision, E.M.S.; project administration, Y.I.R. and E.V.K.; funding acquisition, Y.I.R. All authors have read and agreed to the published version of the manuscript.

**Funding:** This review was conducted within the framework of the project НШ-2595.2020.7 and as part of the budget theme on the state task number АААА-А17-117112850280-2.

**Acknowledgments:** English language was corrected and certified by shevchuk-editing.com.

**Conflicts of Interest:** The authors declare that they have no conflicts of interest associated with the publication of this review.

## References

1. Castellani, L.N.; Costa-Dookhan, K.A.; McIntyre, W.B.; Wright, D.C.; Flowers, S.A.; Hahn, M.; Ward, K.M. Preclinical and Clinical Sex Differences in Antipsychotic-Induced Metabolic Disturbances: A Narrative Review of Adiposity and Glucose Metabolism. *J. Psychiatry Brain Sci.* **2019**, *4*, 190013.
2. Triggiani, A.I.; Valenzano, A.; Trimigno, V.; Di Palma, A.; Moscatelli, F.; Cibelli, G.; Messina, G. Heart rate variability reduction is related to a high amount of visceral adiposity in healthy young women. *PLoS ONE* **2019**, *14*, e0223058.
3. WHO. Fact Sheet. Available online: https://www.who.int/ru/news-room/fact-sheets/detail/obesity-and-overweight (accessed on 16 February 2018).
4. González, N.; Moreno-Villegas, Z.; González-Bris, A.; Egido, J.; Lorenzo, O. Regulation of visceral and epicardial adipose tissue for preventing cardiovascular injuries associated to obesity and diabetes. *Cardiovasc. Diabetol.* **2017**, *16*, 44.

5. Ibrahim, M.M. Subcutaneous and visceral adipose tissue: Structural and functional differences. *Obes. Rev.* **2010**, *11*, 11–18. [CrossRef] [PubMed]
6. Karlsson, T.; Rask-Andersen, M.; Pan, G.; Höglund, J.; Wadelius, C.; Ek, W.E.; Johansson, Å. Contribution of genetics to visceral adiposity and its relation to cardiovascular and metabolic disease. *Nat. Med.* **2019**, *25*, 1390–1395. [CrossRef]
7. Mitchell, J.; Church, T.S.; Rankinen, T.; Earnest, C.P.; Sui, X.; Blair, S.N. FTO Genotype and the Weight Loss Benefits of Moderate Intensity Exercise. *Obesity* **2009**, *18*, 641–643. [CrossRef]
8. McCarthy, M.I. Genomics, Type 2 Diabetes, and Obesity. *New Engl. J. Med.* **2010**, *363*, 2339–2350. [CrossRef]
9. Marcadenti, A.; Fuchs, S.C.; Matte, U.; Sperb, F.; Moreira, L.; Fuchs, S.C. Effects of FTO RS9939906 and MC4R RS17782313 on obesity, type 2 diabetes mellitus and blood pressure in patients with hypertension. *Cardiovasc. Diabetol.* **2013**, *12*, 103. [CrossRef]
10. Da Silva, C.F.; Zandoná, M.R.; Vitolo, M.R.; Campagnolo, P.D.B.; Rotta, L.N.; Almeida, S.; Mattevi, V.S. Association between a frequent variant of the FTO gene and anthropometric phenotypes in Brazilian children. *BMC Med. Genet.* **2013**, *14*, 34. [CrossRef]
11. Klimentidis, Y.C.; Lemas, D.J.; Wiener, H.H.; O'Brien, D.; Havel, P.; Stanhope, K.L.; Hopkins, S.E.; Tiwari, H.K.; Boyer, B.B. CDKAL1 and HHEX are associated with type 2 diabetes-related traits among Yup'ik people. *J. Diabetes* **2013**, *6*, 251–259. [CrossRef]
12. Lemas, D.J.; Klimentidis, Y.C.; Wiener, H.W.; O'Brien, D.; Hopkins, S.; Allison, D.B.; Fernández, J.R.; Tiwari, H.K.; Boyer, B.B. Obesity polymorphisms identified in genome-wide association studies interact with n-3 polyunsaturated fatty acid intake and modify the genetic association with adiposity phenotypes in Yup'ik people. *Genes Nutr.* **2013**, *8*, 495–505. [CrossRef] [PubMed]
13. Chung, W.K.; Patki, A.; Matsuoka, N.; Boyer, B.B.; Liu, N.; Musani, S.K.; Goropashnaya, A.V.; Tan, P.L.; Katsanis, N.; Johnson, S.; et al. Analysis of 30 Genes (355 SNPS) Related to Energy Homeostasis for Association with Adiposity in European-American and Yup'ik Eskimo Populations. *Hum. Hered.* **2008**, *67*, 193–205. [CrossRef] [PubMed]
14. Lyon, H.N.; Emilsson, V.; Hinney, A.; Heid, I.M.; Lasky-Su, J.; Zhu, X.; Thorleifsson, G.; Gunnarsdottir, S.; Walters, G.B.; Thorsteinsdóttir, U.; et al. The Association of a SNP Upstream of INSIG2 with Body Mass Index is Reproduced in Several but Not All Cohorts. *PLoS Genet.* **2007**, *3*, e61. [CrossRef] [PubMed]
15. Cha, S.; Koo, I.; Choi, S.M.; Park, B.L.; Kim, K.S.; Jae-Ryong, K.; Shin, H.D.; Kim, J.Y. Association analyses of the INSIG2 polymorphism in the obesity and cholesterol levels of Korean populations. *BMC Med. Genet.* **2009**, *10*, 96. [CrossRef]
16. Agra, R.M.; Fernández-Trasancos, Á.; Sierra, J.; González-Juanatey, J.R.; Eiras, S. Differential Association of S100A9, an Inflammatory Marker, and p53, a Cell Cycle Marker, Expression with Epicardial Adipocyte Size in Patients with Cardiovascular Disease. *Inflammation* **2014**, *37*, 1504–1512. [CrossRef]
17. Shibasaki, I.; Nishikimi, T.; Mochizuki, Y.; Yamada, Y.; Yoshitatsu, M.; Inoue, Y.; Kuwata, T.; Ogawa, H.; Tsuchiya, G.; Ishimitsu, T.; et al. Greater expression of inflammatory cytokines, adrenomedullin, and natriuretic peptide receptor-C in epicardial adipose tissue in coronary artery disease. *Regul. Pept.* **2010**, *165*, 210–217. [CrossRef]
18. Sacks, H.S.; Fain, J.N.; Cheema, P.; Bahouth, S.W.; Garrett, E.; Wolf, R.Y.; Wolford, D.; Samaha, J. Depot-Specific Overexpression of Proinflammatory, Redox, Endothelial Cell, and Angiogenic Genes in Epicardial Fat Adjacent to Severe Stable Coronary Atherosclerosis. *Metab. Syndr. Relat. Disord.* **2011**, *9*, 433–439. [CrossRef]
19. Gazioglu, S.B.; Akan, G.; Atalar, F.; Erten, G. PAI-1 and TNF-α profiles of adipose tissue in obese cardiovascular disease patients. *Int. J. Clin. Exp. Pathol.* **2015**, *8*, 15919–15925.
20. Chatterjee, T.K.; Aronow, B.J.; Tong, W.S.; Manka, D.; Tang, Y.; Bogdanov, V.Y.; Unruh, D.; Blomkalns, A.L.; Piegore, M.G.; Weintraub, D.S.; et al. Human coronary artery perivascular adipocytes overexpress genes responsible for regulating vascular morphology, inflammation, and hemostasis. *Physiol. Genom.* **2013**, *45*, 697–709. [CrossRef]
21. Gruzdeva, O.; Akbasheva, O.E.; Dyleva, Y.A.; Antonova, L.V.; Matveeva, V.G.; Uchasova, E.G.; Fanaskova, E.V.; Karetnikova, V.N.; Ivanov, S.V.; Barbarash, O. Adipokine and Cytokine Profiles of Epicardial and Subcutaneous Adipose Tissue in Patients with Coronary Heart Disease. *Bull. Exp. Boil. Med.* **2017**, *163*, 608–611. [CrossRef]
22. Uchasova, E.; Gruzdeva, O.; Dyleva, Y.; Belik, E.; Barbarash, O. The role of immune cells in the development of adipose tissue dysfunction in cardiovascular diseases. *Russ. J. Cardiol.* **2019**, *4*, 92–98. [CrossRef]

23. Alexopoulos, N.; Katritsis, D.; Raggi, P. Visceral adipose tissue as a source of inflammation and promoter of atherosclerosis. *Atherosclerosis* **2014**, *233*, 104–112.
24. Galic, S.; Oakhill, J.; Steinberg, G.R. Adipose tissue as an endocrine organ. *Mol. Cell. Endocrinol.* **2010**, *316*, 129–139.
25. Huang, X.; Jiang, X.; Wang, L.; Chen, L.; Wu, Y.; Gao, P.; Hua, F. Visceral adipose accumulation increased the risk of hyperuricemia among middle-aged and elderly adults: A population-based study. *J. Transl. Med.* **2019**, *17*, 341.
26. Jung, J.Y.; Ryoo, J.-H.; Oh, C.-M.; Choi, J.-M.; Chung, P.-W.; Hong, H.P.; Park, S.K. Visceral adiposity index and longitudinal risk of incident metabolic syndrome: Korean genome and epidemiology study (KoGES). *Endocr. J.* **2020**, *67*, 45–52.
27. Hausman, G.J.; Barb, C.R.; Lents, C.A. Leptin and reproductive function. *Biochimie* **2012**, *94*, 2075–2081.
28. Sweeney, G. Cardiovascular effects of leptin. *Nat. Rev. Cardiol.* **2009**, *7*, 22–29.
29. Gruzdeva, O.; Borodkina, D.; Uchasova, E.; Dyleva, Y.; Barbarash, O. Leptin resistance: Underlying mechanisms and diagnosis. *Diabetes, Metab. Syndr. Obesity: Targets Ther.* **2019**, *12*, 191–198.
30. Singh, M.; Bedi, U.S.; Singh, P.P.; Arora, R.; Khosla, S. Leptin and the clinical cardiovascular risk. *Int. J. Cardiol.* **2010**, *140*, 266–271.
31. Toczylowski, K.; Hirnle, T.; Harasiuk, D.; Zabielski, P.; Lewczuk, A.; Dmitruk, I.; Ksiazek, M.; Sulik, A.; Górski, J.; Chabowski, A.; et al. Plasma concentration and expression of adipokines in epicardial and subcutaneous adipose tissue are associated with impaired left ventricular filling pattern. *J. Transl. Med.* **2019**, *17*, 310–311.
32. Tao, P.; Jing, Z.; Shou-Hong, G.; Shu-Juan, P.; Jian-Peng, J.; Wen-Quan, L.; Wan-Sheng, C. Effects of leptin on norepinephrine in acute ischemic stroke. *Pharmazie* **2019**, *74*, 477–480.
33. Ilhan, N.; Susam, S.; Canpolat, O.; Belhan, O. The emerging role of leptin, Adiponectin and Visfatin in Ischemic/Hemorrhagic stroke. *Br. J. Neurosurg.* **2019**, *33*, 504–507.
34. Chen, M.-C.; Wang, J.-H.; Lee, C.-J.; Hsu, B.-G. Association between hyperleptinemia and cardiovascular outcomes in patients with coronary artery disease. *Ther. Clin. Risk Manag.* **2018**, *14*, 1855–1862.
35. Kappelle, P.J.; Dullaart, R.P.; Van Beek, A.P.; Hillege, H.L.; Wolffenbuttel, B.H. The plasma leptin/adiponectin ratio predicts first cardiovascular event in men: A prospective nested case–control study. *Eur. J. Intern. Med.* **2012**, *23*, 755–759.
36. Anaszewicz, M.; Wawrzeńczyk, A.; Czerniak, B.; Banaś, W.; Socha, E.; Lis, K.; Żbikowska-Gotz, M.; Bartuzi, Z.; Budzyński, J. High leptin and low blood adiponectin, TNF-alpha and irisin blood concentrations as factors linking obesity with the risk of atrial fibrillation among inpatients with cardiovascular disorders. *Kardiologia Polska* **2019**.
37. Ebrahimi, R.; Shanaki, M.; Azadi, S.M.; Bahiraee, A.; Radmard, A.R.; Poustchi, H.; Emamgholipour, S. Low level of adiponectin predicts the development of Nonalcoholic fatty liver disease: Is it irrespective to visceral adiposity index, visceral adipose tissue thickness and other obesity indices? *Arch. Physiol. Biochem.* **2019**, *4*, 1–8.
38. Maeda, N.; Funahashi, T.; Matsuzawa, Y.; Shimomura, I. Adiponectin, a unique adipocyte-derived factor beyond hormones. *Atherosclerosis* **2019**, *292*, 1–9.
39. Abdallah, L.R.; De Matos, R.C.; e Souza, Y.P.D.M.; Vieira-Soares, D.; Muller-Machado, G.; Pollo-Flores, P. Non-alcoholic Fatty Liver Disease and Its Links with Inflammation and Atherosclerosis. *Curr. Atheroscler. Rep.* **2020**, *22*, 7.
40. Pischon, T.; Hu, F.B.; Girman, C.J.; Rifai, N.; Manson, J.E.; Rexrode, K.; Rimm, E.B. Plasma total and high molecular weight adiponectin levels and risk of coronary heart disease in women. *Atherosclerosis* **2011**, *219*, 322–329.
41. Kotani, K.; Shimohiro, H.; Sakane, N. The relationship between leptin: Adiponectin ratio and carotid intima-media thickness in asymptomatic females. *Stroke* **2007**, *39*, e32–e33.
42. Kozakova, M.; Muscelli, E.O.A.; Flyvbjerg, A.; Frystyk, J.; Morizzo, C.; Palombo, C.; Ferrannini, E. Adiponectin and Left Ventricular Structure and Function in Healthy Adults. *J. Clin. Endocrinol. Metab.* **2008**, *93*, 2811–2818.

43. Ebinç, H.; Ebinc, F.A.; Özkurt, Z.N.; Doğru, M.T.; Tulmac, M.; Yilmaz, M.; Çağlayan, O.; Yılmaz, M.; Çağlayan, O. Impact of Adiponectin on Left Ventricular Mass Index in Non-complicated Obese Subjects. *Endocr. J.* **2008**, *55*, 523–528. [CrossRef] [PubMed]
44. Van Berendoncks, A.M.; Garnier, A.; Beckers, P.; Hoymans, V.Y.; Possemiers, N.; Fortin, D.; Martinet, W.; Van Hoof, V.; Vrints, C.J.; Ventura-Clapier, R.; et al. Functional Adiponectin Resistance at the Level of the Skeletal Muscle in Mild to Moderate Chronic Heart Failure. *Circ. Hear. Fail.* **2010**, *3*, 185–194. [CrossRef] [PubMed]
45. Smitka, K.; Marešová, D. Adipose Tissue as an Endocrine Organ: An Update on Pro-inflammatory and Anti-inflammatory Microenvironment. *Prague Med. Rep.* **2015**, *116*, 87–111. [CrossRef] [PubMed]
46. Muse, E.D.; Feldman, D.; Blaha, M.J.; Dardari, Z.; Blumenthal, R.S.; Budoff, M.J.; Nasir, K.; Criqui, M.H.; Cushman, M.; McClelland, R.L.; et al. The association of resistin with cardiovascular disease in the Multi-Ethnic Study of Atherosclerosis. *Atherosclerosis* **2014**, *239*, 101–108. [CrossRef]
47. Zhang, J.-Z.; Gao, Y.; Zheng, Y.-Y.; Liu, F.; Yang, Y.-N.; Li, X.-M.; Ma, X.; Ma, Y.-T.; Xie, X. Increased serum resistin level is associated with coronary heart disease. *Oncotarget* **2017**, *8*, 50148–50154. [CrossRef]
48. Gencer, B.; Auer, R.; De Rekeneire, N.; Butler, J.; Kalogeropoulos, A.; Bauer, U.C.; Kritchevsky, S.B.; Miljkovic, I.; Vittinghoff, E.; Harris, T.; et al. Association between resistin levels and cardiovascular disease events in older adults: The health, aging and body composition study. *Atherosclerosis* **2015**, *245*, 181–186. [CrossRef]
49. Wang, H.; Chen, D.-Y.; Cao, J.; He, Z.-Y.; Zhu, B.-P.; Long, M. High Serum Resistin Level may be an Indicator of the Severity of Coronary Disease in Acute Coronary Syndrome. *Chin. Med. Sci. J.* **2009**, *24*, 161–166. [CrossRef]
50. Kapłon-Cieślicka, A.; Tyminska, A.; Rosiak, M.; Ozierański, K.; Peller, M.; Eyileten, C.; Kondracka, A.; Pordzik, J.; Mirowska-Guzel, D.; Opolski, G.; et al. Resistin is a prognostic factor for death in type 2 diabetes. *Diabetes/Metabolism Res. Rev.* **2018**, *35*, e3098. [CrossRef]
51. Corsetti, J.P.; Gansevoort, R.T.; Bakker, S.J.; Navis, G.; Sparks, C.E.; Dullaart, R.P. Apolipoprotein E predicts incident cardiovascular disease risk in women but not in men with concurrently high levels of high-density lipoprotein cholesterol and C-reactive protein. *Metabolism* **2012**, *61*, 996–1002. [CrossRef]
52. Corsetti, J.P.; Gansevoort, R.T.; Bakker, S.J.L.; Dullaart, R.P. Apolipoprotein E levels and apolipoprotein E genotypes in incident cardiovascular disease risk in subjects of the Prevention of Renal and Vascular End-stage disease study. *J. Clin. Lipidol.* **2016**, *10*, 842–850. [CrossRef] [PubMed]
53. Weikert, C.; Spranger, J.; Willich, S.N.; Boeing, H.; Westphal, S.; Berger, K.; Dierkes, J.; Möhlig, M.; Rimm, E.B.; Pischon, T. Plasma Resistin Levels and Risk of Myocardial Infarction and Ischemic Stroke. *J. Clin. Endocrinol. Metab.* **2008**, *93*, 2647–2653. [CrossRef] [PubMed]
54. Bergh, N.; Ulfhammer, E.; Glise, K.; Jern, S.; Karlsson, L. Influence of TNF-α and biomechanical stress on endothelial anti- and prothrombotic genes. *Biochem. Biophys. Res. Commun.* **2009**, *385*, 314–318. [CrossRef] [PubMed]
55. Jung, H.S.; Shimizu-Albergine, M.; Shen, X.; Kramer, F.; Shao, D.; Vivekanandan-Giri, A.; Pennathur, S.; Tian, R.; Kanter, J.E.; Bornfeldt, K.E. TNF-α induces acyl-CoA synthetase 3 to promote lipid droplet formation in human endothelial cells. *J. Lipid Res.* **2019**, *61*, 33–44. [CrossRef]
56. D'Agostino, R.B.; Vasan, R.S.; Pencina, M.J.; Wolf, P.; Cobain, M.; Massaro, J.; Kannel, W.B. General Cardiovascular Risk Profile for Use in Primary Care: The Framingham Heart Study. *Circulation* **2008**, *117*, 743–753. [CrossRef]
57. Gao, X.; Belmadani, S.; Picchi, A.; Xu, X.; Potter, B.J.; Tewari-Singh, N.; Capobianco, S.; Chilian, W.M.; Zhang, C. Tumor necrosis factor-alpha induces endothelial dysfunction in Lepr(db) mice. *Circ. Res.* **2007**, *115*, 245–254. [CrossRef]
58. Dinarello, C.A.; Simon, A.; Van Der Meer, J.W.M. Treating inflammation by blocking interleukin-1 in a broad spectrum of diseases. *Nat. Rev. Drug Discov.* **2012**, *11*, 633–652. [CrossRef]
59. Dinarello, C.A. The history of fever, leukocytic pyrogen and interleukin-1. *Temperature* **2015**, *2*, 8–16. [CrossRef]
60. Dinarello, C.A. Interleukin-1 in the pathogenesis and treatment of inflammatory diseases. *Blood* **2011**, *117*, 3720–3732. [CrossRef]
61. Amaral, G.A.; Alves, J.D.; Honorio-França, A.C.; Fagundes, D.L.; Araujo, G.G.; Lobato, N.S.; Lima, V.V.; Giachini, F.R. Interleukin 1-beta is Linked to Chronic Low-grade Inflammation and Cardiovascular Risk Factors in Overweight Adolescents. *Endocrine, Metab. Immune Disord.—Drug Targets* **2019**, *19*, 1. [CrossRef]

62. Almog, T.; Kfir, M.K.; Levkovich, H.; Shlomai, G.; Barshack, I.; Stienstra, R.; Lustig, Y.; Frenkel, A.L.; Harari, A.; Bujanover, Y.; et al. Interleukin-1α deficiency reduces adiposity, glucose intolerance and hepatic de-novo lipogenesis in diet-induced obese mice. *BMJ Open Diabetes Res. Care* **2019**, *7*, e000650. [CrossRef]
63. Lamkanfi, M.; Kanneganti, T.-D. Nlrp3: An immune sensor of cellular stress and infection. *Int. J. Biochem. Cell Boil.* **2010**, *42*, 792–795. [CrossRef]
64. Terkeltaub, R.; Sundy, J.S.; Schumacher, H.R.; Murphy, F.; Bookbinder, S.; Biedermann, S.; Wu, R.; Mellis, S.; Radin, A. The interleukin 1 inhibitor rilonacept in treatment of chronic gouty arthritis: Results of a placebo-controlled, monosequence crossover, non-randomised, single-blind pilot study. *Ann. Rheum. Dis.* **2009**, *68*, 1613–1617. [CrossRef] [PubMed]
65. Scheller, J.; Chalaris, A.; Schmidt-Arras, D.; Rose-John, S. The pro- and anti-inflammatory properties of the cytokine interleukin-6. *Biochim. Biophys. Acta (BBA)—Bioenerg.* **2011**, *1813*, 878–888. [CrossRef] [PubMed]
66. Libby, P.; Rocha, V.Z. All roads lead to IL-6: A central hub of cardiometabolic signaling. *Int. J. Cardiol.* **2018**, *259*, 213–215. [CrossRef] [PubMed]
67. Interleukin-6 Receptor Mendelian Randomisation Analysis (IL6R MR) Consortium; Swerdlow, D.; Holmes, M.V.; Kuchenbaecker, K.B.; Engmann, J.; Shah, T.; Sofat, R.; Guo, Y.; Chung, C.; Peasey, A.; et al. The interleukin-6 receptor as a target for prevention of coronary heart disease: A mendelian randomisation analysis. *Lancet* **2012**, *379*, 1214–1224. [CrossRef]
68. Velásquez, I.M.; Gajulapuri, A.; Leander, K.; Berglund, A.; De Faire, U.; Gigante, B. Serum IL8 is not associated with cardiovascular events but with all-cause mortality. *BMC Cardiovasc. Disord.* **2019**, *19*, 34. [CrossRef] [PubMed]
69. Inoue, T.; Komoda, H.; Nonaka, M.; Kameda, M.; Uchida, T.; Node, K. Interleukin-8 as an independent predictor of long-term clinical outcome in patients with coronary artery disease. *Int. J. Cardiol.* **2008**, *124*, 319–325. [CrossRef]
70. Wu, Z.-K.; Laurikka, J.; Vikman, S.; Nieminen, R.; Moilanen, E.; Tarkka, M.R. High Postoperative Interleukin-8 Levels Related to Atrial Fibrillation in Patients Undergoing Coronary Artery Bypass Surgery. *World J. Surg.* **2008**, *32*, 2643–2649. [CrossRef]
71. Sikka, G.; Miller, K.L.; Steppan, J.; Pandey, D.; Jung, S.M.; Fraser, C.D.; Ellis, C.; Ross, D.; Vandegaer, K.; Bedja, D.; et al. Interleukin 10 knockout frail mice develop cardiac and vascular dysfunction with increased age. *Exp. Gerontol.* **2012**, *48*, 128–135. [CrossRef]
72. Didion, S.P.; Kinzenbaw, D.A.; Schrader, L.I.; Chu, Y.; Faraci, F.M. Endogenous interleukin-10 inhibits angiotensin II-induced vascular dysfunction. *Hypertension* **2009**, *54*, 619–624. [CrossRef] [PubMed]
73. Cavusoglu, E.; Marmur, J.D.; Hojjati, M.R.; Chopra, V.; Butala, M.; Subnani, R.; Huda, M.S.; Yanamadala, S.; Ruwende, C.; Eng, C.; et al. Plasma Interleukin-10 Levels and Adverse Outcomes in Acute Coronary Syndrome. *Am. J. Med.* **2011**, *124*, 724–730. [CrossRef] [PubMed]
74. Izumi, T.; Nishii, M. Diagnostic and prognostic biomarkers in acute myocarditis. *Herz* **2012**, *37*, 627–631. [CrossRef] [PubMed]
75. Santoro, F.; Tarantino, N.; Ferraretti, A.; Ieva, R.; Musaico, F.; Guastafierro, F.; Di Martino, L.; Di Biase, M.; Correale, M. Serum interleukin 6 and 10 levels in Takotsubo cardiomyopathy: Increased admission levels may predict adverse events at follow-up. *Atherosclerosis* **2016**, *254*, 28–34. [CrossRef]
76. Cugno, M.; Borghi, A.; Garcovich, S.; Marzano, A.V. Coagulation and Skin Autoimmunity. *Front. Immunol.* **2019**, *10*, 1407. [CrossRef]
77. Mälarstig, A.; Tenno, T.; Johnston, N.; Lagerqvist, B.; Axelsson, T.; Syvänen, A.-C.; Wallentin, L.; Siegbahn, A. Genetic Variations in the Tissue Factor Gene Are Associated with Clinical Outcome in Acute Coronary Syndrome and Expression Levels in Human Monocytes. *Arter. Thromb. Vasc. Boil.* **2005**, *25*, 2667–2672. [CrossRef]
78. Khera, A.V.; Won, H.-H.; Peloso, G.M.; O'Dushlaine, C.; Liu, D.; Stitziel, N.O.; Natarajan, P.; Nomura, A.; Emdin, C.A.; Gupta, N.; et al. Association of Rare and Common Variation in the Lipoprotein Lipase Gene with Coronary Artery Disease. *JAMA* **2017**, *317*, 937–946. [CrossRef]
79. Lotta, L.; Stewart, I.D.; Sharp, S.J.; Day, F.R.; Burgess, S.; Luan, J.; Bowker, N.; Cai, L.; Li, C.; Wittemans, L.B.L.; et al. Association of Genetically Enhanced Lipoprotein Lipase–Mediated Lipolysis and Low-Density Lipoprotein Cholesterol–Lowering Alleles with Risk of Coronary Disease and Type 2 Diabetes. *JAMA Cardiol.* **2018**, *3*, 957–966. [CrossRef]

80. Xie, L.; Li, Y.-M. Lipoprotein Lipase (LPL) Polymorphism and the Risk of Coronary Artery Disease: A Meta-Analysis. *Int. J. Environ. Res. Public Heal.* **2017**, *14*, 84. [CrossRef]
81. Jiang, L.; Zhong, J.; Dou, X.; Cheng, C.; Huang, Z.; Sun, X. Effects of ApoE on intracellular calcium levels and apoptosis of neurons after mechanical injury. *Neuroscience* **2015**, *301*, 375–383. [CrossRef]
82. Rasmussen, K.L.; Tybjaerg-Hansen, A.; Nordestgaard, B.G.; Frikke-Schmidt, R. Plasma levels of apolipoprotein E and risk of ischemic heart disease in the general population. *Atherosclerosis* **2016**, *246*, 63–70. [CrossRef]
83. Sofat, R.; Cooper, J.A.; Kumari, M.; Casas, J.P.; Mitchell, J.P.; Acharya, J.; Thom, S.; Hughes, A.; Humphries, S.E.; Hingorani, A. Circulating Apolipoprotein E Concentration and Cardiovascular Disease Risk: Meta-analysis of Results from Three Studies. *PLoS Med.* **2016**, *13*, e1002146. [CrossRef]
84. Barratt-Due, A.; Pischke, S.; Brekke, O.-L.; Thorgersen, E.B.; Nielsen, E.W.; Espevik, T.; Huber-Lang, M.; Mollnes, T.E. Bride and groom in systemic inflammation—The bells ring for complement and Toll in cooperation. *Immunobiology* **2012**, *217*, 1047–1056. [CrossRef]
85. Patzelt, J.; Verschoor, A.; Langer, H.F. Platelets and the complement cascade in atherosclerosis. *Front. Physiol.* **2015**, *6*, 49. [CrossRef]
86. Busche, M.N.; Pavlov, V.; Takahashi, K.; Stahl, G.L. Myocardial ischemia and reperfusion injury is dependent on both IgM and mannose-binding lectin. *Am. J. Physiol. Circ. Physiol.* **2009**, *297*, H1853–H1859. [CrossRef]
87. Trendelenburg, M.; Theroux, P.; Stebbins, A.; Granger, C.; Armstrong, P.; Pfisterer, M. Influence of functional deficiency of complement mannose-binding lectin on outcome of patients with acute ST-elevation myocardial infarction undergoing primary percutaneous coronary intervention. *Eur. Hear. J.* **2010**, *31*, 1181–1187. [CrossRef]
88. Zhang, M.; Hou, Y.J.; Cavusoglu, E.; Lee, D.C.; Steffensen, R.; Yang, L.; Bashari, D.; Villamil, J.; Moussa, M.; Fernaine, G.; et al. MASP-2 activation is involved in ischemia-related necrotic myocardial injury in humans. *Int. J. Cardiol.* **2011**, *166*, 499–504. [CrossRef]
89. Gombos, T.; Förhécz, Z.; Pozsonyi, Z.; Széplaki, G.; Kunde, J.; Füst, G.; Jánoskuti, L.; Karádi, I.; Prohászka, Z. Complement anaphylatoxin C3a as a novel independent prognostic marker in heart failure. *Clin. Res. Cardiol.* **2012**, *101*, 607–615. [CrossRef]
90. Yarmolinsky, J.; Barbieri, N.B.; Weinmann, T.; Ziegelmann, P.K.; Duncan, B.B.; Schmidt, M.I. Plasminogen activator inhibitor-1 and type 2 diabetes: A systematic review and meta-analysis of observational studies. *Sci. Rep.* **2016**, *6*, 17714. [CrossRef]
91. Smits, M.; Woudstra, P.; Utzschneider, K.M.; Tong, J.; Gerchman, F.; Faulenbach, M.; Carr, D.B.; Aston-Mourney, K.; Chait, A.; Knopp, R.H.; et al. Adipocytokines as features of the metabolic syndrome determined using confirmatory factor analysis. *Ann. Epidemiology* **2013**, *23*, 415–421. [CrossRef]
92. Meltzer, M.E.; Doggen, C.J.M.; De Groot, P.G.; Rosendaal, F.R.; Lisman, T. Plasma levels of fibrinolytic proteins and the risk of myocardial infarction in men. *Blood* **2010**, *116*, 529–536. [CrossRef]
93. Tofler, G.H.; Massaro, J.; O'Donnell, C.; Wilson, P.; Vasan, R.; Sutherland, P.; Meigs, J.; Levy, D.; D'Agostino, R. Plasminogen activator inhibitor and the risk of cardiovascular disease: The Framingham Heart Study. *Thromb. Res.* **2016**, *140*, 30–35. [CrossRef]
94. Knudsen, A.; Katzenstein, T.L.; Benfield, T.; Jørgensen, N.R.; Kronborg, G.; Gerstoft, J.; Obel, N.; Kjær, A.; Lebech, A.-M.; Kjaer, A. Plasma plasminogen activator inhibitor-1 predicts myocardial infarction in HIV-1-infected individuals. *AIDS* **2014**, *28*, 1171–1179. [CrossRef]
95. Yu, F.; Li, J.; Huang, Q.; Cai, H. Increased Peripheral Blood Visfatin Concentrations May Be a Risk Marker of Coronary Artery Disease: A Meta-Analysis of Observational Studies. *Angiology* **2018**, *69*, 825–834. [CrossRef]
96. Auguet, T.; Aragonès, G.; Guiu-Jurado, E.; Berlanga, A.; Curriu, M.; Martinez, S.; Alibalic, A.; Aguilar, C.; Camara, M.-L.; Hernández, E.; et al. Adipo/cytokines in atherosclerotic secretomes: Increased visfatin levels in unstable carotid plaque. *BMC Cardiovasc. Disord.* **2016**, *16*, 149. [CrossRef]
97. Zheng, L.-Y.; Xu, X.; Wan, R.-H.; Xia, S.; Lu, J.; Huang, Q. Association between serum visfatin levels and atherosclerotic plaque in patients with type 2 diabetes. *Diabetol. Metab. Syndr.* **2019**, *11*, 60–67. [CrossRef]
98. Yvan-Charvet, L.; Massiera, F.; Lamandé, N.; Ailhaud, G.; Teboul, M.; Moustaid-Moussa, N.; Gasc, J.-M.; Quignard-Boulange, A. Deficiency of Angiotensin Type 2 Receptor Rescues Obesity but Not Hypertension Induced by Overexpression of Angiotensinogen in Adipose Tissue. *Endocrinology* **2009**, *150*, 1421–1428. [CrossRef]
99. Lemieux, M.; Ramalingam, L.; Mynatt, R.L.; Kalupahana, N.S.; Kim, J.H.; Moustaid-Moussa, N. Inactivation of adipose angiotensinogen reduces adipose tissue macrophages and increases metabolic activity. *Obesity* **2015**, *24*, 359–367. [CrossRef]

100. Yiannikouris, F.; Gupte, M.; Putnam, K.; Thatcher, S.; Charnigo, R.; Rateri, D.L.; Daugherty, A.; Cassis, L.A. Adipocyte deficiency of angiotensinogen prevents obesity-induced hypertension in male mice. *Hypertension* **2012**, *60*, 1524–1530.
101. Falcone, C.; Buzzi, M.; D'Angelo, A.; Schirinzi, S.; Falcone, R.; Rordorf, R.; Capettini, A.C.; Landolina, M.; Storti, C.; Pelissero, G. Apelin Plasma Levels Predict Arrhythmia Recurrence in Patients with Persistent Atrial Fibrillation. *Int. J. Immunopathol. Pharmacol.* **2010**, *23*, 917–925.
102. Sato, T.; Kadowaki, A.; Suzuki, T.; Ito, H.; Watanabe, H.; Imai, Y.; Kuba, K. Loss of Apelin Augments Angiotensin II-Induced Cardiac Dysfunction and Pathological Remodeling. *Int. J. Mol. Sci.* **2019**, *20*, 239.
103. Kuklińska, A.M.; Sobkowicz, B.; Sawicki, R.; Musial, W.J.; Waszkiewicz, E.; Bolinska, S.; Małyszko, J. Apelin: A novel marker for the patients with first ST-elevation myocardial infarction. *Heart Vessel.* **2010**, *25*, 363–367.
104. Tycinska, A.; Sobkowicz, B.; Mroczko, B.; Sawicki, R.; Musial, W.J.; Dobrzycki, S.; Waszkiewicz, E.; Knapp, M.; Szmitkowski, M. The value of apelin-36 and brain natriuretic peptide measurements in patients with first ST-elevation myocardial infarction. *Clin. Chim. Acta* **2010**, *411*, 2014–2018.
105. Kadoglou, N.P.; Lampropoulos, S.; Kapelouzou, A.; Gkontopoulos, A.; Theofilogiannakos, E.K.; Fotiadis, G.; Kottas, G. Serum levels of apelin and ghrelin in patients with acute coronary syndromes and established coronary artery disease—KOZANI STUDY. *Transl. Res.* **2010**, *155*, 238–246.
106. Shibata, R.; Ouchi, N.; Kikuchi, R.; Takahashi, R.; Takeshita, K.; Kataoka, Y.; Ohashi, K.; Ikeda, N.; Kihara, S.; Murohara, T. Circulating omentin is associated with coronary artery disease in men. *Atherosclerosis* **2011**, *219*, 811–814.
107. Niersmann, C.; Carstensen-Kirberg, M.; Maalmi, H.; Holleczek, B.; Roden, M.; Brenner, H.; Herder, C.; Schöttker, B. Higher circulating omentin is associated with increased risk of primary cardiovascular events in individuals with diabetes. *Diabetologia* **2019**, *63*, 410–418.
108. Narumi, T.; Watanabe, T.; Kadowaki, S.; Kinoshita, D.; Yokoyama, M.; Honda, Y.; Otaki, Y.; Nishiyama, S.; Takahashi, H.; Arimoto, T.; et al. Impact of serum omentin-1 levels on cardiac prognosis in patients with heart failure. *Cardiovasc. Diabetol.* **2014**, *13*, 84.
109. Lee, Y.-H.; Lee, S.-H.; Jung, E.S.; Kim, J.S.; Shim, C.Y.; Ko, Y.; Choi, D.; Jang, Y.; Chung, N.; Ha, J.-W. Visceral adiposity and the severity of coronary artery disease in middle-aged subjects with normal waist circumference and its relation with lipocalin-2 and MCP-1. *Atherosclerosis* **2010**, *213*, 592–597.
110. Huang, Q.; Fei, X.; Li, S.; Xu, C.; Tu, C.; Jiang, L.; Wo, M. Predicting significance of COX-2 expression of peripheral blood monocyte in patients with coronary artery disease. *Ann. Transl. Med.* **2019**, *7*, 483.
111. Park, S.E.; Lee, N.S.; Park, J.W.; Rhee, E.-J.; Lee, W.-Y.; Oh, K.-W.; Park, S.-W.; Park, C.-Y.; Youn, B.-S. Association of urinary RBP4 with insulin resistance, inflammation, and microalbuminuria. *Eur. J. Endocrinol.* **2014**, *171*, 443–449.
112. Wessel, H.; Saeed, A.; Heegsma, J.; Connelly, M.A.; Faber, K.N.; Dullaart, R.P. Plasma Levels of Retinol Binding Protein 4 Relate to Large VLDL and Small LDL Particles in Subjects with and without Type 2 Diabetes. *J. Clin. Med.* **2019**, *8*, 1792.
113. Kadoglou, N.P.; Lambadiari, V.; Gastounioti, A.; Gkekas, C.; Giannakopoulos, T.; Koulia, K.; Maratou, E.; Alepaki, M.; Kakisis, J.; Karakitsos, P.; et al. The relationship of novel adipokines, RBP4 and omentin-1, with carotid atherosclerosis severity and vulnerability. *Atherosclerosis* **2014**, *235*, 606–612.
114. Liu, G.; Ding, M.; Chiuve, S.E.; Rimm, E.B.; Franks, P.W.; Meigs, J.B.; Hu, F.B.; Sun, Q. Plasma Levels of Fatty Acid-Binding Protein 4, Retinol-Binding Protein 4, High-Molecular-Weight Adiponectin, and Cardiovascular Mortality Among Men with Type 2 Diabetes: A 22-Year Prospective Study. *Arter. Thromb. Vasc. Boil.* **2016**, *36*, 2259–2267.
115. Ingelsson, E.; Sundström, J.; Melhus, H.; Michaelsson, K.; Berne, C.; Vasan, R.S.; Riserus, U.; Blomhoff, R.; Lind, L.; Ärnlöv, J. Circulating retinol-binding protein 4, cardiovascular risk factors and prevalent cardiovascular disease in elderly. *Atherosclerosis* **2009**, *206*, 239–244.
116. Alkharfy, K.M.; Al-Daghri, N.M.; Vanhoutte, P.M.; Krishnaswamy, S.; Xu, A. Serum Retinol-Binding Protein 4 as a Marker for Cardiovascular Disease in Women. *PLoS ONE* **2012**, *7*, e48612.

117. Dyleva, Y.; Gruzdeva, O.; Belik, E.; Akbasheva, O.; Uchasova, E.; Borodkina, D.; Sinitsky, M.; Sotnikov, A.; Kozyrin, K.; Karetnikova, V.; et al. Expression of gene and content of adiponectin in fatty tissue in patients with ischemic heart disease. *Biomeditsinskaya Khimiya* **2019**, *65*, 239–244. [CrossRef]
118. Sinitskiy, M.Y.; Ponasenko, A.V.; Gruzdeva, O.V. Genetic Profile and Secretome Of Adipocytes from Visceral and Subcutaneous Adipose Tissue in Patients with Cardiovascular Diseases. *Complex Issues Cardiovasc. Dis.* **2017**, *3*, 155–165. [CrossRef]
119. Bambace, C.; Telesca, M.; Zoico, E.; Sepe, A.; Olioso, D.; Rossi, A.; Corzato, F.; Di Francesco, V.; Mazzucco, A.; Santini, F.; et al. Adiponectin gene expression and adipocyte diameter: A comparison between epicardial and subcutaneous adipose tissue in men. *Cardiovasc. Pathol.* **2011**, *20*, e153–e156. [CrossRef]
120. Bambace, C.; Sepe, A.; Zoico, E.; Telesca, M.; Olioso, D.; Venturi, S.; Rossi, A.; Corzato, F.; Faccioli, S.; Cominacini, L.; et al. Inflammatory profile in subcutaneous and epicardial adipose tissue in men with and without diabetes. *Heart Vessel.* **2013**, *29*, 42–48. [CrossRef]
121. Gormez, S.; Demirkan, A.; Atalar, F.; Caynak, B.; Erdim, R.; Sözer, V.; Gunay, D.; Akpinar, B.; Ozbek, U.; Buyukdevrim, A.S.; et al. Adipose Tissue Gene Expression of Adiponectin, Tumor Necrosis Factor-α and Leptin in Metabolic Syndrome Patients with Coronary Artery Disease. *Intern. Med.* **2011**, *50*, 805–810. [CrossRef]
122. Teijeira-Fernández, E.; Eiras, S.; Grigorian-Shamagian, L.; Fernández, A.L.; Adrio, B.; González-Juanatey, J.R. Epicardial adipose tissue expression of adiponectin is lower in patients with hypertension. *J. Hum. Hypertens.* **2008**, *22*, 856–863. [CrossRef]
123. Eiras, S.; Teijeira-Fernández, E.; Shamagian, L.G.; Fernández, A.L.; Vazquez-Boquete, A.; Gonzalez-Juanatey, J.R. Extension of coronary artery disease is associated with increased IL-6 and decreased adiponectin gene expression in epicardial adipose tissue. *Cytokine* **2008**, *43*, 174–180. [CrossRef]
124. Iacobellis, G.; Pistilli, D.; Gucciardo, M.; Leonetti, F.; Miraldi, F.; Brancaccio, G.; Gallo, P.; Di Gioia, C.R.T. Adiponectin expression in human epicardial adipose tissue in vivo is lower in patients with coronary artery disease. *Cytokine* **2005**, *29*, 251–255. [CrossRef]
125. Fernández-Trasancos, Á.; Guerola-Segura, R.; Paradela-Dobarro, B.; Álvarez, E.; Acuña, J.M.G.; Fernández, A.L.; González-Juanatey, J.R.; Eiras, S. Glucose and Inflammatory Cells Decrease Adiponectin in Epicardial Adipose Tissue Cells: Paracrine Consequences on Vascular Endothelium. *J. Cell. Physiol.* **2015**, *231*, 1015–1023.
126. Smekal, A.; Vaclavik, J. Adipokines and cardiovascular disease: A comprehensive review. *Biomed. Pap.* **2017**, *161*, 31–40. [CrossRef]

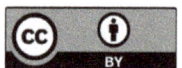

© 2020 by the authors. Licensee MDPI, Basel, Switzerland. This article is an open access article distributed under the terms and conditions of the Creative Commons Attribution (CC BY) license (http://creativecommons.org/licenses/by/4.0/).

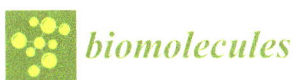 

*Review*

# Galectin-3: A Potential Prognostic and Diagnostic Marker for Heart Disease and Detection of Early Stage Pathology

Akira Hara [1,*], Masayuki Niwa [2], Tomohiro Kanayama [1], Kei Noguchi [1], Ayumi Niwa [1], Mikiko Matsuo [1], Takahiro Kuroda [1], Yuichiro Hatano [1], Hideshi Okada [3] and Hiroyuki Tomita [1]

1. Department of Tumor Pathology, Gifu University Graduate School of Medicine, Gifu 501-1194, Japan; t_knym@gifu-u.ac.jp (T.K.); gucchan1013@gmail.com (K.N.); mulmirry@yahoo.co.jp (A.N.); kyokui100202@gmail.com (M.M.); longhong.heitian@gmail.com (T.K.); yuha@gifu-u.ac.jp (Y.H.); h_tomita@gifu-u.ac.jp (H.T.)
2. Medical Education Development Center, Gifu University School of Medicine, Gifu 501-1194, Japan; mniwa@gifu-u.ac.jp
3. Department of Emergency and Disaster Medicine, Gifu University Graduate School of Medicine, Gifu 501-1194, Japan; hideshi@gifu-u.ac.jp
* Correspondence: ahara@gifu-u.ac.jp; Tel.: +81-58-230-6225

Received: 8 July 2020; Accepted: 2 September 2020; Published: 4 September 2020

**Abstract:** The use of molecular biomarkers for the early detection of heart disease, before their onset of symptoms, is an attractive novel approach. Ideal molecular biomarkers, those that are both sensitive and specific to heart disease, are likely to provide a much earlier diagnosis, thereby providing better treatment outcomes. Galectin-3 is expressed by various immune cells, including mast cells, histiocytes and macrophages, and plays an important role in diverse physiological functions. Since galectin-3 is readily expressed on the cell surface, and is readily secreted by injured and inflammatory cells, it has been suggested that cardiac galectin-3 could be a marker for cardiac disorders such as cardiac inflammation and fibrosis, depending on the specific pathogenesis. Thus, galectin-3 may be a novel candidate biomarker for the diagnosis, analysis and prognosis of various cardiac diseases, including heart failure. The goals of heart disease treatment are to prevent acute onset and to predict their occurrence by using the ideal molecular biomarkers. In this review, we discuss and summarize recent developments of galectin-3 as a next-generation molecular biomarker of heart disease. Furthermore, we describe how galectin-3 may be useful as a diagnostic marker for detecting the early stages of various heart diseases, which may contribute to improved early therapeutic interventions.

**Keywords:** galectin-3; biomarker; diagnostic; prognostic; early stage; heart disease; animal model

## 1. Introduction

Heart diseases are a leading cause of death worldwide, killing approximately 17.9 million people each year. Individuals at risk of heart disease may demonstrate an elevated body weight, blood pressure, plasma cholesterol and blood glucose, as well as obesity. These factors can be easily measured in primary healthcare services. In addition to these standard measures, the use of molecular biomarkers may provide a much earlier detection of heart disease, thereby providing earlier and more efficacious therapeutic interventions. The detection of ideal molecular biomarkers, those that are both sensitive and specific to heart disease, are likely to provide an early diagnosis and suggest specific targeted therapy. However, to date, such ideal biomarkers of heart disease have yet to be identified, despite advances in technologies such as multiplex molecular and genetic biomarkers [1,2]. Thus, the aim of this review is to provide an overview of a candidate molecular heart disease biomarker, galectin-3 (Gal-3).

Galectins are composed of a family of widely expressed β-galactoside-binding lectins and can modulate basic cellular functions such as "cell-to-cell" and "cell-to-matrix" interactions, cell growth and differentiation, tissue regeneration and the regulation of immune cell activities [3–5]. Galectins have been classified according to their carbohydrate recognition domain (CRD) number and function. The CRDs recognize β-galactoside residues that form complexes that crosslink glycosylated ligands [6–8]. The following three types of galectin members are widely accepted (Figure 1): (1) prototype galectins (galectin-1, -2, -5, -7, -10, -11, -13, -14, and -15), containing a single CRD that form noncovalent homodimers; (2) tandem-repeat galectins (galectin-4, -6, -8, -9, and -12), carrying two CRD motifs connected by a peptide linker and (3) a chimera-type galectin (Gal-3), which is characterized by having a single CRD and an amino-terminal polypeptide tail region [4,7,8]. The members of galectins, numbered consecutively by order of discovery, are ubiquitously present in vertebrates, invertebrates and, also, protists [3].

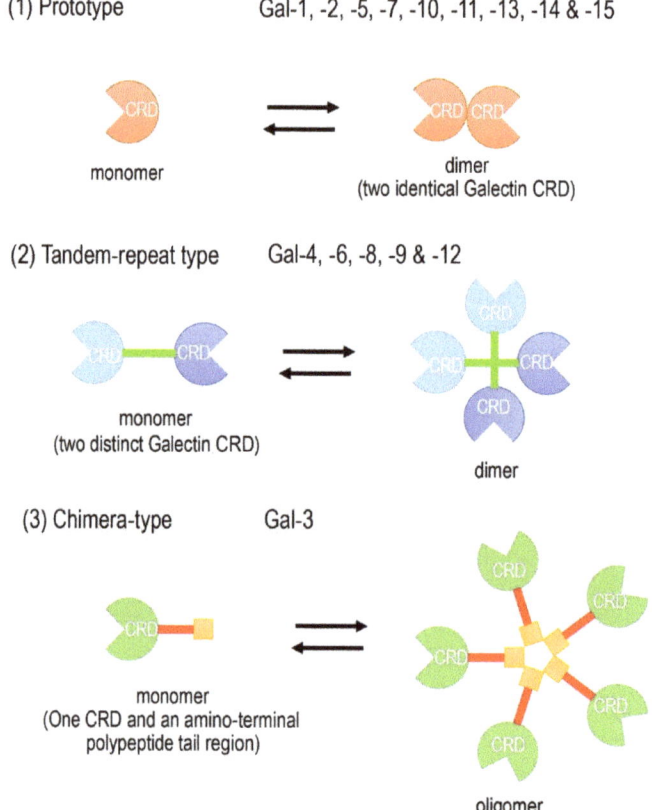

**Figure 1.** Schematic diagram of the galectin family members. Galectin members are divided into three types based on the organization of the galectin carbohydrate recognition domain (CRD).

One member of the family, Gal-3, an approximately 30-kDa chimera-type galectin, is expressed by various immune cells, including mast cells, histiocytes and macrophages, which are associated with the mononuclear phagocytic system in various tissues [9]. Although Gal-3 is predominantly present as a cytosolic protein for cellular function and a nuclei protein for splicing, it is also expressed on cell surfaces and secreted into the plasma by various cells [10]. It has been shown that Gal-3 plays an important role in diverse physiological functions, such as cell growth and differentiation, macrophage activation, angiogenesis, apoptosis and antimicrobial activity, as well as acting as a mediator of local inflammatory responses in many pathological conditions [ ].

Since Gal-3 is readily expressed on the cell surface, and easily secreted into biological fluids (e.g., serum and urine) from injured cells and inflammatory cells, recent studies suggest that cardiac Gal-3 could be a marker for cardiac disorders such as cardiac inflammation and fibrosis, depending on the specific pathogenesis of human heart diseases [ , ]. Therefore, Gal-3 may be a novel candidate biomarker for the diagnosis, analysis and prognosis of various cardiac diseases, including heart failure [ – ].

Furthermore, Gal-3 may also be useful for detecting the early stages of some diseases. Gal-3 has already been used as a possible clinical biomarker in the early detection of myocardial dysfunction, including acute heart failure [ ]. In experimental acute myocarditis following viral infection, Gal-3 has been validated as a biomarker of cardiac fibrotic degeneration in animal models [ , ]. Serum Gal-3 levels have been used as an early diagnostic biomarker for detecting cardiac degeneration in acute myocarditis [ ] and acute myocardial infarction [ ].

Established cardiovascular biomarkers, other than Gal-3, have been investigated for many years for their ability to differentiate different pathophysiological processes, such as inflammation, injury and fibrosis. These biomarkers have been used in clinical practices to reveal the pathophysiological characteristics of heart failure, myocyte injury, ventricular wall stress, fibrosis and cardiac remodeling. Natriuretic peptides (NPs), soluble ST2 (suppression of tumourigenicity2) (sST2), myocardial troponin I (cTnI), myocardial troponin T (cTnT), C-reactive protein (CRP) and growth and differentiation factor-15 (GDF-15) are the cardiovascular biomarkers discussed in this review.

In this review, we discuss and summarize the recent developments of Gal-3 as a next-generation molecular biomarker in not only the patients with various types of heart diseases but, also, the disease-associated animal models. Furthermore, we provide a possibility of Gal-3 as a diagnostic or prognostic marker for detecting the early stages of various heart diseases.

## 2. Current Clinical Studies of Gal-3 as a Possible Biomarker in Heart Disease

Clinically, Gal-3 is studied most intensively in heart disease as a diagnostic or prognostic marker [ – ]. In addition to heart disease, Gal-3 has also been considered as a biomarker in other human diseases, such as viral infections [ – ], autoimmune diseases [ – ], diabetes [ – ], kidney disease [ , , , ] and even tumor formations, including thyroid tumors [ – ]. The diverse clinical involvement of galectins in many diseases has been suggested as a role for the regulators of acute and chronic inflammation, which is linking inflammation-related macrophages to the promotion of fibrosis [ ]. The evidence suggests that Gal-3 is not an organ-specific marker but a specific marker of individual pathogenesis, such as inflammation or fibrosis. Therefore, the primary sources for circulating Gal-3 are not always identified.

Many clinical studies of heart failure suggest that plasma and cardiac Gal-3 levels reflect cardiac inflammatory responses and can be considered as a possible marker for both cardiac inflammation and fibrosis, depending on the pathogenesis of heart failure [ ]. However, the mechanism responsible for increased blood levels of Gal-3 remains incompletely defined. Several studies have been conducted on Gal-3 to assess its prognostic effect in heart failure populations. In general, a high concentration of plasma Gal-3 correlates with a clinical outcome in heart failure associated with cardiac fibrosis [ , ]. The increased plasma levels of Gal-3 are associated with adverse long-term cardiovascular outcomes in both patients with acute [ , ] and chronic [ , ] heart failure. However, some studies have generated conflicting results and suggested that Gal-3 is a poor predictor of mortality [ ]. In addition, some studies have reported contradictory results on the association between plasma and cardiac Gal-3 levels and cardiac fibrosis in heart failure [ – ]. These clinical studies were limited by their small sample sizes and nondetailed evaluations. However, a large-scale meta-analysis of the plasma Gal-3 in the general population has revealed that elevated plasma galectin-3 is associated with a high risk of cardiovascular mortality and heart failure, in addition to all-cause mortality, and has suggested that galectin-3 is an important prognostic factor for patients with heart disease [ ].

Various heart diseases, such as myocardial infarction, myocarditis, hypertension and subsequent heart failure, have dynamic interactions between inflammation and fibrosis [52]. Furthermore, recent studies indicate that Gal-3 is involved in cardiovascular fibrosis as a regulatory molecule in heart failure and, thus, that Gal-3 inhibition ameliorates myocardial injury, highlighting its therapeutic potential [53,54]. Atrial fibrillation, the most common arrhythmia presented in clinical practice, can occur in association with electrical and structural remodeling in the atria. Several lines of evidence demonstrate that myocardial strain, fibrosis and inflammation are involved in the pathogenesis of arrhythmia, including atrial fibrillation, in addition to conventional factors such as the increased left atrial size and the presence of heart failure, coronary heart disease or valvular heart disease. Galectin-3 may be involved in atrial structural remodeling, which involves progressive fibrogenesis in atrial fibrillation patients [55]. A meta-analysis of the relationship between baseline circulating Gal-3 levels and the recurrence of atrial fibrillation in patients undergoing catheter ablation showed that baseline circulating Gal-3 levels were significantly higher in patients with a recurrence of atrial fibrillation compared to those without atrial fibrillation [56]. In addition, higher baseline Gal-3 levels were independently associated with a significantly higher risk of recurrence of atrial fibrillation after catheter ablation [56].

Gal-3 is also reported to be elevated in patients with adult congenital heart disease. A significant association of Gal-3 with functional capacity, cardiac function and adverse cardiovascular events in patients with adult congenital heart disease has been reported recently [57]. In pediatric heart surgery, elevated pre-and postoperative levels of Gal-3 are reported to be associated with an increased risk of readmission or mortality after the operation [58]. Thus, the clinically available biomarker Gal-3 can be used for improved risk stratification.

Chronic kidney disease (CKD) is a risk factor for cardiovascular disease (CVD). Many cardiac biomarkers associated with heart diseases may also reflect the progression of kidney disease. It is plausible that CKD and CVD are closely interrelated, and patients with CKD have a strong risk of CVD [59,60]. Gal-3 is associated with myofibroblast proliferation, fibrogenesis, tissue repair and myocardial remodeling and is also associated with kidney fibrosis and an increased risk of CKD. Thus, the wide tissue distribution of Gal-3 associated with fibrosis in both CVD and CKD complicates the utility of Gal-3 as a cardiac biomarker in CKD patients [28]. Furthermore, a strong and negative correlation between circulating Gal-3 levels and the estimated glomerular filtration rate has been reported. Renal dysfunction is a determinant of blood Gal-3 levels, and the Gal-3 levels are markedly elevated in patients with severe renal failure [61–63]. This means that high concentrations of Gal-3 may be associated with the progression of CKD [26]. Furthermore, Gal-3 is reported to play a pivotal role in renal interstitial fibrosis and the progression of CKD [64]. A glomerular Gal-3 expression was observed in 81.8% of patients with systemic lupus erythematosus (SLE) nephritis but not in the control patients [65]. Blood Gal-3 levels were particularly higher in SLE patients with nephritis than in healthy controls. Gal-3 may contribute to the glomerulonephritis in SLE, and thus, the inhibition of Gal-3 may be a promising therapeutic strategy to prevent advanced renal disease.

The potential use of Gal-3 as a diagnostic biomarker and prognostic indicator in various heart diseases is summarized in Table 1.

**Table 1.** The potential use of Gal-3 as a diagnostic biomarker and prognostic indicator in various heart diseases.

|  | Heart Disease | Usage of Biomarker | Potential Use as Biomarkers | Refs. |
|---|---|---|---|---|
| Diagnostic Biomarkers | acute heart failure | plasma level | • combination with natriuretic peptide | [43] |
|  | acute heart failure | plasma level | • promising prognostic marker | [44] |
|  | chronic heart failure | plasma level | • useful in heart failure | [66] |

**Table 1.** *Cont.*

| | Heart Disease | Usage of Biomarker | Potential Use as Biomarkers | Refs. |
|---|---|---|---|---|
| **Prognostic Indicators** | chronic heart failure | myocardial and plasma level | • no association with histology | [ ] |
| | acute myocardial infarction | serum level | • no definite relationship with ventricular remodeling | [ ] |
| | chronic heart failure | myocardial and plasma level | • marker for both cardiac inflammation and fibrosis<br>• circulating Gal-3 do not reflect cardiac fibrosis | [ ] |
| | chronic heart failure | plasma level | • association of Gal-3 with increased risk for incident heart failure and mortality | [ ] |
| | cardiovascular disease | plasma level | • association of Gal-3 with age and risk factors of cardiovascular disease | [ ] |
| | chronic heart failure | plasma level | • not suggested to be a predictor of mortality<br>• candidate marker of a multi-biomarker panel in prognostication | [ ] |
| | chronic heart failure | plasma level | • association of Gal-3 with severe heart failure<br>• no prediction of outcomes after device implantation | [ ] |
| | heart failure undergoing heart transplantation | plasma levelmyocardial Gal-3 expression | • insufficient use of Gal-3 as a marker of heart<br>• local expression of myocardial Gal-3 | [ ] |
| | heart failure of hypertensive origin | biopsies and plasma samples | • cardiac and systemic excess Gal-3 in heart failure patients<br>• no association with histology | [ ] |
| | cardiovascular mortality and heart failure | plasma level | • large-scale meta-analysis<br>• important prognostic value for heart disease | [ ] |
| | atrial fibrillation | circulating Gal-3 level | • significantly higher in patients with recurrence of atrial fibrillation | [ ] |
| | adult congenital heart disease | serum level | • association of Gal-3 with adverse cardiovascular events | [ ] |
| | pediatric congenital heart disease | serum level | • association of Gal-3 with increased risk of readmission or mortality after the operation | [ ] |

## 3. Current Guidelines for the Clinical Use of Biomarkers in Heart Disease

The clinical use of established or recommended biomarkers in the diagnosis and risk management of heart failure has been indicated by some representative guidelines. The Heart Failure Society of America (HFSA), European Society of Cardiology (ESC) and American College of Cardiology Foundation (ACC)/American Heart Association (AHA) have indicated that the NPs, circulating hormones secreted by cardiomyocytes in the heart ventricles, play an important role in the regulation of the intravascular blood volume and vascular tone and act as useful diagnostic biomarkers in patients suspected of heart failure [ , – ]. Guideline management based on biomarkers has brought a new dimension in diagnosis, prognosis and treatment evaluation. However, the utilities of novel biomarkers other than NPs are not well-established in clinical routine analyses. The National Academy of Clinical Biochemistry (NACB) recommended the clinical assessment and analytical perspectives of novel biomarkers in the diagnosis and management of heart failure [71]. The novel biomarkers in these criteria need to be able to recognize the fundamental causes of heart failure, assess their severity and foresee the risk of disease progression. In fact, with regards to Gal-3 as a novel biomarker, the ACC/AHA guidelines recommended the use of Gal-3 for the assessment of cardiac fibrosis in heart failure; however, thus far, the ESC has not recommended the clinical use of Gal-3 [72].

## 4. Established Cardiovascular Biomarkers Other than Gal-3

As mentioned in the above section, beside the recommendation of NPs by several guidelines on heart failure, many other biomarkers have been investigated as to whether they could reflect different pathophysiological processes such as inflammation, injury and fibrosis. In fact, many candidate protein markers reveal the pathophysiological characteristics of heart failure, including inflammation, myocyte injury, biochemical wall stress, fibrosis and cardiac remodeling. Below, we describe established and novel biomarkers for heart disease.

*4.1. NPs*

Since the first discovery of NP structures and functions in humans in 1984, three types of NPs have been identified in mammals: atrial natriuretic diuretic peptide (ANP), cerebral natriuretic peptide (BNP) and C-type natriuretic peptide (CNP). In particular, BNP and N-terminal-proBNP (the prohormone proBNP is cleaved to the active BNP and the inactive amino acid N-terminal proBNP (NT-proBNP)) are the gold standard clinical diagnostic biomarkers as heart failure biomarkers [73]. In healthy adults, BNP blood levels are less than 25 pg/mL, and NT-proBNP levels are less than 70 pg/mL [74].

Heart failure is a complex, progressive clinical condition in which the heart fails to pump enough blood to supply the body with the amount of blood it needs. Heart failure is a progressive condition that is accompanied by sudden dysfunction. The rapid and accurate diagnosis of heart failure is essential when the progression of the disease is rapid. The diagnosis of heart failure is based on a physical examination and the patient's history, and additional diagnostic tests such as electrocardiography, chest radiography, echocardiography and NT-proBNP have been found to be useful as a means of the further detailed diagnosis of heart failure.

According to the 2016 ESC guidelines [69], measuring plasma NPs can help differentiate both nonacute and acute heart from noncardiac conditions. However, high levels of NPs do not definitively confirm heart failure; therefore, the use of NPs is not recommended to establish the final diagnosis.

It is recommended to use plasma NP concentrations as a clinical test at the first visit of patients with nonacute symptoms if echocardiography is not rapidly available: NT- proBNP < 125 pg/ml = a low probability of heart failure.

A similar concept in the case of acute symptoms but with a higher cut-off value: NT-proBNP < 300 pg/mL = less chance of heart failure. The guideline recommends differentiating acute heart failure from acute dyspnea of noncardiac origin by measuring NT-proBNP in emergency patients with suspected acute dyspnea or acute heart failure.

It is widely recognized that the mechanisms that contribute to the development of heart failure include a complex bidirectional interaction between the kidney and the heart, which is expressed in the term cardiac-renal syndrome (CRS). In a wave of new urinary biomarkers associated with CRS, CNP has emerged as an innovative biomarker of renal structural and functional impairment in heart failure and chronic renal disease states. CNP as a diagnostic and prognostic biomarker in heart failure and renal disease states is expected to have future clinical utility [75].

## 4.2. Soluble ST2 (sST2)

ST2 (suppression of tumourigenicity2) is a member of the interleukin (IL)-1 family and has both a membrane-bound receptor type (ST2L) and soluble (sST2) isoform. In the physiological stretch state of the heart, myofibroblasts release IL-33, which binds to ST2L and promotes cell survival and integrity. This ST2L/IL-33 signaling is regulated by the sST2, which is a decoy of IL-33 secreted by cardiac fibroblasts in response to cardiac pressure and volume overload [ ]. However, when local and neighboring cells abnormally increase the release of sST2, it excessively blocks IL-33/ST2L-binding, which is detrimental to the heart. That is, sST2 acts as a decoy receptor for IL-33 to regulate excessive IL33 signaling under normal conditions, but under pathological conditions, it excessively represses IL-33 signaling, resulting in the interruption of ST2L-mediated cardioprotection. This imbalance in sST2 levels in the extracellular space of the heart is strongly associated with major cardiovascular disorders, including coronary artery disease, heart failure and valvular heart disease [ , ]. Thus, sST2 has come to be used as a biomarker of cardiac stress and fibrosis, and its circulating blood levels are now approved as an additional stratification factor for heart failure [ ] and as a biomarker of ventricular remodeling and fibrosis, along with Gal-3 [ ].

Recent studies have demonstrated that elevated ST2 levels in acute heart failure are prognostic for both recurrent hospitalization and mortality [ ] and that ST2 levels in response to drug treatments are associated with improved outcomes in patients with chronic heart failure [ ]. Thus, while sST2 is a biomarker of myocardial wall stress and the activation of the fibrosis pathway, sST2 is also expressed in organs other than the heart and is not specific to heart failure, making its use for diagnostic purposes in non-heart failure patients problematic.

## 4.3. Myocardial Troponin I (cTnI) and Myocardial Troponin T (cTnT)

The troponin complex, consisting of three subunits: Troponin T, I and C, regulates calcium-mediated muscle contractions between actin and myosin in both skeletal and cardiac muscles. The cardiac-specific isoforms of the troponin subunits cTnI and cTnT have very low or barely detectable blood levels in normal myocardium, but the blood levels of cTnI and cTnT are elevated when myocardial infarction damages cardiomyocytes. They are currently considered to be the most specific markers of myocardial damage, and clinical tests of cTnI and cTnT have been found to be clinically useful for the relative mortality risk classification of patients with acute coronary syndrome (ACS). The system for measuring cardiac troponin in the blood uses cardiac-specific antibodies that do not cross-react with skeletal muscle. Cardiac troponin is the diagnostic criteria for acute myocardial infarction [ , ].

## 4.4. C-reactive Protein (CRP)

CRP is a nonspecific blood marker of biological disease. The measurement of plasma CRP levels has proven clinically useful in the diagnosis and management of infectious diseases and the monitoring of a variety of noninfectious inflammatory diseases, including heart disease.

The importance of high-sensitive C-reactive protein (hs-CRP) measurements has also been reported. One small cohort study concluded that about 70% of patients with hs-CRP values above 4.25 mg/L at 90-day hospitalization died, compared to only 6.5% of patients with hs-CRP values below 4.25 mg/L [ ]. Of note, Japanese people are characterized by lower mean CRP levels (one-third to one-fourth) compared to Westerners; however, a large cohort study revealed that higher levels of hs-CRP are associated with an increased risk of cardiovascular death and myocardial infarction, which may be useful in assessing cardiovascular disease risk [ , ].

## 4.5. Growth and Differentiation Factor-15 (GDF-15)

GDF-15, a member of the transforming growth factor-beta superfamily, also known as macrophage inhibitory cytokine-1 (MIC-1) or nonsteroidal anti-inflammatory drug-activating gene (NAG-1), has been implicated in pathologies such as inflammation, cancer, cardiovascular disease, lung disease and kidney disease. Cardiomyocytes produce and secrete GDF-15 in response to oxidative stress, stimulation by angiotensin II or proinflammatory cytokines, ischemia and mechanical stretch. Cell sources other than cardiomyocytes are known to include macrophages, vascular smooth muscle cells, endothelial cells and adipocytes, which secrete GDF-15 in response to oxidative or metabolic stress or stimulation by proinflammatory cytokines. GDF-15 is thought to protect the heart and adipose tissue, as well as endothelial cells, by inhibiting JNK (c-Jun N-terminal kinase), Bad (Bcl-2-associated death promoter) and EGFR (epidermal growth factor receptor) and activating the Smad, eNOS, PI3K and AKT signaling pathways [87].

GDF-15 can be used as a prognostic marker in patients with cardiovascular disorders in combination with conventional prognostic factors such as NT-proBNP and hs-TnT, as it is induced in hypertrophic and dilated cardiomyopathy after volume overload, ischemia and heart failure [88]. GDF-15 has also been shown to predict both the morbidity and mortality of CVD and cancer in apparently healthy older men [89]. It is interesting to suggest here that GDF-15 expression may be a common early indicator of cellular vulnerability to the development of vascular and cancer diseases. Measurements of sST2, hs-TnI and GDF-15 in the general population have also shown that sST2, GDF-15 and hs-TnI, in addition to established biomarkers such as hs-CRP, can predict cardiovascular risks [90]. GDF-15 has also been widely studied for its usefulness as a biomarker of cardiovascular events in diabetic patients, and it is interesting to note that GDF-15 was the only biomarker associated with cardiovascular events in patients with type 2 diabetes [91]. It has also been suggested that GDF-15 may be a new biomarker for identifying high-risk patients with muscle wasting and kidney dysfunction prior to cardiovascular surgery [92].

In a recent study of three biomarkers: Galectin 3, sSt2 and GDF-15 in adult CKD patients, higher circulating concentrations of all of them were associated with higher mortality, but only elevated GDF-15 concentrations were associated with an increased incidence of heart failure [93].

Finally, many biomarkers for heart disease, including Gal-3, have low tissue specificity, so it will be necessary to study them in combination as multiple markers rather than using them alone.

## 5. Gal-3 as a Biomarker of Cardiac Fibrosis

Cardiac inflammation and fibrosis are tightly implicated in the pathophysiological mechanisms for the myocardial tissue remodeling of heart failure regardless of its etiology [52]. As the important cellular and molecular mechanisms contributing to heart failure, the US Food and Drug Administration has approved Gal-3 as a soluble biomarker for cardiac fibrosis to detect cardiac tissue remodeling [94]. Thus, the serum levels of Gal-3 are associated with cardiac tissue remodeling and cardiac function. However, whether and how Gal-3 contributes to pathophysiology in cardiac remodeling remains unclear, especially in clinical settings. Although certain biomarkers involved in extracellular matrix turnover such as matrix metalloproteinase-3 and monocyte chemoattractant protein-1 at baseline were highly associated with the pathophysiology of acute myocardial infarction, the serum levels of Gal-3 were not related to the left ventricular remodeling defined by cardiac MRI in patients showing cardiac dysfunction [67].

The diverse clinical involvement of galectins in many diseases suggests its role as a regulator of acute and chronic inflammation, linking inflammation-related macrophages to the promotion of fibrosis [52,95]. Specifically, Gal-3 expression and secretion by macrophages is a major mechanism linking macrophages to fibrosis. Macrophages are increasingly recognized as a potential therapeutic target in cardiac fibrosis through interactions with connective tissue fibroblasts [96].

## 6. Usefulness of Gal-3 in Animal Models

The use of animal models that reproduce the clinical features of heart failure and heart disease have contributed to new approaches to improve diagnostic techniques and preventive/therapeutic strategies. As mentioned above, the roles of Gal-3 in heart failure and heart disease in humans are still controversial; however, many animal models have greatly improved our understanding of Gal-3 as a novel biomarker of heart disease. On the other hand, a few studies in animal models have generated conflicting results and suggested that Gal-3 is not a critical disease mediator of cardiac disease [ , ].

The overexpression of cardiac Gal-3 during early pre-symptomatic stages has been demonstrated to induce heart failure and heart disease in several studies using animal models. The intrapericardial injection of recombinant Gal-3 in healthy rats significantly increased the prevalence of cardiac fibrosis with cardiac remodeling and dysfunction and the induction of heart failure [ , ]. Gal-3 was also found to be colocalized with cardiac-infiltrating macrophages [ ]. In contrast, cardiac remodeling and dysfunction induced by Gal-3 was prevented by a pharmacological inhibitor of Gal-3, N-acetyl-seryl-aspartyl-lysyl-proline [ ]. An early increase in Gal-3 expression occurs in hypertrophied hearts, prior to the development of heart failure in a rat model of heart failure, with Gal-3 inducing cardiac fibroblast proliferation, collagen deposition and ventricular dysfunction [ ]. This suggests that Gal-3 may be a novel biomarker candidate for the early stages of heart failure and that antagonizing Gal-3 at the early stages of heart failure may be a useful novel heart failure therapy. In a rat model subjected to pulmonary artery banding to induce right ventricular heart failure, Gal-3 was significantly increased in both the right and left ventricles, and protein kinase C promoted cardiac fibrosis and heart failure by stimulating the Gal-3 expression [ ].

A myocardial ischemia/reperfusion (IR) injury is caused by reperfusion to restore the coronary blood flow to the ischemic region. IR also initiates an inflammatory response, contributing to adverse ventricular remodeling, which is possibly promoted by Gal-3. The upregulation of Gal-3, contributing to IR-induced cardiac dysfunction in a mouse model, has been reported [ ]. Gal-3 inhibition ameliorates myocardial injury and suggests its therapeutic potential. In a rat model of IR injury induced by coronary artery ligation, a Gal-3 blockade improved ischemic injury through lower myocardial inflammation and reduced fibrosis [ ]. In a mouse model of IR injury in the heart using wild-type and Gal-3 knockout mice, Gal-3 was shown to influence the redox pathways, control cell survival and death and play a protective role in the myocardium following IR injury [ ].

In order to clarify the important role of cardiac Gal-3 expression during the early stage of heart failure, the time-course analysis of cardiac and serum Gal-3 in viral myocarditis, which was induced at 12, 24, 48, 96, 168 and 240 hours after a specific virus inoculation, was performed using a mouse model [ ]. Gal-3 was demonstrated as a useful histological biomarker of cardiac fibrosis in acute myocarditis following a viral infection, and serum Gal-3 levels could be used as an early diagnostic marker for detecting cardiac fibrotic degeneration in acute myocarditis [ ].

As mentioned earlier, Gal-3 expression and secretion by macrophages is a major function of macrophages not only contributing to excessive macrophage accumulation and their activation in cardiac tissue but, also, promoting fibroblast activation and proliferation, thus leading to cardiac fibrosis and cardiac remodeling [ , ]. In a mouse model of coxsackievirus B3 (CVB3)-induced myocarditis, mice infected with CVB3 and depleted of macrophages by a liposome-encapsulated clodronate treatment presented a reduction of acute myocarditis and chronic fibrosis, compared with untreated CVB3-infected mice [ ]. In a pressure-overloaded mouse model of heart failure, Gal-3 interacted with aldosterone in promoting macrophage infiltration and cardiac fibrosis. The pharmacological inhibition of Gal-3 prevented the expression of genes involved in fibrogenesis (collagen type 1 and collagen type 3) and macrophage infiltration and cardiac remodeling [ ]. Interestingly, in a pressure-overloaded mouse model, induced by transverse aortic constriction, an early upregulation of Gal-3 occurred three days after transverse aortic constriction in subpopulations of macrophages showing interstitial infiltration [ ]. In contrast, large amounts of Gal-3 were localized in a subset of cardiomyocytes adjacent to fibrotic areas after 7–28 days of transverse aortic constriction [ ]. The results indicate that the Gal-3 expressing cells change depending on the stage (early to late) of disease. Furthermore, these results from animal models indicate that cardiac-infiltrating macrophages expressing Gal-3 in the early stage are potential therapeutic targets for cardiac fibrosis and remodeling. Therefore, the early detection of such Gal-3-producing macrophages by a diagnostic marker is important.

Gal-3 is a key modulator of macrophages for differentiation or activation [107]. In a mouse model for acute myocardial infarction, the treatment of intravenous transplantation using human umbilical cord blood mesenchymal stem cells by modulating the conversion of macrophage subtype M1/M2 reduced the inflammatory response, decreased the serum Gal-3 level, improved cardiac function and protected the infarcted myocardium [108]. The serum level of Gal-3 is closely associated with the ratio of M1 macrophages to M2 macrophages, which is an important factor to improve cardiac function and protect the infarcted myocardium [108].

Representative microphotographs in cardiac lesions showing clear Gal-3 expression are demonstrated in Figure 2. The cardiac lesions of dilated cardiomyopathy in the late stage of δ-sarcoglycan (SG) knockout (KO) mice [13] is shown. The cardiac fibrous lesions, including tissue-resident macrophages, which are usually called histiocytes as a histomorphological term, are seen, with fibroblasts and collagen detected as blue in azan staining. Many histiocytes in the lesions are clearly seen as dark brown in Gal-3 immunostaining.

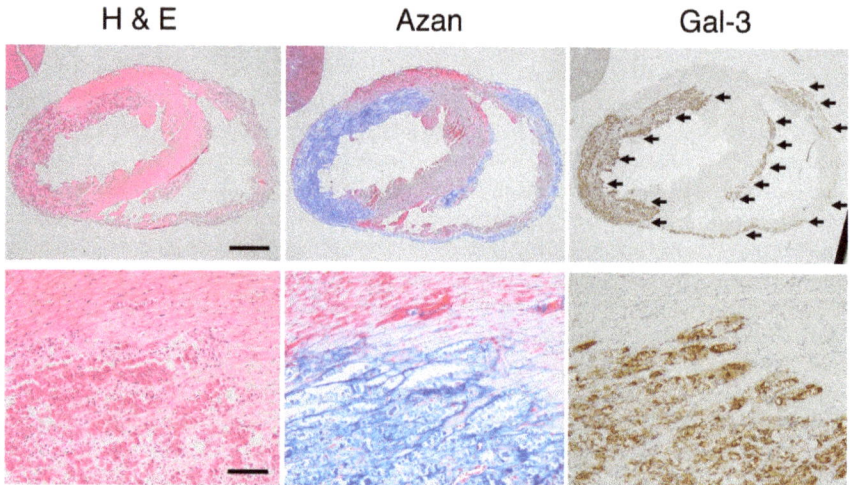

**Figure 2.** The cardiac lesions of dilated cardiomyopathy in the late stage of δ-sarcoglycan (δ-SG) knockout (KO) mice. Microphotographs for hematoxylin and eosin (H&E) staining, Azan staining and immunohistochemistry of Gal-3 are shown. Scale bars in H&E = 1 mm in the upper panel and 100 μm in the lower panel. Gal-3 expression sites indicated by arrows are identical to the fibrotic areas detected as blue in azan staining.

The promising animal models reproducing the clinical features of Gal-3 in heart failure and heart disease are summarized in Table 2.

**Table 2.** Promising animal models reproducing the clinical features of Gal-3 in heart failure and cardiovascular disease. IR: ischemia/reperfusion.

| Animal Species | Experimental Models | Experimental Methods | Experimental Findings | Refs. |
|---|---|---|---|---|
| rat | chronic heart failure | intrapericardial injection of recombinant Gal-3 | • myocardial fibrosis and its pharmacological inhibition • prevention of remodeling by an inhibitor of Gal-3 | [99] |
| rat | chronic heart failure | intrapericardial infusion of low-dose Gal-3 | • increased Gal-3 in hypertrophied hearts • a novel biomarker at the early stages of heart failure | [100] |

Table 2. Cont.

| Animal Species | Experimental Models | Experimental Methods | Experimental Findings | Refs. |
|---|---|---|---|---|
| rat | chronic heart failure | banding of the pulmonary artery | • increase of Gal-3 in ventricles | [ ] |
| rat | ischemia/reperfusion injury | Gal-3 pharmacological inhibition | • Gal-3 blockade improved ischemic injury | [ ] |
| mouse | acute heart failure | viral myocarditis | • time-course analysis of cardiac and serum Gal-3<br>• an early diagnostic marker for cardiac fibrosis | [ ] |
| mouse | myocardial fibrosis | angiotensin-mediated hypertension in AngII/Cx3cr1-/- mice | • macrophages promoting fibroblast differentiation and collagen production | [ ] |
| mouse | acute myocarditis and chronic fibrosis | coxsackievirus B3-induced myocarditis | • disruption of Gal-3 gene reduced acute myocarditis and chronic fibrosis | [ ] |
| mouse | heart failure | isoproterenol-induced left ventricular dysfunction and fibrosis | • interaction of Gal-3 with aldosterone in promoting macrophage infiltration and cardiac fibrosis | [ ] |
| mouse | pressure-overloaded heart | transverse aortic constriction | • early upregulation of Gal-3 in macrophages<br>• large amounts of Gal-3 in cardiomyocytes at the late stage<br>• Loss of Gal-3 did not affect survival, cardiac fibrosis and hypertrophy | [ ] |
| mouse | acute myocardial infarction | intravenous transplantation of human umbilical cord blood mesenchymal stem cells | • close association of Gal-3 with the ratio of M1 macrophages to M2 macrophages | [ ] |
| mouse | ischemia/reperfusion injury | 30 min/24 h in ischemia/ reperfusion model | • contribution of upregulated Gal-3 in cardiac dysfunction<br>• amelioration of myocardial injury by inhibition of Gal-3 | [ ] |
| mouse | ischemia/reperfusion injury | wild-type mice and Gal-3 knockout mice | • protective role of Gal-3 on the myocardium following IR injury | [ ] |
| mouse | several mouse models of heart disease | cardiac and plasma Gal-3-level analysis | • multifold increases in cardiac Gal-3 expression<br>• etiology-dependency of increments in circulating Gal-3 | [ ] |
| mouse | fibrotic cardiomyopathy | cardiac overexpression of b2-adrenoceptors | • upregulation of cardiac Gal-3 expression<br>• Gal-3 may not be a critical disease mediator of cardiac remodeling | [ ] |

## 7. Clinical Use of Gal-3 as a Next-generation Biomarker in the Future

As mentioned earlier, the clinical data has not shown that circulating Gal-3 levels reflect cardiac Gal-3 levels or cardiac fibrosis, although circulating Gal-3 has been demonstrated as a potential predictor for clinical outcomes in several cohort studies [ , ].

In a clinical setting, since various degrees of cardiac inflammation and the progression of fibrosis may be present in a patient with heart disease, blood Gal-3 levels may reflect a sum of different stages of pathophysiological conditions [12]. This is because the circulating blood levels of Gal-3 in a patient with various stages of heart disease cannot adequately reflect cardiac inflammation and fibrosis.

An endomyocardial biopsy is widely used as a diagnostic tool for patients with heart disease, such as myocarditis and secondary cardiomyopathies, which are often difficult to diagnose by conventional imaging alone [109]. There are many variables in human biopsy material by its nature, unlike those obtained from experimental animals. Human biopsies are usually performed under different conditions, variable time periods between biopsy and processing and variations in disease onset or severity. However, the histological examination of an endomyocardial biopsy is still the gold standard for the final diagnosis, despite continued advancements in diagnostic and therapeutic strategies [110–112].

In contrast to the clinical data, the blood levels of Gal-3 reflect the cardiac Gal-3 expression or cardiac fibrosis by using a sophisticated animal model for the time-course histological examination. Especially in the early phase of pathophysiology, there is a close relationship between the infiltration of Gal-3-positive macrophages and fibrotic lesions following myocarditis, and the blood levels of Gal-3 are tightly correlated with the number of cardiac Gal-3-positive cells [13]. The difference between the experimental data from animal studies and clinical findings from individual patients is due to a wide variability in clinical settings, with differences in sample collections and disease stages or severity.

Since experimental data from animal studies clearly indicate that the blood level of Gal-3 might be an early diagnostic biomarker for cardiac degeneration or fibrosis in acute myocarditis [13], further studies are needed to investigate whether such findings are also observed in cardiac degeneration or fibrosis in human patients. Gal-3 can be used reliably as a predictive biomarker for the early stage or new onset of heart disease, especially if it is derived from only the first single pathological lesion, without complicated factors. In addition, Gal-3 can also possibly be used in late stages of the diseases as an additional indicator for detecting a worse prognosis, mortality and readmission.

## 8. Conclusions and Perspectives

The blood levels of Gal-3 are altered by different clinical factors depending on the underlying pathophysiological conditions in patients, and thus, Gal-3 itself is not an organ-specific marker. However, Gal-3 is a specific marker of pathogenesis, such as macrophage-related disease or fibrosis, and the cardiac-infiltrating macrophages expressing Gal-3 in the early stages are potential therapeutic targets for cardiac fibrosis and remodeling. Therefore, the early detection of such Gal-3-producing macrophages by a diagnostic marker is important. Furthermore, Gal-3 is being tested for personalized medicine based on biomarker-guided diagnostics, using new technologies such as genetic biomarkers and multiplex biomarkers, combining multiple markers into a multiplex panel. In pediatric heart surgery, the clinically available biomarker Gal-3 can be used for improved risk stratification, because Gal-3 has recently been reported to be associated with an increased risk of readmission or mortality after the operation. In addition, Gal-3 at the early stages of inflammatory responses may be a potential therapeutic target for diseases, especially in cardiac fibrosis, autoimmune diseases, neurodegenerative diseases and cardio- and cerebrovascular diseases.

**Author Contributions:** Conceptualization, A.H. and H.O.; investigation, T.K. (Tomohiro Kanayama), K.N., A.N., M.M., T.K. (Takahiro Kuroda) and Y.H.; writing—original draft preparation, A.H. and M.N. and writing—review and editing, H.T. All authors have read and agreed to the published version of the manuscript.

**Funding:** This research received no external funding.

**Acknowledgments:** The authors thank Paul Green for his English editing to complete this review.

**Conflicts of Interest:** The authors declare no conflict of interest.

## References

1. Rather, R.A.; Dhawan, V. Genetic markers: Potential candidates for cardiovascular disease. *Int. J. Cardiol.* **2016**, *220*, 914–923. [CrossRef] [PubMed]
2. Adamcova, M.; Šimko, F. Multiplex biomarker approach to cardiovascular diseases perspective. *Acta Pharmacol. Sin.* **2018**, *39*, 1068–1072. [CrossRef]
3. Liu, F.T.; Patterson, R.J.; Wang, J.L. Intracellular functions of galectins. *Biochim. Biophys. Acta Gen. Subj.* **2002**, *1572*, 263–273. [CrossRef]
4. Yang, R.Y.; Rabinovich, G.A.; Liu, F.T. Galectins: Structure, function and therapeutic potential. *Expert Rev. Mol. Med.* **2008**, *10*, e17. [CrossRef]
5. Chen, H.Y.; Weng, I.C.; Hong, M.H.; Liu, F.T. Galectins as bacterial sensors in the host innate response. *Curr. Opin. Microbiol.* **2014**, *17*, 75–81. [CrossRef]
6. Barondes, S.H.; Castronovo, V.; Cooper, D.N.W.; Cummings, R.D.; Drickamer, K.; Felzi, T.; Gitt, M.A.; Hirabayashi, J.; Hughes, C.; Kasai, K.I.; et al. Galectins: A family of animal β-galactoside-binding lectins. *Cell* **1994**, *76*, 597–598. [CrossRef]
7. Nabi, I.R.; Shankar, J.; Dennis, J.W. The galectin lattice at a glance. *J. Cell Sci.* **2015**, *128*, 2213–2219. [CrossRef]
8. Johannes, L.; Jacob, R.; Leffler, H. Galectins at a glance. *J. Cell Sci.* **2018**, *131*, jcs208884. [CrossRef]
9. Cherayil, B.J.; Weiner, S.J.; Pillai, S. The Mac-2 antigen is a galactose-specific lectin that binds IgE. *J. Exp. Med.* **1989**, *170*, 1959–1972. [CrossRef]
10. Hughes, R.C. Mac-2: A versatile galactose-binding protein of mammalian tissues. *Glycobiology* **1994**, *4*, 5–12. [CrossRef]
11. Díaz-Alvarez, L.; Ortega, E. The Many Roles of Galectin-3, a Multifaceted Molecule, in Innate Immune Responses against Pathogens. *Mediators Inflamm.* **2017**, *2017*, 9–12. [CrossRef] [PubMed]
12. Besler, C.; Lang, D.; Urban, D.; Rommel, K.P.; Von Roeder, M.; Fengler, K.; Blazek, S.; Kandolf, R.; Klingel, K.; Thiele, H.; et al. Plasma and cardiac galectin-3 in patients with heart failure reflects both inflammation and fibrosis: Implications for its use as a biomarker. *Circ. Heart Fail.* **2017**, *10*, e003804. [CrossRef] [PubMed]
13. Noguchi, K.; Tomita, H.; Kanayama, T.; Niwa, A.; Hatano, Y.; Hoshi, M.; Sugie, S.; Okada, H.; Niwa, M.; Hara, A. Time-course analysis of cardiac and serum galectin-3 in viral myocarditis after an encephalomyocarditis virus inoculation. *PLoS ONE* **2019**, *14*, e0210971. [CrossRef] [PubMed]
14. Hrynchyshyn, N.; Jourdain, P.; Desnos, M.; Diebold, B.; Funck, F. Galectin-3: A new biomarker for the diagnosis, analysis and prognosis of acute and chronic heart failure. *Arch. Cardiovasc. Dis.* **2013**, *106*, 541–546. [CrossRef]
15. Dong, R.; Zhang, M.; Hu, Q.; Zheng, S.; Soh, A.; Zheng, Y.; Yuan, H. Galectin-3 as a novel biomarker for disease diagnosis and a target for therapy (Review). *Int. J. Mol. Med.* **2018**, *41*, 599–614. [CrossRef] [PubMed]
16. Hashmi, S.; Al-Salam, S. Galectin-3 is expressed in the myocardium very early post-myocardial infarction. *Cardiovasc. Pathol.* **2015**, *24*, 213–223. [CrossRef]
17. De Couto, G.; Ouzounian, M.; Liu, P.P. Early detection of myocardial dysfunction and heart failure. *Nat. Rev. Cardiol.* **2010**, *7*, 334–344. [CrossRef]
18. Sato, S.; Ouellet, M.; St-Pierre, C.; Tremblay, M.J. Glycans, galectins, and HIV-1 infection. *Ann. N. Y. Acad. Sci.* **2012**, *1253*, 133–148. [CrossRef]
19. Nielsen, C.T.; Østergaard, O.; Rasmussen, N.S.; Jacobsen, S.; Heegaard, N.H.H. A review of studies of the proteomes of circulating microparticles: Key roles for galectin-3-binding protein-expressing microparticles in vascular diseases and systemic lupus erythematosus. *Clin. Proteomics* **2017**, *14*, 11. [CrossRef]
20. Kobayashi, K.; Niwa, M.; Hoshi, M.; Saito, K.; Hisamatsu, K.; Hatano, Y.; Tomita, H.; Miyazaki, T.; Hara, A. Early microlesion of viral encephalitis confirmed by galectin-3 expression after a virus inoculation. *Neurosci. Lett.* **2015**, *592*, 107–112. [CrossRef]
21. de Oliveira, F.L.; Gatto, M.; Bassi, N.; Luisetto, R.; Ghirardello, A.; Punzi, L.; Doria, A. Galectin-3 in autoimmunity and autoimmune diseases. *Exp. Biol. Med.* **2015**, *240*, 1019–1028. [CrossRef] [PubMed]
22. Dhirapong, A.; Lleo, A.; Leung, P.; Gershwin, M.E.; Liu, F.T. The immunological potential of galectin-1 and -3. *Autoimmun. Rev.* **2009**, *8*, 360–363. [CrossRef]
23. Shin, T. The pleiotropic effects of galectin-3 in neuroinflammation: A review. *Acta Histochem.* **2013**, *115*, 407–411. [CrossRef] [PubMed]

24. Saccon, F.; Gatto, M.; Ghirardello, A.; Iaccarino, L.; Punzi, L.; Doria, A. Role of galectin-3 in autoimmune and non-autoimmune nephropathies. *Autoimmun. Rev.* **2017**, *16*, 34–47. [CrossRef]
25. Tan, K.C.B.; Cheung, C.-L.; Lee, A.C.H.; Lam, J.K.Y.; Wong, Y.; Shiu, S.W.M. Galectin-3 is independently associated with progression of nephropathy in type 2 diabetes mellitus. *Diabetologia* **2018**, *61*, 1212–1219. [CrossRef] [PubMed]
26. Alam, M.L.; Katz, R.; Bellovich, K.A.; Bhat, Z.Y.; Brosius, F.C.; de Boer, I.H.; Gadegbeku, C.A.; Gipson, D.S.; Hawkins, J.J.; Himmelfarb, J.; et al. Soluble ST2 and Galectin-3 and Progression of CKD. *Kidney Int. Rep.* **2019**, *4*, 103–111. [CrossRef] [PubMed]
27. Gopal, D.M.; Ayalon, N.; Wang, Y.C.; Siwik, D.; Sverdlov, A.; Donohue, C.; Perez, A.; Downing, J.; Apovian, C.; Silva, V.; et al. Galectin-3 is associated with stage B metabolic heart disease and pulmonary hypertension in young obese patients. *J. Am. Heart Assoc.* **2019**, *8*, e011100. [CrossRef] [PubMed]
28. Savoj, J.; Becerra, B.; Kim, J.K.; Fusaro, M.; Gallieni, M.; Lombardo, D.; Lau, W.L. Utility of Cardiac Biomarkers in the Setting of Kidney Disease. *Nephron* **2019**, *141*, 227–235. [CrossRef]
29. Chen, S.C.; Kuo, P.L. The role of galectin-3 in the kidneys. *Int. J. Mol. Sci.* **2016**, *17*, 565. [CrossRef]
30. Binh, N.H.; Satoh, K.; Kobayashi, K.; Takamatsu, M.; Hatano, Y.; Hirata, A.; Tomita, H.; Kuno, T.; Hara, A. Galectin-3 in preneoplastic lesions of glioma. *J. Neurooncol.* **2013**, *111*, 123–132. [CrossRef]
31. Song, L.; Tang, J.W.; Owusu, L.; Sun, M.Z.; Wu, J.; Zhang, J. Galectin-3 in cancer. *Clin. Chim. Acta* **2014**, *431*, 185–191. [CrossRef] [PubMed]
32. Fortuna-Costa, A.; Gomes, A.M.; Kozlowski, E.O.; Stelling, M.P.; Pavão, M.S.G. Extracellular galectin-3 in tumor progression and metastasis. *Front. Oncol.* **2014**, *4*, 138. [CrossRef] [PubMed]
33. Funasaka, T.; Raz, A.; Nangia-Makker, P. Galectin-3 in angiogenesis and metastasis. *Glycobiology* **2014**, *24*, 886–891. [CrossRef] [PubMed]
34. Xin, M.; Dong, X.W.; Guo, X.L. Role of the interaction between galectin-3 and cell adhesion molecules in cancer metastasis. *Biomed. Pharmacother.* **2015**, *69*, 179–185. [CrossRef] [PubMed]
35. Ruvolo, P.P. Galectin 3 as a guardian of the tumor microenvironment. *Biochim. Biophys. Acta-Mol. Cell Res.* **2016**, *1863*, 427–437. [CrossRef]
36. Zeinali, M.; Adelinik, A.; Papian, S.; Khorramdelazad, H.; Abedinzadeh, M. Role of galectin-3 in the pathogenesis of bladder transitional cell carcinoma. *Hum. Immunol.* **2015**, *76*, 770–774. [CrossRef]
37. Wang, L.; Guo, X.L. Molecular regulation of galectin-expression and therapeutic implication in cancer progression. *Biomed. Pharmacother.* **2016**, *78*, 165–171. [CrossRef]
38. Nangia-Makker, P.; Hogan, V.; Raz, A. Galectin-3 and cancer stemness. *Glycobiology* **2018**, *28*, 172–181. [CrossRef]
39. Wang, C.; Zhou, X.; Ma, L.; Zhuang, Y.; Wei, Y.; Zhang, L.; Jin, S.; Liang, W.; Shen, X.; Li, C.; et al. Galectin-3 may serve as a marker for poor prognosis in colorectal cancer: A meta-analysis. *Pathol. Res. Pract.* **2019**, *215*, 152612. [CrossRef]
40. Henderson, N.C.; Mackinnon, A.C.; Farnworth, S.L.; Kipari, T.; Haslett, C.; Iredale, J.P.; Liu, F.T.; Hughes, J.; Sethi, T. Galectin-3 expression and secretion links macrophages to the promotion of renal fibrosis. *Am. J. Pathol.* **2008**, *172*, 288–298. [CrossRef]
41. Ho, J.E.; Liu, C.; Lyass, A.; Courchesne, P.; Pencina, M.J.; Vasan, R.S.; Larson, M.G.; Levy, D. Galectin-3, a marker of cardiac fibrosis, predicts incident heart failure in the community. *J. Am. Coll. Cardiol.* **2012**, *60*, 1249–1256. [CrossRef] [PubMed]
42. de Boer, R.A.; van Veldhuisen, D.J.; Gansevoort, R.T.; Muller Kobold, A.C.; van Gilst, W.H.; Hillege, H.L.; Bakker, S.J.L.; van der Harst, P. The fibrosis marker galectin-3 and outcome in the general population. *J. Intern. Med.* **2012**, *272*, 55–64. [CrossRef] [PubMed]
43. van Kimmenade, R.R.; Januzzi, J.L.; Ellinor, P.T.; Sharma, U.C.; Bakker, J.A.; Low, A.F.; Martinez, A.; Crijns, H.J.; MacRae, C.A.; Menheere, P.P.; et al. Utility of Amino-Terminal Pro-Brain Natriuretic Peptide, Galectin-3, and Apelin for the Evaluation of Patients With Acute Heart Failure. *J. Am. Coll. Cardiol.* **2006**, *48*, 1217–1224. [CrossRef] [PubMed]
44. Agnello, L.; Bivona, G.; Lo Sasso, B.; Scazzone, C.; Bazan, V.; Bellia, C.; Ciaccio, M. Galectin-3 in acute coronary syndrome. *Clin. Biochem.* **2017**, *50*, 797–803. [CrossRef]

45. Lopez-Andrés, N.; Rossignol, P.; Iraqi, W.; Fay, R.; Nuée, J.; Ghio, S.; Cleland, J.G.F.; Zannad, F.; Lacolley, P. Association of galectin-3 and fibrosis markers with long-term cardiovascular outcomes in patients with heart failure, left ventricular dysfunction, and dyssynchrony: Insights from the CARE-HF (Cardiac Resynchronization in Heart Failure) trial. *Eur. J. Heart Fail.* **2012**, *14*, 74–81.

46. Yancy, C.W.; Mariell Jessup, C.; Chair Biykem Bozkurt, V.; Butler, J.; Casey, D.E., Jr.; Colvin, M.M.; Drazner, M.H.; Filippatos, G.S.; Fonarow, G.C.; Givertz, M.M.; et al. 2017 ACC/AHA/HFSA Focused Update of the 2013 ACCF/AHA Guideline for the Management of Heart Failure. *Circulation* **2017**, *136*, 137–161.

47. Srivatsan, V.; George, M.; Shanmugam, E. Utility of galectin-3 as a prognostic biomarker in heart failure: Where do we stand? *Eur. J. Prev. Cardiol.* **2015**, *22*, 1096–1110.

48. Erkilet, G.; Özpeker, C.; Böthig, D.; Kramer, F.; Röfe, D.; Bohms, B.; Morshuis, M.; Gummert, J.; Milting, H. The biomarker plasma galectin-3 in advanced heart failure and survival with mechanical circulatory support devices. *J. Heart Lung Transplant.* **2013**, *32*, 221–230.

49. Beiras-Fernandez, A.; Weis, F.; Rothkopf, J.; Kaczmarek, I.; Ledderose, C.; Dick, A.; Keller, T.; Beiras, A.; Kreth, S. Local expression of myocardial galectin-3 does not correlate with its serum levels in patients undergoing heart transplantation. *Ann. Transplant.* **2013**, *18*, 643–650.

50. López, B.; González, A.; Querejeta, R.; Zubillaga, E.; Larman, M.; Díez, J. Galectin-3 and histological, molecular and biochemical aspects of myocardial fibrosis in heart failure of hypertensive origin. *Eur. J. Heart Fail.* **2015**, *17*, 385–392.

51. Imran, T.F.; Shin, H.J.; Mathenge, N.; Wang, F.; Kim, B.; Joseph, J.; Gaziano, J.M.; Djoussé, L. Meta-Analysis of the Usefulness of Plasma Galectin-3 to Predict the Risk of Mortality in Patients With Heart Failure and in the General Population. *Am. J. Cardiol.* **2017**, *119*, 57–64.

52. Suthahar, N.; Meijers, W.C.; Silljé, H.H.W.; de Boer, R.A. From Inflammation to Fibrosis—Molecular and Cellular Mechanisms of Myocardial Tissue Remodelling and Perspectives on Differential Treatment Opportunities. *Curr. Heart Fail. Rep.* **2017**, *14*, 235–250.

53. Mo, D.; Tian, W.; Zhang, H.N.; Feng, Y.D.; Sun, Y.; Quan, W.; Hao, X.W.; Wang, X.Y.; Liu, X.X.; Li, C.; et al. Cardioprotective effects of galectin-3 inhibition against ischemia/reperfusion injury. *Eur. J. Pharmacol.* **2019**, *863*, 172701.

54. Zhong, X.; Qian, X.; Chen, G.; Song, X. The role of galectin-3 in heart failure and cardiovascular disease. *Clin. Exp. Pharmacol. Physiol.* **2019**, *46*, 197–203.

55. Clementy, N.; Piver, E.; Bisson, A.; Andre, C.; Bernard, A.; Pierre, B.; Fauchier, L.; Babuty, D. Galectin-3 in atrial fibrillation: Mechanisms and therapeutic implications. *Int. J. Mol. Sci.* **2018**, *19*, 976.

56. Zhang, G.; Wu, Y. Circulating galectin-3 and atrial fibrillation recurrence after catheter ablation: A meta-analysis. *Cardiovasc. Ther.* **2019**, *2019*.

57. Baggen, V.J.M.; van den Bosch, A.E.; Eindhoven, J.A.; Menting, M.E.; Witsenburg, M.; Cuypers, J.A.A.E.; Boersma, E.; Roos-Hesselink, J.W. Prognostic value of galectin-3 in adults with congenital heart disease. *Heart* **2018**, *104*, 394–400.

58. Parker, D.M.; Everett, A.D.; Stabler, M.E.; Vricella, L.; Jacobs, M.L.; Jacobs, J.P.; Thiessen-Philbrook, H.; Parikh, C.R.; Brown, J.R. Biomarkers associated with 30-day readmission and mortality after pediatric congenital heart surgery. *J. Card. Surg.* **2019**, *34*, 329–336.

59. Chowdhury, P.; Kehl, D.; Choudhary, R.; Maisel, A. The use of biomarkers in the patient with heart failure. *Curr. Cardiol. Rep.* **2013**, *15*, 372.

60. Mahmood, U.; Johnson, D.W.; Fahim, M.A. Cardiac biomarkers in dialysis. *AIMS Genet.* **2016**, *4*, 1–20.

61. Nguyen, M.N.; Su, Y.; Vizi, D.; Fang, L.; Ellims, A.H.; Zhao, W.B.; Kiriazis, H.; Gao, X.M.; Sadoshima, J.; Taylor, A.J.; et al. Mechanisms responsible for increased circulating levels of galectin-3 in cardiomyopathy and heart failure. *Sci. Rep.* **2018**, *8*, 1–12.

62. Gopal, D.M.; Kommineni, M.; Ayalon, N.; Koelbl, C.; Ayalon, R.; Biolo, A.; Dember, L.M.; Downing, J.; Siwik, D.A.; Liang, C.S.; et al. Relationship of plasma galectin-3 to renal function in patients with heart failure: Effects of clinical status, pathophysiology of heart failure, and presence or absence of heart failure. *J. Am. Heart Assoc.* **2012**, *1*, 1–7.

63. Meijers, W.C.; van der Velde, A.R.; Ruifrok, W.P.; Schroten, N.F.; Dokter, M.M.; Damman, K.; Assa, S.; Franssen, C.F.; Gansevoort, R.T.; van Gilst, W.H.; et al. Renal handling of galectin-3 in the general population, chronic heart failure, and hemodialysis. *J. Am. Heart Assoc.* **2014**, *3*, 1–11. [CrossRef] [PubMed]
64. Desmedt, V.; Desmedt, S.; Delanghe, J.R.; Speeckaert, R.; Speeckaert, M.M. Galectin-3 in Renal Pathology: More Than Just an Innocent Bystander? *Am. J. Nephrol.* **2016**, *43*, 305–317. [CrossRef] [PubMed]
65. Kang, E.H.; Moon, K.C.; Lee, E.Y.; Lee, Y.J.; Lee, E.B.; Ahn, C.; Song, Y.W. Renal expression of galectin-3 in systemic lupus erythematosus patients with nephritis. *Lupus* **2009**, *18*, 22–28. [CrossRef]
66. De Boer, R.A.; Lok, D.J.A.; Jaarsma, T.; Van Der Meer, P.; Voors, A.A.; Hillege, H.L.; Van Veldhuisen, D.J. Predictive value of plasma galectin-3 levels in heart failure with reduced and preserved ejection fraction. *Ann. Med.* **2011**, *43*, 60–68. [CrossRef]
67. Weir, R.A.P.; Petrie, C.J.; Murphy, C.A.; Clements, S.; Steedman, T.; Miller, A.M.; McInnes, I.B.; Squire, I.B.; Ng, L.L.; Dargie, H.J.; et al. Galectin-3 and cardiac function in survivors of acute myocardial infarction. *Circ. Heart Fail.* **2013**, *6*, 492–498. [CrossRef]
68. Paul, S.; Lindenfeld, J.; Mann, D.L.; Albert, N.M.; Boehmer, J.P.; Collins, S.P.; Ezekowitz, J.A.; Givertz, M.M.; Katz, S.D.; Klapholz, M.; et al. Heart Failure Practice Guideline HFSA 2010 Comprehensive Heart Failure Practice Guideline. *J. Card. Fail.* **2010**, *16*, e1–e2.
69. Ponikowski, P.; Voors, A.A.; Anker, S.D.; Bueno, H.; Cleland, J.G.F.; Coats, A.J.S.; Falk, V.; González-Juanatey, J.R.; Harjola, V.P.; Jankowska, E.A.; et al. 2016 ESC Guidelines for the diagnosis and treatment of acute and chronic heart failure. *Eur. Heart J.* **2016**, *37*, 2129–2200. [CrossRef]
70. Yancy, C.W.; Jessup, M.; Bozkurt, B.; Butler, J.; Casey, D.E.; Drazner, M.H.; Fonarow, G.C.; Geraci, S.A.; Horwich, T.; Januzzi, J.L.; et al. 2013 ACCF/AHA Guideline for the Management of Heart Failure. *J. Am. Coll. Cardiol.* **2013**, *62*, e147–e239. [CrossRef]
71. Tang, W.H.W.; Francis, G.S.; Morrow, D.A.; Newby, L.K.; Cannon, C.P.; Jesse, R.L.; Storrow, A.B.; Christenson, R.H.; Christenson, R.H.; Apple, F.S.; et al. National Academy of Clinical Biochemistry Laboratory Medicine Practice Guidelines: Clinical Utilization of Cardiac Biomarker Testing in Heart Failure. *Clin. Biochem.* **2008**, *41*, 210–221. [CrossRef] [PubMed]
72. Sarhene, M.; Wang, Y.; Wei, J.; Huang, Y.; Li, M.; Li, L.; Acheampong, E.; Zhengcan, Z.; Xiaoyan, Q.; Yunsheng, X.; et al. Biomarkers in heart failure: The past, current and future. *Heart Fail. Rev.* **2019**, *24*, 867–903. [CrossRef] [PubMed]
73. Tang, W.H.W.; Francis, G.S.; Morrow, D.A.; Newby, L.K.; Cannon, C.P.; Jesse, R.L.; Storrow, A.B.; Christenson, R.H. National Academy of Clinical Biochemistry Laboratory Medicine Practice Guidelines: Clinical utilization of cardiac biomarker testing in heart failure. *Circulation* **2007**, *116*, e99–e109. [CrossRef]
74. Daniels, L.B.; Allison, M.A.; Clopton, P.; Redwine, L.; Siecke, N.; Taylor, K.; Fitzgerald, R.; Bracker, M.; Maisel, A.S. Use of natriuretic peptides in pre-participation screening of college athletes. *Int. J. Cardiol.* **2008**, *124*, 411–414. [CrossRef] [PubMed]
75. Zakeri, R.; Burnett, J.C.; Sangaralingham, S.J. Urinary C-type natriuretic peptide: An emerging biomarker for heart failure and renal remodeling. *Clin. Chim. Acta* **2015**, *443*, 108–113. [CrossRef]
76. Millar, N.L.; O'Donnell, C.; McInnes, I.B.; Brint, E. Wounds that heal and wounds that don't - The role of the IL-33/ST2 pathway in tissue repair and tumorigenesis. *Semin. Cell Dev. Biol.* **2017**, *61*, 41–50. [CrossRef]
77. Gao, Q.; Li, Y.; Li, M. The potential role of IL-33/ST2 signaling in fibrotic diseases. *J. Leukoc. Biol.* **2015**, *98*, 15–22. [CrossRef]
78. Kotsiou, O.S.; Gourgoulianis, K.I.; Zarogiannis, S.G. IL-33/ST2 Axis in Organ Fibrosis. *Front. Immunol.* **2018**, *9*, 2432. [CrossRef]
79. Januzzi, J.L.; Mebazaa, A.; Di Somma, S. ST2 and prognosis in acutely decompensated heart failure: The International ST2 Consensus Panel. *Am. J. Cardiol.* **2015**, *115*, 26B–31B. [CrossRef]
80. Aimo, A.; Vergaro, G.; Ripoli, A.; Bayes-Genis, A.; Pascual Figal, D.A.; de Boer, R.A.; Lassus, J.; Mebazaa, A.; Gayat, E.; Breidthardt, T.; et al. Meta-Analysis of Soluble Suppression of Tumorigenicity-2 and Prognosis in Acute Heart Failure. *JACC Heart Fail.* **2017**, *5*, 287–296. [CrossRef]
81. O'Meara, E.; Prescott, M.F.; Claggett, B.; Rouleau, J.L.; Chiang, L.-M.; Solomon, S.D.; Packer, M.; McMurray, J.J.V.; Zile, M.R. Independent Prognostic Value of Serum Soluble ST2 Measurements in Patients With Heart Failure and a Reduced Ejection Fraction in the PARADIGM-HF Trial (Prospective Comparison of ARNI With ACEI to Determine Impact on Global Mortality and Morbidity in Heart Failure). *Circ. Heart Fail.* **2018**, *11*, e004446. [CrossRef]

82. Thygesen, K.; Alpert, J.S.; White, H.D. Universal definition of myocardial infarction. *Circulation* **2007**, *116*, 2634–2653. [CrossRef] [PubMed]
83. Thygesen, K.; Alpert, J.S.; White, H.D. Universal definition of myocardial infarction. *Eur. Heart J.* **2007**, *28*, 2525–2538. [CrossRef]
84. Nursyamsiah; Hasan, R. High-sensitivity c-reactive protein (hs-CRP) value with 90 days mortality in patients with heart failure. *IOP Conf. Ser. Earth Environ. Sci.* **2018**, *125*, 012124. [CrossRef]
85. Iso, H.; Cui, R.; Date, C.; Kikuchi, S.; Tamakoshi, A. C-reactive protein levels and risk of mortality from cardiovascular disease in Japanese: The JACC Study. *Atherosclerosis* **2009**, *207*, 291–297. [CrossRef]
86. Iso, H.; Noda, H.; Ikeda, A.; Yamagishi, K.; Inoue, M.; Iwasaki, M.; Tsugane, S. The impact of C-reactive protein on risk of stroke, stroke subtypes, and ischemic heart disease in middle-aged Japanese: The Japan public health center-based study. *J. Atheroscler. Thromb.* **2012**, *19*, 756–766. [CrossRef]
87. Adela, R.; Banerjee, S.K. GDF-15 as a Target and Biomarker for Diabetes and Cardiovascular Diseases: A Translational Prospective. *J. Diabetes Res.* **2015**, *2015*, 490842. [CrossRef]
88. Arkoumani, M.; Papadopoulou-Marketou, N.; Nicolaides, N.C.; Kanaka-Gantenbein, C.; Tentolouris, N.; Papassotiriou, I. The clinical impact of growth differentiation factor-15 in heart disease: A 2019 update. *Crit. Rev. Clin. Lab. Sci.* **2020**, *57*, 114–125. [CrossRef]
89. Wallentin, L.; Zethelius, B.; Berglund, L.; Eggers, K.M.; Lind, L.; Lindahl, B.; Wollert, K.C.; Siegbahn, A. GDF-15 for prognostication of cardiovascular and cancer morbidity and mortality in men. *PLoS ONE* **2013**, *8*, e78797. [CrossRef]
90. Wang, T.J.; Wollert, K.C.; Larson, M.G.; Coglianese, E.; McCabe, E.L.; Cheng, S.; Ho, J.E.; Fradley, M.G.; Ghorbani, A.; Xanthakis, V.; et al. Prognostic utility of novel biomarkers of cardiovascular stress: The Framingham Heart Study. *Circulation* **2012**, *126*, 1596–1604. [CrossRef]
91. Carlsson, A.C.; Nowak, C.; Lind, L.; Östgren, C.J.; Nyström, F.H.; Sundström, J.; Carrero, J.J.; Riserus, U.; Ingelsson, E.; Fall, T.; et al. Growth differentiation factor 15 (GDF-15) is a potential biomarker of both diabetic kidney disease and future cardiovascular events in cohorts of individuals with type 2 diabetes: A proteomics approach. *Upsala J. Med. Sci.* **2020**, *125*, 37–43. [CrossRef] [PubMed]
92. Nakajima, T.; Shibasaki, I.; Sawaguchi, T.; Haruyama, A.; Kaneda, H.; Nakajima, T.; Hasegawa, T.; Arikawa, T.; Obi, S.; Sakuma, M.; et al. Growth Differentiation Factor-15 (GDF-15) is a Biomarker of Muscle Wasting and Renal Dysfunction in Preoperative Cardiovascular Surgery Patients. *J. Clin. Med.* **2019**, *8*, 576. [CrossRef]
93. Tuegel, C.; Katz, R.; Alam, M.; Bhat, Z.; Bellovich, K.; de Boer, I.; Brosius, F.; Gadegbeku, C.; Gipson, D.; Hawkins, J.; et al. GDF-15, Galectin 3, Soluble ST2, and Risk of Mortality and Cardiovascular Events in CKD. *Am. J. kidney Dis. Off. J. Natl. Kidney Found.* **2018**, *72*, 519–528. [CrossRef] [PubMed]
94. Wu, A.H.B. Biomarkers Beyond the Natriuretic Peptides for Chronic Heart Failure: Galectin-3 and Soluble ST2. *Ejifcc* **2012**, *23*, 98–102. [PubMed]
95. MacKinnon, A.C.; Farnworth, S.L.; Hodkinson, P.S.; Henderson, N.C.; Atkinson, K.M.; Leffler, H.; Nilsson, U.J.; Haslett, C.; Forbes, S.J.; Sethi, T. Regulation of Alternative Macrophage Activation by Galectin-3. *J. Immunol.* **2008**, *180*, 2650–2658. [CrossRef]
96. Falkenham, A.; De Antueno, R.; Rosin, N.; Betsch, D.; Lee, T.D.G.; Duncan, R.; Légaré, J.F. Nonclassical resident macrophages are important determinants in the development of myocardial fibrosis. *Am. J. Pathol.* **2015**, *185*, 927–942. [CrossRef]
97. Frunza, O.; Russo, I.; Saxena, A.; Shinde, A.V.; Humeres, C.; Hanif, W.; Rai, V.; Su, Y.; Frangogiannis, N.G. Myocardial Galectin-3 Expression Is Associated with Remodeling of the Pressure-Overloaded Heart and May Delay the Hypertrophic Response without Affecting Survival, Dysfunction, and Cardiac Fibrosis. *Am. J. Pathol.* **2016**, *186*, 1114–1127. [CrossRef]
98. Nguyen, M.N.; Su, Y.; Kiriazis, H.; Yang, Y.; Gao, X.M.; McMullen, J.R.; Dart, A.M.; Du, X.J. Upregulated galectin-3 is not a critical disease mediator of cardiomyopathy induced by β2-adrenoceptor overexpression. *Am. J. Physiol. Heart Circ. Physiol.* **2018**, *314*, H1169–H1178. [CrossRef]
99. Liu, Y.H.; D'Ambrosio, M.; Liao, T.D.; Peng, H.; Rhaleb, N.E.; Sharma, U.; Andre, S.; Gabius, H.J.; Carretero, O.A. N-acetyl-seryl-aspartyl-lysyl-proline prevents cardiac remodeling and dysfunction induced by galectin-3, a mammalian adhesion/growth-regulatory lectin. *Am. J. Physiol. Heart Circ. Physiol.* **2009**, *296*, 404–412. [CrossRef]

100. Sharma, U.C.; Pokharel, S.; Van Brakel, T.J.; Van Berlo, J.H.; Cleutjens, J.P.M.; Schroen, B.; André, S.; Crijns, H.J.G.M.; Gabius, H.J.; Maessen, J.; et al. Galectin-3 marks activated macrophages in failure-prone hypertrophied hearts and contributes to cardiac dysfunction. *Circulation* **2004**, *110*, 3121–3128. [CrossRef]
101. Song, X.; Qian, X.; Shen, M.; Jiang, R.; Wagner, M.B.; Ding, G.; Chen, G.; Shen, B. Protein kinase C promotes cardiac fibrosis and heart failure by modulating galectin-3 expression. *Biochim. Biophys. Acta Mol. Cell Res.* **2015**, *1853*, 513–521. [CrossRef] [PubMed]
102. Ibarrola, J.; Matilla, L.; Martínez-Martínez, E.; Gueret, A.; Fernández-Celis, A.; Henry, J.P.; Nicol, L.; Jaisser, F.; Mulder, P.; Ouvrard-Pascaud, A.; et al. Myocardial Injury After Ischemia/Reperfusion Is Attenuated By Pharmacological Galectin-3 Inhibition. *Sci. Rep.* **2019**, *9*, 1–10. [CrossRef] [PubMed]
103. Al-Salam, S.; Hashmi, S. Myocardial Ischemia Reperfusion Injury: Apoptotic, Inflammatory and Oxidative Stress Role of Galectin-3. *Cell. Physiol. Biochem.* **2018**, *50*, 1055–1067. [CrossRef] [PubMed]
104. Lippi, G.; Cervellin, G.; Sanchis-Gomar, F. Galectin-3 in atrial fibrillation: Simple bystander, player or both? *Clin. Biochem.* **2015**, *48*, 818–822. [CrossRef] [PubMed]
105. De Giusti, C.J.; Ure, A.E.; Rivadeneyra, L.; Schattner, M.; Gomez, R.M. Macrophages and galectin 3 play critical roles in CVB3-induced murine acute myocarditis and chronic fibrosis. *J. Mol. Cell. Cardiol.* **2015**, *85*, 58–70. [CrossRef] [PubMed]
106. Vergaro, G.; Prud'Homme, M.; Fazal, L.; Merval, R.; Passino, C.; Emdin, M.; Samuel, J.L.; Cohen Solal, A.; Delcayre, C. Inhibition of Galectin-3 Pathway Prevents Isoproterenol-Induced Left Ventricular Dysfunction and Fibrosis in Mice. *Hypertension* **2016**, *67*, 606–612. [CrossRef] [PubMed]
107. Novak, R.; Dabelic, S.; Dumic, J. Galectin-1 and galectin-3 expression profiles in classically and alternatively activated human macrophages. *Biochim. Biophys. Acta Gen. Subj.* **2012**, *1820*, 1383–1390. [CrossRef]
108. Peng, Y.; Chen, B.; Zhao, J.; Peng, Z.; Xu, W.; Yu, G. Effect of intravenous transplantation of hUCB-MSCs on M1/M2 subtype conversion in monocyte/macrophages of AMI mice. *Biomed. Pharmacother.* **2019**, *111*, 624–630. [CrossRef]
109. Ishibashi-Ueda, H.; Matsuyama, T.A.; Ohta-Ogo, K.; Ikeda, Y. Significance and value of endomyocardial biopsy based on our own experience. *Circ. J.* **2017**, *81*, 417–426. [CrossRef]
110. Basso, C.; Calabrese, F.; Angelini, A.; Carturan, E.; Thiene, G. Classification and histological, immunohistochemical, and molecular diagnosis of inflammatory myocardial disease. *Heart Fail. Rev.* **2013**, *18*, 673–681. [CrossRef]
111. Stone, J.R.; Basso, C.; Baandrup, U.T.; Bruneval, P.; Butany, J.; Gallagher, P.J.; Haluschka, M.K.; Miller, D.V.; Padera, R.F.; Radio, S.J.; et al. Recommendations for processing cardiovascular surgical pathology specimens: A consensus statement from the Standards and Definitions Committee of the Society for Cardiovascular Pathology and the Association for European Cardiovascular Pathology. *Cardiovasc. Pathol.* **2012**, *21*, 2–16. [CrossRef] [PubMed]
112. Andréoletti, L.; Lévêque, N.; Boulagnon, C.; Brasselet, C.; Fornes, P. Viral causes of human myocarditis. *Arch. Cardiovasc. Dis.* **2009**, *102*, 559–568. [CrossRef] [PubMed]

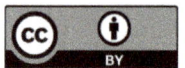

© 2020 by the authors. Licensee MDPI, Basel, Switzerland. This article is an open access article distributed under the terms and conditions of the Creative Commons Attribution (CC BY) license (http://creativecommons.org/licenses/by/4.0/).

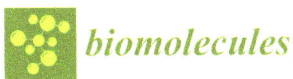 

Article

# Sirt1 Activity in PBMCs as a Biomarker of Different Heart Failure Phenotypes

Valeria Conti [1,†], Graziamaria Corbi [2,†], Maria Vincenza Polito [1], Michele Ciccarelli [1], Valentina Manzo [1,*], Martina Torsiello [1], Emanuela De Bellis [1], Federica D'Auria [1], Gennaro Vitulano [1], Federico Piscione [1], Albino Carrizzo [1,3], Paola Di Pietro [1], Carmine Vecchione [1,3], Nicola Ferrara [4,5] and Amelia Filippelli [1]

1. Department of Medicine, Surgery and Dentistry "Scuola Medica Salernitana", University of Salerno, 84081 Baronissi, Italy; vconti@unisa.it (V.C.); mvpolito@hotmail.it (M.V.P.); mciccarelli@unisa.it (M.C.); m.torsiello5@studenti.unisa.it (M.T.); e.debellis93@gmail.com (E.D.B.); federica.dauria19@gmail.com (F.D.); vitulanogennaro@yahoo.it (G.V.); fpiscione@unisa.it (F.P.); acarrizzo@unisa.it (A.C.); pdipietro@unisa.it (P.D.P.); cvecchione@unisa.it (C.V.); afilippelli@unisa.it (A.F.)
2. Department of Medicine and Health Sciences, University of Molise, 86100 Campobasso, Italy; graziamaria.corbi@unimol.it
3. Department of Vascular Physiopathology, IRCCS Neuromed, 86077 Pozzilli, Italy
4. Department of Translational Medical Sciences, Federico II University of Naples, 80131 Naples, Italy; nicferra@unina.it
5. Istituti Clinici Scientifici Maugeri SPA-Società Benefit, IRCCS, 82037 Telese Terme (BN), Italy
* Correspondence: vmanzo@unisa.it; Tel.: +39-089-672-424
† These authors contributed equally to this work.

Received: 11 October 2020; Accepted: 20 November 2020; Published: 23 November 2020

**Abstract:** Heart Failure (HF) is a syndrome, which implies the existence of different phenotypes. The new categorization includes patients with preserved ejection fraction (HFpEF), mid-range EF (HFmrEF), and reduced EF (HFrEF) but the molecular mechanisms involved in these HF phenotypes have not yet been exhaustively investigated. Sirt1 plays a crucial role in biological processes strongly related to HF. This study aimed to evaluate whether Sirt1 activity was correlated with EF and other parameters in HFpEF, HFmrEF, and HFrEF. Seventy patients, HFpEF ($n = 23$), HFmrEF ($n = 23$) and HFrEF ($n = 24$), were enrolled at the Cardiology Unit of the University Hospital of Salerno. Sirt1 activity was measured in peripheral blood mononuclear cells (PBMCs). Angiotensin-Converting Enzyme 2 (ACE2) activity, Tumor Necrosis Factor-alpha (TNF-α) and Brain Natriuretic Peptide (BNP) levels were quantified in plasma. HFpEF showed lower Sirt1 and ACE2 activities than both HFmrEF and HFrEF ($p < 0.0001$), without difference compared to No HF controls. In HFmrEF and HFrEF a very strong correlation was found between Sirt1 activity and EF ($r^2 = 0.899$ and $r^2 = 0.909$, respectively), and between ACE2 activity and Sirt1 ($r^2 = 0.801$ and $r^2 = 0.802$, respectively). HFrEF showed the highest TNF-α levels without reaching statistical significance. Significant differences in BNP were found among the groups, with the highest levels in the HFrEF. Determining Sirt1 activity in PBMCs is useful to distinguish the HF patients' phenotypes from each other, especially HFmrEF/HFrEF from HFpEF.

**Keywords:** heart failure with preserved ejection fraction; heart failure with mid-range ejection fraction; heart failure with reduced ejection fraction; sirtuins; Sirt1

---

## 1. Introduction

Despite impressive advances in clinical/diagnostic tools and therapies, heart failure (HF) still represents a paramount public health problem being one of the most important causes of death and hospitalization worldwide [ ]. As a syndrome, HF has multifactorial pathogenesis, and its diagnosis and management can be very demanding [2]. Determining the left ventricular ejection fraction (EF) is an essential diagnostic step [3].

The most recent guidelines of the European Society of Cardiology (ESC) consider three patient's categories, Heart Failure (HF) with reduced Ejection Fraction (HFrEF; EF < 40%), HF with preserved ejection fraction (HFpEF; EF ≥ 50%), and HF with mid-range EF (between 40 and 49%) referred to as HFmrEF [4]. While there is an agreement that the categorization of HFrEF requires EF < 40%, the clinical overview of the patients with HFpEF has not been clearly established yet. The same ESC guidelines propose the measurement of the B-type natriuretic peptide (BNP) and/or N-terminal pro-BNP as an additional diagnostic criterion for HFmrEF and HFpEF, specifying that this cannot be useful to discriminate all three HF phenotypes because of its increase in other clinical conditions, including atrial fibrillation and renal failure, that compromise the interpretation of BNP and pro-BNP quantification [4].

Given the clinical implication, especially concerning comorbidities and therapy response, the correct characterization of the HF patients represents a crucial step for the management of this syndrome. One of the most important questions is if the HFmrEF represents a distinct phenotype or a transitional condition from HFrEF to HFpEF, or vice-versa [5]. However, doubtless, such a new category has been introduced to stimulate the research on these particular patients because there is an urgent need to identify new biomarkers and pharmacological targets helpful to choose the best therapy according to the different failing heart phenotypes.

Recent studies have investigated the possible role in the HF of sirtuins, a family of NAD+ dependent deacetylases, among which Sirtuin 1 (Sirt1) is the best-characterized member [6]. Sirt1 is involved in biological processes strongly related to HF, including oxidative stress, cell senescence, and energy production [7]. Moreover, it also plays a crucial role in angiotensin II-induced vascular remodeling [8] and inflammatory response modulating the expression of some cytokines [9]. For instance, tumor necrosis factor-alpha (TNF-α), which is involved in both central and peripheral manifestations of HF, has been found to increase in HFrEF when compared to HFpEF. Therefore, such a proinflammatory cytokine could be useful to separate the HF patients' phenotypes from each other [9].

The overexpression of Sirt1 has been shown to favor the survival of cardiomyocytes, but to be also associated with cardiac hypertrophy and HF [10,11]. Indeed, both expression and activity levels of Sirt1 vary in the response of internal and external stimuli [12,13] and, following a hormetic mechanism, can be either advantageous or injurious [14]. However, until now, no data on Sirt1 activity according to the different HF phenotypes are available. Then, the present study aimed at evaluating in HFpEF, HFmrEF, and HFrEF patients whether the amount of Sirt1 activity was correlated with EF and other characteristics, including circulating TNF-α and angiotensin-converting enzyme 2 (ACE2) activity levels.

## 2. Materials and Methods

### 2.1. Study Population

Seventy patients with chronic HF in NYHA classes 2 and 3 were consecutively enrolled at the Cardiology Unit of the University Hospital of Salerno. Twenty-nine age-matched subjects without heart failure represented the control group (no HF controls). All the enrolled patients underwent a physical examination, blood chemistry tests, electrocardiographic and echocardiographic exams, and a 6-min walking test. Additionally, baseline demographic, clinical, echocardiographic, and functional data were collected on a predefined computerized datasheet. All subjects included in the study were in optimal medical therapy and managed according to ESC guidelines. All participants gave their written informed consent. The study was in accordance with the Declaration of Helsinki and its amendments and was approved by the local Ethical Committee (Comitato Etico Campania Sud Prot.n.4_r.p.s.o.).

### 2.2. Echocardiography

Transthoracic echocardiography (TTE) was performed following the ASE and ESC/EACVI recommendations using a Vivid E95 system with an M5S phased array and probe (GE Healthcare

Vingmed Ultrasound AS, Horten, Norway). All echocardiographic images were digitally recorded. The left ventricular (LV) end-diastolic diameter (LVEDD) and the LV end-systolic diameter (LVESD) were measured using M-mode by the parasternal long-axis view; the LV volumes (LV end-diastolic volume, LVEDV, and LV end-systolic volume, LVESV) and the EF were calculated by the Simpson's method using the apical 2-chamber and 4-chamber view. The LV diastolic function was characterized by the assessment of the ELV/e'LV ratio as a surrogate parameter of LV filling pressure. For the evaluation of the early-diastolic filling (E), the pulsed-wave Doppler sample volume was positioned at the tip of the tenting area of the mitral valve in the apical long-axis view. The mean of e' was assessed in the basal inferoseptal and lateral LV region in the apical 4-chamber view using Tissue Doppler Imaging TDI. The left atrial (LA) volume index was calculated by biplane LA planimetry in the apical 2- and 4-chamber view. The right ventricular function resulted by the measurement of the tricuspid annular plane systolic excursion (TAPSE), and the pulmonary artery systolic pressure was estimated by tricuspid regurgitation velocity in the apical 4-chamber view and the right arterial pressure (RAP), derived from the inferior vena cava diameter and degree of respiratory collapse.

### 2.3. Six-Minute Walking Test

The 6-min walking test (6MWT) was performed according to the American Thoracic Society (ATS) guidelines [ ].

The primary measurement was the total distance (meters, m) walked. The patients were instructed to walk up and down a corridor of 30 m, covering as much ground as possible in 6 min without running. Blood pressure was recorded at the end of the test, and pulse and oxygen saturation. The latter was measured by using a handheld pulse oximeter (G.i.ma. Spa, Milan, Italy) placed on the index finger of patients.

### 2.4. Blood Sampling and SIRT1 Activity

Blood samples were collected in fasting conditions in the BD Vacutainer® containing sodium EDTA (BD, USA). The separation of plasma and peripheral blood mononuclear cells (PBMCs) was obtained by Ficoll density gradient centrifuged at 3000 rcf spin for 30 min at room temperature. Aliquots of plasma and PBMCs were frozen at −80 °C until further analysis.

To measure SIRT1 activity, nuclear extracts (10 µL) were isolated by PBMCs using a nuclear extraction kit (EpiGentek Group Inc., Farmingdale, NY, USA). Then, SIRT1 activity was determinate by a SIRT1/Sir2 Deacetylase Fluorometric Assay (CycLex, Ina, Nagano, Japan), following the manufacturer's instructions. The values were reported as relative fluorescence/micrograms of protein (AU).

### 2.5. Circulating Angiotensin-Converting Enzyme 2 (ACE2) Activity and TNF-Alpha Measurement

The ACE2 activity was measured as previously described [ ] using fluorogenic substrate 7-methoxycoumarin-4-yl) acetyl-Ala-Pro-Lys(2,4-dinitrophenyl)-OH (Mca-APK(Dnp)) Mca-Ala-Pro-Lys(Dnp)-OH (BioVision Inc., CA, USA). Briefly, plasma was diluted 1:10 in ACE2 reaction buffer containing protease inhibitors (10 µM Bestatin-hydrochloride, 10 µM Z-prolyl-prolinal, (Sigma, MO, USA), 5 µM Amastatin-hydrochloride, 10 µM Captopril in a buffer of 500 mM NaCl, 100 µM ZnCl2, and 75 mM TRIS HCl, pH 6.5). All chemicals were from Santa Cruz (CA, USA) if not stated otherwise. The reaction was performed at 37 °C in black 96-well microtiter plates in a total volume of 200 µL using a fluorescence plate reader (TECAN® infinite 200 PRO) at an excitation wavelength of 320 nm and emission wavelength of 405 nm. Enzymatic activity was determined from a fluorescence rate increase over a 10–120 min time course, and the activity was reported as relative fluorescence units (RFU)/min.

The TNF-alpha evaluation was performed on plasma samples according to the manufacturer's instruction (Diaclone, Human TNF-α ELISA Kit; #950.090.192).

The measurements of Sirt1 and ACE2 activities and TNF-alpha levels were performed in a blinded fashion. All data are expressed as the mean ± SD of three independent experiments.

## 2.6. Statistical Analysis

Data were analyzed using the SPSS (v 23.0) software package (SPSS Inc., Chicago, IL, USA). The Shapiro–Wilk test was used to assess the normal distribution of data. Differences between multiple groups were evaluated by the analysis of variance (ANOVA) with the Bonferroni post hoc test and are presented as mean ± SD. The $\chi^2$ test was used to compare categorical variables. A multiple linear analysis was used to investigate the relationship between variables when appropriate. To explore the correlation between variables, Spearman's correlation (r) was used. The statistical significance was established at a $p$-value $< 0.05$.

The sample size was calculated from similar studies where Sirt1 activity determination in PBMCs was assessed in healthy individuals and HF patients (12, 17). We used an estimated standard deviation of 0.5 and the two-tailed alpha set at 0.05. An $n = 9$ per group was determined to provide sufficient power at 0.9 to detect a significant difference among groups.

Then a total of 99 subjects (29 No HF controls; 23 HFpEF; 23 HFmrEF; and 24 HFrEF) were included in the study.

## 3. Results

### 3.1. Study Population

The study population consisted of 99 subjects (66 M, 33 F; mean age $62.6 \pm 9.4$, and range 42–85) including 29 No HF controls and 70 HF patients (Table 1) belonging to the HFpEF ($n = 23$), HFmrEF ($n = 23$), and HFrEF ($n = 24$) categories defined according to the criteria of the ESC guidelines [4]. The main demographic and clinical characteristics of each group are reported in Table 1. Among the groups, no differences were found in age, gender, and body mass index (BMI). The echocardiographic findings confirmed the different types of the HF with the HFpEF group showing lower LVESV and LVEDV compared to both HmrEF and HFrEF (in both $p < 0.0001$), with an increasing trend between the groups through EF reduction.

From a functional point of view, all the HF groups showed a reduction in six-minute walking distance in comparison to the no HF controls ($p < 0.0001$) but no differences were found among the HF groups.

The HF groups were more affected by diabetes mellitus ($p = 0.042$) and used more diuretics ($p < 0.0001$), beta-blockers ($p < 0.0001$), ACE-inhibitors ($p < 0.0001$), and statins ($p = 0.004$) in respect to the no HF controls. No differences were found in comorbidities and therapy among the HF groups.

### 3.2. Sirt1 Activity

The HFpEF subjects showed significant lower Sirt1 activity values than both the HFmrEF and the HFrEF ($p < 0.0001$), without any difference compared to the no HF controls (Figure 1A).

When a multivariate linear regression analysis was performed by using the EF as a dependent variable, after correction for the parameters statistically significant at the univariate analysis, the best predictors of EF were represented by Sirt1 activity ($p < 0.0001$; $\beta = -0.019$; 95%CI $-0.023$–$0.014$), and the use of beta-blockers ($p = 0.001$; $\beta = -7.404$; 95%CI $-11.622$–$3.186$).

The Sirt1 activity (used as dependent variable) was significantly associated to the HF groups ($p = 0.003$; $\beta = -133.960$; 95%CI $-221.708$–$46.212$). Then, because of the different characteristics of the HF in the three groups, to better explore the relationship between EF and Sirt1 activity, other multivariate regression analyses were performed. For each group, setting the EF as the dependent variable, the parameters statistically significant at the univariate analysis were identified, and then they were introduced in the multivariate analysis. In the no HF controls, the best predictors of EF were represented by the gender ($p = 0.011$; $\beta = 4.539$; 95%CI 1.132 7.946) and six-minute walking distance ($p = 0.032$; $\beta = 0.067$; 95%CI 0.006 0.127).

In the HFpEF group the EF was not associated to any variable. In the HFmrEF and HFrEF groups the best predictor of EF was represented only by the Sirt1 activity (for HFmrEF with $p < 0.0001$, $\beta = -0.009$, 95%CI $-0.010$–$0.008$ and for HFrEF with $p < 0.0001$; $\beta = -0.011$; 95%CI $-0.013$–$0.010$).

In Figure A, the correlation between Sirt1 activity and EF is pictured by groups, showing a very strong correlation between the two variables in the HFrEF ($r^2 = 0.909$) and HFmrEF ($r^2 = 0.899$), but not in the HFpEF ($r^2 = 0.001$). Moreover, a logistic regression analysis with the NYHA classes, as the dependent variable, showed that Sirt 1 activity represented the best predictor in the HFrEF ($p = 0.018$, $\beta = 1.006$; 95%CI 1.001 1.010) and HFmrEF ($p = 0.024$; $\beta = 1.005$; 95%CI 1.001 1.009) but not in the HFpEF (Figure B). In particular, the higher NYHA class was significantly associated to the higher Sirt 1 activity levels in the HFrEF and HFmrEF.

These findings suggest the possible role of Sirt1 as a marker useful to distinguish the HF phenotypes.

**Table 1.** Main characteristics of the study population stratified by No HF Controls and on the basis of HF type.

| | Ctr (n = 29) | HFpEF (n = 23) | HFmrEF (n = 23) | HFrEF (n = 24) | p |
|---|---|---|---|---|---|
| Age, years | 60.52 ± 8.91 | 63.87 ± 10.25 | 63.00 ± 9.16 | 63.50 ± 9.57 | 0.558 |
| Sex, (M/F) n (%) | 19/10 (65.5/34.5) | 13/10 (56.5/43.5) | 15/8 (65.2/34.8) | 16/8 (66.7/33.3) | 0.157 |
| BMI, kg/m$^2$ | 27.00 ± 3.14 | 27.89 ± 2.80 | 28.40 ± 3.80 | 28.07 ± 4.73 | 0.545 |
| SBP, mmHg | 126 ± 8 [a] | 123 ± 7 [b] | 121 ± 6 [c] | 106 ± 12 | <0.0001 |
| DBP, mmHg | 81 ± 5 [a] | 80 ± 4 [d] | 79 ± 7 [e] | 72 ± 8 | <0.0001 |
| EF, % | 61.07 ± 4.75 [f,g] | 57.61 ± 5.39 [h] | 44.35 ± 2.93 [i] | 33.03 ± 4.24 | <0.0001 |
| BNP, pg/mL | 31.33 ± 14.00 [f] | 105.00 ± 64.42 [b,j] | 408.08 ± 55.5 [i] | 814.50 ± 193.83 | <0.0001 |
| LVESV, mL | 32.56 ± 4.82 [f] | 44.30 ± 17.48 [b,k] | 72.63 ± 21.69 [i] | 122.17 ± 33.56 | <0.0001 |
| LVEDV, mL | 84.83 ± 10.22 [a] | 103.17 ± 34.06 [k] | 131.68 ± 39.51 [l] | 171.25 ± 44.74 | <0.0001 |
| Cardiac Index, L/min/m$^2$ | 2.94 ± 0.35 | 2.82 ± 0.47 | 2.74 ± 0.43 | 2.64 ± 0.36 | 0.059 |
| SPAP, mmHg | 28.41 ± 3.57 [m,n] | 40.00 ± 17.15 | 32.16 ± 5.83 | 36.33 ± 11.48 | 0.002 |
| E/e' ratio | 6.72 ± 1.56 [a,o] | 12.85 ± 6.75 | 10.87 ± 2.61 [p] | 16.54 ± 8.03 | <0.0001 |
| Walking distance at 6', m | 522.69 ± 26.63 [q] | 387.30 ± 56.14 | 406.65 ± 49.14 | 408.54 ± 73.69 | <0.0001 |
| Walking distance at 6' ≥ 350 m, n (%) | 29 (100.0) | 19 (82.6) | 18 (78.3) | 18 (75.0) | 0.049 |
| CKD, (yes) n (%) | 0 (0) | 5 (22.2) | 6 (26.7) | 8 (35) | 0.116 |
| Hypertension, (yes) n (%) | 10 (34.5) | 16 (69.6) | 14 (60.9) | 14 (58.3) | 0.063 |
| Dyslipidaemia, (yes) n (%) | 7 (24.1) | 12 (52.2) | 12 (52.2) | 14 (58.3) | 0.051 |
| Smoking, (yes) n (%) | 8 (27.6) | 5 (21.7) | 9 (39.1) | 6 (25.0) | 0.582 |
| Diabetes Mellitus, (yes) n (%) | 2 (6.9) | 8 (34.8) | 6 (26.1) | 9 (37.5) | 0.042 |
| COPD, (yes) n (%) | 3 (10.3) | 5 (21.7) | 4 (17.4) | 6 (25.0) | 0.541 |
| Prior MI, (yes) n (%) | 0 (0) | 4 (26.7) | 8 (44.4) | 12 (50.0) | 0.415 |
| HF etiology, (yes) n (%) | | | | | |
| Ischemic cardiomyopathy | 0 (0) | 5 (21.7) | 11 (47.8) | 19 (79.2) | 0.004 |
| Valvular cardiomyopathy | 0 (0) | 6 (26.1) | 5 (21.7) | 2 (8.3) | 0.083 |
| Hypertensive cardiomyopathy | 0 (0) | 5 (21.7) | 4 (17.4) | 1 (4.2) | 0.329 |
| Primary cardiomyopathy | 0 (0) | 7 (30.4) | 3 (13) | 2 (8.3) | 0.195 |
| Diuretics, (yes) n (%) | 1 (3.4) | 8 (34.8) | 27 (73.9) | 20 (83.3) | <0.0001 |
| Beta-blockers, (yes) n (%) | 3 (10.3) | 22 (95.7) | 21 (91.3) | 22 (91.7) | <0.0001 |
| ACE-inhibitors, (yes) n (%) | 4 (13.8) | 14 (60.9) | 15 (65.2) | 15 (62.5) | <0.0001 |
| ARBs, (yes) n (%) | 3 (10.3) | 7 (30.4) | 7 (30.4) | 3 (12.5) | 0.132 |
| Statins, (yes) n (%) | 8 (27.6) | 15 (65.2) | 16 (69.6) | 16 (66.7) | 0.004 |

Ctr, No Heart Failure Controls; HFpEF, Heart Failure with preserved Ejection Fraction; HFmrEF, Heart failure with mid-range Ejection Fraction; HFrEF, Heart Failure with reduced Ejection Fraction; BMI, Body Mass Index; SBP, Systolic Blood Pressure; DBP, Diastolic Blood Pressure; EF, Ejection Fraction; BNP, Brain Natriuretic Peptide; LVESV, Left Ventricle End Systolic Volume; LVEDV, Left Ventricle End Diastolic Volume; SPAP, Systolic Pulmonary Artery Pressure; CKD, Chronic Kidney Disease; COPD, Chronic Obstructive Pulmonary Disease; MI, Myocardial Infarction; ARBs, Angiotensin Receptor Blockers. [a] Ctr vs. HFrEF $p < 0.0001$; [b] HFpEF vs. HFrEF $p < 0.0001$; [c] HFmrEF vs. HFrEF $p = 0.002$; [d] HFpEF vs. HFrEF $p = 0.001$; [e] HFmrEF vs. HFrEF $p = 0.035$; [f] Ctr vs. HFmrEF and HFrEF group $p < 0.0001$; [g] Ctr vs. HFpEF $p = 0.038$; [h] HFpEF vs. HFmrEF and HFrEF group $p < 0.0001$; [i] HFmrEF vs. HFrEF $p < 0.0001$; [j] HFpEF vs. HFmrEF $p = 0.010$; [k] HFpEF vs. HFmrEF $p = 0.002$; [l] HFmrEF vs. HFrEF $p = 0.001$; [m] Ctr vs. HFpEF $p = 0.002$; [n] Ctr vs. HFmrEF $p = 0.028$; [o] Ctr vs. HFpEF $p = 0.003$; [p] HFmrEF vs. HFrEF $p = 0.004$; [q] Ctr vs. all other groups $p < 0.0001$.

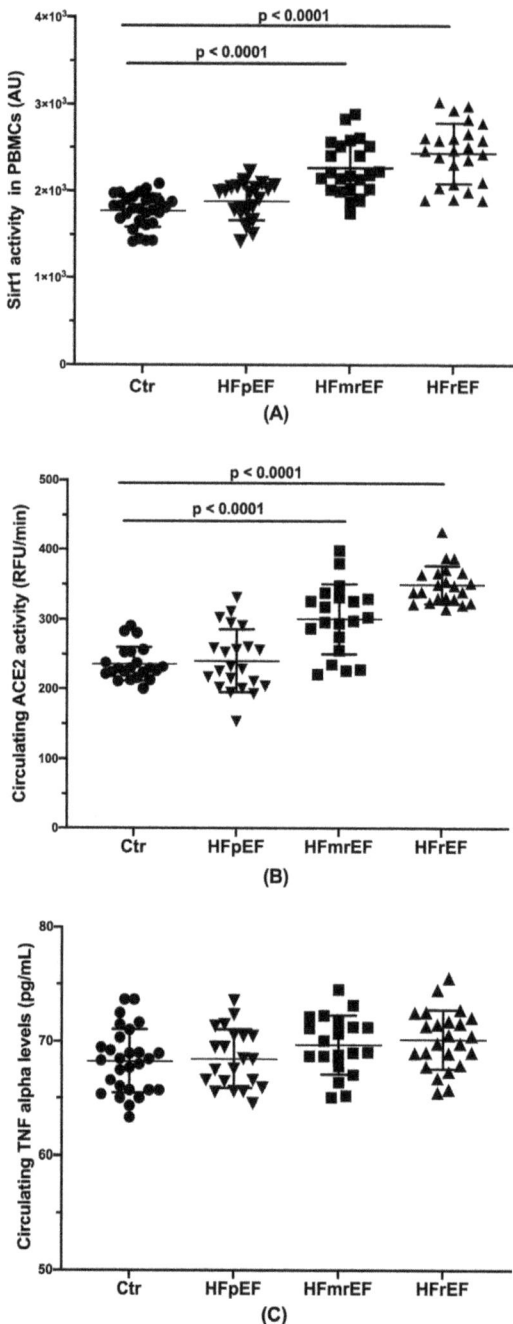

**Figure 1.** (**A**) Sirt1 activity levels by groups in the study population. Subjects with heart failure with preserved ejection fraction showed significant lower Sirt1 activity values than both subjects with heart failure with mid-range EF (HFmrEF) and those with heart failure with reduced EF (HFrEF) ($p < 0.0001$), without any difference compared to the no heart failure (HF) controls (Ctr). (**B**) Circulating ACE2 activity

by groups in the study population. The HFpEF subjects showed significant lower ACE2 activity values than both HFmrEF and HFrEF ($p < 0.0001$), without any difference compared to the no HF controls (Ctr). (**C**) Circulating TNF-alpha levels by groups in the study population. An increasing trend of plasma TNF-alpha levels from the HFpEF through the HFmrEF to the HFrEF patients without reaching statistical significance was found.

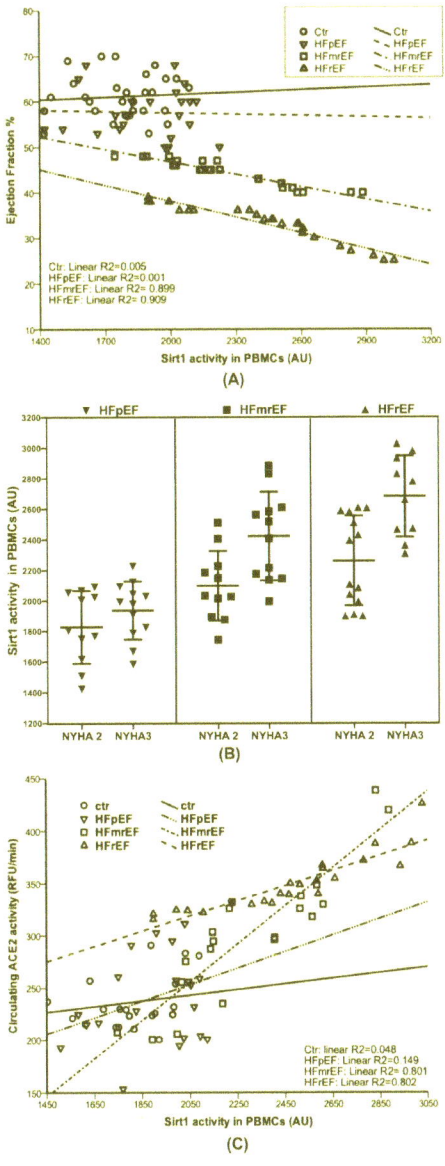

**Figure 2.** (**A**) Correlation between EF and Sirt 1 activity stratified by HF groups and no HF controls (Ctr). In the HFmrEF and HFrEF groups a very strong correlation was found between Sirt 1 activity levels and EF values ($r^2 = 0.899$ and $r^2 = 0.909$, respectively). Otherwise, in the HFpEF as in the no HF controls no correlation was found. (**B**) Association between NYHA classes and Sirt 1 activity stratified by HF groups.

Sirt 1 activity represented the best predictor of NYHA classes in the HFrEF ($p = 0.018$, $\beta = 1.006$; 95%CI 1.001 1.010) and HFmrEF ($p = 0.024$; $\beta = 1.005$; 95%CI 1.001 1.009) but not in the HFpEF. (**C**) Correlation between ACE2 and Sirt 1 activities stratified by HF groups and no HF controls (Ctr). In the HFmrEF and HFrEF groups a very strong correlation was found between Sirt 1 activity and ACE2 activity levels ($r^2 = 0.801$ and $r^2 = 0.802$, respectively). Otherwise, in the HFpEF as in the no HF controls no correlation was found.

### 3.3. Circulating Angiotensin-Converting Enzyme 2 (ACE2) Activity

The HFpEF subjects showed significant lower ACE2 activity values than both the HFmrEF and HFrEF ($p < 0.0001$) without any difference compared to the no HF controls (Figure 1B).

In Figure 2C, the correlation between the Sirt1 activity and ACE2 activity is pictured by groups, showing a very strong correlation between the two variables in the HFrEF ($r^2 = 0.802$) and HFmrEF ($r^2 = 0.801$), but not in the HFpEF ($r^2 = 0.149$).

### 3.4. Circulating Tumor Necrosis Factor-Alpha (TNF-α) Levels

As shown in Figure 1C, no statistically significant differences in plasma levels of TNF-α were found among the groups. An increasing trend was observed from the HFpEF through HFmrEF to HFrEF. The No HF control subjects showed values closed to the HFpEF patients.

### 3.5. Circulating Brain Natriuretic Peptide (BNP) levels

At the univariate analysis, statistically significant differences in plasma levels of BNP were found among the groups, with the highest levels in the HFrEF group (Table 1). An increasing trend was observed from the HFpEF through HFmrEF to HFrEF. The no HF control subjects showed values close to the HFpEF patients. However, a multivariate linear regression analysis demonstrated no correlation between BNP and Sirt1 activity levels in all groups (for Ctr $p = 0.434$, $r^2 = 0.097$, $\beta = -0.026$, 95%CI $-0.104$ $0.052$; for HFpEF $p = 0.566$, $r^2 = 0.024$, $\beta = -0.206$, 95%CI $-3.428$ $3.016$; for HFmrEF $p = 0.752$, $r^2 = 0.025$, $\beta = -0.073$; 95%CI $-0.580$ $0.434$; for HFrEF $p = 0.388$, $r^2 = 0.050$, $\beta = 0.126$; 95%CI $-0.175$ $0.427$).

## 4. Discussion

The introduction in the recent ESC guidelines of the HFmrEF category [4] has given the impulse for investigations aiming at a better characterization of the patients suffering from HF. What emerges from the trials performed until now has highlighted that the clinical overview of the patients with HFpEF has not been adequately studied and, consequently, there are few effective treatments for them. Moreover, the HFmrEF represents a borderline group scarcely investigated, even less than HFpEF [3].

The processes and mechanisms involved in the cardiac failing phenotypes have not been exhaustively investigated, nonetheless elucidating the molecular card of the different HF patients might be of great help to better manage the disease and personalize the therapy.

Sirt1 represents a good candidate in this field because of its involvement in cardiac pathophysiology [17]. Indeed, historically Sirt1 has been recognized as an enzyme crucial to assure lifespan prolonging from yeasts to humans, and, in general, its decreased levels have been linked to endothelial dysfunction and the pathogenesis of metabolic and cardiovascular diseases [7,17–19]. Therefore, interventions aiming at increasing Sirt1 levels have been considered beneficial in aging and aging-associated diseases [20,21].

Sirt 1 expression and activity are often measured in PBMCs, which represent a model helpful to provide a comprehensive overview of the cellular system status together with measurement of circulating serum or plasma markers [22]. PBMCs are cells easy to isolate by a non-invasive and inexpensive method. This model has been used to study Sirt1 in several disorders such as diabetes mellitus [23], chronic obstructive pulmonary disease (COPD) [24,25], and in patients assuming a specific diet [26], or underwent cardiac rehabilitation [27].

Herein, we found that Sirt1 activity was much higher in PBMCs isolated from the HFrEF patients when compared to the HFmrEF and even more HFpEF. Importantly, the levels were so different making it possible to distinguish the HFmrEF/HFrEF from the HFpEF that, conversely, had Sirt1 activity very similar to the no HF control subjects. A very strong correlation between Sirt1 activity and EF values was found in the HFrEF ($r^2 = 0.909$) and HFmrEF ($r^2 = 0.899$), while no correlation in the HFpEF and no HF control subjects was observed. Additionally, the higher Sirt 1 activity levels were significantly associated with the higher NYHA class in the HFrEF and HFmrEF but not in the HFpEF.

Concerning the involvement of Sirt1 in cardiac remodeling, literature data show contrasting evidence. Some data report a relationship between increased Sirt1 levels and cardiac hypertrophy [ ], while other data suggest that low-moderate Sirt1 overexpression has beneficial effects in contrasting fibrosis and hypertrophy [ ]. Currently, several studies, while confirming a link between these conditions and Sirt1 increased levels, stressed the importance of a Sirt1 overexpression degree in determining beneficial or detrimental effects [ , ]. It is unsurprising when you consider that the intensity of caloric restriction and exercise training, interventions well recognized to activate Sirt1, makes the difference between their positive and negative effects [ – ]. Moreover, accumulating evidence has corroborated the idea that both expression and activity of Sirt1 vary in the response of internal and external stimuli, and the outcomes strongly depend on the cell type and condition [ ]. Furthermore, understanding the role and the effects of Sirt1 in different contexts is essential, given the indubitable involvement of this enzyme in cardiovascular homeostasis and diseases [ ]. In our opinion, the results of the present study go in such a direction. We found different Sirt1 activity levels with the highest value in the HFrEF patients, by measuring this parameter in HF patients classified (according to the recent ESC guidelines) in three different categories.

A possible explanation may be related to a link existing between Sirt1 and the renin angiotensin aldosterone system (RAAS) [ – ]. RAAS is one of the most important components of the so-called 'neurohormonal' system, designed to maintain cardiovascular homeostasis through a series of compensatory mechanisms. While this system is beneficial in the short term, its prolonged activation causes hemodynamic stress, cardiac and vessel structural modifications, and ultimately progression of HF, especially in HFrEF patients [ ]. As a matter of fact, it is well known the better therapeutic response of HFrEF patients to beta-blockers, RAAS inhibitors, and angiotensin receptor–neprilysin inhibitors (ARNI), the latter licensed only in these subjects [ , ]. Furthermore, the lack of an optimal therapeutic response in HFpEF subjects represented one of the fundamental reasons to stimulate a better pathophysiology understanding of this HF phenotype [ ].

It has been demonstrated both in vivo and in vitro that resveratrol, a polyphenol able to activate Sirt1, leads to a decrease of angiotensin II receptor AT1 through Sirt1 activation [ ]. Another important result is that overexpression of Sirt1 exerts beneficial effects contrasting the angiotensin II-induced vascular remodeling and attenuating hypertension in mice [ ]. In addition, an interesting study by Davis et al. performed in patients with Bartter's/Gitelman's (BS/GS) syndromes, who have a persistent RAAS activation with increased circulating levels of angiotensin II, showed that Sirt1 protein levels were higher in patients' PBMCs than in those of healthy subjects [ ]. Noteworthy, circulating AngII-degrading enzyme (ACE2) activity is much higher in the HFrEF in comparison with the HFpEF subjects. This finding indicates circulating ACE2 activity as a potential biomarker to differentiate these two cardiac failing phenotypes [ ]. Moreover, Epelman et al. demonstrated that elevated plasma ACE2 activity was associated with greater severity of myocardial dysfunction, without a relationship between circulating ACE2 activity and markers of systemic inflammation [ ]. On the contrary, Niethammer et al. found increased circulating levels of TNF-alpha in HFrEF in comparison to HFpEF patients and showed that such higher levels were negatively correlated to EF [ ].

Here, we found an increasing trend of plasma TNF-alpha levels from the HFpEF through the HFmrEF to the HFrEF patients without reaching statistical significance.

Our results show that the HFrEF group had levels of ACE2 activity significantly higher than those measured in the HFmrEF and even more in the HFpEF subjects, with the latter showing no difference when compared with the No HF controls. Notably, a positive correlation between Sirt1 activity and ACE2 activity in the HFrEF ($r^2 = 0.802$) and the HFmrEF ($r^2 = 0.801$) but not in the HFpEF ($r^2 = 0.149$) was found (Figure 2C).

Altogether these findings suggest a role for Sirt1 activity as a biomarker to distinguish the three HF phenotypes.

The highest Sirt1 activity in the HFrEF patients might reflect the high neurohormonal activation, including RAAS, which in turn characterizes systolic HF [33].

As already stated, the HFmrEF remains insufficiently characterized compared with the other groups. We found that the HFmrEF and HFrEF patients have similar Sirt1 levels, both much higher than the HFpEF and the correlation between Sirt1 activity and EF values in the HFmrEF was as relevant as in the HFrEF, even if less strong. However, the intermediate mean value of the Sirt1 activity found in the HFmrEF group (Figure 1A) seems to confirm the arising idea that the HFmrEF could represent an intermediate condition rather than a different HF category.

Sirt1 activity induced by pharmacological and non-pharmacological activators has been demonstrated to ameliorate the health status of HF patients [13,21,27]. Indeed, mild and moderate overexpression of Sirt1 might favor resistance to stress, thereby leading to cardiac positive outcomes, while further increased levels might be associated with cardiac damages [14]. Possibly, Sirt1 activity values, linked to beneficial effects, depending on the individual baseline levels, and their assessment could be useful in the management of the different HF patients.

In our opinion, the most important result of the present investigation is the existence, observed for the first time, of the relationship between the EF and Sirt1 activity with a very strong correlation between Sirt1 activity and EF in the HFmrEF and HFrEF. Of note, this correlation does not exist in the HFpEF patients.

This study is subject to some limitations. One of them is the lack of the cardiopulmonary stress test because it was performed not in all enrolled patients and no HF controls. Another limitation is the small number of patients included in each group.

As discussed, the high levels of Sirt1 might reflect an adaptive activation of the sympathetic system and RAAS characterizing the systolic HF. The relationship between Sirt1 and circulating ACE2 activity found in the HFrEF and HFmrEF but not in the HFpEF patients corroborates this hypothesis. Measuring factors other than ACE2 activity involved in the neurohormonal modulation could be helpful to better classify patients with HF.

Another limitation is the absence of Sirt1 activity levels definition in healthy subjects as a reference.

Undoubtedly, further and larger studies are necessary to measure such and other inflammatory parameters, other than TNF alpha, and verify whether they correlate with Sirt1 activity.

## 5. Conclusions

In our study, Sirt1 activity levels increased from the HFpEF through HFmrEF to the HFrEF.

Sirt1 activity in the HFmrEF, showing an average value between the HFrEF and HFpEF subjects, suggests the hypothesis that the HFmrEF represents an intermediate phenotype. This is supported by the finding of the strong correlation between Sirt1 activity and EF values observed also in HFmrEF patients.

The correlation between Sirt1 and ACE2 also reinforces the hypothesis that Sirt1 activity could be used as a biomarker to better differentiate the patients with different HF phenotypes, especially to separate HFmrEF/HFrEF from HFpEF.

Further studies with a larger sample size are needed to confirm or deny these results and clarify whether monitoring Sirt1 activity levels can effectively help the management of the patients suffering from HF. Moreover, more trials should also be performed to better understand the mechanisms underlining the HF phenotypes that could explain the different Sirt1 activation and to define the range of Sirt1 activity levels associated with beneficial effects.

**Author Contributions:** Conceptualization, V.C., G.C., M.C. and A.F.; Data curation, V.C., G.C., V.M. and A.C.; Funding acquisition, V.C.; Investigation, V.M., M.T., E.D.B. and P.D.P.; Methodology, V.M., M.T., E.D.B. and P.D.P.; Project administration, V.C., G.C. and A.F.; Resources, M.V.P., F.D. and G.V.; Supervision, V.C., M.C. and A.F.; Writing—original draft, V.C., G.C., M.C. and A.F.; Writing—review and editing, F.P., A.C., C.V. and N.F., V.C. and G.C. contributed equally to this work. All authors have read and agreed to the published version of the manuscript.

**Funding:** ORSA153180 fund (University of Salerno, Italy) to V.C.

**Acknowledgments:** We thank the English mother tongue Jan Festa who revised the manuscript.

**Conflicts of Interest:** The authors declare no conflict of interest.

## References

1. Savarese, G.; Lund, L.H. Global Public Health Burden of Heart Failure. *Card. Fail. Rev.* **2017**, *3*, 7–11.
2. Tschöpe, C.; Birner, C.; Böhm, M.; Bruder, O.; Frantz, S.; Luchner, A.; Maier, L.; Störk, S.; Kherad, B.; Laufs, U. Heart failure with preserved ejection fraction: Current management and future strategies: Expert opinion on the behalf of the Nucleus of the "Heart Failure Working Group" of the German Society of Cardiology (DKG). *Clin. Res. Cardiol.* **2018**, *107*, 1–19.
3. Hsu, J.J.; Ziaeian, B.; Fonarow, G.C. Heart Failure with Mid-Range (Borderline) Ejection Fraction: Clinical Implications and Future Directions. *JACC Heart Fail.* **2017**, *5*, 763–771.
4. Ponikowski, P.; Voors, A.A.; Anker, S.D.; Bueno, H.; Cleland, J.G.; Coats, A.J.; Falk, V.; Gonzalez-Juanatey, J.R.; Harjola, V.P.; Jankowska, E.A.; et al. ESC Guidelines for the diagnosis and treatment of acute and chronic heart failure: The Task Force for the diagnosis and treatment of acute and chronic heart failure of the European Society of Cardiology (ESC). Developed with the special contribution of the Heart Failure Association (HFA) of the ESC. *Eur. J. Heart Fail.* **2016**, *18*, 891–975.
5. Lopatin, Y. Heart Failure with Mid-Range Ejection Fraction and How to Treat It. *Card. Fail. Rev.* **2018**, *4*, 9–13.
6. Tanno, M.; Kuno, A.; Horio, Y.; Miura, T. Emerging beneficial roles of sirtuins in heart failure. *Basic Res. Cardiol.* **2012**, *107*, 273.
7. Conti, V.; Forte, M.; Corbi, G.; Russomanno, G.; Formisano, L.; Landolfi, A.; Izzo, V.; Filippelli, A.; Vecchione, C.; Carrizzo, A. Sirtuins: Possible Clinical Implications in Cardio and Cerebrovascular Diseases. *Curr. Drug Targets* **2017**, *18*, 473–484.
8. Gao, P.; Xu, T.T.; Lu, J.; Li, L.; Xu, J.; Hao, D.L.; Chen, H.Z.; Liu, D.P. Overexpression of SIRT1 in vascular smooth muscle cells attenuates angiotensin II-induced vascular remodeling and hypertension in mice. *J. Mol. Med. (Berl.)* **2014**, *92*, 347–357.
9. Niethammer, M.; Sieber, M.; von Haehling, S.; Anker, S.D.; Munzel, T.; Horstick, G.; Genth-Zotz, S. Inflammatory pathways in patients with heart failure and preserved ejection fraction. *J. Cardiol.* **2008**, *129*, 111–117.
10. Vahtola, E.; Louhelainen, M.; Merasto, S.; Martonen, E.; Penttinen, S.; Aahos, I.; Kytö, V.; Virtanen, I.; Mervaala, E. Forkhead class O transcription factor 3a activation and Sirtuin1 overexpression in the hypertrophied myocardium of the diabetic Goto-Kakizaki rat. *J. Hypertens.* **2008**, *26*, 334–344.
11. Li, L.; Zhao, L.; Yi-Ming, W.; Yu, Y.S.; Xia, C.Y.; Duan, J.L.; Su, D.F. Sirt1 hyperexpression in SHR heart related to left ventricular hypertrophy. *Can. J. Physiol. Pharmacol.* **2009**, *87*, 56–62.
12. Conti, V.; Corbi, G.; Simeon, V.; Russomanno, G.; Manzo, V.; Ferrara, N.; Filippelli, A. Aging-related changes in oxidative stress response of human endothelial cells. *Aging Clin. Exp. Res.* **2015**, *27*, 547–553.
13. Yu, W.; Qin, J.; Chen, C.; Fu, Y.; Wang, W. Moderate calorie restriction attenuates age-associated alterations and improves cardiac function by increasing SIRT1 and SIRT3 expression. *Mol. Med. Rep.* **2018**, *18*, 4087–4094.
14. Alcendor, R.R.; Gao, S.; Zhai, P.; Zablocki, D.; Holle, E.; Yu, X.; Tian, B.; Wagner, T.; Vatner, S.F.; Sadoshima, J. Sirt1 regulates aging and resistance to oxidative stress in the heart. *Circ. Res.* **2007**, *100*, 1512–1521.
15. ATS Committee on Proficiency Standards for Clinical Pulmonary Function Laboratories. ATS statement: Guidelines for the six-minute walk test. *Am. J. Respir. Crit. Care Med.* **2002**, *166*, 111–117.

16. Qi, Y.; Zhang, J.; Cole-Jeffrey, C.T.; Shenoy, V.; Espejo, A.; Hanna, M.; Song, C.; Pepine, C.J.; Katovich, M.J.; Raizada, M.K. Diminazene aceturate enhances angiotensin-converting enzyme 2 activity and attenuates ischemia-induced cardiac pathophysiology. *Hypertension* **2013**, *62*, 746–752. [CrossRef] [PubMed]
17. Kane, A.E.; Sinclair, D.A. Sirtuins and NAD$^+$ in the Development and Treatment of Metabolic and Cardiovascular Diseases. *Circ. Res.* **2018**, *123*, 868–885. [CrossRef]
18. Corbi, G.; Conti, V.; Scapagnini, G.; Filippelli, A.; Ferrara, N. Role of sirtuins, calorie restriction and physical activity in aging. *Front. Biosci. Elite Ed.* **2012**, *4*, 768–778. [CrossRef]
19. Park, S.; Mori, R.; Shimokawa, I. Do sirtuins promote mammalian longevity? A critical review on its relevance to the longevity effect induced by calorie restriction. *Mol. Cells* **2013**, *35*, 474–480. [CrossRef]
20. Ferrara, N.; Rinaldi, B.; Corbi, G.; Conti, V.; Stiuso, P.; Boccuti, S.; Rengo, G.; Rossi, F.; Filippelli, A. Exercise training promotes SIRT1 activity in aged rats. *Rejuvenation Res.* **2008**, *11*, 139–150. [CrossRef]
21. Bonkowski, M.S.; Sinclair, D.A. Slowing ageing by design: The rise of NAD+ and sirtuin-activating compounds. *Nat. Rev. Mol. Cell Biol.* **2016**, *17*, 679–690. [CrossRef] [PubMed]
22. Sen, P.; Kemppainen, E.; Orešič, M. Perspectives on Systems Modeling of Human Peripheral Blood Mononuclear Cells. *Front. Mol. Biosci.* **2018**, *4*, 96. [CrossRef] [PubMed]
23. Bo, S.; Togliatto, G.; Gambino, R.; Ponzo, V.; Lombardo, G.; Rosato, R.; Cassader, M.; Brizzi, M.F. Impact of sirtuin-1 expression on H3K56 acetylation and oxidative stress: A double-blind randomized controlled trial with resveratrol supplementation. *Acta Diabetol.* **2018**, *55*, 331–340. [CrossRef] [PubMed]
24. Taka, C.; Hayashi, R.; Shimokawa, K.; Tokui, K.; Okazawa, S.; Kambara, K.; Inomata, M.; Yamada, T.; Matsui, S.; Tobe, K. SIRT1 and FOXO1 mRNA expression in PBMC correlates to physical activity in COPD patients. *Int. J. Chronic Obstruct. Pulmon. Dis.* **2017**, *12*, 3237–3244. [CrossRef]
25. Conti, V.; Corbi, G.; Manzo, V.; Malangone, P.; Vitale, C.; Maglio, A.; Cotugno, R.; Capaccio, D.; Marino, L.; Selleri, C.; et al. SIRT1 Activity in Peripheral Blood Mononuclear Cells Correlates with Altered Lung Function in Patients with Chronic Obstructive Pulmonary Disease. *Oxid. Med. Cell Longev.* **2018**, *2018*, 9391261. [CrossRef]
26. Santos-Bezerra, D.P.; Machado-Lima, A.; Monteiro, M.B.; Admoni, S.N.; Perez, R.V.; Machado, C.G.; Shimizu, M.H.; Cavaleiro, A.M.; Thieme, K.; Queiroz, M.S.; et al. Dietary advanced glycated end-products and medicines influence the expression of SIRT1 and DDOST in peripheral mononuclear cells from long-term type 1 diabetes patients. *Diabetes Vasc. Dis. Res.* **2018**, *15*, 81–89. [CrossRef]
27. Russomanno, G.; Corbi, G.; Manzo, V.; Ferrara, N.; Rengo, G.; Puca, A.A.; Latte, S.; Carrizzo, A.; Calabrese, M.C.; Andriantsitohaina, R.; et al. The anti-ageing molecule sirt1 mediates beneficial effects of cardiac rehabilitation. *Immun. Ageing* **2017**, *14*, 7. [CrossRef]
28. Sundaresan, N.R.; Pillai, V.B.; Gupta, M.P. Emerging roles of SIRT1 deacetylase in regulating cardiomyocyte survival and hypertrophy. *J. Mol. Cell Cardiol.* **2011**, *51*, 614–618. [CrossRef]
29. Kawashima, T.; Inuzuka, Y.; Okuda, J.; Kato, T.; Niizuma, S.; Tamaki, Y.; Iwanaga, Y.; Kawamoto, A.; Narazaki, M.; Matsuda, T.; et al. Constitutive SIRT1 overexpression impairs mitochondria and reduces cardiac function in mice. *J. Mol. Cell Cardiol.* **2011**, *51*, 1026–1036. [CrossRef]
30. Conti, V.; Russomanno, G.; Corbi, G.; Guerra, G.; Grasso, C.; Filippelli, W.; Paribello, V.; Ferrara, N.; Filippelli, A. Aerobic training workload affects human endothelial cells redox homeostasis. *Med. Sci. Sports Exerc.* **2013**, *45*, 644–653. [CrossRef]
31. Zullo, A.; Simone, E.; Grimaldi, M.; Musto, V.; Mancini, F.P. Sirtuins as Mediator of the Anti-Ageing Effects of Calorie Restriction in Skeletal and Cardiac Muscle. *Int. J. Mol. Sci.* **2018**, *19*, 928. [CrossRef] [PubMed]
32. Hansen, D.; Bonné, K.; Alders, T.; Hermans, A.; Copermans, K.; Swinnen, H.; Maris, V.; Jansegers, T.; Mathijs, W.; Haenen, L.; et al. Exercise training intensity determination in cardiovascular rehabilitation: Should the guidelines be reconsidered? *Eur. J. Prev. Cardiol.* **2019**, *26*, 1921–1928. [CrossRef] [PubMed]
33. Hartupee, J.; Mann, D.L. Neurohormonal activation in heart failure with reduced ejection fraction. *Nat. Rev. Cardiol.* **2017**, *14*, 30–38. [CrossRef] [PubMed]
34. Miyazaki, R.; Ichiki, T.; Hashimoto, T.; Inanaga, K.; Imayama, I.; Sadoshima, J.; Sunagawa, K. SIRT1, a longevity gene, downregulates angiotensin II type 1 receptor expression in vascular smooth muscle cells. *Arterioscler. Thromb. Vasc. Biol.* **2008**, *28*, 1263–1269. [CrossRef] [PubMed]
35. Davis, P.A.; Pagnin, E.; Dal Maso, L.; Caielli, P.; Maiolino, G.; Fusaro, M.; Paolo Rossi, G.; Calò, L.A. SIRT1, heme oxygenase-1 and NO-mediated vasodilation in a human model of endogenous angiotensin II type 1 receptor antagonism: Implications for hypertension. *Hypertens. Res.* **2013**, *36*, 873–878. [CrossRef]

36. Forte, M.; Conti, V.; Damato, A.; Ambrosio, M.; Puca, A.A.; Sciarretta, S.; Frati, G.; Vecchione, C.; Carrizzo, A. Targeting Nitric Oxide with Natural Derived Compounds as a Therapeutic Strategy in Vascular Diseases. *Oxid. Med. Cell Longev.* **2016**, 7364138. [CrossRef]
37. Liu, R.C. Focused Treatment of Heart Failure with Reduced Ejection Fraction Using Sacubitril/Valsartan. *Am. J. Cardiovasc. Drugs* **2018**, *18*, 473–482. [CrossRef]
38. Komajda, M.; Lam, C.S. Heart failure with preserved ejection fraction: A clinical dilemma. *Eur. Heart J.* **2014**, *35*, 1022–1032. [CrossRef]
39. Úri, K.; Fagyas, M.; Kertész, A.; Borbély, A.; Jenei, C.; Bene, O.; Csanádi, Z.; Paulus, W.J.; Édes, I.; Papp, Z.; et al. Circulating ACE2 activity correlates with cardiovascular disease development. *J. Renin-Angiotensin-Aldosterone Syst.* **2016**, *17*. [CrossRef]
40. Epelman, S.; Shrestha, K.; Troughton, R.W.; Francis, G.S.; Sen, S.; Klein, A.L.; Tang, W. Soluble Angiotensin Converting Enzyme 2 in Human Heart Failure: Relation with Myocardial Function and Clinical Outcomes. *J. Card. Fail.* **2009**, *15*, 565–571. [CrossRef]

**Publisher's Note:** MDPI stays neutral with regard to jurisdictional claims in published maps and institutional affiliations.

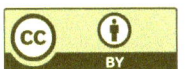

© 2020 by the authors. Licensee MDPI, Basel, Switzerland. This article is an open access article distributed under the terms and conditions of the Creative Commons Attribution (CC BY) license (http://creativecommons.org/licenses/by/4.0/).

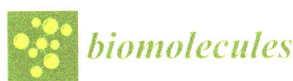 

*Review*

# Post-Myocardial Infarction Ventricular Remodeling Biomarkers—The Key Link between Pathophysiology and Clinic

**Maria-Madălina Bostan [1,2], Cristian Stătescu [1,2,\*], Larisa Anghel [1,2,\*], Ionela-Lăcrămioara Șerban [3], Elena Cojocaru [4] and Radu Sascău [1,2]**

1. Internal Medicine Department, "Grigore T. Popa" University of Medicine and Pharmacy, 700503 Iasi, Romania; madalina_farima@yahoo.com (M.-M.B.); radu.sascau@gmail.com (R.S.)
2. Cardiology Department, Cardiovascular Diseases Institute "Prof. Dr. George I.M.Georgescu", 700503 Iasi, Romania
3. Physiology Department, "Grigore T. Popa" University of Medicine and Pharmacy, 700503 Iasi, Romania; ionela.serban@umfiasi.ro
4. Department of Morphofunctional Sciences I—Pathology, "Grigore T. Popa" University of Medicine and Pharmacy, 700503 Iasi, Romania; elena2.cojocaru@umfiasi.ro
* Correspondence: cstatescu@gmail.com (C.S.); larisa.anghel@umfiasi.ro (L.A.); Tel.: +40-0232-211834 (C.S. & L.A.)

Received: 28 October 2020; Accepted: 18 November 2020; Published: 23 November 2020

**Abstract:** Studies in recent years have shown increased interest in developing new methods of evaluation, but also in limiting post infarction ventricular remodeling, hoping to improve ventricular function and the further evolution of the patient. This is the point where biomarkers have proven effective in early detection of remodeling phenomena. There are six main processes that promote the remodeling and each of them has specific biomarkers that can be used in predicting the evolution (myocardial necrosis, neurohormonal activation, inflammatory reaction, hypertrophy and fibrosis, apoptosis, mixed processes). Some of the biomarkers such as creatine kinase–myocardial band (CK-MB), troponin, and N-terminal-pro type B natriuretic peptide (NT-proBNP) were so convincing that they immediately found their place in the post infarction patient evaluation protocol. Others that are related to more complex processes such as inflammatory biomarkers, atheroma plaque destabilization biomarkers, and microRNA are still being studied, but the results so far are promising. This article aims to review the markers used so far, but also the existing data on new markers that could be considered, taking into consideration the most important studies that have been conducted so far.

**Keywords:** post-myocardial infarction ventricular remodeling; prognosis; myocardial necrosis biomarkers; neurohormonal activation biomarkers; inflammatory reaction biomarkers; fibrosis biomarkers; apoptosis biomarkers; new generation biomarkers

## 1. Introduction

Cardiovascular diseases represent a leading cause of death, accounting for 30% of deaths worldwide. Of these, up to 7 million deaths a year are caused by coronary ischemic disease, accounting for 12.8% of the total. Therefore, the statistics speak of a sad reality: every sixth patient in Europe dies from a heart attack [ ]. This explains the increased interest in this pathology and the increased interest that the evaluation of these patients enjoys lately. Increasing access to cardiac catheterization laboratories and, implicitly, to percutaneous myocardial revascularization techniques, has significantly reduced both short-term and long-term mortality in patients with heart attacks.

Therefore, in the context of current knowledge, studies in recent years have shown increased interest in developing new methods of evaluation, but also in limiting post-infarction ventricular remodeling, hoping to improve ventricular function and the further evolution of the patient. This is the point where biomarkers have proven effective in early detection of remodeling phenomena, some of them being so convincing that they immediately found their place in the post-infarction patient evaluation protocol. This article aims to review the markers used so far, and also, the existing data on new markers that could be considered, in order to see the biomarkers that approach the characteristics of an ideal biomarker.

## 2. Ventricular Remodeling—Pathophysiology

Despite this medical progress, in the case of patients who suffered a myocardial infarction, there is more and more concerns about the phenomenon of ventricular remodeling that deeply affects ventricular function and implicitly resonates with the patient's prognosis. Experimentally, it has been shown that acute ischemia causes important changes in the ventricular architecture, localized changes both in the infarct area and in other segments.

From a physiopathological point of view, the ventricular remodeling manifests under two directions: macroscopic changes that occur after 3 months of onset and microscopic changes that begin from the first moment of the coronary occlusion.

At the macroscopic level, despite complete and successful coronary angioplasty, studies have shown that both in the infarcted area and in the adjacent areas, there is a remodeling process translated into the loss of shortening and contraction with asynchronous abnormalities, hypokinesia, akinesia, and dyskinesia at the level of the ischemic zone and of the initial hyperkinesia followed by the subsequent hypokinesia at the level of the neighboring areas and the final result is a decrease in cardiac pump function, in the cardiac output, and in blood pressure and an increase in ventricular volumes [2,3]. In parallel, the ventricular cavity dilates as a compensatory response to its dysfunction, a process directly related to the magnitude of the infarction area. Its purpose is to maintain a constant beating volume as the percentage of viable contractile myocardium decreases. In the long run, however, this dilation increases the systolic and diastolic parietal stress, thus creating a vicious circle in which the initial dilation generates additional dilation [4].

In addition to myocardial ischemia, at least two other processes participate in this process: the phenomenon of no reflow and the epigenetically mediating disturbance of endogenous repair system.

The no reflow phenomenon is associated with early remodeling and is determined by the microvascular obstruction and dysfunction that disrupts regional perfusion [5]. Studies have shown that the phenomenon of no reflow correlates with the higher incidence of ventricular remodeling and increased risk of cardiovascular events and sudden death [6].

On the other hand, epigenetically mediating disturbance of endogenous repair system translates to altered vascular repair, with maintenance of vasoconstriction and vascular dysfunction in the area adjacent to myocardial infarction [7,8].

At the microscopic level, from the moment of coronary obstruction, a series of nitric oxide disrupting processes are initiated, the vascular signaling systems endothelial growth factors signaling systems are activated, the cytokines are released and this is how the apoptosis and necrosis pathways are activated, generating an increase in oxidative stress, mitochondrial dysfunction, alteration of myocyte metabolism, promotion of fibrosis, and cell remodeling. Therefore, microvascular inflammation, small vessel obstruction, and endothelial dysfunction maintain the remodeling phenomenon [9].

Sequentially, in the first 72 h hours of ischemia, myocytic necrosis appears accompanied by edema and inflammation of the area affected by the infarction. Subsequently, a process of fibroblastic proliferation and collagen storage is installed, which results in the occurrence of the scar. In the period between the resorption of necrotic tissue and scarring, the infarct area undergoes a process of thinning and elongation which is called "infarction expansion" [10]. Proteases and the activation of matrix metalloproteinases (MMPs) released by neutrophils that cause degradation of collagen fibers participate in this process. The final effect is an increased parietal stress which stimulates the mechanoreceptors and generates angiotensin II-releasing intracellular signals. After 72 h, there is a process mediated by the renin–angiotensin–aldosterone system and by neurohormonal activation, which causes changes in ventricular geometry, with dilation of the cavities and myocardial hypertrophy [ , ].

The remodeling process can take from a few weeks to a few months, until a balance between the forces of distension and the resistance offered by the collagen fibers is obtained [ ]. This balance is decisively influenced by [ ]:

- Characteristics of myocardial infarction: its size, location, and transmurality;
- Extension of the sidereal myocardium;
- Re-permeabilization of the artery responsible for infarction [ ];
- Local trophic factors [ ].

In summary, within the ventricular remodeling, four types of processes take place that are closely related to the types of biomarkers that can be detected (Figure ):

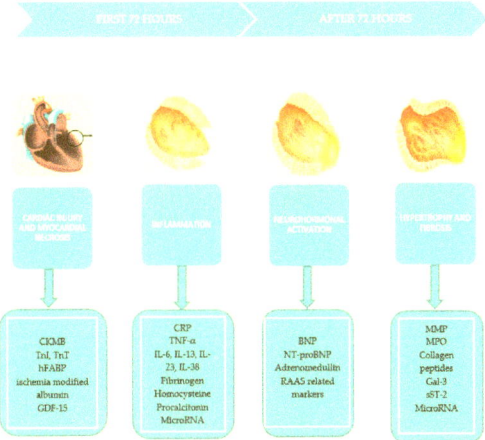

**Figure 1.** The processes that promote the ventricular remodeling and their specific biomarkers. CK-MB: creatine kinase–myocardial band; hFABP: heart fatty acids binding protein; NT-proBNP: N-terminal-pro type B natriuretic peptide; BNP: type B natriuretic peptide; RAAS: renin–angiotensin–aldosterone system; TNF: tumor necrosis factor; IL: interleukin; MPO: myeloperoxidase; ST-2: suppression of tumorgenicity; GDF-15: growth differentiation factor-15; VEGFR: vascular endothelial growth factor receptor.

1. Myocardial necrosis: creatine kinase–myocardial band (CK-MB), troponin I and T (TnI, TnT), myoglobin, heart fatty acids binding protein (hFABP), ischemia modified albumin, GDF-15.
2. Neurohormonal activation: N-terminal-pro type B natriuretic peptide (NT-proBNP), type B natriuretic peptide (BNP), adrenomedullin, renin–angiotensin–aldosterone system (RAAS)-related biomarkers.
3. Inflammatory reaction closely related to the release of C-reactive protein (CRP), tumor necrosis factor α (TNF-α), interleukins 6, 13, 23, and 38 (IL-6, IL-13, IL-23, IL-38), homocysteine, procalcitonin.
4. Hypertrophy and fibrosis involving MMP, collagen propeptidases, galectin-3 (Gal-3), soluble ST-2 (sST-2) [ ].

There are also some novel biomarkers that are involved in several processes and they cannot be categorized. The main exponents are microRNA (miRNA), which epigenetically regulates the cardiac myocytes apoptosis and increases oxidative stress and inflammation by triggering proinflammatory cytokine release [16,17].

## 3. Biomarkers

The use of biomarkers in the evaluation of patients after acute myocardial infarction has a history of 40 years (the initial term was that of biological marker and was first introduced in 1989), and the scientific trend seems to favor such an approach, which will clearly lead to new studies and new biomarkers.

The characteristics of a biomarker concern three central aspects: the mode of synthesis and release, specificity, and sensitivity [18,19]. The outline of an ideal biomarker is therefore outlined (Table 1).

Table 1. Characteristics of the ideal biomarker.

| Characteristics of the Ideal Biomarker |
|---|
| *High sensitivity* |
| Increased myocardial concentrations after heart attack |
| Rapid release to allow early diagnosis |
| Long half-life to allow late diagnosis |
| *High specificity* |
| Its absence in tissues other than the myocardial one |
| Its absence in healthy patients |
| *Assay-related characteristics* |
| Good cost-effectiveness ratio |
| Easy to assay |
| Short processing time |
| High precision |
| *Clinical characteristics* |
| Useful in guiding therapy |
| Useful in predicting the prognosis |

### 3.1. Biomarkers of Cardiac Injury and Myocardial Necrosis

The first question that arose was whether biomarkers used in the diagnosis of myocardial ischemia could also be interpreted as prognostic markers, so these were the first to be investigated in this respect.

#### 3.1.1. Creatine Kinase MB

CK-MB is an enzyme found in the myocardium, its role being related to the generation of contraction [20]. Its discharge into the circulatory stream is related to myocytolysis and not only to the process of ischemia [21]. It is one of the most used biomarkers in the diagnosis of myocardial injury, being detectable in plasma 4–8 h after the onset of pain and reaching a peak at 18–24 h [20,21]. Studies have placed it above myoglobin in terms of diagnostic value, but recognize its poor specificity in patients with multiple comorbidities such as kidney disease, non-cardiac surgery, chest trauma, muscle disorders, hypothyroidism, hypoventilation, and pulmonary embolism [22,23].

Predictively, studies have shown that a low CK-MB value at the time of diagnosis of AMI means a small amount of affected myocardium and therefore, the success of reperfusion therapy can be maximum, this translating into a lower rate of morbidity and mortality [24]. Clinical data from previous years' studies have shown the importance of CK-MB at admission as an independent predictor in both the short and long term [25–27]. Other studies have shown that not serial CK-MB values, but its increased value for a longer period (values above 124 mg/dL more than 18 h after the onset of myocardial infarction, despite the successful PCI) is correlated with subsequent cardiovascular events (reinfarctions, hospitalizations for cardiac decompensation, death) [28]. Another study was able to correlate the CK-MB peak ratio value (the ratio between the maximum value of CK-MB reached by the patient and the higher value of normal) with a higher mortality at two years post infarction [29]. Some retrospective studies have suggested a correlation between increased CK-MB and long-term mortality [ – ], while others have established that only a significant increase, of 5 to 8 times the upper limit, could have prognostic implications [ – ]. Yee KC et al. evaluated, in a study, the independent prognostic value of CK-MB in patients with acute coronary syndrome and negative troponin [ ] and showed that an increase in CK-MB, even in the absence of troponin dynamics, is correlated with an increase in morbidity and mortality at 6 months. Although these results failed to create a consensus on the use of CK-MB as a prognostic factor, the accessibility and low cost of this analysis could be additional arguments for further studies.

3.1.2. Troponin

Troponin is a protein found in both the heart and skeletal muscles, but I and T isoforms have a higher specificity for the myocardium. This is also the reason why in 2000, the European Society of Cardiology (ESC) and the American College of Cardiology (ACC) introduced in the Universal Definition of Myocardial Infarction, the need for biochemical evidence of myocardial necrosis and indicated as a biomarker of choice, troponin [ ]. The sensitivity of myocytolysis detection is significantly higher in the case of troponin as compared to CK-MB, due to a higher percentage of discharge in the circulatory torrent after an acute coronary event, which makes it detectable after a short period of time from the onset of events [ ]. Troponin is involved in the binding of actin to myosin and in the regulation of contraction in response to calcium overflow and phosphorylation of contractile proteins. Starting from this mechanism, there was an experimental study that found an inverse correlation of the level of phosphorylation of troponin T dosed in plasma with the risk of ventricular remodeling after acute myocardial infarction [ ]. A prospective observational study [ ] determined the CK-MB and troponin levels in the first 24 h after onset and correlated them with the evolution of patients one year after the acute coronary event. The results showed that an increase in isolated troponin, in the absence of CK-MB increase, was associated with a higher mortality (6.5% vs. 12.5%), but also in the situation where there was a CK-MB dynamic, the association of increased troponin values led to an increased mortality rate (6.8% vs. 11.7%). In the case of a normal troponin value, in this study, the increase in CK-MB was correlated with a higher mortality, but without statistical significance. Similar data were obtained in a relatively small study conducted in Pakistan that compared the predictive value of creatine kinase with that of troponin T from admission for acute myocardial infarction [ ]. They showed that TnT is a better predictor of mortality. Some studies shown that admission troponin is directly related to the incidence of cardiovascular events (cardiac death, non-fatal myocardial infarction, coronary revascularization) and to the mortality rate [ ].

3.1.3. Myoglobin

Myoglobin is a heme protein that is found in all types of muscle tissue, but with a higher concentration in the skeletal and myocardial one [ ]. This is exactly what makes it a biomarker with low specificity, which is why, at least in the diagnosis of myocardial infarction, the recommendations are to be used in relation to the clinical context, electrocardiography (ECG), and other biomarkers. An important feature, however, is the early growth in plasma (approximately 2 h after the onset of pain), given its small size and high cytoplasmic concentration [ ]. However, its sensitivity in the first 2 h after the onset of the acute coronary event is of 70%, which means a good diagnostic performance during this time. It reaches a peak in 6–9 h and disappears from the torrent in the first 24 h [ ]. Despite these characteristics, the combined analysis of myoglobin with troponin significantly increased the ability to identify patients with myocardial infarction with increased mortality comparing to either of the two biomarkers evaluated separately [ , ]). Myoglobin is mainly renal eliminated and as kidney disease is a well-known predictor of cardiovascular events, including mortality in patients with a myocardial infarction [ ], it has been suggested that the predictive power of myoglobin mortality is due to its ability to identify patients with associated renal failure [ ].

### 3.1.4. Ischemia Modified Albumin

In acute ischemia, the N-terminal end of albumin is damaged, reducing its ability to bind. It has been used in several studies that have shown its usefulness in the diagnosis of acute coronary syndromes in conjunction with tropine values and ECG changes [52]. It has been shown that this combination of biomarkers (troponin and modified albumin) has a predictive value higher than any of them taken separately [53]. However, high values are also found in patients with neoplasms, kidney disease, strokes, and liver disease, which significantly limits its specificity.

### 3.1.5. hFABP (Heart-Type Fatty Acid Binding Protein)

hFABP is a small protein, located cytosolically, and the role of which is related to the transport and metabolism of fatty acids. The largest amount is found in the myocardium, but we find it in lower percentages in the kidneys, brain, and skeletal muscles [54]. In serum, it appears early after coronary occlusion, at about 30 min, with a peak at 6–8 h and with a return to baseline level after 24–30 h. After 6–8 h from the acute event, its diagnostic value decreases and becomes useless due to accelerated renal clearance [55–57]. Studies have also shown an individual predictive value of this biomarker in terms of mortality in patients with acute coronary syndrome [58]. Other studies have hypothesized an even better predictive value than other markers of myocardial necrosis (TnI, CK-MB) for cardiovascular events occurring more than 1 year after an ACS [59]. For patients with chronic heart failure, elevated hFABP levels on admission and discharge were correlated with an increased number of cardiovascular events, including reinfarction and death [60].

### 3.1.6. GDF-15

Growth differentiation factors (GDF) are a subfamily of proteins belonging to the TGF-beta (transforming growth factor-beta) family. GDF-15 increases with myocardial injury and the inflammation process, suggesting an increased cardiovascular risk [61]. Therefore, studies have shown its increase in myocardial infarction [62] and propose it as an independent predictor of mortality in these patients. Cumulative dosing of TnT/NT-proBNP and GDF-15 has been shown to be very useful in stratifying the risk of these patients [63].

## 3.2. Biomarkers of Neurohormonal Activity

### 3.2.1. Natriuretic Peptides

BNP is a neurohormone released by myocardial cells following parietal stress associated with the condition of increased intraventricular pressure. As atrial natriuretic peptides, their role is the vasodilation, natriuresis, and inhibition of both the sympathetic nervous system and the renin–angiotensin–aldosterone system [64]. Therefore, both the active form, BNP, and the inactive form, NT-proBNP, can be considered markers of hemodynamic stress. There have been studies that have shown that although these markers may represent predictors for the development of heart failure and death, they do not play an important role as indicators of recurrent infarction [65,66]. Their role in the diagnosis and prognosis of heart failure of any etiology has long been established by extensive studies [67,68]. Regarding their predictive role in patients with myocardial infarction, other studies, such as DETECT, have shown that increased admission levels of NT-proBNP are correlated with higher mortality rates and cardiovascular events at 5 years [69]. Additionally, in these patients, the level of BNP seems to correlate with the size of the myocardial infarction [70]. Their levels at 2–4 days after the acute coronary event may be an independent predictor of left ventricular function and survival after one year [71]. In fibrinolysis-treated infarction, the initial elevated BNP level was correlated with worse reperfusion and 30-day mortality, being considered an independent prognostic factor for mortality, heart failure, and death [72]. There have also been studies comparing the predictive ability of NT-proBNP and BNP with that of TIMI and GRACE scores, with natriuretic peptides proving superior, and their combination with these scores did not significantly increase their predictive value [73,74].

Both BNP and NT-proBNP are therefore excellent biomarkers for cardiovascular events, but their specificity is low, being increased in other forms of heart failure, pulmonary embolism, and kidney damage. Further studies are needed to evaluate their use in various protocols in order to guide the treatment of these patients accordingly to their prognosis.

3.2.2. Adrenomedullin

Adrenomedullin is a regulatory cardiovascular peptide which is increased in the context of the acute coronary event, its role being related to the limitation of infarction and myocardial remodeling. Therefore, although few studies have targeted it, they have shown a role in predicting post infarction remodeling, as well as in stratifying the risk in patients with heart failure and myocardial infarction [ , ].

3.2.3. Renin–Angiotensin–Aldosterone System-Related Biomarkers

RAAS is a hormonal system designed to regulate blood pressure and water balance. After a myocardial infarction, its activation occurs mediated by the increase in ventricular volumes and by vasoconstriction. Aldosterone is associated with a wide range of undesirable effects in the coronary event (endothelial dysfunction, increased oxidative stress, promotion of myocyte necrosis, hypertrophy, and myocardial fibrosis) [ ]. Although no other neuropeptide besides BNP and NT-proBNP is routinely used in practical evaluation, there is indirect evidence of their ability to predict morbidity and mortality in patients with infarction by decreasing it in patients treated with RAAS inhibitors [ , ] Some studies have also shown that a higher renin/aldosterone ratio is correlated with higher chances of developing ventricular remodeling [ ].

3.3. Inflammatory Biomarkers

3.3.1. C-Reactive Protein

This is an acute phase inflammatory protein that causes macrophage activation and is correlated with oxidative stress. The idea of studying it within the pathophysiology of acute myocardial infarction is related to the role of inflammation in atherothrombosis and to CRP synthesis by hepatocytes, as a result of stimulation by inflammatory cytokines, primarily by IL-6. It has long been considered a marker of cardiovascular disease, being correlated with ventricular dysfunction and increased mortality rates among patients with heart failure [ ]. Its role in fibrosis and inflammation associated with angiotensin II-induced myocardial remodeling is also known [ ]. Some studies tried to recommend CRP as a diagnostic biomarker for myocardial infarction, but low sensitivity and specificity have ruled it out [ ]. Studies have shown a direct correlation of CRP dosed at 2 days post PCI with the level of NT-proBNP, infarct size, and ejection fraction and an inverse correlation with non-infarcted myocardial volume, but no association with ventricular volumes was found. The described relationships are observed at 1 week after the acute cardiovascular event, but are lost at 2 months [ ]. Similar data were obtained in other studies that managed to correlate CRP not only with infarct size and ejection fraction, but also with the telesystolic volume of the left ventricle measured at admission and at 6 months [ ]. Cardiovascular events after an acute myocardial infarction appear to be associated with an initially increased CRP value [ – ].

There were also studies that proved the opposite, cancelling by the obtained results, the predictive value of CRP [ ]. Its high sensitivity as an indicator of inflammation has been proposed as an independent prognostic marker in patients with acute coronary syndromes [ , ], but without the same ability of troponin to detect patients who may benefit from reperfusion therapy [ , ].

3.3.2. Other Inflammatory Markers

The idea of studying inflammatory markers as predictors for ventricular remodeling after infarction starts from some well-known pathophysiological mechanisms. Coronary heart disease is seen as the product of an inflammatory process. The formation of the atheroma plaque starts from the endothelial injury caused by risk factors (smoking, diabetes, hypertension, dyslipidemia), as it has an important contribution in the process of atherosclerosis. Elevated serum LDL-cholesterol concentrations play a proatherogenic role by stimulating inflammation and oxidative processes in the endothelium. The latter's response results in the activation of adhesion molecules and the synthesis of inflammatory cytokines [93,94], which thus attracts monocytes and T lymphocytes. The atheroma plaque consists of a lipid center wrapped in a fibrous cap with inflammatory infiltrate. In the development of myocardial infarction, inflammation again plays an important role, the rupture of the plaque triggering a proinflammatory and procoagulant status that ultimately leads to acute thrombotic occlusion. Therefore, it can be stated that inflammation not only promotes the initiation and progression of atherosclerosis, but also contributes to all thrombotic complications [19].

Perhaps the most important inflammatory markers associated with ischemia and reperfusion lesions in acute myocardial infarction are IL-6 and TNF-α. IL-6 is involved in the process of recruitment and activation of inflammatory cells, as well as in CRP synthesis in the liver, having a negative inotropic effect mediated by nitric oxide synthesis [95].

TNF-α is a cytokine with a cardio-inhibitory role that we find in the endothelium, smooth muscle cell, or macrophages and that causes a decrease in myocardial contractility either by direct action or by nitric oxide. There have been studies that have shown the prognostic value in terms of IL-6 mortality in patients with infarction [82,89], while being also able to identify those who could benefit more from an invasive treatment than from a drug treatment [96]. What limits the use of IL-6 as a biomarker for both diagnosis and prognosis is its circadian variation and the small number of studies on this topic [97]. Regarding TNF-α, studies that evaluated its correlation with mortality at 6 months were able to prove its prognostic value together with CRP [98].

Other studies have shown that deficiency of inflammatory factors such as interleukin-13 (IL-13) and interleukin-23 (IL-23) are associated with post infarction ventricular remodeling and a worse long-term prognosis [99,100].

A recent in vitro study showed that interleukin-38 (IL-38) has an increased level of peri-myocardial infarction and that the phenomenon of myocardial remodeling has been markedly improved after the administration of recombinant IL-38. The mechanism involved is related to the decrease in the inflammatory response in dendritic cells [101].

Fibrinogen, an acute phase reactant with direct procoagulant action, is known to be associated with a worse prognosis in the short and long term [87,102,103]. Homocysteine, on the other hand, is associated with the presence of thrombotic material and a greater tendency to reinfarction [104]. However, their individual predictive value is low.

Procalcitonin is a precursor of calcitonin, involved in calcium homeostasis and the synthesis of which is linked to inflammatory processes. There are studies that have shown both its diagnostic value for myocardial infarction [105] and its predictive ability on mortality and the recurrence of ischemic events [106,107].

*3.4. Biomarkers of Myocardial Fibrosis*

3.4.1. Myeloperoxidase

Myeloperoxidase (MPO) is a hemoprotein produced by PMN and macrophages, with a role in converting chlorite and hydrogen peroxide to hypochlorite released in the inflammatory context and involved in the oxidation of LDL-cholesterol particles. This stage is the promoter of foam cell formation in atherosclerosis, which makes MPO a marker of atheroma plaque instability correlated with the risk of developing myocardial infarction in the future. Even if until recently, MPO was thought to be linked only to immune defense [108], recent studies showed its properties as a vascular pro-inflammatory promoter by facilitating the consumption of nitric oxide or by increasing the reactive oxygen species [109]. Particularly, in ventricular remodeling following a myocardial infarction, MPO was proved to increase the collagen deposition in an experimental study that used the ligation of the left anterior descending artery [ ] and the MPO-deficient mice exhibited less left ventricular dilatation and attenuated impairment in systolic left ventricular functions [ , ].

Its value increases from the patient with stable coronary heart disease to unstable angina and reaches a maximum value in the patient with infarction [ ]. Studies have shown that its diagnostic value is lower than that of the other biomarkers, but elevated values may be independent predictors for cardiovascular events in both acute coronary syndrome patients and healthy individuals [ ]. The combined values of MPO, CK-MB, and TnI have shown a more accurate diagnosis of myocardial infarction [ ]. A study that evaluated the prognostic capacity of troponin, CRP, and MPO showed that each of them can be used as a biomarker, but the first two had higher values [ ].

### 3.4.2. Metalloproteinases

MMPs are a whole family of endoproteins with many roles in cardiovascular pathophysiology [ ], involved in tissue remodeling and degradation of the extracellular matrix and therefore, of collagen, elastin, glycoproteins, proteoglycans, and gelatins. These are controlled by hormonal discharges, growth factors, and cytokines secreted by inflammatory cells and also by tissue inhibitors of metalloproteinase (TIMPs), which are the main regulators for the proteolytic activity [ ]. There are four types of TIMPs, three that are present in normal, healthy hearts and one that is more specific to heart diseases [ – ]. Although the main roles of the MMPs and TIMPs are in the extracellular matrix homeostasis, they have also other important functions linked to ventricular remodeling [ , ]. Cardiac fibroblasts (CFBs) can produce a number of MMPs and TIMPs, as a response to the cytokine and chemokines release [ – ]. TNFα and IL-1β [ ], as well as BNP [ ], have been reported to induce their production through CFBs. MMPs can also impact on CFBs' function, as there were studies that have shown that they can trigger fibrosis by cleaving and activating the latent ECM-bound TGFβ, activate the Smad pathway in CFBs, and trigger collagen production [ ]. MMP-2 and MMP-9 have particular roles in collagen synthesis [ , ]. Of these, MMP-9 was shown to be correlated with [ ].

### 3.4.3. Collagen Peptides

A 2013 study [ ] tried to test a number of markers of fibrosis as elements of post infarction prognosis. Their previous determinations had already shown a correlation of the cardiac extracellular matrix turnover and evolution after the acute coronary event in terms of heart failure development and left ventricle ejection fraction (LVEF) reduction, independent of congestion estimated by using BNP [ ]. Prolonging this phenomenon weeks after the infarction increased the risk of decreased LVEF and progression to heart failure, and the combined determination of BNP and TnI after one month refined the prediction of cardiovascular events [ – , – ]. The study wanted to test the predictive value of collagen peptides dosed at 1 month after infarction. Therefore, they dosed the telopeptide of type I collagen, the aminoterminal propeptide of procollagen type I, and the aminoterminal propeptide of procollagen type III. The results showed that the ratio between type I procollagen aminoterminal propeptide and type III procollagen aminoterminal propeptide over 1, in combination with BNP and LVEF values, may be correlated with a negative prognostic in terms of ventricular remodeling, heart failure, and death.

### 3.4.4. Galectin-3

Galectin-3 is a lectin that binds to beta-galactosidase. It is secreted by activated macrophages and is involved in cardiac fibrosis, the process of inflammation, and the process of myocardial healing, mechanisms closely related to ventricular remodeling. Increased serum levels in myocardial infarction have long been studied in multiple clinical trials [ , ]. The novelty brought by the latest research is the correlation of Gal-3 with ventricular remodeling and decreased LVEF after myocardial infarction [ ]. Additionally, elevated levels of Gal-3 are associated with a higher KILLIP class, hemodynamic instability with intra-aortic balloon pump (IABP) requirements, higher NYHA class, and increased CADILLAC score, and in evolution, these patients are prone to a higher rate of major cardiovascular events, despite effective primary angioplasty [143]. A contradictory result was obtained by Weir et al. [144], which showed the link between galectin-3 and decreased LVEF at 24 months, but without a significant correlation in terms of remodeling per se. In a subgroup of patients, Di Tano et al. showed that in patients with previous myocardial infarction and primary angioplasty, Gal-3 was associated with a higher rate of ventricular remodeling at 1 and 6 months [145], while Gal-3 dosing at 30 days in patients with a first myocardial infarction, treated by angioplasty, showed an increased predictive value in terms of systolic and diastolic ventricular dysfunction [146].

3.4.5. ST2

ST2 is a cardiac biomarker associated with parietal stress and the fibrosis process, with important dynamics in patients with myocardial infarction or acute heart failure [147]. Because of its lack of cardiac specificity, it has been ruled out as a diagnostic tool for myocardial infarction, but other studies have shown promising results on its prognostic value related to mortality and heart failure development for these patients [148,149].

*3.5. New Generation Biomarkers*

MicroRNA

MicroRNAs are small RNA molecules without coding function, expressed endogenously, very stable and detectable in plasma, their serum concentration being variable depending on the different pathologies in which these are associated, which makes them suitable as diagnostic or prognostic biomarkers. Studies in recent years have identified multiple cardio-specific microRNAs that appear to play an important role in the development of cardiovascular disease [150] and they have been shown to be linked to almost all the processes that lead to ventricular remodeling [10] (Figure 2). Of these, four appear to be more common in patients with myocardial infarction (miRNA-208a, miRNA-499, miRNA-1, and miRNA-133) [151,152]. Regarding the diagnosis of myocardial infarction, some studies [153,154] indicate as biomarkers miRNA-92 and miRNA-181, while others recommend the combined use of miRNA-1, miRNA-21, and miRNA-499, as having an even higher diagnostic value as hsTnI [155]. Regarding the prognostic value of these biomarkers, miRNA-197a and miRNA-223a were identified as correlated with an increased risk of cardiovascular death [156], while miRNA-134, miRNA-328, miRNA-34a, and miRNA-208b seem to be predictive factors for heart failure development and for an increased risk of post infarction mortality [157,158].

The study conducted by Pin et al. concluded that elevated plasma values of miRNA-208b and miRNA-34a can be considered predictors of left ventricular remodeling after myocardial infarction, associated with higher mortality at 6 months and a 23.1% higher rate of heart failure development. miRNA-208b thus appears to be a cardiac-specific microRNA, with high values in the acute phase of infarction and with a predictive role regarding the development of ventricular dysfunction. Although the miRNA-34 family is considered to have a protective role against pathological remodeling, by overexpression, these prove their ability to induce endothelial cell aging and, implicitly, atherosclerosis [159].

A study led by Devaux et al. [160] found a correlation between miRNA-150 and left ventricular remodeling after a first myocardial infarction. They also showed that miRNA-150, miRNA-101, miRNA-16, and miRNA-27a are linked to a decrease in ventricular contractility.

Some studies have tested the prognostic value of microRNA in patients with primary angioplasty [161]. These identified molecules that are present in plasma even before angioplasty, with rapid dynamics (miRNA-29a, miRNA-29b, miRNA-324, miRNA-208, miRNA-423, miRNA-522, and miRNA-545) and others (miRNA-320a) that are correlated with ventricular remodeling, despite procedural success.

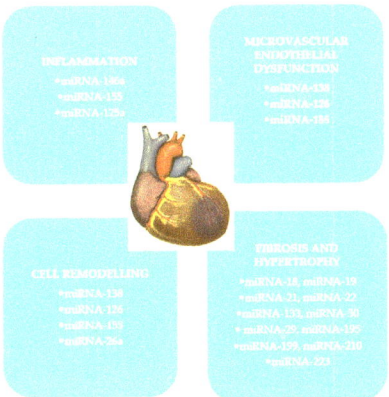

**Figure 2.** The role of different types of miRNA in the ventricular remodeling. miRNA: microRNA.

Studies targeting microRNAs have evaluated their prognostic value in terms of two important aspects of post infarction evolution: the ability to predict cardiovascular mortality and left ventricular remodeling.

In terms of mortality, the first molecules identified as having prognostic value were miRNA-133a and miRNA-208b, which were correlated with a significant increase in all-cause mortality at 6 months post infarction [ ]. miRNA-208b was studied in other research works too and they identified the same link [ , ]. Subsequently, other microRNA molecules, such as miRNA-499, have been shown to be effective in predicting mortality at 30 days, 4 months, and 1, 2, and 6 years [ , , ]. Increased levels of miRNA-155 and miRNA-380 have also been shown to be correlated with cardiovascular mortality [ ], and miRNA-192, miRNA-194, and miRNA-34 were significantly high in the serum of patients who later developed heart failure [ ]. The ability to predict cumulatively both cardiovascular mortality and heart failure development has been attributed to miRNA-145 [ ]. A ratio of serum level of miRNA-122-5p/133b measured at the time of cardiac catheterization has also been proposed as a predictor of mortality [ ].

In terms of predictive capacity regarding post infarction ventricular remodeling, miRNA-133a has also proven to be a useful tool, being associated with large infarcts with large areas of residual ischemia even after reperfusion [ ]. In patients treated with primary angioplasty, increased levels of miRNA-1, miRNA-208b, and miRNA-499 had a negative impact on left ventricular ejection fraction [ ]. The same aspect was identified in the case of long chains of RNA lncRNA MALAT1 associated with the decrease in the ejection fraction at 4 months after the infarction [ ]. Extensive studies have, in fact, shown the role of long RNA chains in the development of myocardial fibrosis [ , ]. On the other hand, low levels of miRNA-150, miRNA-16, miRNA-27a, and miRNA-101 seem to predict ventricular remodeling [ , ], while increased values of miRNA-208b, miRNA-34a, miRNA-21, and miRNA-155 correlate inversely with the same complication of myocardial infarction [ , ]. Circular microRNA was also not omitted from the studies, as it was associated with left ventricular dysfunction after infarction [ ].

Therefore, circulating microRNAs have shown promising results as post-infarction prognostic biomarkers, so other studies should be conducted in order to find a risk stratification formula based on their serum values.

Concluding the results of the previously presented studies, Table  presents the prognostic characteristics of each biomarker analyzed in the review, while Table S1 presents detailed data regarding every study protocol.

**Table 2.** Summarized data about each biomarker's prognostic value.

| Category | Biomarker | Prognostic Value |
|---|---|---|
| Cardiac injury and myocardial necrosis | CK-MB [25,27–38] | Predictive of mortality and cardiovascular events |
| | Troponin [42–45] | Independent predictor of ventricular remodeling and cardiovascular events |
| | Myoglobin [49] | Predictive only in association with troponin |
| | Ischemia modified albumin [52,53] | Raises the predictive value of troponin when measured together |
| | hFABP [58,59] | Predictive of mortality and major cardiovascular events after 1 year |
| | GDF-15 [61–63] | Independent predictor of mortality |
| Neurohormonal activity | BNP, NT-proBNP [65,66,69–73] | Highly predictive of heart failure, cardiovascular events, and mortality |
| | Adrenomedullin [76] | Predictive of cardiovascular events and severity of heart failure |
| | RAAS-related biomarkers [77,78] | The use of its inhibitors is associated with a mortality and morbidity decrease |
| Inflammatory biomarkers | C-reactive protein [83–88] | Predictive of ventricular remodeling and only when associated with other biomarkers, it becomes predictive of mortality |
| | IL-6 [89,96] | Predictive of mortality and cardiovascular events |
| | TNF-α [98] | Might be predictive for survival in association with C-reactive protein |
| | IL-13, IL-23, IL-38, fibrinogen, homocysteine [99–104] | Might be predictive of ventricular remodeling |
| | Procalcitonin [106,107] | Predictive of mortality, cardiovascular events, and ventricular remodeling |
| Fibrosis biomarkers | MMP, MPO [116,133] | Might be predictive of ventricular remodeling |
| | Collagen peptides [134,135] | Predictive of cardiovascular events and mortality |
| | Galectin-3 [143,144,146] | Predictive of major cardiovascular events. Might be predictive of ventricular remodeling |
| | ST-2 [149] | Predictive of survival |
| Novel biomarkers | microRNA [156–158,160,162,168–170,173,174] | Predictive of mortality, heart failure, cardiovascular events, and ventricular remodeling |

CK-MB: creatine kinase–myocardial band; hFABP: heart-type fatty acids binding protein; GDF-15: growth differentiation; RAAS: renin–angiotensin–aldosterone system; IL: interleukin; BNP: brain-type natriuretic peptide; NT-proBNP: N-terminal-prohormone brain-type natriuretic peptide; MPO: myeloperoxidase; MMP: metalloproteinase; TNF-α: tumor necrosis factor α, ST-2: suppression of tumourigenicity-2.

## 4. Multi Testing

The desire for early ventricular remodeling detection led to the idea of multi-testing, by combining biomarkers generated by different pathophysiological mechanisms. Thus, starting from the premise that TnI, CRP, and BNP are independent markers for post infarction cardiovascular events, a series of studies with promising results were made. Kim et al. [176] tested hsCRP and NT-proBNP, thus showing that the cumulative predictive value is superior to any of them taken separately. At the same time, the use of biomarkers of myocardial stress, inflammation, and myocyte necrosis has increased the predictive capacity for heart failure development [177].

Some studies have even managed to stratify the risk of mortality based on the cumulative dosage of cTnI/CK-MB/myoglobin [178]. Similar data were obtained in patients with STEMI in whom NT-proBNP, hs-TnT, aspartate transaminase (AST), alanine transaminase (ALT), hs-CRP, and lactate-dehydrogenase (LDH) were dosed, showing an increase in their predictive capacity [179]. ST2/GDF-15/hFABP/hs-TnT multi-testing has also shown promising results as a prognostic value [180].

There were also opinions that contradicted the value of multi-testing. Feistritzer et al. [181] showed that the predictive value of hs-cTnT is not improved by adding CK, hs-CRP, LDH, ALT, and AST. Other research has shown that once a biomarker with a high predictive value such as troponin is included in multi-testing, it is difficult to quantify the contribution of other biomarkers added to it.

## 5. Conclusions

The multiple characteristics related to the specificity, sensitivity, early growth, and accessibility that the ideal biomarker should meet have made it difficult to identify a single parameter that meets them all.

Considering the results of our study, we think that the biomarkers that are closest to the characteristics of an ideal biomarker are hsTnI, hsCRP, and NT-proBNP, which have a high level of sensitivity, a high prognostic power, and in addition, the advantage of a low cost and of great accessibility. Out of the desire to refine the prediction, multi-testing was used, which, in most cases, proved to have the specificity and sensitivity of the stronger biomarker, without increasing the power of prediction in this way.

In terms of specificity, fibrosis markers stand out in particular, most having a direct role in the process of ventricular remodeling. The main disadvantage of their use is given by the difficulty of dosing in terms of accessibility and costs, which makes them difficult to use in practice, being reserved especially for clinical trials.

Particular attention must be paid to the new biomarkers; microRNAs that participate in several stages of the ventricular remodeling process are noted as important early markers of remodeling, but also of mortality. We believe that they should be studied in the coming years.

**Supplementary Materials:** The following are available online at , Table S1: Detailed data of every study protocol.

**Author Contributions:** Conceptualization, M.-M.B.; methodology, M.-M.B.; validation, C.S., R.S. and L.A.; formal analysis, C.S., R.S. and L.A.; investigation, M.-M.B.; resources, M.-M.B. and I.-L.S.; data curation, C.S., R.S. and L.A.; writing—original draft preparation, M.-M.B.; writing—review and editing, C.S., R.S., E.C. and L.A. All authors have read and agreed to the published version of the manuscript.

**Funding:** This research received no external funding.

**Conflicts of Interest:** The authors declare no conflict of interest.

## References

1. Antman, E.M.; Braunwald, E. ST-Elevation Myocardial Infarction: Pathology, Pathophysiology, and Clinical Features. In *Braunwald's Heart Disease: A Textbook of Cardiovascular Medicine*, 9th ed.; Zipes, D.P., Libby, P., Bonow, R.O., Braunwald, E., Eds.; Elsevier Saunders: Philadelphia, PA, USA, 2012; pp. 1207–1230.
2. Patel, K.V.; Mauricio, R.; Grodin, J.L.; Ayers, C.; Fonarow, G.C.; Berry, J.D.; Pandey, A. Identifying a low-flow phenotype in heart failure with preserved ejection fraction: A secondary analysis of the RELAX trial. *ESC Heart Fail.* **2019**, *6*, 613–620.
3. Halade, G.V.; Kain, V.; Tourki, B.; Jadapalli, J.K. Lipoxygenase drives lipidomic and metabolic reprogramming in ischemic heart failure. *Metabolism* **2019**, *96*, 22–32.
4. Sutton, M.S.J.; Ferrari, V.A. Prevention of Left Ventricular Remodeling After Myocardial Infarction. *Circulation* **2000**, *101*, 2981–2988.
5. Rezkalla, S.H.; Stankowski, R.V.; Hanna, J.; Kloner, R.A. Management of No-Reflow Phenomenon in the Catheterization Laboratory. *JACC Cardiovasc. Interv.* **2017**, *10*, 215–223.
6. Barrabes, J.A. Comments on the 2015 ESC Guidelines for the Management of Acute Coronary Syndromes in Patients Presenting without Persistent ST-segment Elevation. *Rev. Española de Cardiol. (Engl. Ed.)* **2015**, *68*, 1061–1067.
7. Berezin, A.E. Endogenous vascular repair system in cardiovascular disease: The role of endothelial progenitor cells. *Australas. Med. J.* **2019**, *12*, 42–48.
8. Berezin, A.E. Epigenetics in heart failure phenotypes. *BBA Clin.* **2016**, *6*, 31–37.
9. Neri, M.; Riezzo, I.; Pascale, N.; Pomara, C.; Turillazzi, E. Ischemia/Reperfusion Injury following Acute Myocardial Infarction: A Critical Issue for Clinicians and Forensic Pathologists. *Mediat. Inflamm.* **2017**, *2017*, 14.
10. Berezin, A.E.; Berezin, A.A. Adverse cardiac remodeling after acute myocardial infarction: Old and new biomarkers. *Dis. Markers* **2020**, *2020*, 21.

11. Libby, P. The vascular biology of atherosclerosis. In *Braunwald's Heart Disease. A Textbook of Cardiovascular Medicine*, 9th ed.; Zipes, D.P., Libby, P., Bonow, R.O., Braunwald, E., Eds.; Elsevier Saunders: Philadelphia, PA, USA, 2012; pp. 1087–1110.
12. Peksiene, D.Z.; Portacenko, J. Left Ventricular Remodeling after Acute Myocardial Infarction and Biomarkers. *J. Cardiovasc. Dis. Diagn.* **2017**, *5*, 5. [CrossRef]
13. Anzai, T. Post-Infarction Inflammation and Left Ventricular Remodeling. *Circ. J.* **2013**, *77*, 580–587. [CrossRef] [PubMed]
14. Sgueglia, G.A.; D'Errico, F.; Gioffrè, G.; De Santis, A.; Summaria, F.; Piccioni, F.; Gaspardone, A. Angiographic and clinical performance of polymer-free biolimus-eluting stent in patients with ST-segment elevation acute myocardial infarction in a metropolitan public hospital: The BESAMI MUCHO study. *Catheter. Cardiovasc. Interv.* **2018**, *91*, 851–858. [PubMed]
15. Scarsini, R.; De Maria, G.L.; Borlotti, A.; Kotronias, R.A.; Langrish, J.P.; Lucking, A.J.; Choudhury, R.P.; Ferreira, V.M.; Ribichini, F.; Channon, K.M.; et al. Incremental Value of Coronary Microcirculation Resistive Reserve Ratio in Predicting the Extent of Myocardial Infarction in Patients with STEMI. Insights from the Oxford Acute Myocardial Infarction (OxAMI) Study. *Cardiovasc. Revascularization Med.* **2019**, *20*, 1148–1155. [CrossRef]
16. Long, B.; Li, N.; Xu, X.-X.; Li, X.-X.; Xu, X.-J.; Guo, D.; Zhang, D.; Wu, Z.-H.; Zhang, S.-Y. Long noncoding RNA FTX regulates cardiomyocyte apoptosis by targeting miR-29b-1-5p and Bcl2l2. *Biochem. Biophys. Res. Commun.* **2018**, *495*, 312–318. [CrossRef] [PubMed]
17. Zhang, N.; Meng, X.; Mei, L.; Hu, J.; Zhao, C.; Chen, W. The Long Non-Coding RNA SNHG1 Attenuates Cell Apoptosis by Regulating miR-195 and BCL2-Like Protein 2 in Human Cardiomyocytes. *Cell. Physiol. Biochem.* **2018**, *50*, 1029–1040. [CrossRef] [PubMed]
18. Christenson, R.H.; Azzazy, H.M. Biochemical markers of the acute coronary syndromes. *Clin. Chem.* **1998**, *44*, 1855–1864. [CrossRef] [PubMed]
19. Ahmad, M.I.; Sharma, N. Biomarkers in Acute Myocardial Infarction. *J. Clin. Exp. Cardiol.* **2012**, *3*, 222. [CrossRef]
20. Bloomberg, D.J.; Kimber, W.D.; Burke, M.D. Cretin kinase isoenzymes. Predictive value in the early diagnosis of acute myocardial infarction. *Am. J. Med.* **1975**, *59*, 464–469.
21. Ishikawa, Y.; Saffitz, J.E.; Mealman, T.L. Reversible myocardial ischemic injury is not associated with increased cretine kinase activity in plasma. *Clin. Chem.* **1997**, *43*, 467–475.
22. Jeffe, A.S. Biochemical detection of acute myocardial infarction. In *Acute Myocardial Infarction*; Gersh, B., Rahimtoola, S., Eds.; Elsevier Saunders: Philadelphia, PA, USA, 1991; pp. 110–127.
23. Wu, A.H.; Wang, X.M.; Gornet, T.G.; Ordonez-Llanos, J. Cretine kinase MB isoforms in patients with skeletal muscle injury: Ramifications for early detection of acute myocardial infarction. *Clin. Chem.* **1992**, *38*, 2396–2400.
24. Fioretti, P.; Sclavo, M.; Brower, R.W.; Simoons, M.L.; Hugenholtz, P.G. Prognosis of patients with different peak serum creatine kinase levels after first myocardial infarction. *Eur. Heart J.* **1985**, *6*, 473–478. [CrossRef]
25. Savonitto, S.; Granger, S.B.; Ardissino, D.; Gardner, L.; Cavallini, C.; Galvani, M.; Ottani, F.; White, H.D.; Armstrong, P.W.; Ohman, E.M.; et al. The prognostic value of cretine kinase elevations extends across the whole spectrum of acute coronary syndromes. *J. Am. Coll. Cardiol.* **2002**, *39*, 22–29.
26. Glezer, M.G.; Syrkin, A.L.; Gitel, E.P.; Sulimov, V.A.; Persiianov-Dubrov, I.V. Acute coronary syndrome without elevation of the ST segment: Prognostic significance of determining the levels of troponin I and CPK-MBmass. *Ter Arkh* **2002**, *74*, 26–30.
27. Szymanski, F.M.; Grabowski, M.; Filipiak, K.J.; Karpiński, G.; Hrynkiewicz, A.; Stolarz, P.; Oręziak, A.; Rudowski, R.; Opolski, G. Prognostic implications of myocardial necrosis triad markers' concentration measured at admission in patients with suspected acute coronary syndrome. *Am. J. Emerg. Med.* **2007**, *25*, 65–68. [CrossRef]
28. Carvalho, G.; Rassi, S. The Prognostic Value of CK-MB in Acute Myocardial Infarction in Developing Countries: A Descriptive Study. *Angiol. Open Access* **2016**, *4*, 3. [CrossRef]
29. Cavallini, C.; Savonitto, S.; Violini, R.; Arraiz, G.; Plebani, M.; Olivari, Z.; Rubartelli, P.; Battaglia, S.; Niccoli, L.; Steffenino, G.; et al. Impact of the elevation of biochemical markers of myocardial damage on long-term mortality after percutaneous coronary intervention: Results of the CK-MB and PCI study. *Eur. Heart J.* **2005**, *26*, 1494–1498. [CrossRef]
30. Abdelmeguid, A.E.; Topol, E.J.; Whitlow, P.L.; Sapp, S.K.; Ellis, S.G. Significance of mild transient release of creatinine kinase-MB fraction after percutaneous coronary intervention. *Circulation* **1996**, *94*, 1528–1536.

31. Kong, T.Q.; Davidson, C.J.; Meyers, S.N.; Tauke, J.T.; Parker, M.A.; Bonow, R.O. Prognostic implication of creatine kinase elevation following elective coronary artery interventions. *JAMA* **1997**, *277*, 461–466.
32. Akkerhuis, K.M.; Alexander, J.H.; Tardiff, B.E.; Boersma, E.; Harrington, R.A.; Lincoff, A.M.; Simmons, M.L. Minor myocardial damage and prognosis. Are spontaneous and percutaneous coronary intervention- related events different? *Circulation* **2002**, *105*, 554–556.
33. Ioannidis, J.P.; Karvouni, E.; Katritsis, D.G. Mortality risk conferred by small elevations of creatine kinase-MB isoenzyme after percutaneous coronary intervention. *J. Am. Coll. Cardiol.* **2003**, *42*, 1406–1411.
34. Roe, M.T.; Mahaffey, K.; Kilaru, R.; Alexander, J.; Akkerhuis, K.; Simoons, M.; Harrington, R.; Tardiff, B.; Granger, C.; Ohman, E.; et al. Creatine kinase-MB elevation after percutaneous coronary intervention predicts adverse outcomes in patients with acute coronary syndromes. *Eur. Heart J.* **2004**, *25*, 313–321.
35. Kini, A.; Marmur, J.D.; Kini, S.; Dangas, G.; Cocke, T.P.; Wallenstein, S.; Brown, E.; Ambrose, J.A.; Sharma, S.K. Creatine kinase-MB elevation after coronary intervention correlates with diffuse atherosclerosis, and low-to-medium level elevation has a benign clinical course. *J. Am. Coll. Cardiol.* **1999**, *34*, 663–671.
36. Baim, D.S.; Cutlip, D.E.; Sharma, S.; Ho, K.K.L.; Fortuna, R.; Schreiber, T.L.; Feldman, R.L.; Shani, J.; Senerchia, C.; Zhang, Y.; et al. Final Results of the Balloon vs Optimal Atherectomy Trial (BOAT). *Circulation* **1998**, *97*, 322–331.
37. Stone, G.W.; Mehran, R.; Dangas, G.; Lansky, A.J.; Kornowski, R.; Leon, M.B. Differential impact on survival of electrocardiographic Q-wave versus enzymatic myocardial infarction after percutaneous intervention: A device-specific analysis of 7147 patients. *Circulation* **2001**, *104*, 642–647.
38. Brener, S.; Ellis, S.; Schneider, J.; Topol, E.J. Frequency and long-term impact of myonecrosis after coronary stenting. *Eur. Heart J.* **2002**, *23*, 869–876.
39. Yee, K.C.; Mukherjee, D.; Smith, D.E.; Kline-Rogers, E.M.; Fang, J.; Mehta, R.H.; Almanaseer, Y.; Akhras, E.; Cooper, J.V.; Eagle, K.A. Prognostic significance of an elevated creatine kinase in the absence of an elevated troponin I during an acute coronary syndrome. *Am. J. Cardiol.* **2003**, *92*, 1442–1444.
40. Danne, O.; Lueders, C.; Storm, C.; Frei, U.; Möckel, M. Whole blood choline and plasma choline in acute coronary syndromes: Prognostic and pathophysiological implications. *Clin. Chim. Acta* **2007**, *383*, 103–109.
41. Rosenblat, J.; Zhang, A.; Fear, T. Biomarkers of myocardial infarction: Past, present and future. *UWOMJ* **2012**, *81*, 23–26.
42. Dubois-Deruy, E.; Richard, V.; Mulder, P.; Lamblin, N.; Drobecq, H.; Henry, J.-P.; Amouyel, P.; Thuillez, C.; Bauters, C.; Pinet, F. Decreased Serine207 phosphorylation of troponin T as a biomarker for left ventricular remodelling after myocardial infarction. *Eur. Heart J.* **2010**, *32*, 115–123.
43. Yan, A.T.; Yan, R.T.; Tan, M.; Chow, C.-M.; Fitchett, D.; Stanton, E.; Langer, A.; Goodman, S.G. Troponin is more useful than creatine kinase in predicting one-year mortality among acute coronary syndrome patients. *Eur. Heart J.* **2004**, *25*, 2006–2012.
44. Kazmi, K.A.; Bakr, A.; Perwaiz Iqbal, S.; Perwaiz Iqbal, M. Admission cretinkinase as a prognostic marker in acute myocardial infaction. *J. Pak. Med. Assoc.* **2009**, *59*, 819–822.
45. Matetzky, S.; Sharir, T.; Domingo, M.; Noc, M.; Chyu, K.-Y.; Kaul, S.; Eigler, N.; Shah, P.K.; Cercek, B. Elevated troponin I level on admission is associated with adverse outcome of primary angioplasty in acute myocardial infarction. *Circulation* **2000**, *102*, 1611–1616.
46. Rajappa, M.; Sharma, A. Biomarkers of Cardiac Injury: An Update. *Angiology* **2005**, *56*, 677–691.
47. Melanson, S.F.; Lewandrowski, E.L.; Januzzi, J.L.; Lewandrowski, K.B. Reevaluation of myoglobin for acute chest pain evaluation: Would false positive results on "first-draw" specimens lead to increased hospital admissions? *Am. J. Clin. Pathol.* **2004**, *121*, 804–808.
48. Newby, L.K.; Storrow, A.B.; Gibler, W.B.; Garvey, J.L.; Tucker, J.F.; Kaplan, A.L.; Schreiber, D.H.; Tuttle, R.H.; McNulty, S.E.; Ohman, E.M. Bedside multimarker testing for risk stratification in chest pain units: The chest pain evaluation by creatine kinase-MB, myoglobin, and troponin I (CHECKMATE) study. *Circulation* **2001**, *103*, 1832–1837.
49. Mccord, J.; Nowak, R.M.; Hudson, M.P.; McCullough, P.A.; Tomlanovich, M.C.; Jacobsen, G.; Tokarski, G.; Khoury, N.; Weaver, W. The prognostic significance of serial myoglobin, troponin I, and creatine kinase–MB measurements in patients evaluated in the emergency department for acute coronary syndrome. *Ann. Emerg. Med.* **2003**, *42*, 343–350.

50. Kontos, M.C.; Garg, R.; Anderson, F.P.; Roberts, C.S.; Ornato, J.P.; Tatum, J.L.; Jesse, R.L. Ability of myoglobin to predict mortality in patients admitted for exclusion of myocardial infarction. *Am. J. Emerg. Med.* **2007**, *25*, 873–879. [CrossRef]
51. Chen, Y.; Tao, Y.; Zhang, L.; Xu, W.; Zhou, X. Diagnostic and prognostic value of biomarkers in acute myocardial infarction. *Postgrad. Med. J.* **2019**, *95*, 210–216. [CrossRef]
52. Mehta, M.D.; Marwah, S.A.; Ghosh, S.; Shah, H.N.; Trivedi, A.P.; Haridas, N. A synergistic role of ischemia modified albumin and high-sensitivity troponin T in the early diagnosis of acute coronary syndrome. *J. Fam. Med. Prim. Care* **2015**, *4*, 570–575. [CrossRef]
53. Manini, A.F.; Ilgen, J.; E Noble, V.; Bamberg, F.; Koenig, W.; Bohan, J.S.; Hoffmann, U. Derivation and validation of a sensitive IMA cutpoint to predict cardiac events in patients with chest pain. *Emerg. Med. J.* **2009**, *26*, 791–796. [CrossRef]
54. Chan, D.C.S.; Ng, L.L. Biomarkers in acute myocardial infarction. *BMC Med.* **2010**, *8*, 34. [CrossRef]
55. Haltern, G.; Peiniger, S.; Bufe, A.; Reiss, G.; Gülker, H.; Scheffold, T. Comparison of Usefulness of Heart-Type Fatty Acid Binding Protein Versus Cardiac Troponin T for Diagnosis of Acute Myocardial Infarction. *Am. J. Cardiol.* **2010**, *105*, 1–9. [CrossRef] [PubMed]
56. Mad, P.; Domanovits, H.; Fazelnia, C.; Stiassny, K.; Russmüller, G.; Cseh, A.; Sodeck, G.; Binder, T.; Christ, G.; Szekeres, T.; et al. Human heart-type fatty-acid-binding protein as a point-of-care test in the early diagnosis of acute myocardial infarction. *QJM* **2007**, *100*, 203–210. [CrossRef]
57. Ryzgar, O.; Blige, A.K.; Bugra, Z. The use of human heart-type fatty-acid binding proteinas an early diagnostic biochemical marker of myocardial necrosis in patients with acute coronary syndrome, and its comparison with troponin T and creatine kinase-myocardial band. *Heart Vessel.* **2006**, *21*, 309–314.
58. Jolly, S.S.; Shenkman, H.; Brieger, D.; Fox, K.A.A.; Yan, A.T.; Eagle, K.A.; Steg, P.G.; Lim, K.-D.; Quill, A.L.; Goodman, S.G.; et al. Quantitative troponin and death, cardiogenic shock, cardiac arrest and new heart failure in patients with non-ST-segment elevation acute coronary syndromes (NSTE ACS): Insights from the Global Registry of Acute Coronary Events. *Heart* **2010**, *97*, 197–202. [CrossRef]
59. Erlikh, A.D.; Katrukha, A.G.; Trifonov, I.R.; Bereznikova, A.V.; A Gratsianskiĭ, N. Prognostic significance of heart fatty acid binding protein in patients with non-ST elevation acute coronary syndrome: Results of follow-up for twelve months. *Kardiologiia* **2005**, *45*, 13–21.
60. Jones, J.D.; Chew, P.G.; Dobson, R.; Wootton, A.; Ashrafi, R.; Khand, A. The Prognostic Value of Heart Type Fatty Acid Binding Protein in Patients with Suspected Acute Coronary Syndrome: A Systematic Review. *Curr. Cardiol. Rev.* **2017**, *13*, 189–198. [CrossRef]
61. Adela, R.; Banerjee, S.K. GDF-15 as a Target and Biomarker for Diabetes and Cardiovascular Diseases: A Translational Prospective. *J. Diabetes Res.* **2015**, *2015*, 1–14. [CrossRef]
62. Schaub, N.; Reichlin, T.; Twerenbold, R.; Reiter, M.; Steuer, S.; Bassetti, S.; Stelzig, C.; Wolf, C.; Winkler, K.; Haaf, P.; et al. Growth Differentiation Factor-15 in the Early Diagnosis and Risk Stratification of Patients with Acute Chest Pain. *Clin. Chem.* **2012**, *58*, 441–449. [CrossRef]
63. Kempf, T.; Björklund, E.; Olofsson, S.; Lindahl, B.; Allhoff, T.; Peter, T.; Tongers, J.; Wollert, K.C.; Wallentin, L. Growth-differentiation factor-15 improves risk stratification in ST-segment elevation myocardial infarction. *Eur. Heart J.* **2007**, *28*, 2858–2865. [CrossRef]
64. De Lemos, J.A.; Morrow, D.A. Brain Natriuretic Peptide Measurement in Acute Coronary Syndromes. *Circulation* **2002**, *106*, 2868–2870. [CrossRef] [PubMed]
65. Möckel, M.; Danne, O.; Muller, R.; Vollert, J.O.; Müller, C.; Lueders, C.; Stork, T.; Frei, U.; Koenig, W.; Dietz, R.; et al. Development of an optimized multimarker strategy for early risk assessment of patients with acute coronary syndromes. *Clin. Chim. Acta* **2008**, *393*, 103–109. [CrossRef] [PubMed]
66. Morrow, D.; De Lemos, J.; Sabatine, M. Evaluation of B-type natriuretic peptide for risk assessment in unstable angina/non-ST-elevation myocardial infarction B-type natriuretic peptide and prognosis in TACTICS-TIMI 18. *J. Am. Cardiol.* **2003**, *41*, 1264–1272.
67. Maisel, A.; Krishnawswamy, P.; Nowak, R. Rapid measurement of B-Type natriuretic peptide in the mergency diagnosis of heart failure. *N. Engl. J. Med.* **2002**, *11*, 55.
68. Neuhold, S.; Huelsmann, M.; Strunk, G.; Stoiser, B.; Struck, J.; Morgenthaler, N.; Bergmann, A.; Gouya, G.; Elhenicky, M.; Pacher, R. Comparison of copeptin B-type natriuretic peptide and amino-terminal pro-B-Type natriuretic peptide in patients with Chronic Heart Failure: Prediction of death at different stages of the disease. *J. Am. Coll. Cardiol.* **2008**, *52*, 266–272. [PubMed]

69. Leistner, D.M.; Klotsche, J.; Pieper, L.; Palm, S.; Stalla, G.K.; Lehnert, H.; Silber, S.; März, W.; Wittchen, H.-U.; Zeiher, A.M. Prognostic value of NT-pro-BNP and hs-CRP for risk stratification in primary care: Results from the population-based DETECT study. *Clin. Res. Cardiol.* **2013**, *102*, 259–268.
70. Niu, J.; Ma, Z.; Xie, C.; Zhang, Z. Association of plasma B-type natriuretic peptide concentration with myocardial infarct size in patients with acute myocardial infarction. *Genet. Mol. Res.* **2014**, *13*, 6177–6183.
71. Drewniak, W.; Szybka, W.; Bielecki, D.; Malinowski, M.; Kotlarska, J.; Krol-Jaskulska, A.; Popielarz-Grygalewicz, A.; Konwicka, A.; Dąbrowski, M. Prognostic Significance of NT-proBNP Levels in Patients over 65 Presenting Acute Myocardial Infarction Treated Invasively or Conservatively. *BioMed Res. Int.* **2015**, *2015*, 782026.
72. Islam, M.N.; Alam, M.F.; Debnath, R.C.; Aditya, G.P.; Ali, M.H.; Hossain, M.A.; Siddique, S.R. Correlation between Troponin-I and B-Type Natriuretic Peptide Level in Acute Myocardial Infarction Patients with Heart Failure. *Mymensingh Med. J.* **2016**, *25*, 226–231.
73. Reesukumal, K.; Pratumvinit, B. B-type natriuretic peptide not TIMI risk score predicts death after acute coronary syndrome. *Clin. Lab.* **2012**, *58*, 1017–1022.
74. Khan, S.Q.; Quinn, P.; Davies, J.E.; Ng, L.L. N-terminal pro-B-type natriuretic peptide is better than TIMI risk score at predicting death after acute myocardial infarction. *Heart* **2008**, *94*, 40–43.
75. Hamid, S.A.; Baxter, G.F. Adrenomedullin: Regulator of systemic and cardiac homeostasis in acute myocardial infarction. *Pharmacol. Ther.* **2005**, *105*, 95–112.
76. Yuyun, M.F.; Narayan, H.K.; Ng, L.L. Prognostic Significance of Adrenomedullin in Patients with Heart Failure and with Myocardial Infarction. *Am. J. Cardiol.* **2015**, *115*, 986–991.
77. Liu, J.; Masoudi, F.A.; Spertus, J.A.; Wang, Q.; Murugiah, K.; Spatz, E.S.; Li, J.; Li, X.; Ross, J.S.; Krumholz, H.M.; et al. Patterns of Use of Angiotensin-Converting Enzyme Inhibitors/Angiotensin Receptor Blockers Among Patients with Acute Myocardial Infarction in China From 2001 to 2011: China PEACE-Retrospective AMI Study. *J. Am. Heart Assoc.* **2015**, *4*, e001343.
78. Pitt, B.; Bakris, G.; Ruilope, L.M.; Dicarlo, L.; Mukherjee, R. On behalf of the EPHESUS Investigators Serum Potassium and Clinical Outcomes in the Eplerenone Post–Acute Myocardial Infarction Heart Failure Efficacy and Survival Study (EPHESUS). *Circulation* **2008**, *118*, 1643–1650.
79. Velagaleti, R.S.; Gona, P.; Levy, D.; Aragam, J.; Larson, M.G.; Tofler, G.H.; Lieb, W.; Wang, T.J.; Benjamin, E.J.; Vasan, R.S. Relations of Biomarkers Representing Distinct Biological Pathways to Left Ventricular Geometry. *Circulation* **2008**, *118*, 2252–2258.
80. Nagai, T.; Anzai, T.; Kaneko, H.; Mano, Y.; Anzai, A.; Maekawa, Y.; Takahashi, T.; Meguro, T.; Yoshikawa, T.; Fukuda, K. C-Reactive Protein Overexpression Exacerbates Pressure Overload–Induced Cardiac Remodeling Through Enhanced Inflammatory Response. *Hypertension* **2011**, *57*, 208–215.
81. Zhang, R.; Zhang, Y.Y.; Huang, X.R.; Wu, Y.; Chung, A.C.; Wu, E.X.; Szalai, A.J.; Wong, B.C.; Lau, C.-P.; Lan, H.Y. C-Reactive Protein Promotes Cardiac Fibrosis and Inflammation in Angiotensin II–Induced Hypertensive Cardiac Disease. *Hypertension* **2010**, *55*, 953–960.
82. Wang, J.; Tang, B.; Liu, X.; Wu, X.; Wang, H.; Xu, D.; Guo, Y. Increased monomeric CRP levels in acute myocardial infarction: A possible new and specific biomarker for diagnosis and severity assessment of disease. *Atherosclerosis* **2015**, *239*, 343–349.
83. Ørn, S.; Manhenke, C.; Ueland, T.; Damås, J.K.; Mollnes, T.E.; Edvardsen, T.; Aukrust, P.; Dickstein, K. C-reactive protein, infarct size, microvascular obstruction, and left-ventricular remodelling following acute myocardial infarction. *Eur. Heart J.* **2009**, *30*, 1180–1186.
84. Schoos, M.M.; Munthe-Fog, L.; Skjoedt, M.-O.; Ripa, R.S.; Lønborg, J.; Kastrup, J.; Kelbæk, H.; Laursen, P.N.; Garred, P. Association between lectin complement pathway initiators, C-reactive protein and left ventricular remodeling in myocardial infarction—A magnetic resonance study. *Mol. Immunol.* **2013**, *54*, 408–414.
85. Puljak, L.; Lukin, A.; Novak, K.; Polić, S. Prognostic value of low and moderately elevated C-reactive protein in acute coronary syndrome: A 2-year follow-up study. *Med. Sci. Monit.* **2013**, *19*, 777–786.
86. He, L.-P.; Tang, X.-Y.; Ling, W.-H.; Chen, W.-Q.; Chen, Y.-M. Early C-reactive protein in the prediction of long-term outcomes after acute coronary syndromes: A meta-analysis of longitudinal studies. *Heart* **2010**, *96*, 339–346.
87. Bodi, V.; Sanchis, J.; Llácer, A.; Facila, L.; Núñez, J.; Pellicer, M.; Bertomeu, V.; Ruiz, V.; Chorro, F.J. Prognostic markers of non-ST elevation acute coronary syndromes. *Rev. Española de Cardiol.* **2003**, *56*, 857.

88. Fertin, M.; Hennache, B.; Hamon, M.; Ennezat, P.V.; Biausque, F.; Elkohen, M.; Nugue, O.; Tricot, O.; Lamblin, N.; Pinet, F.; et al. Usefulness of Serial Assessment of B-Type Natriuretic Peptide, Troponin I, and C-Reactive Protein to Predict Left Ventricular Remodeling After Acute Myocardial Infarction (from the REVE-2 Study). *Am. J. Cardiol.* **2010**, *106*, 1410–1416. [CrossRef]
89. Hamzic-Mehmedbasic, A. Inflammatory Cytokines as Risk Factors for Mortality After Acute Cardiac Events. *Med. Arch.* **2016**, *70*, 252–255. [CrossRef]
90. Yousuf, O.; Mohanty, B.D.; Martin, S.S.; Joshi, P.H.; Blaha, M.J.; Nasir, K.; Blumenthal, R.S.; Budoff, M.J. High-Sensitivity C-Reactive Protein and Cardiovascular Disease. *J. Am. Coll. Cardiol.* **2013**, *62*, 397–408. [CrossRef]
91. Puri, R.; Nissen, S.E.; Shao, M.; Uno, K.; Kataoka, Y.; Kapadia, S.R.; Tuzcu, E.M.; Nicholls, S.J. Impact of Baseline Lipoprotein and C-Reactive Protein Levels on Coronary Atheroma Regression Following High-Intensity Statin Therapy. *Am. J. Cardiol.* **2014**, *114*, 1465–1472. [CrossRef]
92. Mueller, C. Biomarkers and acute coronary syndromes: An update. *Eur. Heart J.* **2014**, *35*, 552–556. [CrossRef]
93. Duffy, J.R.; Salerno, M. New Blood Test to Measure Heart Attack Risk. *J. Cardiovasc. Nurs.* **2004**, *19*, 425–429. [CrossRef]
94. De Servi, S.; Mariani, M.; Mariani, G.; Mazzone, A. C-reactive protein increase in unstable coronary disease cause or effect? *J. Am. Cardiol.* **2005**, *456*, 1496–1502.
95. Bodi, V.; Sanchis, J.; Lopez Llereu, M.P.; Losada, A.; Nunez, J.; Pellicer, M.; Bertomeu, V.; Chorro, F.J.; Llacer, A. Usefullness of comprehensive cardiovascular magnetic resonance imaging assessment for predicting recovery of left ventricular wall motion in the setting of myocardial stunning. *J. Am. Cardiol.* **2005**, *46*, 1747–1752.
96. García-Salas, J.M.; Tello-Montoliu, A.; Manzano-Fernández, S.; Casas-Pina, T.; López-Cuenca, A.; Pérez-Berbel, P.; Puche-Morenilla, C.; Martínez-Hernández, P.; Valdés, M.; Marín, F. Interleukin-6 as a predictor of cardiovascular events in troponin-negative non-ST elevation acute coronary syndrome patients. *Int. J. Clin. Pract.* **2014**, *68*, 294–303. [CrossRef]
97. Kubková, L.; Spinar, J.; Goldbergová, M.P.; Jarkovský, J.; Pařenica, J. Inflammatory response and C-reactive protein value in patient with acute coronary syndrome. *Vnitrni Lek.* **2013**, *59*, 981–988.
98. Cherneva, Z.V.; Denchev, S.V.; Gospodinova, M.V.; Cakova, A.; Cherneva, R.V. Inflammatory cytokines at admission-independent prognostic markers in patients with acute coronary syndrome and hyperglycemia. *Acute Card Care* **2012**, *14*, 13–19.
99. Hofmann, U.; Knorr, S.; Vogel, B.; Weirather, J.; Frey, A.; Ertl, G.; Frantz, S. Interleukin-13 Deficiency Aggravates Healing and Remodeling in Male Mice After Experimental Myocardial Infarction. *Circ. Heart Fail.* **2014**, *7*, 822–830. [CrossRef]
100. Savvatis, K.; Pappritz, K.; Becher, P.M.; Lindner, D.; Zietsch, C.; Volk, H.-D.; Westermann, D.; Schultheiss, H.-P.; Tschöpe, C. Interleukin-23 Deficiency Leads to Impaired Wound Healing and Adverse Prognosis After Myocardial Infarction. *Circ. Heart Fail.* **2014**, *7*, 161–171. [CrossRef]
101. Wei, Y.; Lan, Y.; Zhong, Y.; Yu, K.; Xu, W.; Zhu, R.; Sun, H.; Ding, Y.; Wang, Y.; Zeng, Q. Interleukin-38 alleviates cardiac remodelling after myocardial infarction. *J. Cell. Mol. Med.* **2020**, *24*, 371–384. [CrossRef]
102. Toss, H.; Lindahl, B.; Siegbahn, A.; Wallentin, L. Prognostic Influence of Increased Fibrinogen and C-Reactive Protein Levels in Unstable Coronary Artery Disease. *Circulation* **1997**, *96*, 4204–4210. [CrossRef]
103. Sanchis, J.; Bodi, V.; Navarro, A.; Llacer, A.; Nunez, J.; Blasco, M.; Mainar, L.; Monmeneu, J.V.; Insa, L.; Ferrero, J.A.; et al. Factores prognosticos en la angina inestable con cambios dinamicos del electrocardiograma. Valor del fibrinogeno. *Rev. Esp. Cardiol.* **2002**, *55*, 921–927.
104. Bozkurt, E.; Erol, M.K.; Keleş, S.; Acikel, M.; Yilmaz, M.; Gurlertop, Y.; Yilmaz, M. Relation of plasma homocysteine levels to intracoronary thrombus in unstable angina pectoris and in non–Q-wave acute myocardial infarction. *Am. J. Cardiol.* **2002**, *90*, 413–415. [CrossRef] [PubMed]
105. Kafkas, N.; Venetsanou, K.; Patsilinakos, S.; Voudris, V.; Antonatos, D.; Kelesidis, K.; Baltopoulos, G.; Maniatis, P.; Cokkinos, D.V. Procalcitonin in acute myocardial infarction. *Acute Card. Care* **2008**, *10*, 30–36. [CrossRef] [PubMed]
106. Ataoğlu, H.E.; Yilmaz, F.; Uzunhasan, I.; Çetin, F.; Temiz, L.; Döventaş, Y.E.; Kaya, A.; Yenigün, M. Procalcitonin: A Novel Cardiac Marker with Prognostic Value in Acute Coronary Syndrome. *J. Int. Med. Res.* **2010**, *38*, 52–61. [CrossRef] [PubMed]
107. Kelly, D.; Khan, S.Q.; Dhillon, O.; Quinn, P.; Struck, J.; Squire, I.B.; Davies, J.E.; Ng, L.L. Procalcitonin as a prognostic marker in patients with acute myocardial infarction. *Biomarkers* **2010**, *15*, 325–331. [CrossRef]

108. Lau, D.; Baldus, S. Myeloperoxidase and its contributory role in inflammatory vascular disease. *Pharmacol. Ther.* **2006**, *111*, 16–26.
109. Abu-Soud, H.M.; Hazen, S.L. Nitric Oxide Is a Physiological Substrate for Mammalian Peroxidases. *J. Biol. Chem.* **2000**, *275*, 37524–37532.
110. Vasilyev, N.; Williams, T.; Brennan, M.-L.; Unzek, S.; Zhou, X.; Heinecke, J.W.; Spitz, D.R.; Topol, E.J.; Hazen, S.L.; Penn, M.S. Myeloperoxidase-Generated Oxidants Modulate Left Ventricular Remodeling but Not Infarct Size After Myocardial Infarction. *Circulation* **2005**, *112*, 2812–2820.
111. Askari, A.T.; Brennan, M.-L.; Zhou, X.; Drinko, J.; Morehead, A.; Thomas, J.D.; Topol, E.J.; Hazen, S.L.; Penn, M.S. Myeloperoxidase and Plasminogen Activator Inhibitor 1 Play a Central Role in Ventricular Remodeling after Myocardial Infarction. *J. Exp. Med.* **2003**, *197*, 615–624.
112. Mollenhauer, M.; Firedrichs, K.; Lange, K.; Gesenberg, J.; Remane, L.; Kerkenpas, C.; Krause, J.; Schneider, J.; Ravekes, T.; Maass, M.; et al. Myeloperoxidase mediates postischemic arrhytmogenic ventricular remodeling. *Circ. Res.* **2017**, *121*, 56–70.
113. Eggers, K.M.; Dellborg, M.; Johnston, N.; Oldgren, J.; Swahn, E.; Venge, P.; Lindahl, B. Myeloperoxidase is not useful for the early assessment of patients with chest pain. *Clin. Biochem.* **2010**, *43*, 240–245.
114. Hochholzer, W.; Morrow, D.A.; Giugliano, R.P. Novel biomarkers in cardiovascular disease: Update 2010. *Am. Heart J.* **2010**, *160*, 583–594.
115. Omran, M.M.; Zahran, F.M.; Kadry, M.; Belal, A.A.M.; Emran, T.M. Role of myeloperoxidase in early diagnosis of acute myocardial infarction in patients admitted with chest pain. *J. Immunoass. Immunochem.* **2018**, *39*, 337–347.
116. Urbano-Moral, J.A.; Lopez-Haldon, J.E.; Fernandez, M.; Mancha, F.; Sanchez, A.; Rodriguez-Puras, M.J.; Villa, M.; Lopez-Pardo, F.; De La Llera, L.D.; Valle, J.I.; et al. Prognostic value of different serum biomarkers for left ventricular remodelling after ST-elevation myocardial infarction treated with primary percutaneous coronary intervention. *BMJ* **2012**, *48*, 15–18.
117. Mittal, B.; Mishra, A.; Srivastava, A.; Kumar, S.; Garg, N. Matrix Metalloproteinases in Coronary Artery Disease. *Int. Rev. Cytol.* **2014**, *64*, 1–72.
118. Moore, L.; Fan, D.; Basu, R.; Kandalam, V.; Kassiri, Z. Tissue inhibitor of metalloproteinases (TIMPs) in heart failure. *Heart Fail. Rev.* **2011**, *17*, 693–706.
119. Nuttall, R.K.; Sampieri, C.L.; Pennington, C.J.; E Gill, S.; A Schultz, G.; Edwards, D.R. Expression analysis of the entire MMP and TIMP gene families during mouse tissue development. *FEBS Lett.* **2004**, *563*, 129–134.
120. Visse, R.; Nagase, H. Matrix Metalloproteinases and Tissue Inhibitors of Metalloproteinases. *Circ. Res.* **2003**, *92*, 827–839.
121. Kandalam, V.; Basu, R.; Abraham, T.; Wang, X.; Soloway, P.D.; Jaworski, D.M.; Oudit, G.Y.; Kassiri, Z. TIMP2 Deficiency Accelerates Adverse Post–Myocardial Infarction Remodeling Because of Enhanced MT1-MMP Activity Despite Lack of MMP2 Activation. *Circ. Res.* **2010**, *106*, 796–808.
122. Li, Y.Y.; Feng, Y.; McTiernan, C.F.; Pei, W.; Moravec, C.S.; Wang, P.; Rosenblum, W.; Kormos, R.L.; Feldman, A.M. Downregulation of Matrix Metalloproteinases and Reduction in Collagen Damage in the Failing Human Heart After Support With Left Ventricular Assist Devices. *Circulation* **2001**, *104*, 1147–1152.
123. Heymans, S.; Schroen, B.; Vermeersch, P.; Milting, H.; Gao, F.; Kassner, A.; Gillijns, H.; Herijgers, P.; Flameng, W.; Carmeliet, P.; et al. Increased Cardiac Expression of Tissue Inhibitor of Metalloproteinase-1 and Tissue Inhibitor of Metalloproteinase-2 Is Related to Cardiac Fibrosis and Dysfunction in the Chronic Pressure-Overloaded Human Heart. *Circulation* **2005**, *112*, 1136–1144.
124. Vanhoutte, D.; Heymans, S. TIMPs and cardiac remodeling: Embracing the MMP-independent-side of the family. *J. Mol. Cell. Cardiol.* **2010**, *48*, 445–453.
125. Page-McCaw, A.; Ewald, A.J.; Werb, Z. Matrix metalloproteinases and the regulation of tissue remodelling. *Nat. Rev. Mol. Cell Biol.* **2007**, *8*, 221–233.
126. Shi, Q.; Liu, X.; Bai, Y.; Cui, C.; Li, J.; Li, Y.; Hu, S.; Wei, Y.-J. In Vitro Effects of Pirfenidone on Cardiac Fibroblasts: Proliferation, Myofibroblast Differentiation, Migration and Cytokine Secretion. *PLoS ONE* **2011**, *6*, e28134.
127. Tyagi, S.C.; Kumar, S.G.; Banks, J.; Fortson, W. Co-expression of tissue inhibitor and matrix metalloproteinase in myocardium. *J. Mol. Cell. Cardiol.* **1995**, *27*, 2177–2189.

128. Awad, A.E.; Kandalam, V.; Chakrabarti, S.; Wang, X.; Penninger, J.M.; Davidge, S.T.; Oudit, G.Y.; Kassiri, Z. Tumor necrosis factor induces matrix metalloproteinases in cardiomyocytes and cardiofibroblasts differentially via superoxide production in a PI3Kγ-dependent manner. *Am. J. Physiol. Physiol.* **2010**, *298*, C679–C692. [CrossRef]
129. Deschamps, A.M.; Spinale, F.G. Pathways of matrix metalloproteinase induction in heart failure: Bioactive molecules and transcriptional regulation. *Cardiovasc. Res.* **2006**, *69*, 666–676. [CrossRef] [PubMed]
130. Tsuruda, T.; Boerrigter, G.; Huntley, B.K.; Noser, J.A.; Cataliotti, A.; Costello-Boerrigter, L.C.; Chen, H.H.; Burnett, J.C. Brain Natriuretic Peptide Is Produced in Cardiac Fibroblasts and Induces Matrix Metalloproteinases. *Circ. Res.* **2002**, *91*, 1127–1134. [CrossRef] [PubMed]
131. Zavadzkas, J.A.; Mukherjee, R.; Rivers, W.T.; Patel, R.K.; Meyer, E.C.; Black, L.E.; McKinney, R.A.; Oelsen, J.M.; Stroud, R.E.; Spinale, F.G. Direct regulation of membrane type 1 matrix metalloproteinase following myocardial infarction causes changes in survival, cardiac function, and remodeling. *Am. J. Physiol. Circ. Physiol.* **2011**, *301*, H1656–H1666. [CrossRef]
132. Spinale, F.G.; Escobar, G.P.; Mukherjee, R.; Zavadzkas, J.A.; Saunders, S.M.; Jeffords, L.B.; Leone, A.M.; Beck, C.; Bouges, S.; Stroud, R.E. Cardiac-restricted overexpression of membrane type-1 matrix metalloproteinase in mice: Effects on myocardial remodeling with aging. *Circ. Heart Fail.* **2009**, *2*, 351–360. [CrossRef]
133. Halade, G.V.; Jin, Y.-F.; Lindsey, M.L. Matrix metalloproteinase (MMP)-9: A proximal biomarker for cardiac remodeling and a distal biomarker for inflammation. *Pharmacol. Ther.* **2013**, *139*, 32–40. [CrossRef]
134. Eschalier, R.; Fertin, M.; Fay, R.; Bauters, C.; Zannad, F.; Pinet, F.; Rossignol, P. Extracellular Matrix Turnover Biomarkers Predict Long-Term Left Ventricular Remodeling After Myocardial Infarction Insights From the REVE-2 Study. *Circ. Heart Fail.* **2013**, *6*, 1199–1205. [PubMed]
135. Iraqi, W.; Rossignol, P.; Angioi, M.; Fay, R.; Nuée, J.; Ketelslegers, J.-M.; Vincent, J.; Pitt, B.; Zannad, F. Extracellular Cardiac Matrix Biomarkers in Patients with Acute Myocardial Infarction Complicated by Left Ventricular Dysfunction and Heart Failure. *Circulation* **2009**, *119*, 2471–2479. [CrossRef] [PubMed]
136. Sun, Y. Infarct scar: A dynamic tissue. *Cardiovasc. Res.* **2000**, *46*, 250–256. [CrossRef] [PubMed]
137. Lindsey, M.L.; Mann, D.L.; Entman, M.L.; Spinale, F.G. Extracellular matrix remodeling following myocardial injury. *Ann. Med.* **2003**, *35*, 316–326. [CrossRef] [PubMed]
138. Bowers, S.L.; Banerjee, I.; Baudino, T.A. The extracellular matrix: At the center of it all. *J. Mol. Cell. Cardiol.* **2010**, *48*, 474–482. [CrossRef] [PubMed]
139. Jourdan-LeSaux, C.; Zhang, J.; Lindsey, M.L. Extracellular matrix roles during cardiac repair. *Life Sci.* **2010**, *87*, 391–400. [CrossRef]
140. Kang, Q.; Li, X.; Yang, M.; Fernando, T.; Wan, Z. Galectin-3 in patients with coronary heart disease and atrial fibrillation. *Clin. Chim. Acta* **2018**, *478*, 166–170. [CrossRef]
141. Bivona, G.; Bellia, C.; Sasso, B.L.; Agnello, L.; Scazzone, C.; Novo, G.; Ciaccio, M. Short-term Changes in Gal 3 Circulating Levels After Acute Myocardial Infarction. *Arch. Med. Res.* **2016**, *47*, 521–525. [CrossRef]
142. Gonzalez, G.E.; Cassaglia, P.; Truant, S.N.; Fernández, M.M.; Wilensky, L.; Volberg, V.; Malchiodi, E.L.; Morales, C.; Gelpi, R.J. Galectin-3 is essential for early wound healing and ventricular remodeling after myocardial infarction in mice. *Int. J. Cardiol.* **2014**, *176*, 1423–1425. [CrossRef]
143. Tsai, T.-H.; Sung, P.-H.; Chang, L.-T.; Sun, C.-K.; Yeh, K.-H.; Chung, S.-Y.; Chua, S.; Chen, Y.-L.; Wu, C.-J.; Chang, H.-W.; et al. Value and level of galectin-3 in acute myocardial infarction patients undergoing primary percutaneous coronary intervention. *J. Atheroscler. Thromb.* **2012**, *19*, 1073–1082. [CrossRef]
144. Weir, R.A.; Petrie, C.J.; Murphy, C.A.; Clements, S.; Steedman, T.; Miller, A.M.; McInnes, I.B.; Squire, I.B.; Ng, L.L.; Dargie, H.J.; et al. Galectin-3 and Cardiac Function in Survivors of Acute Myocardial Infarction. *Circ. Heart Fail.* **2013**, *6*, 492–498. [CrossRef] [PubMed]
145. Di Tano, G.; Caretta, G.; De Maria, R.; Parolini, M.; Bassi, L.; Testa, S.; Pirelli, S. Galectin-3 predicts left ventricular remodelling after anterior-wall myocardial infarction treated by primary percutaneous coronary intervention. *Heart* **2014**, *103*, 1–5.
146. Andrejic, O.M.; Vucic, R.M.; Pavlovic, M.; McClements, L.; Stokanovic, D.; Jevtovic–Stoimenov, T.; Nikolic, V.N. Association between Galectin-3 levels within central and peripheral venous blood, and adverse left ventricular remodelling after first acute myocardial infarction. *Sci. Rep.* **2019**, *9*, 131–145. [CrossRef]
147. Kohli, P.; Bonaca, M.P.; Kakkar, R.; Kudinova, A.Y.; Scirica, B.M.; Sabatine, M.S.; Murphy, S.A.; Braunwald, E.; Lee, R.T.; Morrow, D.A. Role of ST2 in Non–ST-Elevation Acute Coronary Syndrome in the MERLIN-TIMI 36 Trial. *Clin. Chem.* **2012**, *58*, 257–266. [CrossRef]

148. Salvagno, G.L.; Pavan, C. Prognostic biomarkers in acute coronary syndrome. *Ann. Transl. Med.* **2016**, *4*, 258.
149. Zhang, K.; Zhang, X.-C.; Mi, Y.-H.; Liu, J. Predicting value of serum soluble ST2 and interleukin-33 for risk stratification and prognosis in patients with acute myocardial infarction. *Chin. Med. J.* **2013**, *126*, 3628–3631.
150. Sun, T.; Dong, Y.-H.; Du, W.; Shi, C.-Y.; Wang, K.; Akram, J.; Wang, J.; Li, P. The Role of MicroRNAs in Myocardial Infarction: From Molecular Mechanism to Clinical Application. *Int. J. Mol. Sci.* **2017**, *18*, 745.
151. Gidlöf, O.; Smith, J.G.; Miyazu, K.; Gilje, P.; Spencer, A.; Blomquist, S.; Erlinge, D. Circulating cardio-enriched microRNAs are associated with long-term prognosis following myocardial infarction. *BMC Cardiovasc. Disord.* **2013**, *13*, 12.
152. Xiao, J.; Shen, B.; Li, J.; Lv, D.; Zhao, Y.; Wang, F.; Xu, J. Serum microRNA-499 and microRNA-208a as biomarkers of acute myocardial infarction. *Int. J. Clin. Exp. Med.* **2014**, *7*, 136–141.
153. Zhu, J.; Yao, K.; Wang, Q.; Guo, J.; Shi, H.; Ma, L. Circulating miRNA-181a as a potential novel biomarker for diagnosis of acute myocardial infarction. *Cell Physiol. Biochem.* **2016**, *40*, 1591–1602.
154. Zhang, Y.; Cheng, J.; Chen, F.; Wu, C.; Zhang, J.; Ren, X.; Pan, Y.; Nie, B.; Li, Q.; Li, Y. Circulating endothelial microparticles and miR-92a in acute myocardial infarction. *Biosci. Rep.* **2017**, *37*, 37.
155. Oerlemans, M.I.F.J.; Mosterd, A.; Dekker, M.S.; De Vrey, E.A.; Van Mil, A.; Pasterkamp, G.; Doevendans, P.A.; Hoes, A.W.; Sluijter, J.P.G. Early assessment of acute coronary syndromes in the emergency department: The potential diagnostic value of circulating microRNAs. *EMBO Mol. Med.* **2012**, *4*, 1176–1185.
156. Schulte, C.; Molz, S.; Appelbaum, S.; Karakas, M.; Ojeda, F.; Lau, D.M.; Hartmann, T.; Lackner, K.J.; Westermann, D.; Schnabel, R.B.; et al. miRNANA-197 and miRNANA-223 predict cardiovascular death in a cohort of patients with symptomatic coronary artery disease. *PLoS ONE* **2015**, *10*, e0145930.
157. He, F.; Lv, P.; Zhao, X.; Wang, X.; Ma, X.; Meng, W.; Meng, X.; Dong, S. Predictive value of circulating miR-328 and miR-134 for acute myocardial infarction. *Mol. Cell. Biochem.* **2014**, *394*, 137–144.
158. Lv, P.; Zhou, M.; He, J.; Meng, W.; Ma, X.; Dong, S.; Meng, X.; Zhao, X.; Wang, X.; He, F. Circulating miR-208b and miR-34a are Associated with Left Ventricular Remodeling after Acute Myocardial Infarction. *Int. J. Mol. Sci.* **2014**, *15*, 5774–5788.
159. Wang, C.; Jing, Q. Non-coding RNAs as biomarkers for acute myocardial infarction. *Acta Pharmacol. Sin.* **2018**, *39*, 1110–1119.
160. Devaux, Y.; Vausort, M.; McCann, G.P.; Zangrando, J.; Kelly, D.; Razvi, N.; Zhang, L.; Ng, L.L.; Wagner, D.R.; Squire, I.B. MicroRNA-150: A novel marker of left ventricular remodeling after acute myocardial infarction. *Circ. Cardiovasc. Genet.* **2013**, *6*, 290–298.
161. Galeano-Otero, I.; Del Toro, R.; Rasco, A.G.; Díaz, I.; Mayoral-González, I.; Guerrero-Márquez, F.; Gutiérrez-Carretero, E.; Casquero-Domínguez, S.; De La Llera, L.S.D.; Barón-Esquivias, G.; et al. Circulating miR-320a as a Predictive Biomarker for Left Ventricular Remodelling in STEMI Patients Undergoing Primary Percutaneous Coronary Intervention. *J. Clin. Med.* **2020**, *9*, 1051.
162. Widera, C.; Gupta, S.K.; Lorenzen, J.M.; Bang, C.; Bauersachs, J.; Bethmann, K.; Kempf, T.; Wollert, K.C.; Thum, T. Diagnostic and prognostic impact of six circulating microRNAs in acute coronary syndrome. *J. Mol. Cell. Cardiol.* **2011**, *51*, 872–875.
163. Goretti, E.; Vausort, M.; Wagner, D.R.; Devaux, Y. Association between circulating microRNAs, cardiovascular risk factors and outcome in patients with acute myocardial infarction. *Int. J. Cardiol.* **2013**, *t168*, 4548–4550.
164. Olivieri, F.; Antonicelli, R.; Spazzafumo, L.; Santini, G.; Rippo, M.R.; Galeazzi, R.; Giovagnetti, S.; D'Alessandra, Y.; Marcheselli, F.; Capogrossi, M.C.; et al. Admission levels of circulating miRNA-499-5p and risk of death in elderly patients after acute non-ST elevation myocardial infarction. *Int. J. Cardiol.* **2014**, *172*, 276–278.
165. Matsumoto, S.; Sakata, Y.; Nakatani, D.; Suna, S.; Mizuno, H.; Shimizu, M.; Usami, M.; Sasaki, T.; Sato, H.; Kawahara, Y.; et al. A subset of circulating microRNAs are predictive for cardiac death after discharge for acute myocardial infarction. *Biochem. Biophys. Res. Commun.* **2012**, *427*, 280–284.
166. Matsumoto, S.; Sakata, Y.; Suna, S.; Nakatani, D.; Usami, M.; Hara, M.; Kitamura, T.; Hamasaki, T.; Nanto, S.; Kawahara, Y.; et al. Circulating p53-responsive microRNAs are predictive indicators of heart failure after acute myocardial infaction. *Circ. Res.* **2013**, *113*, 322–326.
167. Dong, Y.M.; Liu, X.X.; Wei, G.Q.; Da, Y.N.; Cha, L.; Ma, C.S. Prediction of long-term outcome after acute myocardial infaction using circulating miRNA-145. *Scand. J. Clin. Lab. Investig.* **2015**, *75*, 85–91.

168. Cortez-Dias, N.; Costa, M.C.; Carrilho-Ferreira, P.; Silva, D.; Jorge, C.; Calisto, C.; Pessoa, T.; Martins, S.R.; De Sousa, J.C.; Da Silva, P.C.; et al. Circulating miR-122-5p/miR-133b Ratio Is a Specific Early Prognostic Biomarker in Acute Myocardial Infarction. *Circ. J.* **2016**, *80*, 2183–2191. [CrossRef]
169. Eitel, L.; Adams, V.; Dieterich, P.; Fuernau, G.; de Waha, S.; Desch, S.; Schuler, G.; Thiele, H. Relation of circular microRNS-133a concentrations with myocardial damage and clinical prognosis in ST-elevation myocardial infaction. *Am. Heart J.* **2012**, *164*, 706–714.
170. Vausort, M.; Wagner, D.R.; Devaux, Y. Long Noncoding RNAs in Patients with Acute Myocardial Infarction. *Circ. Res.* **2014**, *115*, 668–677. [CrossRef]
171. Zhai, H.; Li, X.-M.; Liu, F.; Chen, B.-D.; Zheng, H.; Wang, X.-M.; Liao, W.; Chen, Q.-J.; Ma, Y.-T.; Yang, Y.-N. Expression pattern of genome-scale long noncoding RNA following acute myocardial infarction in Chinese Uyghur patients. *Oncotarget* **2017**, *8*, 31449–31464. [CrossRef]
172. Qu, X.; Song, X.; Yuan, W.; Shu, Y.; Wang, Y.; Zhao, X.; Gao, M.; Lu, R.; Luo, S.; Zhao, W.; et al. Expression signature of lncRNAs and their potential roles in cardiac fibrosis of post-infarct mice. *Biosci. Rep.* **2016**, *36*, 00337. [CrossRef]
173. Devaux, Y.; Vausort, M.; McCann, G.P.; Kelly, D.; Collignon, O.; Ng, L.L.; Wagner, R.D.; Squire, I.B. A panel of 4 microRNAs facilitates the prediction of left ventricular contractility after acute myocardial infarction. *PLoS ONE* **2013**, *8*, e70644.
174. Liu, X.; Dong, Y.; Chen, S.; Zhang, G.; Zhang, M.; Gong, Y.; Li, X. Circulating MicroRNA-146a and MicroRNA-21 Predict Left Ventricular Remodeling after ST-Elevation Myocardial Infarction. *Cardiology* **2015**, *132*, 233–241. [CrossRef] [PubMed]
175. Vausort, M.; Salgado-Somoza, A.; Zhang, L.; Leszek, P.; Scholz, M.; Teren, A.; Burkhardt, R.; Thiery, J.; Wagner, D.R.; Devaux, Y. Myocardial Infarction-Associated Circular RNA Predicting Left Ventricular Dysfunction. *J. Am. Coll. Cardiol.* **2016**, *68*, 1247–1248. [CrossRef] [PubMed]
176. Kim, H.; Yang, D.H.; Park, Y.; Han, J.; Lee, H.; Kang, H.; Park, H.S.; Cho, Y.; Chae, S.C.; Jun, J.-E.; et al. Incremental Prognostic Value of C-Reactive Protein and N-Terminal ProB-Type Natriuretic Peptide in Acute Coronary Syndrome. *Circ. J.* **2006**, *70*, 1379–1384. [CrossRef] [PubMed]
177. O'Donoghue, M.L.; Morrow, D.A.; Cannon, C.P.; Jarolim, P.; Desai, N.R.; Sherwood, M.W.; Murphy, S.A.; Gerszten, R.E.; Sabatine, M.S. Multimarker Risk Stratification in Patients with Acute Myocardial Infarction. *J. Am. Heart Assoc.* **2016**, *5*, e002586. [CrossRef]
178. Aldous, S.J. Cardiac biomarkers in acute myocardial infarction. *Int. J. Cardiol.* **2013**, *164*, 282–294. [CrossRef]
179. Reinstadler, S.J.; Feistritzer, H.-J.; Reindl, M.; Klug, G.; Mayr, A.; Mair, J.; Jaschke, W.; Metzler, B. Combined biomarker testing for the prediction of left ventricular remodelling in ST-elevation myocardial infarction. *Open Heart* **2016**, *3*, e000485. [CrossRef]
180. Schernthaner, C.; Lichtenauer, M.; Wernly, B.; Paar, V.; Pistulli, R.; Rohm, I.; Jung, C.; Figulla, H.-R.; Yilmaz, A.; Cadamuro, J.; et al. Multibiomarker analysis in patients with acute myocardial infarction. *Eur. J. Clin. Investig.* **2017**, *47*, 638–648. [CrossRef]
181. Feistritzer, H.-J.; Reinstadler, S.J.; Klug, G.; Reindl, M.; Wöhrer, S.; Brenner, C.; Mayr, A.; Mair, J.; Metzler, B. Multimarker approach for the prediction of microvascular obstruction after acute ST-segment elevation myocardial infarction: A prospective, observational study. *BMC Cardiovasc. Disord.* **2016**, *16*, 239. [CrossRef]

**Publisher's Note:** MDPI stays neutral with regard to jurisdictional claims in published maps and institutional affiliations.

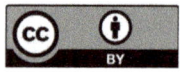

© 2020 by the authors. Licensee MDPI, Basel, Switzerland. This article is an open access article distributed under the terms and conditions of the Creative Commons Attribution (CC BY) license (http://creativecommons.org/licenses/by/4.0/).

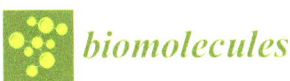

*Review*

# Galectin-3 and sST2 as Prognosticators for Heart Failure Requiring Extracorporeal Life Support: Jack n' Jill

Jianli Bi [1,2], Vidu Garg [1,2,3,4] and Andrew R. Yates [1,2,3,*]

1 Center for Cardiovascular Research, Nationwide Children's Hospital, Columbus, OH 43205, USA; jianli.bi@nationwidechildrens.org (J.B.); vidu.garg@nationwidechildrens.org (V.G.)
2 The Heart Center, Nationwide Children's Hospital, Columbus, OH 43205, USA
3 Department of Pediatrics, The Ohio State University, Columbus, OH 43205, USA
4 Department of Molecular Genetics, The Ohio State University, Columbus, OH 43205, USA
* Correspondence: ANDREW.YATES@nationwidechildrens.org

**Abstract:** Extracorporeal life support provides perfusion for patients with heart failure to allow time for recovery, function as a bridge for patients to heart transplantation, or serve as destination therapy for long term mechanical device support. Several biomarkers have been employed in attempt to predict these outcomes, but it remains to be determined which are suitable to guide clinical practice relevant to extracorporeal life support. Galectin-3 and soluble suppression of tumorigenicity-2 (sST2) are two of the more promising candidates with the greatest supporting evidence. In this review, we address the similarities and differences between galectin-3 and sST2 for prognostic prediction in adults and children with heart failure requiring extracorporeal life support and highlight the significant lack of progress in pediatric biomarker discovery and utilization.

**Keywords:** extracorporeal life support; mechanical circulatory support; ECMO; VAD; galectin-3; sST2; heart failure

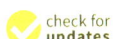

**Citation:** Bi, J.; Garg, V.; Yates, A.R Galectin-3 and sST2 as Prognosticators for Heart Failure Requiring Extracorporeal Life Support: Jack n' Jill. *Biomolecules* 2021, 11, 166. https://doi.org/10.3390/biom11020166

Received: 8 January 2021
Accepted: 22 January 2021
Published: 27 January 2021

**Publisher's Note:** MDPI stays neutral with regard to jurisdictional claims in published maps and institutional affiliations.

**Copyright:** © 2021 by the authors. Licensee MDPI, Basel, Switzerland. This article is an open access article distributed under the terms and conditions of the Creative Commons Attribution (CC BY) license (https://creativecommons.org/licenses/by/4.0/).

## 1. Introduction

Heart failure is a life-threatening condition in both adults and children and is associated with high mortality, morbidity and cost of care. The incidence of heart failure in the general population is 2000/100,000 in adults [ , ] and 0.87–7.4/100,000 in children [ ]. Extracorporeal life support (ECLS) including ventricular assist device (VAD) implantation and extracorporeal membrane oxygenation (ECMO) is required for patients with advanced or end-staged heart failure either as destination therapy or as a bridge-to-transplantation therapy. Over 25,000 adult and 21,000 children (including neonatal and pediatric patients) cases of ECLS were required globally, for cardiac indications, in the past 30 years. The overall survival rate was 59% in adults and 68% in children [ ]. Limited literature is available to document prognostic markers for myocardial recovery in patients with refractory heart failure requiring circulatory support after decades of research. Early attempts to identify a biomarker to predict outcomes of ECLS have followed the evolution of cardiac biomarker testing utilizing brain natriuretic peptide (BNP) [ ] and its N-terminal fragment, NT-proBNP [ ] in the early 2000s through the recognition of cardiac troponin 10 years later [ ]. The early decrease in BNP level is indicative of ventricular unloading during ECLS but the rebound in BNP level after decannulation suggests BNP is not an ideal biomarker to predict complete normalization of cardiac function [ ]. Other heart failure related biomarkers which have been explored in patients who underwent ECLS include dynamic BNP [ ], galectin-3 [ ], ST2 [ ], matrix metalloproteinase-9 (MMP-9) [ ], tissue inhibitors of metalloproteinase-1 (TIMP-1) [ ], MMP-2 [ , ], osteopontin [ ], MR-proANP [ ], proADM [ ], and copeptin [ ]. The above-depicted biomarkers may assist to predict outcomes of heart failure requiring ECLS under limited circumstances and their identifications are summarized in Table . Nevertheless, no single blood biomarker has demonstrated superiority to predict outcomes of heart failure requiring ECLS, but galectin-3 and ST2 have been promising and may be worthwhile to study further [15]. Unfortunately, a decade has passed with no significant progress in our ability to predict outcomes in patients with heart failure requiring ECLS. The failure of a single biomarker and/or single time-point measurement suggest that one may need to employ a combination of biomarkers with associated dynamic changes to predict outcomes in this context. Recently, there is growing interest in the use of galectin-3 and soluble suppression of tumorigenicity-2 (sST2) as potentially reliable prognostic markers [16]. These recent studies have demonstrated that sST2 provides independent predictive value beyond NT-proBNP and cardiac troponin for all-cause cardiovascular mortality in adult patients with chronic heart failure, which may be one explanation for this evolution [17]. Additionally, high levels of galectin-3 and BNP are often found before implantation of a ventricular assist device in patients with terminal heart failure, but elevated BNP failed to identify patients who would not survive VAD support. This prompted interest in galectin-3 levels which could better predict outcomes [18]. If proved in additional studies, the early prognostic value of gelactin-3 and sST2 to accurately identify patients destined for unfavorable recovery after ECLS implementation could provide a critical opportunity to modify treatment algorithms to a more personalized therapeutic approach to improve outcomes. Galectin-3 and sST2 are linked to the development of fibrosis which prevents recovery of myocardial function and may indicate severity of the disease state. In this review, we provide an overview of the recent clinical interpretation of galectin-3 and sST2 and emphasize their similarities and differences for the prognostic prediction of heart failure requiring ECLS. We also address the significant lack of data on galectin-3 and sST2 in pediatric patients undergoing ECLS and attempt to raise awareness about the novel utilization of galection-3 and sST2 as prognosticators in the pediatric population.

**Table 1.** Identification of heart failure-related biomarkers for patients undergoing ECLS.

| Biomarkers | Identification |
|---|---|
| Brain natriuretic peptide (BNP) | cyclic peptide hormone containing disulfide bridge |
| NT-proBNP | N-terminal fragment of BNP |
| Troponin | calcium-regulatory protein |
| Galectin-3 | carbohydrate-binding protein with a single carbohydrate recognition domain and a unique N-terminus |
| MMP-2 and 9 | one of member of Matrix metalloproteinases (zinc- and calcium-dependent endopeptidases) |
| sST2 | soluble suppression of tumorigenicity 2 |
| Tissue inhibitors of metalloproteinases-1 (TIMP-1) | protein containing an N- and C-terminal domain of 125 and 65 amino acids, respectively, with each containing three conserved disulfide bonds |
| Osteopontin | extracellular structural protein |
| MR-proANP | mid-regional fragment of proANP (ANP precursor) |
| proADM | long-acting vasodilatory peptide |
| Copeptin | 39-amino-acid glycopeptide and the C-terminal portion of provasopressin |

## 2. Galectin-3

Galectin-3 is a member of the galectins family of carbohydrate-binding proteins with specificity for N-acetyllactosamine (LacNAc)-containing glycoproteins, and the only known one with a single carbohydrate recognition domain and a unique N-terminus [19,20]. It is a 30 kDa molecule encoded by the LGALS3 gene that is located on chromosome 14, locus q21–q22 [21]. It is mainly secreted by macrophages and regulates basic cellular functions including growth, proliferation, differentiation and inflammation [22–25] and importantly has been found to play a role in cardiac fibrosis [26,27]. Evidence that links Galectin-3 to pathogenesis of heart failure has not been fully elucidated. However, recent studies have suggested that galectin-3 can help to predict prognosis of heart failure and adverse events in various clinical settings such as ST elevation myocardial infraction [28], congenital heart disease patients with a Fontan circulation [29] and survivors of out-of-hospital cardiac arrest [ ]. In addition, its levels have correlated with morbidity and mortality in patients with heart failure [ – ]. Higher values (>15.3 ng/mL) of galectin-3 have been reported to show a correlation with the severity of heart failure [ ].

VAD implantation is a standard ECLS modality for adult patients with end-staged heart failure. A retrospective study [ ] including 57 adult patients with severe heart failure (NYHA Class IIIB–IV) who underwent VAD implantation found that a lower galectin-3 concentration (<30 ng) at the time of VAD implantation was associated with better prognosis when compared to an elevated concentration (>30 ng/mL) 2 years after VAD implantation. Similarly, the plasma galectin-3 concentration immediately before VAD implantation in patients who did not survive ECLS was significantly higher than that in those who were weaned from VAD support or received heart transplantation (18.8 ng/mL vs. 15.3 ng/mL). An additional study in adults noted that a higher galectin-3 concentration (>17 ng/mL) was associated with poor survival in low- or medium-risk VAD patients. However, the galectin-3 concentration was not a predictor in high-risk VAD patients [ ]. These controversial results suggest that a single biomarker is limited in its ability to predict a clinically significant outcome, which is likely the result of multiple factors. A combination of the biomarkers may be required to eliminate this limitation. It is important to note that there is discrepancy in defining the clinically important cut-off values for galectin-3 in the above-mentioned studies, where the at-risk population was reported to be greater than 17 or 30 ng/mL [ , ]. The underlying reasons for this are unknown but may be related to differences in patient populations or techniques. Importantly, the galectin-3 concentrations were determined by different commercial kits in the studies above.

There is significantly less literature regarding galectin-3 in pediatric patients as compared to adults. Similar to adults, the galectin-3 concentration has been reported to be higher in children (median age: 9 years) with chronic heart failure than those (median age: 8.5 years) with normal heart function ($9.46 \pm 5.43$ vs. $1.5 \pm 0.66$ ng/mL, $p < 0.001$). The increased galectin-3 concentration is associated with the severity of heart failure and can be reduced by spironolactone treatment [ ]. The reduction of galectin-3 after spironolactone administration may be related to improvement of heart function. This suggests that galactin-3 may be used as a marker of disease severity in children with chronic heart failure and could potentially guide response to treatment in pediatric patients. In terms of the clinical value of galectin-3 for prognosis prediction in pediatric patients, a prospective study including 76 children with chronic heart disease has demonstrated that galectin-3 is positively associated with the Ross classification score for pediatric heart failure and plays an important role in early diagnosis and prognosis prediction [ ]. The studies regarding application of galectin-3 in pediatric patients with heart failure requiring ECLS are quite scarce compared to adult patient populations and all the studies only evaluate VAD patients (Table ).

Table 2. Application of galectin-3 in adult and pediatric patients with heart failure requiring ECLS.

| Reference | Year | Adult/Peds | N = | Population | Major Finding |
|---|---|---|---|---|---|
| [ ] | 2008 | Adult | 40 | VAD | Higher Gal-3 pre implant associated with mortality (n = 15) compared to bridged to transplant (n = 25) (13.4 + 3.6 ng/mL vs. 9.6 + 5.2 ng/mL, $p < 0.02$) |
| [ ] | 2013 | Adult | 175 | VAD | Higher Galectin-3 levels (>17 ng/mL) increased mortality for low/medium risk VAD patients |
| [ ] | 2015 | Adult | 25 | VAD | Gal-3 remains elevated after continuous flow VAD placed |
| [ ] | 2015 | Adult | 37 | VAD | Gal-3 decreases during LVAD support |
| [ ] | 2016 | Adult | 57 | VAD | Galectin-3 levels >30 ng/mL are associated with lower survival post-LVAD placement (76.5% versus 95.0% at 2 years, $p = 0.009$) |
| [ ] | 2018 | Both | 7 adult 12 pediatric | VAD | Children similar Galectin-3 levels as adults post VAD |

## 3. sST2

sST2 is a circulating form of suppression of tumorigenicity-2 (ST2) glycoprotein that is a member of the interleukin 1 receptor family. The ST2 glycoprotein is encoded by the IL1RL1 gene located in the chromosome 2q12. It serves as the receptor for IL-33, an IL-1–like cytokine that can be secreted by living cells in response to cell damage [42]. IL-33 exerts its cardioprotective function by reducing cardiac fibrosis and inflammation [43]. sST2 can eliminate this cardioprotective function by acting as a decoy to IL-33 [43] and thus is considered an indicator of adverse outcome [44] and a prognostic predictor for heart disease without ECLS [45–47]. Moreover, a pooled study including 1800 elderly patients who underwent cardiac surgery has demonstrated that a higher sST2 level is a soothsayer for an increased incidence of cardiovascular events or mortality [48]. The prognostic value of sST2 in heart failure may benefit physicians by allowing them a way to identify patients with a high risk of adverse events early in their course of care.

sST2 has been much less studied in ECLS than galactin-3. One study by Tseng et al. [49] showed that the sST2 level was significantly increased in 95% of adult patients, aged 17 to 68 years before VAD implantation (the median sST2 level was 74.2 ng/mL with the normal value defined as <35 ng/mL). sST2 then significantly decreased during VAD support and normalized after 6 months (29.5 ng/mL), with the maximum drop occurring by 3 months (no significant decrease thereafter). They concluded that the high sST2 levels predicted poorer outcomes in patients on conventional treatments and was a consequence of end-stage heart failure. Their data suggest that the sST2 level was a useful parameter to monitor therapy. However, they failed to show whether high sST2 levels at any timepoint can predict outcomes post implantation. Similar to galectin 3, there are limited studies (Table 3) in children and will be discussed in a later section.

Table 3. Application of sST2 in adult and pediatric patients with heart failure requiring ECLS.

| Reference | Year | Adult/Peds | N = | Population | Major Finding |
|---|---|---|---|---|---|
| [41] | 2015 | Adult | 37 | VAD | sST2 decreases during LVAD support |
| [48] | 2018 | Adult | 38 | VAD | sST2 elevated in VAD patients and normalized after 6 months; not predictive of outcomes |
| [15] | 2018 | Both | 7 adult 12 pediatric | VAD | sST2 level in children is different than adults following VAD implant |

## 4. Dynamic Changes of Galectin-3 and sST2 in Adult and Children Undergoing ECLS: Similarities and Differences

As described above, galectin-3 and sST2 have been used alone or concomitantly as biomarkers in several studies regarding heart failure with or without ECLS [28,31,46]. Galectin-3 and sST2 are similar in that both can reflect severity of myocardial damage (presumably related to fibrosis) to thereby predict prognosis. However, they act differently in the development of heart failure. As shown in Figure 1, in response to cardiac injury, activated macrophages produce galectin-3 which is then thought to regulate phenotypic change of cardiac fibroblasts from the resting to the activated status [50], whereas sST2 binds to IL33 to block the binding of IL33 to ST2 on cardiomyocytes. Binding of IL33 to cardiomyocyte membrane ST2 results in the initiation of IL33/ST2 pathway which then evokes an antihypertrophic and antifibrotic function [51].

Data regarding the similarities and differences of galectin-3 and sST2 between adults and children at baseline and while undergoing ECLS are extremely limited. To date, only one study [16] is available to compare the dynamic changes of galectin-3 and sST2 in adults and children with heart failure requiring VAD. The investigators demonstrated that the galectin-3 and sST2 from adults and children show a similar trend, climbing up one day after VAD implant, and plunging down two days after VAD implant and to baseline levels in 30 days (Figure 2, redrawn based on the data in the study). The circulating level of sST2 is significantly higher in children than in adults at every time points (Figure 2A). In contrast, the circulating level of galectin-3 is not different (Figure 2B). These data indicate differing responses of galectin-3 and sST2 with VAD implant in children compared to adults. The changes of galectin-3 and sST2 in day 1 and 2 may be a result of macrophage activation related to inflammatory processes surrounding surgical implantation of a VAD. Their differences may indicate varying degree of macrophage activation between children and adults.

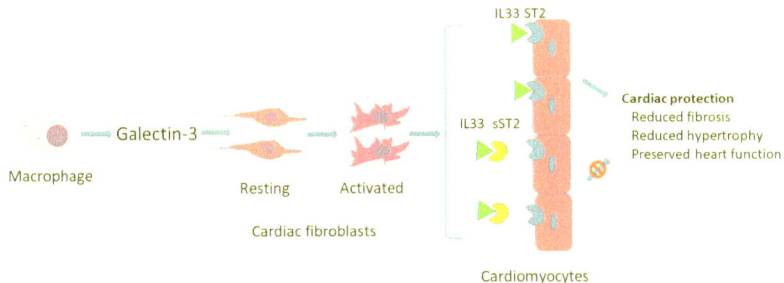

Figure 1. Schematic of possible mechanism of galectin 3 and sST2 in heart failure.

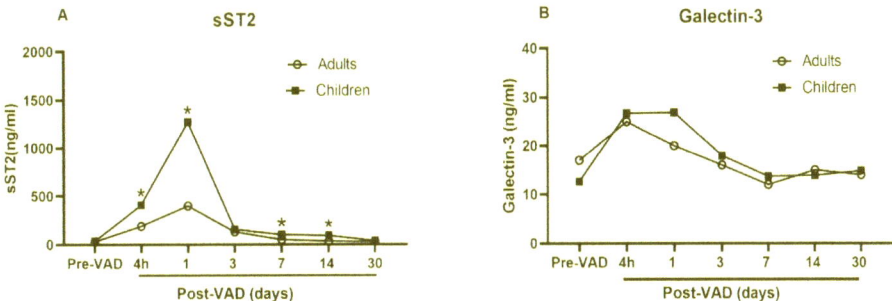

Figure 2. Comparison of sST2 and galectin-3 between adults and children undergoing VAD. Redrawn based upon data reported in [ ]. (A) Significantly higher circulating level of sST2 in children than in adults at every time points; (B) No difference in the circulating level of galectin-3.

To the best of our knowledge, no data are available to describe the trend and prognostic value of plasma or serum galectin-3 and sST2 in children or adults undergoing VA-ECMO for cardiac failure. VA-ECMO use is much more common in pediatric patients than VAD implantation compared to adults, and this deficit requires further studies to fill this gap of our knowledge.

## 5. Feasibility of Using Galectin-3 and sST2 as Prognosticators

The general principles to evaluate feasibility of a biomarker include the following: (a) it is easily obtained, (b) highly reproducible, (c) it is biologically plausible and (d) impacts care. Obtaining a blood sample is part of the postoperative routine and does not involve technically complicated procedures. The measurement of plasma or serum galectin-3 and sST2 would not be a significant burden to a current clinical protocol. Second, a biomarker should be scientifically reproducible and financially affordable. The assays for human plasma/serum galectin-3 and sST2 have been commercially available for clinical and research purposes [ ]. The stability in vitro, biological variation, and reference values for galectin-3 and sST2 have been previously summarized in a comprehensive review [ ] that demonstrates these 2 biomarkers should be clinically reproducible across laboratories. Lastly, studies have highlighted the potential role of galectin-3 and sST2 in the prediction of prognosis in many clinical settings to impact care as discussed above.

Unlike the traditional biomarkers including natriuretic peptides and troponins, sST2 is relatively independent from age, prior diagnosis of HF, body mass index, ischemic type of HF, or atrial fibrillation [53]; galectin-3 is thought to reflect myocardial remodeling and appears to be dynamical biomarker in long-term ECLS. However, galectin-3 is also associated with various fibrotic conditions (liver and lung) [54,55] and this could be a potential confounder in developing treatment strategies.

## 6. Possibility to Use Galectin-3 and sST2 as Indicators to Adjust Medical Regimens or as Therapeutic Targets

Natriuretic peptide-guided therapy in chronic heart failure has been reported in some studies with promising outcomes [56–58], whereas other studies have reported uncertain results [59,60]. The controversies suggest inadequate power to draw a conclusion in biomarker-guided treatment for heart failure. Galectin-3 and sST2 have not yet been sufficiently studied in guiding treatment in patients with heart failure who receive pharmacotherapy, not to mention in patients with heart failure who require ECLS.

As described in Figure 1, galectin-3 is an initiator of the inflammation process in heart failure. Targeting galectin-3 may be a potential therapy to improve the outcomes of heart failure. Extracellular and intracellular small-molecule galectin-3 inhibitors (3,3'-Bis-(4-aryltriazol-1-yl) thiodigalactosides [61] and galectin-3 inhibitor compound 2H [62]) have been investigated [63]. The availability of these inhibitors has laid a foundation for further study of a targeted treatment of galectin-3. Interestingly, modified citrus pectin (a dietary supplement) has been used as an inhibiter of galectin-3 to block cardiac injury that is induced by acute kidney injury via the galectin-3 pathway [64] and may provide an easy initial molecule for clinical trials.

sST2 concentrations have been used to identify patients with chronic heart failure who may particularly benefit from β-adrenergic blocker therapy [47]. At cutoff values of sST2 level of 35 ng/mL and with a metoprolol dose of 50 mg daily (defined as a high dose in the study), patients with low sST2/high-dose BB had the lowest cardiovascular event rate (0.53 events); those with low sST2/low-dose β-adrenergic blocker, or high sST2/high-dose β-adrenergic blocker had intermediate outcomes (0.92 and 1.19 events); patients with high sST2 treated with low-dose β-adrenergic blocker had the highest cardiovascular event rate (2.08 events).

In terms of a targeted therapy on sST2 itself, no chemical compound serving as a sST2 antagonist has been reported. Instead, an anti-ST2 mAb has been used to block the interaction between sST2 and IL33 to release free IL33 [65]. The concern is that the anti-ST2 mAb can block the cell membrane ST2 [66] to thereby suppress the IL33/ST2 pathway that is considered cardioprotective.

Neither galectin-3 and/or sST2 has been examined as guides for adjusting medical management for heart failure in pediatric patients, and thus the role of galectin-3 and /or sST2 as a guide to therapeutic decision-making remains to be established. Additionally, within the pediatric patient population, the use of galectin-3 and/or sST2 as a biomarker for risk stratification in children undergoing ECLS with VAD has not been reported, and the impact of VA-ECMO on galectin-3 and sST2 remains unknown.

## 7. Conclusions

Undergoing ECLS creates a complex clinical situation with challenges related to early and accurate prediction of prognosis, particularly in pediatric patients. To distinguish patients who will improve and those who will not early during ECLS is imperative as would not only assist the medical team to formulate an optimal care plan but may also provide a scientific justification to initiate ethical discussions with the patient's family. Galectin-3 and sST2 have come to prominence as early prognosticators in adult ECLS patients since other biomarkers (BNP [67], NT-proBNP, TnIc, MR-proANP, proADM, and copeptin [14]) have failed to show significance. To discern the complex differences of biomarkers, further studies are needed to investigate the use of a single biomarker (galectin-3 or sST2) versus combined biomarkers (galectin-3, sST2 and/or other markers) which has been done for adult with heart failure but not yet for ECLS patient [ , , ], and sampling at single time point versus multiple time points in ECLS patients.

Beyond protein biomarkers, circulating microRNAs are emerging as intriguing, predictive biomarkers for heart failure. These microRNAs are attractive candidates due to their known biologic roles in reverse remodeling [ , ] and their ability to discriminate heart failure of different etiologies due to their cell-type specific expression [ ]. Akat et al. demonstrated a significant increase in heart-specific circulating microRNAs in patients with advanced heart failure that completely reversed 3 months after initiation of VAD support [ ]. This suggests that the decreased levels of circulating microRNAs are associated with favorable outcomes following VAD support. While no data are available to show a link between circulating microRNAs and prognosis of heart failure requiring ECLS, the potential value of circulating microRNAs in predicting ECLS outcomes in the near future should not be overlooked and requires further investigation in pediatric patients as well.

Based on the currently available published data, we expect that the combined galectin-3 and sST2 biomarkers, followed serially, will be beneficial in guiding management of children undergoing ECLS in the future but additional work is needed to identify other novel biomarkers (e.g., microRNAs), and biomarker response to other forms of ECLS (such as VA-ECMO) that may serve to improve the care of the pediatric patient population.

**Author Contributions:** Conceptualization, A.R.Y., J.B. and V.G.; methodology, A.R.Y. and J.B.; writing—original draft preparation, J.B.; writing—review and editing, A.R.Y., V.G. and J.B. All authors have read and agreed to the published version of the manuscript.

**Funding:** This work was supported by a grant (A.R.Y.) from the Heart Center intramural program (51108-0005-1219) at Nationwide Children's Hospital.

**Institutional Review Board Statement:** Not applicable.

**Informed Consent Statement:** Not applicable.

**Data Availability Statement:** Not applicable.

**Conflicts of Interest:** The authors declare no conflict of interest.

# References

1. Roger, V.L. Epidemiology of heart failure. *Circ. Res.* **2013**, *113*, 646–659. [CrossRef] [PubMed]
2. Ziaeian, B.; Fonarow, G.C. Epidemiology and aetiology of heart failure. *Nat. Rev. Cardiol.* **2016**, *13*, 368–378. [CrossRef]
3. Shaddy, R.E.; George, A.T.; Jaecklin, T.; Lochlainn, E.N.; Thakur, L.; Agrawal, R.; Solar-Yohay, S.; Chen, F.; Rossano, J.W.; Severin, T.; et al. Systematic Literature Review on the Incidence and Prevalence of Heart Failure in Children and Ado-lescents. *Pediatr. Cardiol.* **2018**, *39*, 415–436. [CrossRef]
4. Jenks, C.L.; Raman, L.; Dalton, H.J. Pediatric Extracorporeal Membrane Oxygenation. *Crit. Care Clin.* **2017**, *33*, 825–841. [CrossRef]
5. Huang, S.-C.; Wu, E.-T.; Ko, W.-J.; Lai, L.-P.; Hsu, J.; Chang, C.-I.; Chiu, I.-S.; Wang, S.-S.; Wu, M.-H.; Lin, F.-Y.; et al. Clinical Implication of Blood Levels of B-Type Natriuretic Peptide in Pediatric Patients on Mechanical Circulatory Support. *Ann. Thorac. Surg.* **2006**, *81*, 2267–2272. [CrossRef] [PubMed]
6. Auer, J.; Weber, T. The Diagnostic and Prognostic Value of Brain Natriuretic Peptide and Aminoterminal (nt)-pro Brain Natriuretic Peptide. *Curr. Pharm. Des.* **2005**, *11*, 511–525. [CrossRef]
7. Karam, S.; Moores, R.; Rozycki, H.; Astoria, M. Cardiac Troponin Levels in Neonates Who Require ECMO for Noncardiac Indications Are Elevated in Nonsurvivors. *Am. J. Perinatol.* **2015**, *32*, 859–864. [CrossRef] [PubMed]
8. Papathanasiou, M.; Pizanis, N.; Tsourelis, L.; Koch, A.; Kamler, M.; Rassaf, T.; Luedike, P. Dynamics and prognostic value of B-type natriuretic peptide in left ventricular assist device recipients. *J. Thorac. Dis.* **2019**, *11*, 138–144. [CrossRef]
9. Erkilet, G.; Schulte-Eistrup, S.; Morshuis, M.; Bohms, B.; Roefe, D.; Gummert, J.; Milting, H. Plasma galectin 3 is increased in terminal heart failure patients and is elevated in patients not surviving mechanical circulatory support. *J. Heart Lung Transplant.* **2010**, *29*, S65. [CrossRef]
10. Lee, C.S.; Mudd, J.O.; Lyons, K.S.; Denfeld, Q.E.; Jurgens, C.Y.; Aouizerat, B.E.; Gelow, J.M.; Chien, C.V.; Aarons, E.; Grady, K.L. Heart Failure Symptom Biology in Response to Ventricular Assist Device Implantation. *J. Cardiovasc. Nurs.* **2019**, *34*, 174–182. [CrossRef]
11. Li, Y.; McTiernan, C.F.; Pei, W.; Moravec, C.S.; Wang, P.; Rosenblum, W.; Kormos, R.L.; Feldman, A.M. Downregulation of matrix metalloproteinases and reduction in collagen damage in the failing human heart after support with left ventricular assist devices kmar. *Circulation* **2001**, *104*, 1147–1152. [CrossRef] [PubMed]

12. Bruggink, A.H.; Van Oosterhout, M.F.M.; De Jonge, N.; Cleutjens, J.P.M.; Van Wichen, D.F.; Van Kuik, J.; Tilanus, M.G.J.; Gmelig-Meyling, F.H.J.; Tweel, J.G.V.D.; De Weger, R.A. Type IV collagen degradation in the myocardial basement membrane after unloading of the failing heart by a left ventricular assist device. *Lab. Investig.* **2007**, *87*, 1125–1137. [CrossRef] [PubMed]
13. Schipper, M.E.; Scheenstra, M.R.; Van Kuik, J.; Van Wichen, D.F.; Van Der Weide, P.; Dullens, H.F.; Lahpor, J.; De Jonge, N.; De Weger, R.A. Osteopontin: A potential biomarker for heart failure and reverse remodeling after left ventricular assist device support. *J. Hear. Lung Transpl.* **2011**, *30*, 805–810. [CrossRef] [PubMed]
14. Luyt, C.-E.; Landivier, A.; Leprince, P.; Bernard, M.; Pavie, A.; Chastre, J.; Combes, A. Usefulness of cardiac biomarkers to predict cardiac recovery in patients on extracorporeal membrane oxygenation support for refractory cardiogenic shock. *J. Crit. Care* **2012**, *27*, 524.e7–524.e14. [CrossRef] [PubMed]
15. Kramer, F.; Milting, H. Novel biomarkers in human terminal heart failure and under mechanical circulatory support. *Biomarkers* **2011**, *16*, S31–S41. [CrossRef] [PubMed]
16. Ragusa, R.; Prontera, C.; Di Molfetta, A.; Cabiati, M.; Masotti, S.; Del Ry, S.; Amodeo, A.; Trivella, M.G.; Clerico, A.; Caselli, C. Time-course of circulating cardiac and inflammatory biomarkers after Ventricular Assist Device implan-tation: Comparison between paediatric and adult patients. *Clin. Chim. Acta* **2018**, *486*, 88–93. [CrossRef] [PubMed]
17. Emdin, M.; Aimo, A.; Vergaro, G.; Bayes-Genis, A.; Lupón, J.; Latini, R.; Meessen, J.; Anand, I.S.; Cohn, J.N.; Gravning, J.; et al. sST2 Predicts Outcome in Chronic Heart Failure Beyond NT-proBNP and High-Sensitivity Troponin T. *J. Am. Coll. Cardiol.* **2018**, *72*, 2309–2320. [CrossRef]
18. Milting, H.; Ellinghaus, P.; Seewald, M.; Cakar, H.; Bohms, B.; Kassner, A.; Körfer, R.; Klein, M.; Krahn, T.; Kruska, L.; et al. Plasma biomarkers of myocardial fibrosis and remodeling in terminal heart failure patients supported by mechanical circulatory support devices. *J. Heart Lung Transpl.* **2008**, *27*, 589–596. [CrossRef] [PubMed]
19. Elola, M.T.; Wolfenstein-Todel, C.; Troncoso, M.F.; Vasta, G.R.; Rabinovich, G.A. Galectins: Matricellular glycan-binding proteins linking cell adhesion, migration, and survival. *Cell. Mol. Life Sci.* **2007**, *64*, 1679–1700. [CrossRef]
20. Hughes, R.C. The galectin family of mammalian carbohydrate-binding molecules. *Biochem. Soc. Trans.* **1997**, *25*, 1194–1198. [CrossRef]
21. Meijers, W.C.; Van Der Velde, A.R.; De Boer, R.A. The ARCHITECT galectin-3 assay: Comparison with other automated and manual assays for the measurement of circulating galectin-3 levels in heart failure. *Expert Rev. Mol. Diagn.* **2014**, *14*, 257–266. [CrossRef] [PubMed]
22. Papaspyridonos, M.; McNeill, E.; de Bono, J.P.; Smith, A.; Burnand, K.G.; Channon, K.M.; Greaves, D.R. Galectin-3 is an amplifier of inflammation in atherosclerotic plaque progression through mac-rophage activation and monocyte chemoattraction. *Arterioscler. Thromb. Vasc. Biol* **2008**, *28*, 433–440. [CrossRef] [PubMed]
23. Zhuo, Y.; Chammas, R.; Bellis, S.L. Sialylation of beta1 integrins blocks cell adhesion to galectin-3 and protects cells against galectin-3-induced apoptosis. *J. Biol. Chem.* **2008**, *283*, 22177–22185. [CrossRef] [PubMed]
24. Henderson, N.C.; MacKinnon, A.C.; Farnworth, S.L.; Kipari, T.; Haslett, C.; Iredale, J.P.; Liu, F.-T.; Hughes, J.; Sethi, T. Galectin-3 Expression and Secretion Links Macrophages to the Promotion of Renal Fibrosis. *Am. J. Pathol.* **2008**, *172*, 288–298. [CrossRef] [PubMed]
25. Yang, E.; Shim, J.S.; Woo, H.-J.; Kim, K.-W.; Kwon, H.J. Aminopeptidase N/CD13 induces angiogenesis through interaction with a pro-angiogenic protein, galectin-3. *Biochem. Biophys. Res. Commun.* **2007**, *363*, 336–341. [CrossRef] [PubMed]
26. Martínez-Martínez, E.; Brugnolaro, C.; Ibarrola, J.; Ravassa, S.; Buonafine, M.; López, B.; Fernández-Celis, A.; Querejeta, R.; Santamaria, E.; Fernández-Irigoyen, J.; et al. CT-1 (Cardiotrophin-1)-Gal-3 (Galectin-3) Axis in Cardiac Fibrosis and Inflammation. *Hypertension* **2019**, *73*, 602–611. [CrossRef]
27. Martínez-Martínez, E.; Ibarrola, J.; Fernández-Celis, A.; Santamaria, E.; Fernández-Irigoyen, J.; Rossignol, P.; Jaisser, F.; Lopez-Andres, N. Differential Proteomics Identifies Reticulocalbin-3 as a Novel Negative Mediator of Collagen Production in Human Cardiac Fibroblasts. *Sci. Rep.* **2017**, *7*, 1–10. [CrossRef]
28. Tyminska, A.; Kapłon-Cieślicka, A.; Ozierański, K.; Budnik, M.; Wancerz, A.; Sypień, P.; Peller, M.; Balsam, P.; Opolski, G.; Filipiak, K.J. Association of Galectin-3 and Soluble ST2, and Their Changes, with Echocardiographic Parameters and Development of Heart Failure after ST-Segment Elevation Myocardial Infarction. *Dis. Markers* **2019**, *2019*, 9529053. [CrossRef]
29. Opotowsky, A.; Baraona, F.; Owumi, J.; Loukas, B.; Singh, M.N.; Valente, A.M.; Wu, F.; Cheng, S.; Veldtman, G.; Rimm, E.B.; et al. Galectin-3 Is Elevated and Associated with Adverse Outcomes in Patients with Single-Ventricle Fontan Circulation. *J. Am. Hear. Assoc.* **2016**, *5*, e002706. [CrossRef]
30. Mosleh, W.; Kattel, S.; Bhatt, H.; Al-Jebaje, Z.; Khan, S.; Shah, T.; Dahal, S.; Khalil, C.; Frodey, K.; Elibol, J.; et al. Galectin-3 as a Risk Predictor of Mortality in Survivors of Out-of-Hospital Cardiac Arrest. *Circ. Arrhythmia Electrophysiol.* **2019**, *12*, e007519. [CrossRef]
31. Van Kimmenade, R.R.; Januzzi, J.L., Jr.; Ellinor, P.T.; Sharma, U.C.; Bakker, J.A.; Low, A.F.; Martinez, A.; Crijns, H.J.; MacRae, C.A.; Menheere, P.P.; et al. Utility of amino-terminal pro-brain natriuretic peptide, galectin-3, and apelin for the evaluation of patients with acute heart failure. *J. Am. Coll. Cardiol.* **2006**, *48*, 1217–1224. [CrossRef] [PubMed]
32. Sygitowicz, G.; Tomaniak, M.; Filipiak, K.J.; Kołtowski, Ł.; Sitkiewicz, D. Galectin-3 in Patients with Acute Heart Failure: Preliminary Report on First Polish Experience. *Adv. Clin. Exp. Med.* **2016**, *25*, 617–623. [CrossRef] [PubMed]

33. George, M.; Shanmugam, E.; Srivatsan, V.; Vasanth, K.; Ramraj, B.; Rajaram, M.; Jena, A.; Sridhar, A.; Chaudhury, M.; Kaliappan, I. Value of pentraxin-3 and galectin-3 in acute coronary syndrome: A short-term prospective cohort study. *Ther. Adv. Cardiovasc. Dis.* **2015**, *9*, 275–284. [CrossRef] [PubMed]
34. McEvoy, J.W.; Chen, Y.; Halushka, M.K.; Christenson, E.; Ballantyne, C.M.; Blumenthal, R.S.; Christenson, R.H.; Selvin, E. Galectin-3 and Risk of Heart Failure and Death in Blacks and Whites. *J. Am. Hear Assoc.* **2016**, *5*, e003079. [CrossRef]
35. Ueland, T.; Aukrust, P.; Broch, K.; Aakhus, S.; Skårdal, R.; Muntendam, P.; Gullestad, L. Galectin-3 in heart failure: High levels are associated with all-cause mortality. *Int. J. Cardiol.* **2011**, *150*, 361–364. [CrossRef]
36. Coromilas, E.; Que-Xu, E.-C.; Moore, D.; Kato, T.S.; Wu, C.; Ji, R.; Givens, R.; Jorde, U.P.; Takayama, H.; Naka, Y.; et al. Dynamics and prognostic role of galectin-3 in patients with advanced heart failure, during left ventricular assist device support and following heart transplantation. *BMC Cardiovasc. Disord.* **2016**, *16*, 1–10. [CrossRef]
37. Erkilet, G.; Özpeker, C.; Böthig, D.; Kramer, F.; Röfe, D.; Bohms, B.; Morshuis, M.; Gummert, J.; Milting, H. The biomarker plasma galectin-3 in advanced heart failure and survival with mechanical circulatory support devices. *J. Hear. Lung Transpl.* **2013**, *32*, 221–230. [CrossRef]
38. Kotby, A.A.; Youssef, O.I.; Elmaraghy, M.O.; El Sharkawy, O.S. Galectin-3 in Children with Chronic Heart Failure with Normal and Reduced Ejection Fraction: Rela-tionship to Disease Severity. *Pediatr. Cardiol.* **2017**, *38*, 95–102. [CrossRef]
39. Saleh, N.; Khattab, A.; Rizk, M.; Salem, S.; Abo-Haded, H. Value of Galectin-3 assay in children with heart failure secondary to congenital heart diseases: A prospective study. *BMC Pediatr.* **2020**, *20*, 1–9. [CrossRef]
40. Lok, S.I.; Nous, F.M.; Van Kuik, J.; Van Der Weide, P.; Winkens, B.; Kemperman, H.; Huisman, A.; Lahpor, J.R.; De Weger, R.A.; De Jonge, N. Myocardial fibrosis and pro-fibrotic markers in end-stage heart failure patients during continuous-flow left ventricular assist device support. *Eur. J. Cardiothorac. Surg.* **2015**, *48*, 407–415. [CrossRef]
41. Ahmad, T.; Wang, T.; O'Brien, E.C.; Samsky, M.D.; Pura, J.A.; Lokhnygina, Y.; Rogers, J.G.; Hernandez, A.F.; Craig, D.; Bowles, D.E.; et al. Effects of Left Ventricular Assist Device Support on Biomarkers of Cardiovascular Stress, Fibrosis, Fluid Homeostasis, Inflammation, and Renal Injury. *JACC Hear Fail.* **2015**, *3*, 30–39. [CrossRef]
42. Miller, A.M.; Xu, D.; Asquith, D.L.; Denby, L.; Li, Y.; Sattar, N.; Baker, A.H.; McInnes, I.B.; Liew, F.Y. IL-33 reduces the development of atherosclerosis. *J. Exp. Med.* **2008**, *205*, 339–346. [CrossRef]
43. Pascual-Figal, D.A.; Januzzi, J.L. The Biology of ST2: The International ST2 Consensus Panel. *Am. J. Cardiol.* **2015**, *115*, 3B–7B. [CrossRef] [PubMed]
44. Sabatine, M.S.; Morrow, D.A.; Higgins, L.J.; MacGillivray, C.; Guo, W.; Bode, C.; Rifai, N.; Cannon, C.P.; Gerszten, R.E.; Lee, R.T. Complementary Roles for Biomarkers of Biomechanical Strain ST2 and N-Terminal Prohormone B-Type Natriuretic Peptide in Patients With ST-Elevation Myocardial Infarction. *Circulation* **2008**, *117*, 1936–1944. [CrossRef]
45. Farcaş, A.D.; Mocan, M.; Anton, F.P.; Hognogi, L.D.M.; Chiorescu, R.M.; Stoia, M.A.; Vonica, C.L.; Goidescu, C.M.; Vida-Simiti, L.A. Short-Term Prognosis Value of sST2 for an Unfavorable Outcome in Hypertensive Patients. *Dis. Markers* **2020**, *2020*, 8143737. [CrossRef] [PubMed]
46. Tang, W.W.; Wu, Y.; Grodin, J.L.; Hsu, A.P.; Hernandez, A.F.; Butler, J.; Metra, M.; Voors, A.A.; Felker, G.M.; Troughton, R.W.; et al. Prognostic Value of Baseline and Changes in Circulating Soluble ST2 Levels and the Effects of Nesiritide in Acute Decompensated Heart Failure. *JACC Hear Fail.* **2016**, *4*, 68–77. [CrossRef] [PubMed]
47. Gaggin, H.K.; Motiwala, S.; Bhardwaj, A.; Parks, K.A.; Januzzi, J.L., Jr. Soluble concentrations of the interleukin receptor family member ST2 and beta-blocker therapy in chronic heart failure. *Circ. Heart Fail* **2013**, *6*, 1206–1213. [CrossRef]
48. Patel, D.M.; Thiessen-Philbrook, H.; Brown, J.R.; McArthur, E.; Moledina, D.G.; Mansour, S.G.; Shlipak, M.G.; Koyner, J.L.; Kavsak, P.; Whitlock, R.P.; et al. Association of plasma-soluble ST2 and galectin-3 with cardiovascular events and mortality following cardiac surgery. *Am. Hear. J.* **2020**, *220*, 253–263. [CrossRef]
49. Tseng, C.C.S.; Huibers, M.M.H.; Gaykema, L.H.; Koning, E.S.-D.; Ramjankhan, F.Z.; Maisel, A.S.; De Jonge, N. Soluble ST2 in end-stage heart failure, before and after support with a left ventricular assist device. *Eur. J. Clin. Investig.* **2018**, *48*, e12886. [CrossRef]
50. De Boer, R.A.; Voors, A.A.; Muntendam, P.; van Gilst, W.H.; van Veldhuisen, D.J. Galectin-3: A novel mediator of heart failure development and progression. *Eur. J. Heart Fail.* **2009**, *11*, 811–817. [CrossRef]
51. Chow, S.L.; Maisel, A.S.; Anand, I.; Bozkurt, B.; De Boer, R.A.; Felker, G.M.; Fonarow, G.C.; Greenberg, B.; Januzzi, J.L.; Kiernan, M.S.; et al. Role of Biomarkers for the Prevention, Assessment, and Management of Heart Failure: A Scientific Statement from the American Heart Association. *Circulation* **2017**, *135*, e1054–e1091. [CrossRef] [PubMed]
52. Mueller, T.; Dieplinger, B. Soluble ST2 and Galectin-3: What We Know and Don't Know Analytically. *EJIFCC* **2016**, *27*, 224–237.
53. Rehman, S.U.; Mueller, T.; Januzzi, J.L., Jr. Characteristics of the novel interleukin family biomarker ST2 in atients with acute heart failure. *J Am Coll Cardiol.* **2008**, *52*, 1458–1465. [CrossRef] [PubMed]
54. Henderson, N.C.; MacKinnon, A.C.; Farnworth, S.L.; Poirier, F.; Russo, F.P.; Iredale, J.P.; Haslett, C.; Simpson, K.J.; Sethi, T. Galectin-3 regulates myofibroblast activation and hepatic fibrosis. *Proc. Natl. Acad. Sci. USA* **2006**, *103*, 5060–5065. [CrossRef]
55. Nishi, Y.; Sano, H.; Kawashima, T.; Okada, T.; Kuroda, T.; Kikkawa, K.; Kawashima, S.; Tanabe, M.; Goto, T.; Matsuzawa, Y.; et al. Role of Galectin-3 in Human Pulmonary Fibrosis. *Allergol. Int.* **2007**, *56*, 57–65. [CrossRef] [PubMed]
56. Jourdain, P.; Jondeau, G.; Funck, F.; Gueffet, P.; Le Helloco, A.; Donal, E.; Aupetit, J.F.; Aumont, M.C.; Galinier, M.; Eicher, J.C.; et al. Plasma brain natriuretic peptide-guided therapy to improve outcome in heart failure: The STARS-BNP Multicenter Study. *J. Am. Coll. Cardiol.* **2007**, *49*, 1733–1739. [CrossRef] [PubMed]

57. Sanders-van Wijk, S.; van Asselt, A.D.; Rickli, H.; Estlinbaum, W.; Erne, P.; Rickenbacher, P.; Vuillomenet, A.; Peter, M.; Pfisterer, M.E.; Brunner-La Rocca, H.P. Cost-effectiveness of N-terminal pro-B-type natriuretic-guided therapy in elderly heart failure patients: Results from TIME-CHF (Trial of Intensified versus Standard Medical Therapy in Elderly Patients with Congestive Heart Failure). *JACC Heart Fail* **2013**, *1*, 64–71. [CrossRef]
58. Eurlings, L.W.; van Pol, P.E.; Kok, W.E.; van Wijk, S.; Lodewijks-van der Bolt, C.; Balk, A.H.; Lok, D.J.; Crijns, H.J.; van Kraaij, D.J.; de Jonge, N.; et al. Management of chronic heart failure guided by individual N-terminal pro-B-type natriuretic peptide targets: Results of the PRIMA (Can PRo-brain-natriuretic peptide guided therapy of chronic heart failure IMprove heart fAilure morbidity and mortality?) study. *J. Am. Coll. Cardiol.* **2010**, *56*, 2090–2100.
59. Lainchbury, J.G.; Troughton, R.W.; Strangman, K.M.; Frampton, C.M.; Pilbrow, A.; Yandle, T.G.; Hamid, A.K.; Nicholls, M.G.; Richards, A.M. N-terminal pro-B-type natriuretic peptide-guided treatment for chronic heart failure: Results from the BATTLESCARRED (NT-proBNP-Assisted Treatment to Lessen Serial Cardiac Readmissions and Death) trial. *J. Am. Coll. Cardiol.* **2009**, *55*, 53–60. [CrossRef]
60. Pfisterer, M.; Buser, P.; Rickli, H.; Gutmann, M.; Erne, P.; Rickenbacher, P.; Vuillomenet, A.; Jeker, U.; Dubach, P.; Beer, H.; et al. BNP-guided vs symptom-guided heart failure therapy: The Trial of Intensified vs Standard Medical Therapy in Elderly Patients With Congestive Heart Failure (TIME-CHF) randomized trial. *J. Am. Med. Assoc.* **2009**, *301*, 383–392. [CrossRef]
61. Delaine, T.; Collins, P.; MacKinnon, A.; Sharma, G.; Stegmayr, J.; Rajput, V.K.; Mandal, S.; Cumpstey, I.; Larumbe, A.; Salameh, B.A.; et al. Galectin-3-Binding Glycomimetics that Strongly Reduce Bleomycin-Induced Lung Fibrosis and Modulate Intracellular Glycan Recognition. *ChemBioChem* **2016**, *17*, 1759–1770. [CrossRef] [PubMed]
62. Zetterberg, F.; Peterson, K.; Johnsson, R.E.; Brimert, T.; Håkansson, M.; Logan, D.T.; Leffler, H.; Nilsson, U.J. Monosaccharide Derivatives with Low-Nanomolar Lectin Affinity and High Selectivity Based on Combined Fluorine-Amide, Phenyl-Arginine, Sulfur-$\pi$, and Halogen Bond Interactions. *ChemMedChem* **2018**, *13*, 133–137. [CrossRef] [PubMed]
63. Stegmayr, J.; Zetterberg, F.; Carlsson, M.C.; Huang, X.; Sharma, G.; Kahl-Knutson, B.; Schambye, H.; Nilsson, U.J.; Oredsson, S.; Leffler, H. Extracellular and intracellular small-molecule galectin-3 inhibitors. *Sci. Rep.* **2019**, *9*, 1–12. [CrossRef] [PubMed]
64. Prud'Homme, M.; Coutrot, M.; Michel, T.; Boutin, L.; Genest, M.; Poirier, F.; Launay, J.-M.; Kane, B.; Kinugasa, S.; Prakoura, N.; et al. Acute Kidney Injury Induces Remote Cardiac Damage and Dysfunction Through the Galectin-3 Pathway. *JACC Basic Transl. Sci.* **2019**, *4*, 717–732. [CrossRef] [PubMed]
65. Zhang, J.; Ramadan, A.M.; Griesenauer, B.; Li, W.; Turner, M.J.; Liu, C.; Kapur, R.; Hanenberg, H.; Blazar, B.R.; Tawara, I.; et al. ST2 blockade reduces sST2-producing T cells while maintaining protective mST2-expressing T cells during graft-versus-host disease. *Sci. Transl. Med.* **2015**, *7*, 308ra160. [CrossRef]
66. Fursov, N.; Johnston, E.; Duffy, K.; Cotty, A.; Petley, T.; Fisher, J.; Jiang, H.; Rycyzyn, M.A.; Giles-Komar, J.; Powers, G. Generation and Characterization of Rat Anti-mouse ST2L Monoclonal Antibodies. *Hybrid* **2011**, *30*, 153–162. [CrossRef]
67. Naruke, T.; Inomata, T.; Imai, H.; Yanagisawa, T.; Maekawa, E.; Mizutani, T.; Osaka, T.; Shinagawa, H.; Koitabashi, T.; Nishii, M.; et al. End-tidal carbon dioxide concentration can estimate the appropriate timing for weaning off from extra-corporeal membrane oxygenation for refractory circulatory failure. *Int. Heart J.* **2010**, *51*, 116–120. [CrossRef]
68. Wang, C.-H.; Yang, N.-I.; Liu, M.-H.; Hsu, K.-H.; Kuo, L.-T. Estimating systemic fibrosis by combining galectin-3 and ST2 provides powerful risk stratification value for patients after acute decompensated heart failure. *Cardiol. J.* **2013**, *23*, 563–572. [CrossRef]
69. Rosa, S.; Eposito, F.; Carella, C.; Strangio, A.; Ammirati, G.; Sabatino, J.; Abbate, F.G.; Iaconetti, C.; Liguori, V.; Pergola, V.; et al. Transcoronary concentration gradients of circulating microRNAs in heart failure. *Eur. J. Heart Fail.* **2018**, *20*, 1000–1010. [CrossRef]
70. Barsanti, C.; Trivella, M.G.; D'Aurizio, R.; El Baroudi, M.; Baumgart, M.; Groth, M.; Caruso, R.; Verde, A.; Botta, L.; Cozzi, L.; et al. Differential Regulation of MicroRNAs in End-Stage Failing Hearts Is Associated with Left Ventricular Assist Device Unloading. *BioMed Res. Int.* **2015**, *2015*, 592512. [CrossRef]
71. Lok, S.I.; De Jonge, N.; Van Kuik, J.; Van Geffen, A.J.P.; Huibers, M.M.H.; Van Der Weide, P.; Siera, E.; Winkens, B.; Doevendans, P.A.; De Weger, R.A.; et al. MicroRNA Expression in Myocardial Tissue and Plasma of Patients with End-Stage Heart Failure during LVAD Support: Comparison of Continuous and Pulsatile Devices. *PLoS ONE* **2015**, *10*, e0136404. [CrossRef] [PubMed]
72. Akat, K.M.; Moore-McGriff, D.; Morozov, P.; Brown, M.; Gogakos, T.; Da Rosa, J.C.; Mihailovic, A.; Sauer, M.; Ji, R.; Ramarathnam, A.; et al. Comparative RNA-sequencing analysis of myocardial and circulating small RNAs in human heart failure and their utility as biomarkers. *Proc. Natl. Acad. Sci. USA* **2014**, *111*, 11151–11156. [CrossRef] [PubMed]

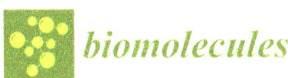 

*Review*

# A Changing Paradigm in Heart Transplantation: An Integrative Approach for Invasive and Non-Invasive Allograft Rejection Monitoring

Alessia Giarraputo [1], Ilaria Barison [1], Marny Fedrigo [1], Jacopo Burrello [2], Chiara Castellani [1], Francesco Tona [3], Tomaso Bottio [3], Gino Gerosa [3], Lucio Barile [2,4,5,†] and Annalisa Angelini [1,*,†]

1. Cardiovascular Pathology and Pathological Anatomy, Department of Cardiac, Thoracic, Vascular Sciences and Public Health, University of Padua, 35128 Padua, Italy; alessia.giarraputo@phd.unipd.it (A.G.); ilaria.barison@unipd.it (I.B.); marny.fedrigo@aopd.veneto.it (M.F.); chiara.castellani@unipd.it (C.C.)
2. Laboratory for Cardiovascular Theranostics, Cardiocentro Ticino Foundation, 6900 Lugano, Switzerland; jacopo.burrello@gmail.com (J.B.); lucio.barile@cardiocentro.org (L.B.)
3. Division of Cardiac Surgery, Department of Cardiac, Thoracic, Vascular Sciences and Public Health, University of Padua, 35128 Padua, Italy; francesco.tona@unipd.it (F.T.); tomaso.bottio@unipd.it (T.B.); gino.gerosa@unipd.it (G.G.)
4. Faculty of Biomedical Sciences, Università Svizzera Italiana, 6900 Lugano, Switzerland
5. Institute of Life Sciences, Scuola Superiore Sant'Anna, 56127 Pisa, Italy
\* Correspondence: annalisa.angelini@unipd.it; Tel.: +39-049-821-1699
† These authors have contributed equally to this work as senior authors.

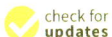

**Citation:** Giarraputo, A.; Barison, I.; Fedrigo, M.; Burrello, J.; Castellani, C.; Tona, F.; Bottio, T.; Gerosa, G.; Barile, L.; Angelini, A. A Changing Paradigm in Heart Transplantation: An Integrative Approach for Invasive and Non-Invasive Allograft Rejection Monitoring. *Biomolecules* **2021**, *11*, 201. https://doi.org/10.3390/biom11020201

Academic Editor: Pietro Scicchitano
Received: 18 December 2020
Accepted: 27 January 2021
Published: 1 February 2021

**Publisher's Note:** MDPI stays neutral with regard to jurisdictional claims in published maps and institutional affiliations.

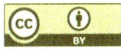

**Copyright:** © 2021 by the authors. Licensee MDPI, Basel, Switzerland. This article is an open access article distributed under the terms and conditions of the Creative Commons Attribution (CC BY) license (https://creativecommons.org/licenses/by/4.0/).

**Abstract:** Cardiac allograft rejection following heart transplantation is challenging to diagnose. Tissue biopsies are the gold standard in monitoring the different types of rejection. The last decade has seen an increased emphasis on identifying non-invasive methods to improve rejection diagnosis and overcome tissue biopsy invasiveness. Liquid biopsy, as an efficient non-invasive diagnostic and prognostic oncological monitoring tool, seems to be applicable in heart transplant follow-ups. Moreover, molecular techniques applied on blood can be translated to tissue samples to provide novel perspectives on tissue and reveal new diagnostic and prognostic biomarkers. This review aims to provide a comprehensive overview of the state-of-the-art of the new methodologies in cardiac allograft rejection monitoring and investigate the future perspectives on invasive and non-invasive rejection biomarkers identification. We reviewed literature from the most used scientific databases, such as PubMed, Google Scholar, and Scopus. We extracted 192 papers and, after a selection and exclusion process, we included in the review 81 papers. The described limitations notwithstanding, this review show how molecular biology techniques and omics science could be deployed complementarily to the histopathological rejection diagnosis on tissue biopsies, thus representing an integrated approach for heart transplant patients monitoring.

**Keywords:** liquid biopsy; tissue biopsy; EMBs; cardiac rejection monitoring; biomarkers; heart transplant; microRNA; mRNA; gene expression profiling; exosomes

## 1. Introduction

The diagnosis of acute and chronic cardiac allograft rejection remains challenging since rejection often occurs in asymptomatic patients, affecting transplanted patients' short- and long-term outcomes [ ]. Endomyocardial biopsies (EMBs) continue to be the gold standard procedure for monitoring and assessing rejection. EMBs were introduced in the cardiac transplant field about 40 years ago in many centers, first in the US and then worldwide. Monitoring EMBs for heart transplants is particularly important for post-transplanted patients, who are subjected to about 14 EMBs during the first year post-transplant [ ]. This procedure provides an open window on the myocardium physiopathologic state but, like many other procedures, is prone to some limitations. First, EMBs are invasive procedures associated with some minor unavoidable clinical complications [3]; secondly, the close correlation between the clinical and histological resolution of rejection is debarred by interobserver variability and sampling errors [4]. Finally, EMBs, systemically used for surveillance during the first year after heart transplantation, represent an expensive medical procedure.

Due to these drawbacks, numerous attempts have recently been made to explore the possibility of identifying a sensitive and non-invasive approach that might be used in combination with tissue histology to reduce the frequency of biopsies [5]. Omics approaches have expanded the number of relevant biomarkers for the diagnosis of allograft rejection [6] and surveillance mainly in asymptomatic patients [7].

Liquid biopsy plays an essential role in this context with regard to the genomics and proteomics performed on blood samples, aiming to identify circulating biomarkers to achieve diagnosis and grading of rejection, bypassing the invasiveness of EMBs [8,9]. Although some of these approaches have already been introduced in several medical centers as EMB-supporting tools to monitor stable patients and reduce the number of required biopsies, the clinical implementation of these markers on a large cohort of patients is still needed. Nevertheless, EMB remains a vital source of graft status information and its potential has only partially been exploited. A specific research line has focused on identifying new molecular approaches, such as miRNomics and gene profiling, which could also be applied to EMBs as supporting technologies to improve and finely dissect histological and immunohistochemical evaluation, as well as to target pharmacological therapy [10,11].

This review covers literature from the last decade from the most used scientific databases, such as PubMed, Google Scholar, and Scopus. Starting from 192 papers, we excluded from the reviewing process all the studies that involved animal models, reviews, meta-analysis, and case studies, as well as conference abstracts/reports. We made a few exceptions however, including for some papers that represent important proofs-of-concept for novel allograft monitoring. We therefore finally included 81 papers related to clinical studies on cohorts of transplanted patients and molecular approaches performed on transplanted patients. This review presents the state-of-the-art (Figure 1) of invasive and non-invasive allograft rejection monitoring in heart transplantation.

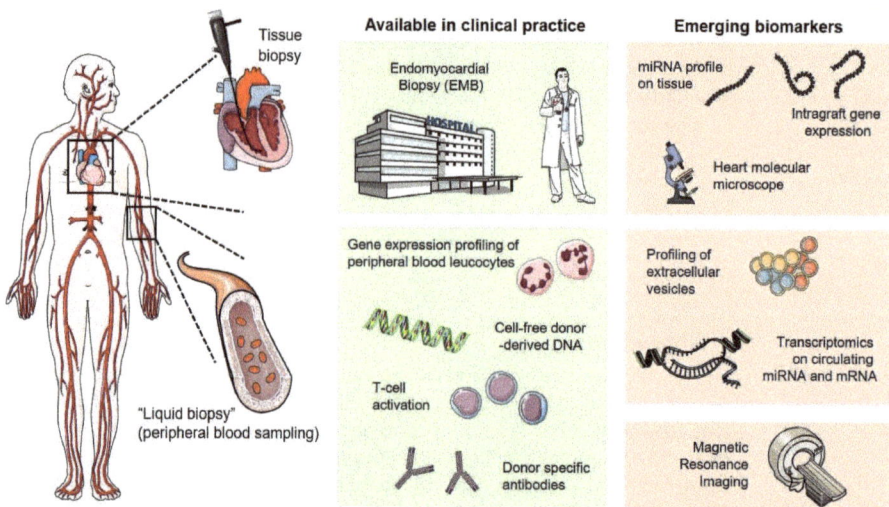

**Figure 1.** Overview of invasive and non-invasive approaches in cardiac allograft rejection monitoring.

## 2. Liquid Biopsy: Clinical Application

Initially, liquid biopsy was applied in the oncological field for diagnosis, monitoring of therapy efficacy, and assessment of progression-free survival [ – ]. Researchers defined it as the analysis of blood and its product to detect cellular and nuclear material derived from a tumor [ ]. Thanks to its capacity to take a genetic picture of the cancer state "from a few blood drops", it was proposed both as a companion diagnostic strategy—but also at the preclinical stage, as a population screening tool—and as a prognostic factor for outcome [ ].Besides this, it showed great potential in other clinical fields, like post-transplant rejection monitoring in solid organs transplants. Good results have been achieved with these non-invasive procedures. Some methodologies, such as gene expression profiling (GEP) [ ], which can detect variations in the cell transcript, have already been applied in the clinical field to monitor stable patients and reduce the number of EMBs.

### 2.1. Gene Expression Profiling of the Peripheral Blood Leucocytes

Various international multicenter studies (Cargo, Image, E-Image, and Cargo II) have investigated the role of the gene expression profiles of the peripheral blood leucocytes as genomic markers of acute rejection [ – , , ]. The first development of such an approach was an algorithm used to process a panel of 20 genes (selected starting from 252 candidates, identified through the literature and studies carried out on other transplanted organs). Eleven out of twenty genes were classifiers that could discriminate between "quiescent" vs. "moderate/severe rejection" in the validation set. Nine genes were chosen as controls. The algorithm reached an agreement of 84% in EMBs in patients with the highest grade of rejection ($\geq$3A), measured according to the International Society for Heart and Lung Transplantation (ISHLT) classification [ ]. Gene analysis converted into a score (0–40) had a negative predictive value (NPV) of 99.6% in patients demonstrating scores lower than 30 within the first year post-transplantation [ ]. The Cargo II study, which included 462 patients, confirmed a GEP score < 34 to identify patients at low risk of rejection, even early after transplantation [ ].

The GEP technology is commercialized as AllopMap and used in many centers in the US and Europe. Patients at >2 months, >6 months, and >1 year with a score inferior to 20, 30, and 34, respectively, were defined as low-risk patients not requiring EMBs monitoring [ , ]. This approach has been systematically compared in a clinical setting with standard routine biopsies in the IMAGE study, comprising 602 patients enrolled between six months and five years post-transplantation [ ] and randomly assigned to the gene-profiling or biopsy group monitoring. Compared with the routine biopsy group, patients monitored by GEP did not experience an increased risk of severe adverse outcomes [ ]. Notably, the study resulted in significantly fewer EMBs. The EImage (Early Image) study [ ] evaluated the sensitivity of GEP technology during the early stage of monitoring (<6 months post-transplantation). Sixty patients were randomly assigned in a 1:1 ratio again to either the GEP or the EMB groups. The threshold for a positive GEP result was set at $\geq$30 for patients two to six months and $\geq$34 for patients six months post-transplantation. Although EImage included a small cohort of relatively low-risk patients on lower doses of corticosteroids (<20 mg), the study showed the safety and efficacy of GEP blood testing as an alternative to routine biopsies within 55 days following cardiac transplantation. There were no significant differences for primary endpoints (death, renewed transplant, hemodynamic compromise, left ventricular ejection fraction, and graft dysfunction) between patients followed-up with Allomap or EMBs [ ].

Additionally, novel biomarkers can be assessed by implementing high-throughput transcriptomics profiling assays without a bias of the target selection on whole-blood samples collected during the EMB monitoring procedure. In this framework, the HEARTBiT initiative, a Canadian multicenter prospective study aimed at improving the non-invasive diagnostic performance of acute cellular rejection (ACR) events at an early stage post-transplant (during the first two months) through transcriptome profiling of nine mRNA transcripts, quantified using NanoString nCounter technology. HEARTBiT achieved a comparable diagnostic performance of non-invasive diagnostic tests currently available in clinical practice with area under the curve (AUC) values of 0.70 (95% CI, 0.57–0.83) and 0.69 (95% CI, 0.56–0.81) and with the expectation of overcoming AlloMap's limitation to application within 55 days post-transplant [19]. A pilot clinical validation study, estimating the robustness and limitation of the previous work, assessed the potential clinical efficacy of HEARTBiT profiling. A promising linear relationship of HEARTBiT's molecular profile with ACR diagnosis was highlighted, as well as the necessity of future longitudinal and large-scale trials [20].

The Canada-wide trial applied the GEP approach, using whole blood as starting material from patients before transplantation and from three years post-transplantation. From 1295 differentially expressed genes between subjects with acute rejection (ISHLT Grade > or = 2R) and no rejection (Grade 0R), a 12-gene biomarker panel, classifying validation samples with 83% sensitivity and 100% specificity, was identified [21]. Hollander et al. expanded and refined the 12-gene biomarker panel with a more heterogeneous cohort of cardiac transplant patients, collecting samples between one week and six months post-heart transplant [22].

Moayedi and colleagues undertook a risk evaluation of the use of GEP in monitoring acute cellular rejection and taking into account the outcomes of the AlloMap® Registry in a prospective observational multicenter study [23]. They assessed short and long-term clinical outcomes in patients that received GEP for routine rejection surveillance after heart transplantation in a cohort of 1504 patients with 7969 clinic visits and records. Despite the limitation of possible selection bias in the study's inclusion criteria, survival outcomes in contemporary heart transplant patients managed with GEP as an ACR surveillance strategy are promising [23].

Using gene-based transcriptional signaling in peripheral blood mononuclear cells in 44 patients, Mehra and Benitez reported that patients could be segregated into low, intermediate, and high risk for future rejection subsets [24]. The informative identified genes represented several biologic pathways, including T-cell activation (PDCD1), T-cell migration (ITGA4), mobilization of hematopoietic precursors (WDR40A and microRNA gene family cMIR), and steroid-responsive genes such as IL1R2, the decoy receptor for IL-2 [24].

*2.2. Cell-Free DNA*

Donor-derived cell-free DNA (dd-cf-DNA) is the DNA of donor origin in heart transplant recipients' blood. During cellular and antibody mediated rejection, in the setting of myocyte necrosis and apoptosis, a more significant amount of dd-cf-DNA from the damaged graft is released into the blood. The detection of dd-cf-DNA is straightforward in female recipients receiving a male donor graft, undertaken by targeting the Y chromosome [25]. A molecular technique that facilitates the identification of graft-derived DNA regardless of the sex of the transplant donor or recipient is shotgun sequencing. This approach is based on sequencing cell-free circulating DNA fragments and exploiting single nucleotide polymorphisms (SNPs) genotyping information to differentiate between donor- and recipient-derived sequences. Hence, this method can identify and quantify circulating dd-cf-DNA and, during computational alignment performance, discriminate human dd-cf-DNA from microbial DNA and other erroneous material [26–28]. Based on this method, Snyder and colleagues introduced a new way to discriminate between donor and recipient DNA molecules, according to which increased dd-cf-DNA levels in recipients after transplantation may suggest the onset of rejection [28]. In patients experiencing acute rejection, augmented dd-cf-DNA assessed by SNPs can occur up to five months before detection on biopsy [26], indicating the potential for early diagnosis. One potential limitation using this approach is the difficulty in distinguishing graft damage due to antibody-mediated rejection (AMR) versus acute cellular rejection, implying the need for supporting follow-up tests to tune therapeutic approaches accordingly. Moreover, the complexity and cost of analyses limit its application as a clinically relevant surveillance tool. Finally, dd-cf-DNA's targeted quantification requires genotyping of both recipient and donors, which is suitable for bone marrow and kidney transplantation but not always possible for heart transplantation. Sharon and colleagues recently addressed this issue by elaborating an algorithm that estimates dd-cf-DNA levels in the absence of a donor genotype [ ]. This analysis was applied in a large, prospective, multicenter clinical trial, including patients with both ACR and AMR who received a heart transplant (HT) at least 55 days before enrolment [ ]. Dd-cf-DNA testing detected acute rejection with an area under the curve of 0.64 and provided an estimated NPV of 97.1% and positive predictive value of 8.9%. The limitation of genotyping donors was also addressed by North et al., who proposed a highly sensitive and quantitative multiplexed PCR test for 94 highly informative bi-allelic SNPs [ ].

North et al. developed a multiplexed allele-specific quantitative PCR method capable of the early detection of mild ACR (ISHLT 1R) in addition to higher grade ACR (ISHLT 2R and 3R), AMR, and graft vasculopathy. Using a specifically defined cut-off, the assay's clinical performance characteristics included an NPV of 100% for grade 2R or higher ACR, with 100% sensitivity and 75.48% specificity. This test's analytical validity facilitates conservative stratification of the probability of moderate to severe ACR as a potential companion tool for EMB in reducing the incidence of invasive biopsies, following the patients' response to therapy [ ].

A recent multicenter prospective blinded study investigated the value the ratio of cf-DNA specific to the transplanted organ, referring to the total amount of cf-DNA present in a blood sample to estimate cardiac allograft rejection. With a statistically optimized cut-off, the authors improved the dd-cf-DNA performance, reaching an NPV > 90.9% for ACR and > 99.7% for a higher grade of rejection, showing its potentiality as a novel surveillance tool thanks to its association with acute allograft rejection and a clinically applicable threshold both in adults and pediatric transplanted patients [ ]. They demonstrate the feasibility of their model in detecting injury to the donor organ and as a potential clinical biomarker for AMR, elucidating new frontiers of investigation to reach statistical significance in this rejection spectrum.

Despite the recent improvement of the dd-cf-DNA technique and its advantages in non-invasive monitoring, there are still some limitations with regard to dd-cf-DNA. Concomitant kidney and liver disease, not a rare situation in heart-transplanted patients, may affect cell-free DNA clearance and may lead to an underestimation of allograft injury. Moreover, the dd-cf-DNA assay could be further limited by the long labor processing time and especially by the need for genotyping [ ].

### 2.3. High-Sensitive Troponins

Cardiac troponins are well-known non-invasive tests used as reliable biological markers for several cardiovascular diseases. They have been investigated and implemented in clinical practice during the last decade. Cardiac troponins are sarcomeric structural proteins released in the bloodstream due to cardiomyocyte disruption, typically during moderate and severe ACR [ ].

Myocyte damage is a mandatory pathological index of ACR for both moderate and severe events. Therefore, it has been evaluated as a potential biomarker of allograft rejection, with the aim of identifying a cutoff value for diagnosis and/or exclusion of ACR to rationalize EMB [ – ].

Recently, Erbel and coworkers established a high-sensitive troponin serum cutoff level of 33.55 ng/l capable of predicting death at 12 months after transplant with a sensitivity of 90.91% and a specificity of 70.97%. Besides this, survival at five years was significantly improved in patients with values below the cutoff [ ]. However, contradictory results exist that show no association between allograft rejection and cardiac troponin levels [ ], suggesting that high-sensitive cardiac troponin cannot be currently recommended as a tool to monitor rejection.

## 2.4. T-Cell Function

A key event in graft rejection is the activation and proliferation of the recipient's lymphocytes, particularly T cells, which are detrimental to the long-term transplant outcome. Pharmacodynamic monitoring by direct measurement of T-cell activation and proliferation can therefore personalize immunosuppression.

The CD4 cell stimulation assay is a technology used to measure cell-mediated immunity and early response to stimulation by detecting intracellular adenosine triphosphate(iATP) synthesis in CD4+ cells selected from the blood by monoclonal antibody-coated magnetic beads. ATP can be measured by the firefly luciferase system and an assay to monitor iATP in CD4+ cells [38]. The CD4 cell stimulation assay has been approved by the US Food and Drug Administration to be applied on solid organ transplantation [38]. The assay has been used to detect iATP level released by activated CD4+ cells and their correlation with the risk of rejection or infection [38]. The significance of iATP measurement in CD4+ cells predicting acute rejection and infection is currently under investigation because different studies have found contradictory results. A published meta-analysis incorporating multiple organ transplants concluded that iATP monitoring is not suitable to identify individuals at risk of rejection or infection [39]. A drawback from the analytical standpoint is that the assay is a time-consuming, indirect cell function test requiring stimulation and a cell isolation step. Furthermore, all the studies analyzed by Ling and colleagues presented an important bias in sample selection: the numbers of rejection and infection episodes were too small to perform a robust correlation [39]. Clinical trials must generate new evidence to support the appropriate interpretation of the results.

## 2.5. Donor-Specific Antibodies

Following the consensus guidelines on the testing and clinical management issue with regard to human leukocyte antigen (HLA) and non-HLA antibodies in 2013 [40], an international consensus conference was organized in 2016 by the ISHLT to discuss current practices for detecting and quantifying circulating antibodies and validating the efficacy of therapeutic approaches [41]. Scientists agreed that equivocal results still exist with regard to the best practices for identifying antibodies of clinical relevance and their treatment. Solid-phase assays, such as the Luminex SAB assay, have been recommended to detect circulating antibodies [41]. Patients with a panel reactive antibody (PRA) <10% or donor-directed antibodies at the time of transplantation are at risk for suboptimal outcomes post-transplantation. The above-mentioned consensus conference recommended performing post-transplant monitoring for donor-specific antibodies (DSAs) at 1, 3, 6, and 12 months post-surgery [42]. For monitoring after 12 months post-surgery, the consensus supports a yearly follow-up, except for high-risk patients, who require stricter surveillance.

## 2.6. Emerging Biomarkers: Micro RNA, mRNA, Exosomes, and Microvesicles

### 2.6.1. RNA

Various RNA molecule classes, such as protein-coding messenger RNAs (mRNA), small non-coding RNAs, long non-coding RNAs (lnc-RNAs), and other non-coding RNA molecules, have been associated with disease phenotypes, raising their potential as minimally invasive biomarkers [43,44].

lnc-RNAs are autonomously transcribed RNAs, usually longer more than 200 nucleotides, affecting significantly gene expression, e.g., with regard to chromatin regulation and T and B cells functions and differentiation. Recently, Gu and colleagues demonstrated, in a mouse model of heart transplantation, that lnc-RNAs regulate Th1 cell response during graft rejection. In this study, they compared the mRNA and lnc-RNA profiles of heart grafts and graft infiltration lymphocytes in both syngeneic and allogenic murine transplanted groups. They not only showed that A930015D03Rik and mouselincRNA1055 are highly upregulated during transplant rejection but also that they are associated with Th1 cell response through the regulation of IL12Rb1 expression. Moreover, they tested, in kidney transplanted human samples, two human lnc-RNAs expression, matching A930015D03Rik and mouselincRNA1055 separately, proving their increased expression in kidney transplant rejection samples rather than controls. This study provides a valuable proof-of-concept: lnc-RNAs can be used as innovative ACR biomarkers and potentially implemented in clinical monitoring of acute rejection episodes [ ].

MicroRNA (miRNA) are small non-coding RNAs that play a role in gene expression regulation by targeting mRNA. Some miRNA are tissue- and cell-type specific and their expression level is linked directly to the pathophysiological state of organs. Extracellular circulating miRNA might be able to give us a "snapshot" of the patient's current health state, thanks to their stability and the possibility of repeating and reproducing the measurement of their levels, which can also be undertaken using multiple frozen/thawed serum/plasma samples. For these reasons, miRNAs are suitable as non-invasive biomarkers, with several groups evaluating their diagnostic and predictor potential for allograft rejection monitoring.

In transplantation and allograft rejection monitoring, two main approaches were followed: in some studies, the authors focused on the analysis of single miRNA, while in others, they chose to analyze a group of different miRNAs that enabled them to define a characteristic pattern and pathway.

In 2013, Dewi and colleagues conducted a small pilot study to assess the potential of using serum miRNAs as acute rejection biomarkers. They investigated ten heart transplant patients, comparing serum miRNA expression levels before, during, and after rejection episodes. The analysis revealed that the levels of seven miRNAs increased during rejection. Among these, only miR-326 and miR-142-3p showed acceptable AUC values (0.86 and 0.80, respectively) (Table 1), demonstrating significant discrimination between normal and pathologic features [ ]. A second study by the same authors validated the selected miRNAs in a different and more extensive cohort of patients with histologically verified acute cellular rejection ($n = 26$) and a control group of heart transplant recipients without allograft rejection ($n = 37$). The diagnostic performance in discriminating rejection vs. absence of rejection in patients using miR-142-3p and miR-101-3p revealed an AUC– ROC (Receiver Operator Characteristic) of 0.78 and 0.75, respectively [ ]. Despite the more extensive and independent cohort, the numerosity was still limited, and the authors could only discriminate ACR from no-rejection status but not identify the AMR cases. However, despite this limitation, this study demonstrated that the use of circulating miRNAs in acute cardiac rejection monitoring could be beneficial [ ].

Duong Van Huyen and colleagues adopted a different approach, demonstrating that miRNAs expression is regulated both on tissue and on serum. They assessed the level of 14 different miRNAs on EMBs, of which seven were differentially expressed between normal and rejecting EMB specimens. After that, the seven miRNAs were analyzed in patients' sera, collected at identical EMB time points [ ]. The analysis showed that miR-10a, miR-31, miR-92a, and miR-155 discriminated accurately between patients with and without rejection, with good yield in the external validation cohort (miR-10a AUC = 0.981, miR-31 AUC = 0.867, miR-92a AUC = 0.959, and miR-155 AUC = 0.974) [ ].

Moreover, these four miRNAs facilitated the potential discriminating issue both for ACR and AMR vs. non-rejection status. However, the study was limited by the lack of an unselected prospective cohort to test miRNAs and the literature-based preselection of the miRNAs tested [ ].

As showed by Van Aelst et al., miRNAs have potential as therapeutic targets for ACR. In their study, through a comparison between miRNA and mRNA expression profiles in human and mouse hearts, they identified a common signature that enabled the discrimination of rejecting and non-rejecting grafts. Hence, they demonstrated that miR-155 is overexpressed in ACR and can be a candidate target for novel therapeutics. Furthermore, they showed in a mouse model that both the knockout and the pharmacological inhibition of miR-155 delay the graft failure by reducing inflammatory infiltrate. Despite some limitations, this study highlighted the potential dual role of miRNAs not only as biomarkers but also as novel therapeutic targets [ ].

### 2.6.2. Extracellular Vesicles

Extracellular vesicles (EVs) are nanospherical membranes formed by a lipid bilayer embedded with transmembrane components, such as proteins, cholesterol, and saccharides. They envelop cytosolic proteins and nucleic acids. Based on biogenesis and size, EV classification includes exosomes, microvesicles, and apoptotic bodies. Exosomes ranging in size between 40 and 150 nm are formed and stored within subcellular compartments termed multivesicular bodies (MVBs). They are released from cells into the extracellular space upon fusion between MVBs and the cell membrane. MVBs or microparticles in the range of 100 to 1000 nm are derived from plasma membrane budding [49–51].

EVs act as vectors of biological information by transferring their content to target cells under basal conditions and in pathological settings. They are emerging as promising biomarker candidates for several reasons. Primarily, this is because EVs can be isolated from peripheral blood through minimally invasive sampling. Furthermore, cells that form tissues finely modulate the sorting of proteins, lipids, and nucleic acids into secretory vesicles in response to specific pathophysiological conditions [52]. Consequently, enrichment in vesicle fractions appears to provide additional diagnostic value in terms of sensitivity and specificity compared to analyses performed on unfractionated body fluids [53]. This enrichment may overcome the limitation of detecting biomarkers circulating in very low concentrations, usually below the test sensitivity routinely used in clinical practice. Our recent study analyzed the phospholipid content of vesicles, demonstrating a specific signature enabling differentiation between patients who underwent myocardial infarction and controls. However, analysis in whole unfractionated plasma resulted in the loss of the specific signature [53].

Vesicles from platelets, endothelial cells, monocytes, and leukocytes form the major component within the circulating exosomal fraction [54]. Furthermore, they are involved in immune responses, inflammation, and coagulation processes [55–57]. Hence, acute and chronic conditions affecting an altered inflammatory response are often associated with a systemic release of EVs containing specific proteins, nucleic acids, and/or lipids, conveying a distinct signature that is potentially relevant as a biomarker [56,57].

In this context, circulating EVs might represent a non-invasive tool for monitoring early post-transplant inflammatory responses in heart transplant recipients, supporting EMBs. We recently proposed and validated a protocol to characterize the surface antigens of circulating vesicles and assess their diagnostic performance in evaluating acute cardiac allograft rejection [58]. The application of a rapid standardized fluorescence bead-based multiplex assay combined with a supervised machine learning approach facilitated the accurate discrimination of patients with allograft rejection compared to patients without rejection. Moreover, we retrospectively confirmed the EMB-based diagnosis of the different cardiac rejection types, with a sensitivity and specificity of 100% and 85.7%, respectively. Given the high diagnostic performance, low cost, and relative usability, this method is highly promising for the characterization, monitoring, and prediction of allograft rejection, potentially reducing the number of EMBs required [58].

Kennel and colleagues performed proteomic analysis by liquid chromatography with tandem mass spectrometry on serum-derived EVs collected from cardiac transplant recipients without rejection, with ACR, and with AMR [59]. Based on relatively complex methods and instruments that analyze the entire protein content, the study demonstrated the predictive and prognostic value of EVs as biomarkers.

The significance of EVs as predictive and diagnostic biomarkers of rejection is even more promising because, besides their role as measurable indicators of distinct biological conditions [60], EVs hold functional biological characteristics in immune response modulation, thus providing consistency as tools to monitor the allograft status and improve post-transplant outcomes [60]. EVs display Major Histocompatibility Complex (MHC) class I and II, as well as adhesion and costimulatory molecules, resembling the role of antigen-presenting vesicles for allospecific T-cell activation [61]. In a murine heart transplant model, exosomes from mature dendritic cells (DCs) mediated their endocrine signaling by migrating to the regional lymph nodes. This process facilitated acute rejection by activating T cells, thus amplifying the effect of the limited number of donor DCs present in the transplanted organ [ ]. In a mechanism implying contact-dependent signaling, MHC peptides carried on the EV surface derived from mature DCs efficiently primed T cells [ ], playing a role in inducing tolerance in a fully MHC-mismatched rat cardiac allograft model [ ]. A further indirect mechanism has been described for follicular DCs unable to synthesize MHC class II proteins. These cells passively acquire the complex by capturing circulating MHC class II-expressing EVs, presenting them to T cells as a vesicle-composed wreath [ ]. In this case, DCs enhanced the stimulatory capacity of EV and the presence of cell-to-EV binding is critical to stimulate specific T cells efficiently [ – ]. Following these findings, which suggest that donor vesicles may play a role as exclusive sources of donor MHC for T-cell activation, Habertheuer et al. recently showed that transplanted hearts release donor-specific EV. In a murine model of a heterotopic heart transplant, the cardiac allograft released a distinct pool of donor MHC-specific EVs into the recipient circulation. The signal peaked during early acute rejection with high accuracy [ ], enabling the developing of a highly specific and sensitive biomarker platform for allograft monitoring [ , ].

Finally, Sharma et al. recognized cardiac myosin and vimentin as tissue-restricted self-antigens that are detectable on the surface of circulating EVs and are associated with primary graft dysfunction [ ]. Hence, the above-cited mechanisms are consistent because the transplanted heart is a vascularized organ at the time of placement and donor vesicles released may leak through the vascular endothelium and be trafficked into the hosts' bloodstream.

## 3. Tissue Biopsy for Molecular Tests

The liquid biopsy is a very attractive non-invasive source of information for monitoring post-heart transplanted patients. However, the opportunity offered by the utilization of tissue biopsy for molecular tests remains pivotal. Different groups have tried to identify new biomarkers in EMBs to improve the diagnosis of rejection. EMB is the gold standard in monitoring cardiac rejection. Generally, the pathologists assess the inflammatory infiltrate and the myocardial injury through histological and immunohistochemical evaluation. This approach makes it possible to define and grade the rejection but also to modify the pharmacological therapy. Thus, EMB is an important source of information about a graft's status, but its potential has only partially been exploited. The opportunity to investigate the rejection mechanisms directly on the tissue offers new insights into the cellular interactions and graft injury evolution over time. Different groups have tried to apply new technologies to understand the molecular pathways involved in rejection, assess the cardiac allograft status, and define new biomarkers to ameliorate the rejection diagnosis on biopsy tissue.

### 3.1. MicroRNA on Tissue

As discussed above, miRNAs are non-coding regulative molecules in numerous signaling pathways also involved in pathophysiological disorders. The investigation of miRNA expression on cardiac tissue could help in the characterization of rejection events [ ].

Recently, we defined an miRNA signature to discriminate ACR, AMR, and mixed rejection (MR) on formalin-fixed and paraffin-embedded (FFPE) EMB specimens through next-generation sequencing (NGS) and reverse transcription quantitative polymerase chain reaction (RT-qPCR). Using logistic regression analysis, we created unique miRNA signatures as predictive models of each type of rejection. More than 2257 mature miRNAs were obtained from all EMBs. Each of the three rejection types showed a different miRNA profile. The logistic regression model formed by miRNAs 208a, 126-5p, and 135a-5p identified MR, whereas ACR was identified by the miRNAs 27b-3p, 29b-3p, and 199a-3p. In contrast, AMR was identified by the miRNAs 208a, 29b-3p, 135a-5p, and 144-3p [ ].

Another interesting work by Nováková and colleagues aimed to identify miRNAs dysregulated on FFPE EMB specimens during ACR [ ]. The authors used a stepwise backward regression method and three principal component analyses (PCA) to create an ACR SCORE model. This model uses the levels of 11 miRNAs (miR-144, -589, -146, -182, -3135b, -3605, -10, -31, -17, -1273, -4506), detected in EMBs through RT-qPCR, to assign an ACR SCORE to the specimens. If the score is above the defined cut-off value, the authors defined ACR as present with a specificity of 91% and a sensitivity of 68% [11].

Furthermore, the RT-qPCR validation of the 11 miRNAs, previously identified in EMBs through NGS, confirmed that miR-144, miR-589, and miR-182 are statistically significantly altered during rejection [11].

As stressed by Nováková et al., a remarkable limitation of studies focused on the use of microRNA as biomarkers is the lack of uniformity (Table 1). Many studies demonstrated that miRNAs are eligible biomarkers of disease; however, they were not unanimous in identifying a unique miRNA or miRNA signature applicable in clinical practice. Various methodological factors could be the source of this heterogeneity, e.g., the different protocols for RNA isolation and analysis or the nature of the EMB specimens, which incorporate many different cell types (cardiomyocytes, lymphocytes, fibroblast and endothelial cells) with different cell-specific levels of miRNA expression. Furthermore, patients' comorbidities and personalized immunosuppressive therapy impact the cohort variability included in multiple studies, leading to a lack of consistency [11].

### 3.2. Molecular Microscope

The molecular microscope, first developed for kidney transplantation (KT), uses rejection-associated transcriptome (RAT) profiling of known kidney biopsies as a reference to generate an automated, objective, and quantitative report to offset intercenter variation [71]. Halloran and colleagues proposed this as a new method to also assess rejection in EMBs. A direct comparison of this system with EMBs guided the development of a molecular microscope heart diagnostic system called the Heart Molecular Microscope Diagnostic System (MMDx-Heart), a microarray-based technology used to evaluate the molecular status of tissue [72]. This approach relies on the hypothesis that the inflammatory lesions and molecular alterations of heart allograft rejection act similarly to KT, closely correlating histologic features of EMBs and KT biopsies [72].

An unsupervised PCA was performed based on RAT expression scores in the 1208 indication kidney biopsies and the 331 EMBs and three archetype scores were assigned in EMBs corresponding to histologic T cell-mediated rejection (TCMR), antibody-mediated rejection (ABMR), and no rejection (NR) groups. Combining the best performing probes, they achieved AUC–ROC values of 0.78, 0.65, and 0.81 for NR, TCMR, and ABMR archetypes, respectively [72]. These results showed that this system has a lower sensibility for EMBs than for kidney biopsies and a higher disagreement level between molecular and histopathologic assessments. According to the authors, this last point reflects the higher interpathological disagreement for EMB assessment highlighted by the Cargo study, particularly for cellular-mediated rejection [72]. Moreover, the authors suggested that the molecular discrepancy observed in TCMR diagnosis could be due to the Quilty effect's presence and that the further investigation of its molecular similarities with TCMR could be very enlightening. Overall, this study demonstrated that molecular tissue analysis reflects the complexity of EMB assessment, with further investigations required to overcome the present limitations [72].

### 3.3. MRI for Non-Invasive Monitoring in Tissue

At the tissue level, graft rejection presents infiltrative inflammatory cells with an expansion of the extracellular space and necrosis. These morphostructural changes have been investigated in several studies with a cardiovascular magnetic resonance (CMR) methodology, enabling non-invasive imaging with qualitative and quantitative tissue characterization. CMR can evaluate histopathologic changes due to rejection, associated with distinct myocardial T1 and T2 relaxation times [73]. Using a multiparametric sequential approach, by combining basal T2 mapping with the basal extracellular volume fraction, improved diagnostic accuracy for transplant rejection can be achieved [ ]. Therefore, a multisequential CMR examination could operate as a non-invasive tool for excluding subclinical ACR in heart transplant patients [ ].

*3.4. Gene Expression Profile in the Tissue*

The value of myocardial GEP for diagnosing and identifying the predictive biomarkers of ACR was evaluated in the GET study by Bodez and Damy in 36 EMBs in 30 patients [ ]. They demonstrated that the cardiac gene expression profiles of EMBs only partly matched the histological grading system, suggesting that cardiac GEP may provide earlier and more sensitive performances in diagnosing ACR and can be used as an early screening test for ACR [ ].

GEP for the identification and classification of antibody-mediated heart rejection was evaluated by Loupy et al. In 110 patients [ ]. The authors applied a combination of multi-dimensional molecular assessments to extensive phenotyping allograft biopsies to characterize anti-HLA antibodies and cellular models, demonstrating that antibody-mediated rejection in heart transplantation is driven mainly by the natural killer burden [ ].

Using the NanoString nCounter technology, the expression of a set of 34 literature-derived genes reflecting the molecular correlates of antibody-mediated injury in 106 FFPE EMBs for a training cohort and 57 EMBs for a validating cohort was evaluated in a recent study by the Edmonton group [ ]. The gene set selected by the authors for AMR profiling revealed a good diagnostic accuracy (approximately 70%) in identifying AMR positive cases vs. negative ones, with a sound correlation with other diagnostic methods routinely applied, such as histopathology, anti-HLA DSA, and C4d immunohistochemistry. However, the gene set was unable to differentiate pathological AMR1(I+) from ACR and normal controls, raising the question of the real value of this histopathological grade, which, according to their results, appears more similar to ACR than to AMR [ ]. This very promising study highlights the need for a larger cohort of patients but also more importantly for the identification of a new set of genes capable of differentiating between AMR and other non-immunologic endothelial injuries [ ].

Intragraft gene expression studies can highlight the functional status of the transplanted organ. Arteriolar vasculitis in EMBs may be pivotal in identifying high-risk episodes in transplant recipients. Gene expression analysis could help in understanding alterations in genes profile associated with vasculitis, affecting the heart allograft's survival in long-term transplantation. From this perspective, Lin-Wang et al. conducted a retrospective study of 300 FFPE EMBs of 63 patients to determine the incidence of vasculitis and its association with ACR, AMR, and cardiac allograft vasculopathy. This study performed a gene expression analysis of the chosen transcript involved in inflammation and vascular function as evaluated by q-PCR. Their results showed that vasculitis carried worse prognostic outcomes [ ].

## 4. Conclusions

Allograft rejection is a life-threatening complication of organ transplantation. Its monitoring is a fundamental step in the post-transplant follow-up.

EMBs remain the gold standard for cardiac allograft monitoring; however, the perceived need to complement the histological examination of the tissue with molecular approaches has led to the development of several molecular approaches to implementing diagnosis.

Indeed, the histological evaluation of cardiac tissue assesses the allograft's inflammatory status; nevertheless, EMBs represent such valuable in vivo tissue that much more information needs to be retrieved from them than just the information about the inflammatory status.

Omics may improve comprehension of the allograft's pathophysiological feature and provide pathologists and clinicians with new insights related to the graft that help in developing a personalized therapeutic approach for better management of transplanted patients.

The application of several molecular techniques on cardiac tissue represented a starting point for a new era of allograft rejection diagnosis. As discussed above and described in the evaluated research (Table 1), many studies demonstrated that comprehension of the rejection process is still limited. Research must go on to dissect it. Like any invasive procedure, EMBs can cause some complications and counterbalancing these negative aspects has been researchers' primary intent for years. Many non-invasive approaches have been designed and tested in clinical trials in the hope of identifying an alternative diagnostic tool for rejection monitoring. Several cutting-edge methods that rely on liquid biopsies have implemented procedures and clinical applications that provide the most comprehensive patient heart transplant snapshots. Recent efforts in the transplant research field have also applied these novel methods to the tissue to combine different information from various resources.

Table 1. Emerging biomarkers in the diagnosis of allograft rejection after heart transplantation.

| Study | Diagnostic Tool | n. of Patients | Area Under the Curve | Sensitivity (%) | Specificity (%) |
|---|---|---|---|---|---|
| Pham MX. 2010 [7] | GEP of peripheral specimen (randomized controlled trial: Image study) | 602 | Not inferior to EMB | | |
| Deng MC. 2006 [8] | GEP of peripheral blood leucocytes (11-gene real time PCR: Cargo study) | 170 | 0.686–0.914 | 75.8 * | 41.8 * |
| Di Francesco A. 2018 [10] | Tissue microRNAs (combination of miR-208a-5p, -126-5p, -135-5p) | 33 | 0.951–1.000 | 83.3 | 95.8 |
| Nováková T. 2019 [11] | Tissue microRNAs (combination of miR-144, 589, 146, 182, 3135b, 10, 31, 17, 1273, 3605, 4506) | 38 | 0.72–0.96 | 68 | 91 |
| Kobashigawa J. 2015 [16] | GEP of peripheral specimen (randomized controlled trial) | 60 | Not inferior to EMB | | |
| Crespo-Leiro MG. 2016 [17] | GEP of peripheral specimen (observational study: Cargo II study) | 462 | 0.690–0.700 | 86.4 * | 46.5 * |
| Shannon CP, 2020 [19] | Whole blood transcriptome profile (nine mRNA transcript Nanostring nCounter) | 177 | 0.69 \| 0.70 | 89 | 47 |
| Lin D. 2009 [21] | Whole blood genomic profile (12-gene biomarker panel) | 28 | N.A. | 83.0 | 100.0 |
| Hollander Z. 2010 [22] | Whole blood genomic profile (Affymetrix Human Genome U133 Plus 2.0 chips) | 31 | 0.600–0.830 | N.A. | N.A. |
| De Vlaminck I. 2014 [26] | Quantification of circulating cell-free donor-derived DNA | 65 | 0.830 | 58.0 | 93 |
| Khush KK. 2019 [30] | Quantification of circulating cell-free donor-derived DNA | 676 | 0.64 | 44.0 | 80 |
| Richmond ME. 2020 [31] | Quantification of donor fraction of cell-free DNA (0R vs. ≥ 1R) | 174 | 0.86 | 80 | 88 |
| Sukma Dewi I. 2013 [45] | Identification of single serum microRNA (miR-326, miR-142-3p) | 10 | 0.800–0.860 | N.A. | N.A. |
| Sukma Dewi I. 2017 [46] | Identification of single serum microRNA (miR-101-3p, miR-142-3p) | 63 | 0.750–0.780 | N.A. | N.A. |
| Duong VH JP. 2014 [47] | Identification of single serum microRNA (miR-10a, -31, -92a, -155) | 113 | 0.867–981 * | N.A. | N.A. |
| Castellani C. 2020 [58] | Characterization of circulating extracellular vesicles surface antigens | 90 | 0.727–0.939 | 100.0 * | 85.7 * |
| Kennel PJ. 2018 [59] | Serum exosomal protein profiling | 48 | N.A. | N.A. | N.A. |
| Halloran PF. 2017 [72] | Microarray-based molecular microscope (MMDx System) | 221 | 0.650–0.810 | N.A. | N.A. |

Table 1. Cont.

| Study | Diagnostic Tool | n. of Patients | Area Under the Curve | Sensitivity (%) | Specificity (%) |
|---|---|---|---|---|---|
| Bodez D. 2016 [ ] | GEP of myocardial tissue (combination of 15 genes—the GET study) | 30 | N.A. | 100.0 | 100.0 |
| Loupy A. 2017 [ ] | GEP of myocardial tissue (four different gene sets) | 110 | 0.800–0.870 * | N.A. | N.A. |
| Afzali B. 2017 [ ] | GEP of myocardial tissue (three different gene sets) | 163 | 0.778 * | 46.5 * | 80.0 * |

* Performance at validation. N.A., not assessed; GEP, gene expression profiling.

Approaches for defining the specific signature of circulating EVs from liquid biopsies show promising results but require further studies to validate their robustness and reliability through large-scale trials introduced in clinical practice.

Despite their contributions to highlighting novel and not-yet-investigated points of view in heart allograft rejection monitoring, the studies cited in this review share several common limitations: the relatively limited size of the patient cohorts and the lack of convergence towards a standard molecular profile of cardiac rejection. The GEP, CARGO, and IMAGE projects have overcome these issues. Their genetic approach can be proposed as a companion tool in diagnosis to reduce the number of EMBs performed. These kinds of processes often leverage sophisticated technologies not yet available for a large segment of transplanted patients.

Hence, the potential of genomics and transcriptomics is well-recognized and the identification of a transcriptome profile without a bias of selection could help in the definition of a shared panel of biomarkers for both the recognition of rejection and the discrimination between ACR, pathological AMR, MR, infections, and other injuries [ , ].

It is therefore crucial to recognize the need for wide-ranging studies, clinical exploiting the potential of big data analysis and machine learning techniques. As seen in the prediction system for kidney allograft loss in the iBox study [ ], there is a raised awareness with regard to the personalization of follow-up procedures and therapies for future heart transplanted patients.

The improvement of novel molecular approaches in tissue and liquid biopsies shows promising results that require further studies to validate their robustness and reliability through large-scale trials introduced in clinical practice. Even though liquid biopsy cannot wholly replace EMB, these two diagnostic approaches can be combined in clinical practice.

The synergic power of these two approaches can increase the accuracy of cardiac allograft rejection diagnosis. Defining the most effective rejection monitoring strategy could be the driving force for the settlement of a multimodal approach toward HT patient management.

The dynamic landscape of rejection surveillance, described in this review, highlights the evolution of the concept of EMB from a necessary procedure for histopathological evaluation of the transplanted heart state towards a comprehensive molecular resource accompanied by liquid biopsy. This holistic view of the follow-up patient's pathway brings to light a consistent multimodal personalized approach with the direct integration in clinical practice of invasive and non-invasive procedures, leading to a progressive change of paradigm in heart transplant monitoring.

**Author Contributions:** Conceptualization, A.A.; writing—original draft preparation, A.G., I.B., L.B. and A.A.; writing—review and editing, A.G., I.B., M.F., J.B., C.C., F.T., T.B., G.G., L.B. and A.A.; visualization, J.B., A.G., and I.B.; supervision, A.A., and L.B.; project administration, A.A., and L.B.; funding acquisition, A.A. All authors have read and agreed to the published version of the manuscript.

**Funding:** This research was funded by the University of Padua, grant numbers BIRD191573, BIRD199570, BIRD204045, and the APC was funded by BIRD199570.

**Institutional Review Board Statement:** Not applicable, it is a review of studies available in scientific literature.

**Informed Consent Statement:** Not applicable, it is a review of studies available in scientific literature.

**Data Availability Statement:** No new data were created or analyzed in this study. Data sharing is not applicable to this article.

**Acknowledgments:** Graphic abstract was produced using Servier Medical Art (https://smart.servier.com/).

**Conflicts of Interest:** The authors declare no conflict of interest. The funders had no role in the design of the study; in the collection, analyses, or interpretation of data; in the writing of the manuscript, or in the decision to publish the results.

## References

1. Lund, L.H.; Edwards, L.B.; Kucheryavaya, A.Y.; Benden, C.; Christie, J.D.; Dipchand, A.I.; Dobbels, F.; Goldfarb, S.B.; Levvey, B.J.; Meiser, B.; et al. The registry of the international society for heart and lung transplantation: Thirty-first official adult heart transplant report-2014; Focus theme: Retransplantation. *J. Hear. Lung Transplant.* **2014**, *33*, 996–1008. [CrossRef] [PubMed]
2. Billingham, M.E. Endomyocardial biopsy detection of acute rejection in cardiac allograft recipients. *Heart Vessels* **1985**, *1*, 86–90. [CrossRef] [PubMed]
3. From, A.M.; Maleszewski, J.J.; Rihal, C.S. Current status of endomyocardial biopsy. *Mayo Clin. Proc.* **2011**, *86*, 1095–1102. [CrossRef] [PubMed]
4. Saraiva, F.; Matos, V.; Gonalves, L.; Antunes, M.; Providência, L.A. Complications of endomyocardial biopsy in heart transplant patients: A retrospective study of 2117 consecutive procedures. *Transplant. Proc.* **2011**, *43*, 1908–1912. [CrossRef]
5. Crespo-Leiro, M.G.; Barge-Caballero, G.; Couto-Mallon, D. Noninvasive monitoring of acute and chronic rejection in heart transplantation. *Curr. Opin. Cardiol.* **2017**, *32*, 308–315. [CrossRef]
6. North, P.E.; Ziegler, E.; Mahnke, D.K.; Stamm, K.D.; Thomm, A.; Daft, P.; Goetsch, M.; Liang, H.L.; Baker, M.A.; Vepraskas, A.; et al. Cell-free DNA donor fraction analysis in pediatric and adult heart transplant patients by multiplexed allele-specific quantitative PCR: Validation of a rapid and highly sensitive clinical test for stratification of rejection probability. *PLoS ONE* **2020**, *15*, e0227385. [CrossRef]
7. Pham, M.X.; Teuteberg, J.J.; Kfoury, A.G.; Starling, R.C.; Deng, M.C.; Cappola, T.P.; Kao, A.; Anderson, A.S.; Cotts, W.G.; Ewald, G.A.; et al. Gene-expression profiling for rejection surveillance after cardiac transplantation. *N. Engl. J. Med.* **2010**, *362*, 1890–1900. [CrossRef]
8. Deng, M.C.; Eisen, H.J.; Mehra, M.R.; Billingham, M.; Marboe, C.C.; Berry, G.; Kobashigawa, J.; Johnson, F.L.; Starling, R.C.; Murali, S.; et al. Noninvasive discrimination of rejection in cardiac allograft recipients using gene expression profiling. *Am. J. Transplant.* **2006**, *6*, 150–160. [CrossRef]
9. Starling, R.C.; Pham, M.; Valantine, H.; Miller, L.; Eisen, H.; Rodriguez, E.R.; Taylor, D.O.; Yamani, M.H.; Kobashigawa, J.; McCurry, K.; et al. Molecular Testing in the Management of Cardiac Transplant Recipients: Initial Clinical Experience. *J. Hear. Lung Transplant.* **2006**, *25*, 1389–1395. [CrossRef]
10. Di Francesco, A.; Fedrigo, M.; Santovito, D.; Natarelli, L.; Castellani, C.; De Pascale, F.; Toscano, G.; Fraiese, A.; Feltrin, G.; Benazzi, E.; et al. MicroRNA signatures in cardiac biopsies and detection of allograft rejection. *J. Hear. Lung Transplant.* **2018**, *37*, 1329–1340. [CrossRef]
11. Nováková, T.; Macháčková, T.; Novák, J.; Hude, P.; Godava, J.; Žampachová, V.; Oppelt, J.; Zlámal, F.; Němec, P.; Bedáňová, H.; et al. Identification of a Diagnostic Set of Endomyocardial Biopsy microRNAs for Acute Cellular Rejection Diagnostics in Patients after Heart Transplantation Using Next-Generation Sequencing. *Cells* **2019**, *8*, 1400. [CrossRef] [PubMed]
12. Reichard, C.A.; Stephenson, A.J.; Klein, E.A. Applying precision medicine to the active surveillance of prostate cancer. *Cancer* **2015**, *121*, 3403–3411. [CrossRef] [PubMed]
13. Rijavec, E.; Coco, S.; Genova, C.; Rossi, G.; Longo, L.; Grossi, F. Liquid biopsy in non-small cell lung cancer: Highlights and challenges. *Cancers* **2020**, *12*, 17. [CrossRef]
14. Cristofanilli, M. Circulating Tumor Cells, Disease Progression, and Survival in Metastatic Breast Cancer. *Semin. Oncol.* **2006**, *33*, 9–14. [CrossRef]
15. Chatterjee, D. Liquid Biopsies: Handle With Care. *Pathol. Lab. Med. Open J.* **2016**, *1*, 3–6.
16. Kobashigawa, J.; Patel, J.; Azarbal, B.; Kittleson, M.; Chang, D.; Czer, L.; Daun, T.; Luu, M.; Trento, A.; Cheng, R.; et al. Randomized Pilot Trial of Gene Expression Profiling Versus Heart Biopsy in the First Year after Heart Transplant: Early Invasive Monitoring Attenuation Through Gene Expression Trial. *Circ. Hear. Fail.* **2015**, *8*, 557–564. [CrossRef]
17. Crespo-Leiro, M.G.; Stypmann, J.; Schulz, U.; Zuckermann, A.; Mohacsi, P.; Bara, C.; Ross, H.; Parameshwar, J.; Zakliczyński, M.; Fiocchi, R.; et al. Clinical usefulness of gene-expression profile to rule out acute rejection after heart transplantation: CARGO II. *Eur. Heart J.* **2016**, *37*, 2591–2601. [CrossRef]

18. Stewart, S.; Winters, G.L.; Fishbein, M.C.; Tazelaar, H.D.; Kobashigawa, J.; Abrams, J.; Andersen, C.B.; Angelini, A.; Berry, G.J.; Burke, M.M.; et al. Revision of the 1990 working formulation for the standardization of nomenclature in the diagnosis of heart rejection. *J. Hear. Lung Transplant.* **2005**, *24*, 1710–1720.
19. Shannon, C.P.; Hollander, Z.; Dai, D.L.Y.; Chen, V.; Assadian, S.; Lam, K.K.; McManus, J.E.; Zarzycki, M.; Kim, Y.W.; Kim, J.Y.V.; et al. HEARTBiT: A Transcriptomic Signature for Excluding Acute Cellular Rejection in Adult Heart Allograft Patients. *Can. J. Cardiol.* **2020**, *36*, 1217–1227.
20. Kim, J.Y.V.; Lee, B.; Koitsopoulos, P.; Shannon, C.P.; Chen, V.; Hollander, Z.; Assadian, S.; Lam, K.; Ritchie, G.; McManus, J.; et al. Analytical Validation of HEARTBiT: A Blood-Based Multiplex Gene Expression Profiling Assay for Exclusionary Diagnosis of Acute Cellular Rejection in Heart Transplant Patients. *Clin. Chem.* **2020**, *66*, 1063–1071.
21. Lin, D.; Hollander, Z.; Ng, R.T.; Imai, C.; Ignaszewski, A.; Balshaw, R.; Freue, G.C.; Wilson-McManus, J.E.; Qasimi, P.; Meredith, A.; et al. Whole Blood Genomic Biomarkers of Acute Cardiac Allograft Rejection. *J. Hear. Lung Transplant.* **2009**, *28*, 927–935.
22. Hollander, Z.; Lin, D.; Chen, V.; Ng, R.; Wilson-Mcmanus, J.; Ignaszewski, A.; Cohen Freue, G.; Balshaw, R.; Mui, A.; McMaster, R.; et al. Whole blood biomarkers of acute cardiac allograft rejection: Double-crossing the biopsy. *Transplantation* **2010**, *90*, 1388–1393.
23. Moayedi, Y.; Foroutan, F.; Miller, R.J.H.; Fan, C.P.S.; Posada, J.G.D.; Alhussein, M.; Tremblay-Gravel, M.; Oro, G.; Luikart, H.I.; Yee, J.; et al. Risk evaluation using gene expression screening to monitor for acute cellular rejection in heart transplant recipients. *J. Hear. Lung Transplant.* **2019**, *38*, 51–58.
24. Mehra, M.R.; Uber, P.A.; Benitez, R.M. Gene-Based Bio-Signature Patterns and Cardiac Allograft Rejection. *Heart Fail. Clin.* **2010**, *6*, 87–92.
25. Lo, Y.M.D.; Tein, M.S.C.; Pang, C.C.P.; Yeung, C.K.; Tong, K.L.; Magnus Hjelm, N. Presence of donor-specific DNA in plasma of kidney and liver-transplant recipients. *Lancet* **1998**, *351*, 1329–1330.
26. De Vlaminck, I.; Valantine, H.A.; Snyder, T.M.; Strehl, C.; Cohen, G.; Luikart, H.; Neff, N.F.; Okamoto, J.; Bernstein, D.; Weisshaar, D.; et al. Circulating cell-free DNA enables noninvasive diagnosis of heart transplant rejection. *Sci. Transl. Med.* **2014**, *6*.
27. Beck, J.; Oellerich, M.; Schulz, U.; Schauerte, V.; Reinhard, L.; Fuchs, U.; Knabbe, C.; Zittermann, A.; Olbricht, C.; Gummert, J.F.; et al. Donor-Derived Cell-Free DNA is a Novel Universal Biomarker for Allograft Rejection in Solid Organ Transplantation. *Transplant. Proc.* **2015**, *47*, 2400–2403.
28. Snyder, T.M.; Khush, K.K.; Valantine, H.A.; Quake, S.R. Universal noninvasive detection of solid organ transplant rejection. *Proc. Natl. Acad. Sci. USA* **2011**, *108*, 6229–6234.
29. Sharon, E.; Shi, H.; Kharbanda, S.; Koh, W.; Martin, L.R.; Khush, K.K.; Valantine, H.; Pritchard, J.K.; De Vlaminck, I. Quantification of transplant-derived circulating cell-free DNA in absence of a donor genotype. *PLoS Comput. Biol.* **2017**, *13*, e1005629.
30. Khush, K.K.; Patel, J.; Pinney, S.; Kao, A.; Alharethi, R.; DePasquale, E.; Ewald, G.; Berman, P.; Kanwar, M.; Hiller, D.; et al. Noninvasive detection of graft injury after heart transplant using donor-derived cell-free DNA: A prospective multicenter study. *Am. J. Transplant.* **2019**, *19*, 2889–2899.
31. Richmond, M.E.; Zangwill, S.D.; Kindel, S.J.; Deshpande, S.R.; Schroder, J.N.; Bichell, D.P.; Knecht, K.R.; Mahle, W.T.; Wigger, M.A.; Gaglianello, N.A.; et al. Donor fraction cell-free DNA and rejection in adult and pediatric heart transplantation. *J. Hear. Lung Transplant.* **2020**, *39*, 454–463.
32. Agbor-Enoh, S.; Tunc, I.; De Vlaminck, I.; Fideli, U.; Davis, A.; Cuttin, K.; Bhatti, K.; Marishta, A.; Solomon, M.A.; Jackson, A. Applying rigor and reproducibility standards to assay donor-derived cell-free DNA as a non-invasive method for detection of acute rejection and graft injury after heart transplantation. *J. Hear. Lung Transplant.* **2020**, *36*, 1004–1012.
33. Fitzsimons, S.; Evans, J.; Parameshwar, J.; Pettit, S.J. Utility of troponin assays for exclusion of acute cellular rejection after heart transplantation: A systematic review. *J. Hear. Lung Transplant.* **2018**, *37*, 631–638.
34. Patel, P.C.; Hill, D.A.; Ayers, C.R.; Lavingia, B.; Kaiser, P.; Dyer, A.K.; Barnes, A.P.; Thibodeau, J.T.; Mishkin, J.D.; Mammen, P.P.A.; et al. High-sensitivity cardiac troponin i assay to screen for acute rejection in patients with heart transplant. *Circ. Hear. Fail.* **2014**, *7*, 463–469.
35. Méndez, A.B.; Cardona, M.; Ordóñez-Llanos, J.; Mirabet, S.; Perez-Villa, F.; Roig, E. Predictive Value of High-sensitive Troponin T to Rule Out Acute Rejection After Heart Transplantation. *Rev. Española Cardiol.* **2014**, *67*, 775–776.
36. Erbel, C.; Taskin, R.; Doesch, A.; Dengler, T.J.; Wangler, S.; Akhavanpoor, M.; Ruhparwar, A.; Giannitsis, E.; Katus, H.A.; Gleissner, C.A. High-sensitive Troponin T measurements early after heart transplantation predict short- and long-term survival. *Transpl. Int.* **2013**, *26*, 267–272.
37. Battes, L.C.; Caliskan, K.; Rizopoulos, D.; Constantinescu, A.A.; Robertus, J.L.; Akkerhuis, M.; Manintveld, O.C.; Boersma, E.; Kardys, I. Repeated measurements of NT-pro-B-Type natriuretic peptide, troponin T or C-reactive protein do not predict future allograft rejection in heart transplant recipients. *Transplantation* **2015**, *99*, 580–585.
38. Andrikopoulou, E.; Mather, P.J. Current insights: Use of Immuknow in heart transplant recipients. *Prog. Transplant.* **2014**, *24*, 44–50.
39. Ling, X.; Xiong, J.; Liang, W.; Schroder, P.M.; Wu, L.; Ju, W.; Kong, Y.; Shang, Y.; Guo, Z.; He, X. Can immune cell function assay identify patients at risk of infection or rejection? A meta-analysis. *Transplantation* **2012**, *93*, 737–743.

40. Tait, B.D.; Süsal, C.; Gebel, H.M.; Nickerson, P.W.; Zachary, A.A.; Claas, F.H.J.; Reed, E.F.; Bray, R.A.; Campbell, P.; Chapman, J.R.; et al. Consensus guidelines on the testing and clinical management issues associated with HLA and Non-HLA antibodies in transplantation. *Transplantation* **2013**, *95*, 19–47. [CrossRef]
41. Kobashigawa, J.; Colvin, M.; Potena, L.; Dragun, D.; Crespo-Leiro, M.G.; Delgado, J.F.; Olymbios, M.; Parameshwar, J.; Patel, J.; Reed, E.; et al. The management of antibodies in heart transplantation: An ISHLT consensus document. *J. Hear. Lung Transplant.* **2018**, *37*, 537–547. [CrossRef] [PubMed]
42. Kobashigawa, J.; Crespo-Leiro, M.G.; Ensminger, S.M.; Reichenspurner, H.; Angelini, A.; Berry, G.; Burke, M.; Czer, L.; Hiemann, N.; Kfoury, A.G.; et al. Report from a consensus conference on antibody-mediated rejection in heart transplantation. *J. Hear. Lung Transplant.* **2011**, *30*, 252–269. [CrossRef] [PubMed]
43. Langseth, H.; Bucher-johannessen, C.; Fromm, B.; Keller, A. A comprehensive profile of circulating RNAs in human serum. *RNA Biol.* **2018**, *15*, 242–250.
44. Gu, G.; Huang, Y.; Wu, C.; Guo, Z.; Ma, Y.; Xia, Q.; Awasthi, A.; He, X. Differential expression of long noncoding RNAs during cardiac allograft rejection. *Transplantation* **2017**, *101*, 83–91. [CrossRef]
45. Sukma Dewi, I.; Torngren, K.; Gidlöf, O.; Kornhall, B.; Öhman, J. Altered serum miRNA profiles during acute rejection after heart transplantation: Potential for non-invasive allograft surveillance. *J. Hear. Lung Transplant.* **2013**, *32*, 463–466. [CrossRef]
46. Sukma Dewi, I.; Hollander, Z.; Lam, K.K.; McManus, J.W.; Tebbutt, S.J.; Ng, R.T.; Keown, P.A.; McMaster, R.W.; McManus, B.M.; Gidlöf, O.; et al. Association of serum MiR-142-3p and MiR-101-3p levels with acute cellular rejection after heart transplantation. *PLoS ONE* **2017**, *12*, e0170842. [CrossRef]
47. Van Huyen, J.P.D.; Tible, M.; Gay, A.; Guillemain, R.; Aubert, O.; Varnous, S.; Iserin, F.; Rouvier, P.; François, A.; Vernerey, D.; et al. MicroRNAs as non-invasive biomarkers of heart transplant rejection. *Eur. Heart J.* **2014**, *35*, 3194–3202. [CrossRef]
48. Van Aelst, L.N.L.; Summer, G.; Li, S.; Gupta, S.K.; Heggermont, W.; De Vusser, F.; Carai, P.; Naesens, M.; Van Cleemput, J.; Van De Werf, F.; et al. RNA profiling in human and murine transplanted hearts: Identification and validation of therapeutic targets for acute cardiac and renal allograft rejection. *Am. J. Transplant.* **2016**, *16*, 99–110. [CrossRef]
49. Bernardi, S.; Balbi, C. Extracellular vesicles: From biomarkers to therapeutic tools. *Biology* **2020**, *9*, 258. [CrossRef]
50. Barile, L.; Gherghiceanu, M.; Popescu, L.M.; Moccetti, T.; Vassalli, G. Ultrastructural evidence of exosome secretion by progenitor cells in adult mouse myocardium and adult human cardiospheres. *J. Biomed. Biotechnol.* **2012**, *2012*, 1–10. [CrossRef]
51. Théry, C.; Witwer, K.W.; Aikawa, E.; Alcaraz, M.J.; Anderson, J.D.; Andriantsitohaina, R.; Antoniou, A.; Arab, T.; Archer, F.; Atkin-Smith, G.K.; et al. Minimal information for studies of extracellular vesicles 2018 (MISEV2018): A position statement of the International Society for Extracellular Vesicles and update of the MISEV2014 guidelines. *J. Extracell. Vesicles* **2018**, *7*, 1535750. [CrossRef] [PubMed]
52. Barile, L.; Vassalli, G. Exosomes: Therapy delivery tools and biomarkers of diseases. *Pharmacol. Ther.* **2017**, *174*, 63–78. [CrossRef] [PubMed]
53. Burrello, J.; Biemmi, V.; Cas, M.D.; Amongero, M.; Bolis, S.; Lazzarini, E.; Bollini, S. Sphingolipid composition of circulating extracellular vesicles after myocardial ischemia. *Sci. Rep.* **2020**, *10*, 1–14. [CrossRef] [PubMed]
54. Li, Y.; He, X.; Li, Q.; Lai, H.; Zhang, H.; Hu, Z.; Li, Y.; Huang, S. EV-origin: Enumerating the tissue-cellular origin of circulating extracellular vesicles using exLR profile. *Comput. Struct. Biotechnol. J.* **2020**, *18*, 2851–2859. [CrossRef] [PubMed]
55. Boulanger, C.M.; Loyer, X.; Rautou, P.E.; Amabile, N. Extracellular vesicles in coronary artery disease. *Nat. Rev. Cardiol.* **2017**, *14*, 259–272. [CrossRef]
56. Vacchi, E.; Burrello, J.; Di Silvestre, D.; Burrello, A.; Bolis, S.; Mauri, P.; Vassalli, G.; Cereda, C.W.; Farina, C.; Barile, L.; et al. Immune profiling of plasma-derived extracellular vesicles identifies Parkinson disease. *Neurol. Neuroimmunol. Neuroinflamm.* **2020**, *7*, e866. [CrossRef] [PubMed]
57. Burrello, J.; Bolis, S.; Balbi, C.; Burrello, A.; Provasi, E.; Caporali, E.; Gauthier, L.G.; Peirone, A.; D'Ascenzo, F.; Monticone, S.; et al. An extracellular vesicle epitope profile is associated with acute myocardial infarction. *J. Cell. Mol. Med.* **2020**, *24*, 9945–9957. [CrossRef]
58. Castellani, C.; Burrello, J.; Fedrigo, M.; Burrello, A.; Bolis, S.; Di Silvestre, D.; Tona, F.; Bottio, T.; Biemmi, V.; Toscano, G.; et al. Circulating extracellular vesicles as non-invasive biomarker of rejection in heart transplant. *J. Hear. Lung Transplant.* **2020**, *39*, 1136–1148. [CrossRef]
59. Kennel, P.J.; Saha, A.; Maldonado, D.A.; Givens, R.; Brunjes, D.L.; Castillero, E.; Zhang, X.; Ji, R.; Yahi, A.; George, I.; et al. Serum exosomal protein profiling for the non-invasive detection of cardiac allograft rejection. *J. Hear. Lung Transplant.* **2018**, *37*, 409–417. [CrossRef]
60. Li, Q.; Wang, H.; Peng, H.; Huyan, T.; Cacalano, N.A. Exosomes: Versatile nano mediators of immune regulation. *Cancers* **2019**, *11*, 1557. [CrossRef]
61. Mirzakhani, M.; Mohammadnia-Afrouzi, M.; Shahbazi, M.; Mirhosseini, S.A.; Hosseini, H.M.; Amani, J. The exosome as a novel predictive/diagnostic biomarker of rejection in the field of transplantation. *Clin. Immunol.* **2019**, *203*, 134–141. [CrossRef] [PubMed]
62. Liu, Q.; Rojas-canales, D.M.; Divito, S.J.; Shufesky, W.J.; Stolz, D.B.; Erdos, G.; Sullivan, M.L.G.; Gibson, G.A.; Watkins, S.C.; Larregina, A.T.; et al. Donor Dendritic cell–derived Exosomes Promote Allograft-Targeting Immune Response. *J. Clin. Investig.* **2016**, *126*, 2805–2820. [CrossRef] [PubMed]

63. Segura, E.; Amigorena, S.; Théry, C. Mature dendritic cells secrete exosomes with strong ability to induce antigen-specific effector immune responses. *Blood Cells, Mol. Dis.* **2005**, *35*, 89–93. [CrossRef]
64. Pêche, H.; Renaudin, K.; Beriou, G.; Merieau, E.; Amigorena, S.; Cuturi, M.C. Induction of tolerance by exosomes and short-term immunosuppression in a fully MHC-mismatched rat cardiac allograft model. *Am. J. Transplant.* **2006**, *6*, 1541–1550. [CrossRef] [PubMed]
65. Denzer, K.; Van Eijk, M.; Kleijmeer, M.J.; Jakobson, E.; De Groot, C.J.; Geuze, H. Follicular Dendritic Cells Carry MHC Class II-Expressing Microvesicles at Their Surface. *J. Immunol.* **2000**, *165*, 1259–1265. [CrossRef]
66. Vincent-Schneider, H.; Stumptner-Cuvelette, P.; Lankar, D.; Pain, S.; Raposo, G.; Benaroch, P.; Bonnerot, C. Exosomes bearing HLA-DR1 molecules needs dendritic cells to efficiently stimulate specific T cells. *Int. Immunol.* **2002**, *14*, 713–722. [CrossRef]
67. Habertheuer, A.; Korutla, L.; Rostami, S.; Reddy, S.; Lal, P.; Naji, A.; Vallabhajosyula, P. Donor tissue-specific exosome profiling enables noninvasive monitoring of acute rejection in mouse allogeneic heart transplantation. *J. Thorac. Cardiovasc. Surg.* **2018**, *155*, 2479–2489. [CrossRef]
68. Vallabhajosyula, P.; Korutla, L.; Habertheuer, A.; Yu, M.; Rostami, S.; Yuan, C.X.; Reddy, S.; Liu, C.; Korutla, V.; Koeberlein, B.; et al. Tissue-specific exosome biomarkers for noninvasively monitoring immunologic rejection of transplanted tissue. *J. Clin. Investig.* **2017**, *127*, 1375–1391. [CrossRef]
69. Sharma, M.; Liu, W.; Perincheri, S.; Gunasekaran, M.; Mohanakumar, T. Exosomes expressing the self-antigens myosin and vimentin play an important role in syngeneic cardiac transplant rejection induced by antibodies to cardiac myosin. *Am. J. Transplant.* **2018**, *18*, 1626–1635. [CrossRef]
70. Shah, P.; Bristow, M.R.; Port, J.D. MicroRNAs in Heart Failure, Cardiac Transplantation, and Myocardial Recovery: Biomarkers with Therapeutic Potential. *Curr. Heart Fail. Rep.* **2017**, *14*, 454–464. [CrossRef]
71. Halloran, P.F.; Famulski, K.; Reeve, J. The molecular phenotypes of rejection in kidney transplant biopsies. *Curr. Opin. Organ Transplant.* **2015**, *20*, 359–367. [CrossRef] [PubMed]
72. Halloran, P.F.; Potena, L.; Van Huyen, J.P.D.; Bruneval, P.; Leone, O.; Kim, D.H.; Jouven, X.; Reeve, J.; Loupy, A. Building a tissue-based molecular diagnostic system in heart transplant rejection: The heart Molecular Microscope Diagnostic (MMDx) System. *J. Hear. Lung Transplant.* **2017**, *36*, 1192–1200. [CrossRef] [PubMed]
73. Miller, R.J.H.; Thomson, L.; Levine, R.; Dimbil, S.J.; Patel, J.; Kobashigawa, J.A.; Kransdorf, E.; Li, D.; Berman, D.S.; Tamarappoo, B. Quantitative myocardial tissue characterization by cardiac magnetic resonance in heart transplant patients with suspected cardiac rejection. *Clin. Transplant.* **2019**, *33*, e13704. [CrossRef] [PubMed]
74. Vermes, E.; Pantaléon, C.; Auvet, A.; Cazeneuve, N.; Machet, M.C.; Delhommais, A.; Bourguignon, T.; Aupart, M.; Brunereau, L. Cardiovascular magnetic resonance in heart transplant patients: Diagnostic value of quantitative tissue markers: T2 mapping and extracellular volume fraction, for acute rejection diagnosis. *J. Cardiovasc. Magn. Reson.* **2018**, *20*, 1–11. [CrossRef]
75. Krieghoff, C.; Barten, M.J.; Hildebrand, L.; Grothoff, M.; Lehmkuhl, L.; Lücke, C.; Andres, C.; Nitzsche, S.; Riese, F.; Strüber, M.; et al. Assessment of sub-clinical acute cellular rejection after heart transplantation: Comparison of cardiac magnetic resonance imaging and endomyocardial biopsy. *Eur. Radiol.* **2014**, *24*, 2360–2371. [CrossRef] [PubMed]
76. Bodez, D.; Hocini, H.; Tchitchek, N.; Tisserand, P.; Benhaiem, N.; Barau, C.; Kharoubi, M.; Guellich, A.; Guendouz, S.; Radu, C.; et al. Myocardial Gene Expression Profiling to predict and identify cardiac allograft acute cellular rejection: The get-study. *PLoS ONE* **2016**, *11*, e0167213. [CrossRef] [PubMed]
77. Loupy, A.; Duong Van Huyen, J.P.; Hidalgo, L.; Reeve, J.; Racapé, M.; Aubert, O.; Venner, J.M.; Falmuski, K.; Cécile Bories, M.; Beuscart, T.; et al. Gene expression profiling for the identification and classification of antibody-mediated heart rejection. *Circulation* **2017**, *135*, 917–935. [CrossRef] [PubMed]
78. Afzali, B.; Chapman, E.; Racapé, M.; Adam, B.; Bruneval, P.; Gil, F.; Kim, D.; Hidalgo, L.; Campbell, P.; Sis, B.; et al. Molecular Assessment of Microcirculation Injury in Formalin-Fixed Human Cardiac Allograft Biopsies With Antibody-Mediated Rejection. *Am. J. Transplant.* **2017**, *17*, 496–505. [CrossRef]
79. Berry, G.J.; Burke, M.M.; Andersen, C.; Bruneval, P.; Fedrigo, M.; Fishbein, M.C.; Goddard, M.; Hammond, E.H.; Leone, O.; Marboe, C.; et al. The 2013 international society for heart and lung transplantation working formulation for the standardization of nomenclature in the pathologic diagnosis of antibody-mediated rejection in heart transplantation. *J. Hear. Lung Transplant.* **2013**, *32*, 1147–1162. [CrossRef]
80. Lin-Wang, H.T.; Cipullo, R.; Dias França, J.I.; Finger, M.A.; Rossi Neto, J.M.; Correia, E.D.B.; Dinkhuysen, J.J.; Hirata, M.H. Intragraft vasculitis and gene expression analysis: Association with acute rejection and prediction of mortality in long-term heart transplantation. *Clin. Transplant.* **2018**, *32*, e13373. [CrossRef]
81. Loupy, A.; Aubert, O.; Orandi, B.J.; Naesens, M.; Bouatou, Y.; Raynaud, M.; Divard, G.; Jackson, A.M.; Viglietti, D.; Giral, M.; et al. Prediction system for risk of allograft loss in patients receiving kidney transplants: International derivation and validation study. *BMJ* **2019**, *366*, 4923. [CrossRef] [PubMed]

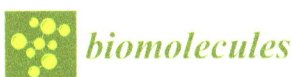 

Article

# Endothelial Dysfunction May Link Interatrial Septal Abnormalities and MTHFR-Inherited Defects to Cryptogenic Stroke Predisposition

Luca Sgarra [1,†], Alessandro Santo Bortone [2,†], Maria Assunta Potenza [1], Carmela Nacci [1], Maria Antonietta De Salvia [1], Tommaso Acquaviva [2], Emanuela De Cillis [2], Marco Matteo Ciccone [2], Massimo Grimaldi [3] and Monica Montagnani [1,*]

1. Department of Biomedical Sciences and Human Oncology—Section of Pharmacology, Medical School, University of Bari "Aldo Moro", 70124 Bari, Italy; sgarraluca@gmail.com (L.S.); mariaassunta.potenza@uniba.it (M.A.P.); carmela.nacci@uniba.it (C.N.); mariaantonietta.desalvia@uniba.it (M.A.D.S.)
2. Department of Emergency and Organ Transplantation—Section of Cardiovascular Diseases, Medical School, University of Bari "Aldo Moro", 70124 Bari, Italy; alessandrosanto.bortone@uniba.it (A.S.B.); tommasoacquaviva68@libero.it (T.A.); emanuela.decillis@gmail.com (E.D.C.); marcomatteo.ciccone@uniba.it (M.M.C.)
3. General Hospital "F. Miulli" Acquaviva delle Fonti, 70021 Bari, Italy; fiatric@hotmail.com
* Correspondence: monica.montagnani@uniba.it
† These authors contributed equally to this work.

Received: 28 March 2020; Accepted: 2 June 2020; Published: 4 June 2020

**Abstract:** We explored the significance of the L-Arginine/asymmetric dimethylarginine (L-Arg/ADMA) ratio as a biomarker of endothelial dysfunction in stroke patients. To this aim, we evaluated the correlation, in terms of severity, between the degree of endothelial dysfunction (by L-Arg/ADMA ratio), the methylene tetrahydrofolate reductase (MTHFR) genotype, and the interatrial septum (IAS) phenotype in subject with a history of stroke. **Methods and Results:** L-Arg, ADMA, and MTHFR genotypes were evaluated; the IAS phenotype was assessed by transesophageal echocardiography. Patients were grouped according to the severity of IAS defects and the residual enzymatic activity of MTHFR-mutated variants, and values of L-Arg/ADMA ratio were measured in each subgroup. Of 57 patients, 10 had a septum integrum (SI), 38 a patent foramen ovale (PFO), and 9 an ostium secundum (OS). The L-Arg/ADMA ratio differed across septum phenotypes ($p \leq 0.01$), and was higher in SI than in PFO or OS patients ($p \leq 0.05$, $p \leq 0.01$, respectively). In the PFO subgroup a negative correlation was found between the L-Arg/ADMA ratio and PFO tunnel length/height ratio ($p \leq 0.05$; r = $-0.37$; R2 = 0.14). Interestingly, the L-Arg/ADMA ratio varied across MTHFR genotypes ($p \leq 0.0001$) and was lower in subgroups carrying the most impaired enzyme with respect to patients carrying the conservative MTHFR ($p \leq 0.0001$, $p \leq 0.05$, respectively). Consistently, OS patients carried the most dysfunctional MTHFR genotypes, whereas SI patients the least ones. **Conclusions:** A low L-Arg/ADMA ratio correlates with impaired activity of MTHFR and with the jeopardized IAS phenotype along a severity spectrum encompassing OS, PFO with long/tight tunnel, PFO with short/large tunnel, and SI. This infers that genetic MTHFR defects may underlie endothelial dysfunction-related IAS abnormalities, and predispose to a cryptogenic stroke. Our findings emphasize the role of the L-Arg/ADMA ratio as a reliable marker of stroke susceptibility in carriers of IAS abnormalities, and suggest its potential use both as a diagnostic tool and as a decision aid for therapy.

**Keywords:** endothelial dysfunction; L-Arg/ADMA; PFO; MTHFR; cryptogenic stroke

## 1. Introduction

The search for causes and mechanisms underlying strokes is particularly important in young patients, where the absence of significant small- and large-vessel disease, and/or dissection accounts for the higher number of strokes diagnosed as cryptogenic [1]. The role of interatrial septum (IAS) defect features [2,3] in the so-called paradoxical embolism is currently investigated. Patent foramen ovale (PFO) is a frequent IAS abnormality, and the potential advantages in secondary prevention of surgical closure over medical therapy are unclear [4–9]. Echocardiographic assessment of PFO interatrial tunnel length has produced conflicting results as well, initially suggesting a greater risk to cryptogenic stroke in patients with larger defects [10], and recently re-evaluating such a statement on the basis of RoPE database analysis [11]. Similarly, the correlative risk of embolism and stroke based on interatrial shunt extent has generated inconclusive, if not controversial, indications [12,13]. In this scenario of diagnostic and therapeutic uncertainty, additional evidence for risk stratification is highly pursued, and the search for potential biomarkers is strongly encouraged.

A position paper from the Italian SICI-GISE Society suggests that thrombophilia is an additional risk factor for stroke predisposition, sufficient to replace pharmacological therapy with PFO percutaneous surgery [14]. Indeed, PFO closure is more effective than medical therapy to mitigate stroke recurrence in thrombophilic subjects [15]; similarly, $PT_{G20210A}$ and $FV_{G1691A}$ mutations are more frequently associated in patients with PFO-related cerebral infarcts than in a control population [16,17]. In the potential relationship linking thrombophilia to cryptogenic stroke, the predisposition conferred by genetic defects in the methylene tetrahydrofolate reductase (MTHFR) is one under-investigated condition.

MTHFR is a key enzyme in the folate cycle, whose vitamin B12-dependent conversion of homocysteine to methionine produces the main cellular carrier for methylation [18]. Polymorphisms of the MTHFR include the 677 C > T and the 1298 A > C substitutions, associated to a progressive loss of enzymatic activity from A1298C heterozygosity to C677T homozygosity [19,20]. Defective MTHFR genes increase homocysteine levels, and hyperhomocysteinemia has been associated to higher risk for atherosclerosis, cardiovascular events, venous thrombosis, and microangiopathy [21]. Similarly, MTHFR C677T and A1298C polymorphisms have been associated with multiple small-artery occlusion [22], a subcortical pattern of potential embolic origin [23,24], and with stroke in patients with large-vessel disease [25].

While sharing stroke aptitude and epidemiology, MTHFR polymorphisms and PFO are regarded as unrelated conditions that can overlap rather than interact. However, it is noteworthy that PFO carriers show higher plasma homocysteine levels than patients without PFO [26]. Thus, from the observations described above, genetic MTHFR defects may lie beneath both inherited thrombophilia and the IAS phenotype, and the missing link explaining both conditions might be endothelial dysfunction. We hypothesize that, by impairing endothelial activity, MTHFR malfunctioning may influence the physiological structure of IAS; in addition to disturbances in the coagulation process, this might represent one mechanism underlying nonobvious sources of cardiovascular embolism, and therefore help to explain the etiology of cryptogenic strokes.

To test this hypothesis, we evaluated the potential correlation between the severity of MTHFR mutation (considering both MTHFR polymorphism and homocysteinemia levels), the degree of endothelial dysfunction (indirectly measured as L-Arg/ADMA levels), and the IAS phenotype (by echocardiographic assessment) in patients diagnosed with Embolic Stroke of Undetemined Source (ESUS).If confirmed, this hypothesis might also help to legitimize L-Arg/ADMA as a marker of endothelial dysfunction.

## 2. Materials and Methods

### 2.1. Study Population and Enrolment Criteria

This retrospective observational study was carried in accordance with the guiding principles of the Declaration of Helsinki, with the approval of the local Ethical Committee on Human Research for non-interventional studies (Comitato Etico Indipendente, CE n. 4398, 03/12/2014). Fifty-seven subjects were consecutively enrolled among patients admitted between January 2017 and March 2019 to our Cardiology Unit with a diagnosis of ESUS [ ]. Multiple and/or bilateral patterns were considered of embolic origin provided that, irrespective of its cerebral location, at least one lesion would be ≥ 15 mm, in the absence of a previous injury at the same site. All patients received standard, individually adjusted, cardiovascular therapy. In each patient, a 12-lead ECG, precordial and transesophageal echocardiography, Holter cardiac monitoring, MR and/or CT angiography of the brain ischemic area, and epiaortic and transcranial Doppler ultrasonography were performed. Patients were not included in the study if their age was ≥ 60 years, had a history of Congestive Heart Failure (CHF), atrial fibrillation (AF) or similar supraventricular arrhythmias, or left ventricular dysfunction, cancer, acute and/or chronic inflammatory disease, were on immunosuppressive therapy, or concomitantly taking vitamin or protein supplements. Each participant gave written informed consent before entering the study.

*2.2. Laboratory Test*

MTHFR polymorphisms were evaluated by RT-PCR on genomic DNA from peripheral blood samples according to standard protocols. Serum folate and vitamin B12 levels were measured by a chemiluminescent immunoassay (Tosoh Bioscience, AIA-PACK, Tessenderlo, Belgium). Homocysteine levels were measured by nephelometric analysis. Plasma asymmetric dimethylarginine (ADMA) and L-Arginine (L-Arg) levels were measured by enzyme-linked immunoassay (DLD Diagnostika GMBH, Hamburg, Germany) [ ].

*2.3. Echocardiographic Imaging*

Echocardiographic analysis was performed (Philips EPIQ 7, Philips Healthcare, Andover, Philips S.p.A. Milan, Italy) using transducer frequencies of 5 to 7.5 MHz. Color Doppler mapping was set on Nyquist velocities from 28 to 55 cm/s during atrial septal examination. Transcranial and epiaortic Doppler sonography was aimed at ruling out concomitant stenosis/occlusion in the cerebral and/or precerebral vasculature, to ascertain the integrity of diastolic and systolic flow in the middle cerebral artery, and to detect and quantify the existence of shunts. Transthoracic echocardiography was aimed at ruling out valve calcification, myxomatous valvulopathies, aortic stenosis, mural and atrial thrombi, cardiac masses, ventricular dysfunction, ventricular non-compaction, endomyocardial fibrosis, endocarditic processes, and aortic arch atherosclerotic plaques, as well as to measure the size of the hearts' right chambers. Transesophageal echocardiography was performed to confirm the existence of interatrial shunt, to detect and quantify shunt extent, and to provide morphologic features of PFO tunnel or OS defects [ ]. In order to assess interobserver reproducibility of echographic measures, a second sonographer experienced in the field performed a second blind measurement of previously acquired images.

*2.4. Statistical Analysis*

All data were expressed as the mean ± error standard or the mean ± standard deviation, as indicated in the figures and tables. Kruskal–Wallis analysis of one-way ANOVA data was used to assess statistical significance across groups; the very same analysis followed by Dunn's multiple comparisons correction was used for multiple testing. The correlation between the Arg/ADMA ratio and length/height of the PFO tunnel was assessed by the Pearson correlation coefficient. The Bland–Altman plots with 95% CIs for correlations were utilized to assess interobserver reproducibility of PFO tunnel morphology (Figure 4). Statistical significance ($p \leq 0.05$) measured with GraphPad Prism 6.0 (GraphPad Inc., La Jolla, CA, USA) software is indicated in figure legends.

## 3. Results

### 3.1. Clinical and Laboratory Characteristics of Enrolled Patients

In 57 patients, a diagnosis of ESUS was made [27]. Baseline demographic, laboratory, and clinical characteristics of subjects are shown according to their IAS phenotype (Table 1) or MTHFR genotype (Table 2). The mean age of all participants was 41.2 years (range 27–57), with no significant difference among subgroups. Likewise, no difference in glucose levels, lipid profile, or blood pressure values were observed among patients (Tables 1 and 2).

Table 1. Clinical characteristics of patients according to septum phenotype.

|  | SEPTUM INTEGRUM | PATENT FORAMEN OVALE | OSTIUM SECUNDUM |
|---|---|---|---|
| PATIENTS (N) | 10 | 38 | 9 |
| Age (year) | 37 ± 10 | 42 ± 11 | 40 ± 17 |
| Fibrinogen (mg/dL) | 264 ± 36 | 249 ± 41 | 239 ± 43 |
| D-dimers (ng/dL) | 488 ± 421 | 463 ± 370 | 387 ± 122 |
| P-Hcy ($\mu$mol/L) | 7.2 ± 3.6 | 12.1 ± 7.6 * | 12.7 ± 3.2 * |
| Folates (ng/mL) | 5.0 ± 4.2 | 7.7 ± 4.5 | 17.7 ± 9.9 * |
| B12 Vit (pg/mL) | 438.4 ± 82.3 | 417.9 ± 166.1 | 341 ± 104.3 |
| Creatinine (mg/dL) | 0.65 ± 0.13 | 0.75 ± 0.13 | 0.70 ± 0.19 |
| eGFR (mL/min) | 103 ± 15 | 102 ±13 | 108 ± 19 |
| Glucose (mg/dL) | 96 ± 13.5 | 88.6 ± 9.5 | 76 ± 11.2 |
| Cholesterol (mg/dL) | 209 ± 27 | 182 ± 26 | 201 ± 12 |
| HDL (mg/dL) | 53 ± 9 | 59 ± 14 | 55 ± 5 |
| LDL (mg/dL) | 125 ± 45 | 103 ± 21 | 116 ± 12 |
| Triglicerides (mg/dL) | 110 ± 34.5 | 75 ± 24.2 | 60 ± 18.2 |
| Systolic BP (mmHg) | 118 ± 5.2 | 121 ± 4.78 | 119 ± 12.2 |
| Diastolic BP (mmHg) | 74 ± 9.5 | 75 ± 3.3 | 70 ± 9.4 |

\* $p < 0.05$ vs. respective values in the SI group.

Table 2. Clinical characteristics of patients according to MTHFR genotype.

|  | 677 T/T | 677 C/T + 1298 A/C | 677 C/T | 1298 C/C | 1298 A/C + WT |
|---|---|---|---|---|---|
| PATIENTS (N) | 16 | 14 | 6 | 5 | 16 |
| Age (year) | 39 ± 12 | 40 ± 9 | 46 ± 18 | 40 ± 16 | 42 ± 9 |
| Fibrinogen (mg/dL) | 225 ± 24 | 268 ± 39 | 260 ± 37 | 264 ± 65 | 263 ± 44 |
| D-dimers (ng/dL) | 356 ± 153 | 466 ± 438 | 462 ± 298 | 653 ± 585 | 349 ± 322 |
| P-Hcy ($\mu$mol/L) | 16.3 ± 5.8 * | 9.8 ± 2.9 | 8.0 ± 2.1 | 7.9 ± 1.1 | 9.1 ± 2.9 |
| Folates (ng/mL) | 10.6 ± 4.4 | 7.9 ± 2.7 | 7.9 ± 5.6 | 11.4 ± 4.1 | 6.6 ± 3.3 |
| B12 Vit. (pg/mL) | 383.8 ± 150.3 | 376.3 ± 88.9 | 385.5 ± 112.5 | 541 ± 202.5 | 440.9 ± 199.4 |
| Creatinine (mg/dL) | 0.60 ± 0.06 | 0.79 ± 0.18 | 0.73 ± 0.21 | 0.72 ± 0.09 | 0.77 ± 0.09 |
| eGFR (mL/min) | 110.5 ± 6.4 | 102 ± 2.8 | 92 ± 26.8 | 109.5 ± 10.6 | 101.75 ± 12.3 |
| Glucose (mg/dL) | 87 ± 8.04 | 107.5 ± 12.02 | 86 ± 4.24 | 93.5 ± 23.33 | 95 ± 10.61 |
| Cholesterol (mg/dL) | 181 ± 24.3 | 172 ± 45.9 | 195 ± 30.4 | 182 ± 17.7 | 188 ± 54.1 |
| HDL (mg/dL) | 56 ± 7.5 | 53 ± 2.8 | 83 ± 4.9 | 46 ± 5.6 | 51 ± 16.2 |
| LDL (mg/dL) | 110 ± 28.2 | 101 ± 38.9 | 101 ± 24.4 | 112 ± 7.8 | 113 ± 40.9 |
| Triglicerides (mg/dL) | 78 ± 27.5 | 91 ± 49.5 | 54 ± 8.5 | 83 ± 21.2 | 69 ± 16.3 |
| Systolic BP (mmHg) | 117 ± 6.2 | 120 ± 7.8 | 122 ± 2.2 | 118 ± 5.6 | 119 ± 8.1 |
| Diastolic BP (mmHg) | 76 ± 5.5 | 78 ± 4.3 | 79 +6.4 | 79 ± 2.5 | 76 ± 10.2 |

\* $p < 0.01$ vs. respective value in all other MTHFR subgroups.

### 3.2. Morphologic Features of the IAS Defects and Folate-Related Metabolism

Out of 57 subjects, 10 had a septum integrum (SI, 17.5%), 38 carried a patency of foramen ovale (PFO, 66.7%), and 9 an ostium secundum defect (OS, 15.8%). For PFO, the average length/height tunnel was 10.6/3.47 mm, with a mean length/height ratio of 3.48 ± 0.22. For OS defect, the mean superior-inferior diameter was 16.5 mm and anterior-posterior diameter of 13.5 mm. Baseline characteristics of patients sub-grouped according to their IAS phenotype are shown in Table 1. Folic acid and homocysteine levels tended to be higher, whereas vitamin B12 tended to be lower among patients with PFO or OS than in SI patients ($p = 0.049$ and $p = 0.039$, respectively).

## 3.3. Distribution of MTHFR Genetic Variants and Folate-Related Metabolism

Sixteen participants carried the 677 T/T homozygous genotype (28.1%), 14 carried the 677 C/T + 1298 A/C double heterozygous mutation (24.6%), 6 carried a 677 C/T heterozygous genotype (10.5%), 5 were carriers of the homozygous 1298 C/C mutation (8.7%), and 16 were carriers of the 1298 A/C variant or wild-type MTHFR (28.1%). As shown in Table 2, levels of vitamin B12 and folic acid did not significantly differ among patients. Conversely, homocysteine levels were higher in the 677 T/T subgroup with respect to all other genotype subgroups (* $p < 0.01$).

## 3.4. L-Arg/ADMA Ratio Related to IAS Phenotype and MTHFR Genotype

The L-Arg/ADMA ratio significantly differed across groups ($p < 0.01$) and was significantly higher in SI patients (mean 119.3 ± 8.6) than in patients carrying a PFO (89 ± 5.3) and/or an OS defect (74.6 ± 4.6) ($p \leq 0.05$ and $p \leq 0.01$, respectively) (Figure 1).

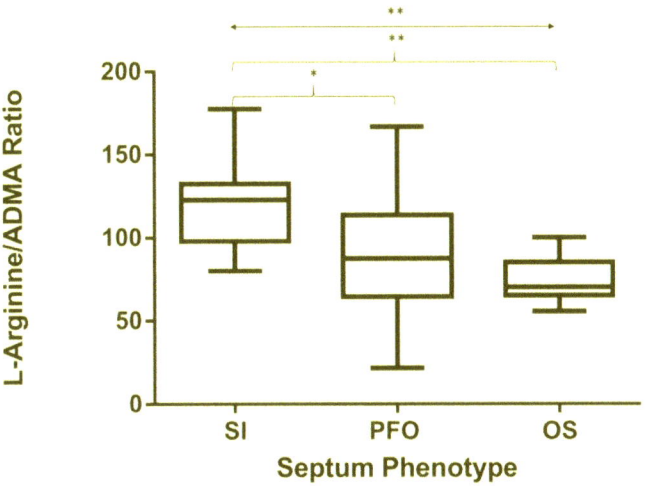

**Figure 1.** L-Arginine/asymmetric dimethylarginine (L-Arg/ADMA) ratios according to septum phenotype subclassification. Box plots indicate the median, maximum, and minimum values. The p-value across groups (double arrow line) was calculated by a Kruskall–Wallis non-parametric test of one-way ANOVA data. The p-value between groups (curly brackets) was calculated by Dunn's multiple correction. * $p \leq 0.05$; ** $p \leq 0.01$.

The L-Arg/ADMA mean values were 67.5 ± 4.6 in patients of the MTHFR 677 T/T subgroup; 81 ± 9.4 in the 677 C/T + 1298 A/C subgroup; 102 ± 4.5 in the 677 C/T subgroup; 105.4 ± 9.5 in the 1298 C/C subgroup; and 116.4 ± 9.6 for patients of the 1298 A/C + WT subgroup. The L-Arg/ADMA ratio was significantly lower in both the most detrimental 677 T/T subgroup and in the 677 C/T + 1298 A/C heterozygous subgroup with respect to the healthiest 1298 A/C and WT subgroup ($p \leq 0.0001$ and $p \leq 0.05$, respectively) (Figure 2).

When combined (irrespective of MTHFR mutation or IAS phenotype), the mean L-Arg/ADMA ratio was lower in the whole group of our cryptogenic stroke patients than in healthy subjects, although still higher if compared to the L-Arg/ADMA ratio obtained in patients with acute myocardial infarction (Figure S1).

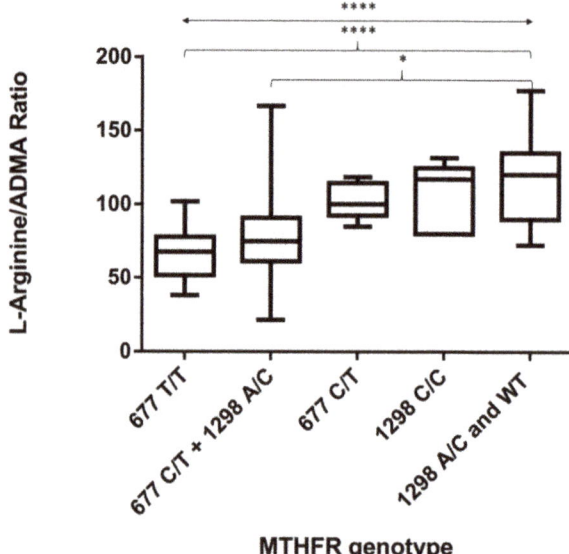

**Figure 2.** L-Arg/ADMA ratios according to MTHFR genotype subclassification. Box plots indicate the median, maximum, and minimum values. The p-value across groups (double arrow line) was calculated by a Kruskall–Wallis non-parametric test of one-way ANOVA data. The *p*-value between groups (curly brackets) was calculated by Dunn's multiple correction. * $p \leq 0.05$; **** $p \leq 0.0001$.

Figure 3 shows a negative linear correlation between the L-Arg/ADMA ratio and the tunnel-like valve length/height ratio in patients carrying a PFO defect ($p < 0.05$; r = −0.37; $R^2 = 0.14$).

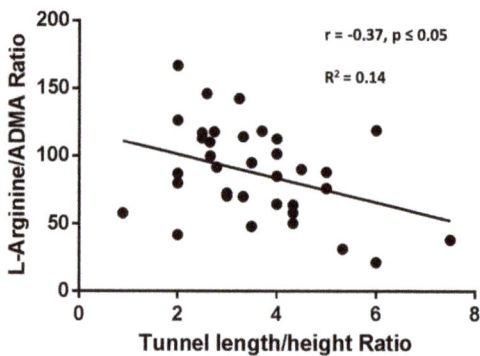

**Figure 3.** Pearson correlation and linear regression model between L-Arg/ADMA ratios and tunnel length/height ratios in patients carrying a patent foramen ovale (PFO) defect.

Inter-observer variability of tunnel length/height ratio assessed by Bland–Altman analysis revealed a mean bias of −0.023, with 95% limits of agreement of −0.52 to 0.47 (Figure 4).

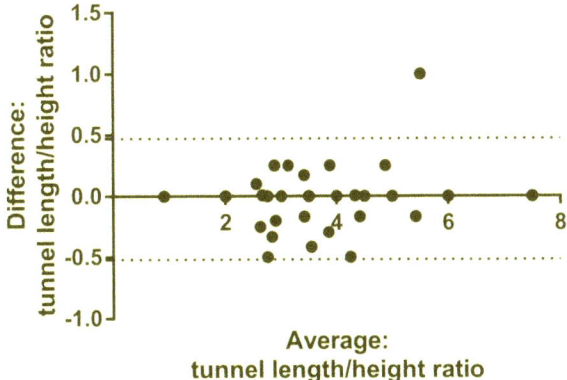

**Figure 4.** Bland–Altman analysis showing a mean bias of −0.023, with 95% limits of agreement between −0.52 and 0.47.

### 3.5. Distribution of MTHFR Genetic Variants and IAS Phenotype

According to the IAS morphology and MTHFR genotype, the following distribution was observed (Figure ): Among patients with an OS defect ($n = 9$), 5 were carrying the 677 T/T mutation, 3 were carrying the 677 C/T + 1298 A/C double heterozygous mutation, and 1 patient was carrying the 677 C/T heterozygous genotype.

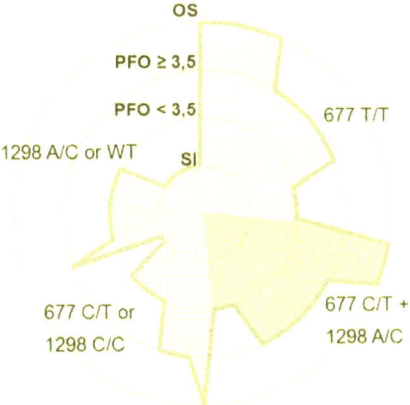

**Figure 5.** Schematic diagram illustrating the distribution of interatrial septum (IAS) phenotypes (concentric circles) with respect to the MTHFR genotypes among all patients. Subjects carrying either the 677 C/T or the 1298 C/C MTHFR genotype as well as 1298 A/C or WT genotype (mutations with similar residual enzymatic activity, respectively) were grouped together for clarity. SI = septum integrum; PFO = patent foramen ovale with tunnel length/height value below or above 3.48 (± 1.43 SD); OS = ostium secundum.

PFO carriers were sub-grouped according to tunnel length/height ratio above or below the average value of 3.5. Of the PFO subjects with a tunnel length/height ratio above 3.5 ($n = 18$), 7 patients carried the 677 T/T mutation, 7 patients carried the 677 C/T + 1298 A/C double heterozygous mutation, 3 patients carried the 677 C/T heterozygous genotype, and 1 patient carried the 1298 A/C genotype. Among PFO subjects with tunnel length/height ratio below 3.5 ($n = 20$), 4 patients carried the 677 T/T mutation, 4 patients carried the 677 C/T + 1298 A/C double heterozygous mutation, 1 patient carried the 677 C/T heterozygous genotype, 4 patients carried the 1298 C/C homozygous genotype, and 7 patients carried the 1298 A/C MTHFR genotype. All patients with SI ($n = 10$) carried either the 1298 A/C ($n = 4$) variant or the wild-type ($n = 4$) MTHFR enzyme, except for 1 patient carrying the 677 C/T heterozygosis and another one carrying the 1298 C/C homozygosis.

## 4. Discussion

Genetic defects in MTHFR have been reportedly coupled to hyperhomocysteinemia, a marker for atherosclerosis, cardiovascular events, and microangiopathy risk [21]. Undeniably, methyl overload and disorders in the folate cycle subsequent to MTHFR mutations disturb the synthesis/function of multiple factors involved in cell regulation: In endothelium, the impaired availability of substrates (as L-Arg) and co-factors (such as tetrahydrobiopterine, BH4) of the nitric oxide (NO) synthase (eNOS) reduces production of NO, the most reliable indicator of endothelial function. We investigated whether abnormal activity of MTHFR may impair the endothelium-driven development/repair of the interatrial septum, with the hypothesis that the concomitant occurrence of these conditions may represent a stroke predisposition. In this scenario, the significance of the L-Arg/ADMA ratio as an indirect marker of endothelial function may acquire clinical importance for its potential use as both a diagnostic tool and a decision aid for therapeutic strategies.

### 4.1. Correlation between the Severity of MTHFR Activity and the Degree of Endothelial Dysfunction

Not surprisingly, higher levels of homocysteine were found in patients with the most impaired MTHFR variants; concomitantly, the L-Arg/ADMA ratio decreased proportionally to the severity of the MTHFR mutation. Several interrelated mechanisms support the idea that MTHFR-mediated disruption in the folate cycle may trigger endothelial dysfunction: Under methylic surcharge and methionine deficiency, L-Arg may be directly converted to ADMA [29], a powerful endogenous inhibitor of eNOS; moreover, homocysteine-dependent downregulation of dimethylarginine dimethyl-aminohydrolase (DDAH) results in increased ADMA levels and endothelial dysfunction [30,31], as observed in patients exposed to methionine loading tests [32]. In addition, low levels of both BH4 and NO, with subsequent endothelial dysfunction, have been observed in patients with hyperhomocysteinemia [33]. Even if easy to be suggested from a molecular perspective, the clinical demonstration of a pathogenic relationship between MTHFR mutations and ADMA still remains an unexplored field [34,35]. On this basis, the present findings represent the first attempt to demonstrate an existing relationship between MTHFR activity and the L-Arg/ADMA ratio, therefore supporting the hypothesis that MTHFR mutations influence endothelial function. Interestingly, in our study, the L-Arg/ADMA ratio behaves as a more sensitive indicator of a folate cycle disruption with respect to homocysteine levels. This last observation further reinforces the proposed idea that the L-Arg/ADMA ratio may serve as a handful marker of endothelial function, whose values may contribute to better characterize specific patient subgroups.

### 4.2. Correlation between the Degree of Endothelial Dysfunction and the IAS Phenotype

Based on the aforementioned considerations—along with its role as an independent marker of ischemic stroke [36], cardiovascular events [37], risk factor for microangiopathy-related cerebral damage [38], and silent brain infarction [39]—the L-Arg/ADMA ratio (as a surrogate of endothelial dysfunction) might be proposed as an indicator of IAS defects. In accordance with Ozdemir et al. [26], we observed that, with respect to patients with SI, levels of homocysteine were proportionally higher in patients with PFO or OS phenotypes. In parallel, the L-Arg/ADMA ratio progressively declined among a spectrum encompassing SI, PFO with shorter and larger tunnel, PFO with longer and tighter tunnel, and complete OS defects. The idea that MTHFR-mediated disorders in the folate cycle trigger endothelial dysfunction, and that this condition may in turn influence the IAS phenotype, grounds on several clinic, translational, and basic research studies: An appropriate L-Arg/ADMA ratio, indicative of a physiological NO production, is required for the proper post-natal cardiomyocyte proliferation and differentiation [40], suggesting that a fully performing eNOS is mandatory for postnatal heart development [ ]. In line with this, congenital atrial septal defects have been observed in eNOS-deficient mice [ ]; interestingly, impaired NO production subsequent to reduced BH4 bioavailability has been reported in mesenteric vessels from MTHFR deficient mice [ ]. The importance of the C677T MTHFR mutation to promote neural tube defects is also well recognized [ , ]; similarly, the preventative effect of low-dose folate administration on stroke onset has been repeatedly confirmed [ ]; these findings are consistent with the higher plasma levels of homocysteine found in PFO carriers [ ]. Taken together, all these ideas contribute to the support of the possibility that MTHFR-related disorders might account for IAS defects in humans [ , ].

The correlation between features of the PFO tunnel-like valve and the L-Arg/ADMA ratio might help to reconcile current controversies concerning tunnel size and risk of cryptogenic stroke [ , ]. According to our findings, the hypothetical major contribution of larger tunnels to paradoxical embolism might be counterbalanced by the more severe endothelial dysfunction in PFO with tighter and longer tunnels. Consistent with this hypothesis, the L-Arg/ADMA ratio was similar in patients carrying either an OS or PFO defect.

*4.3. Relationship between the Severity of MTHFR Activity, the Characteristics of IAS Defects, and Cryptogenic Strokes*

Our findings strongly suggest that the most severe septum defects are found in patients carrying high-dysfunctional MTHFR variants. The relationship found between the L-Arg/ADMA ratio and the PFO tunnel morphology might partially explain why PFO prevalence decreases with age, whereas its size increases [ ]; this idea is consistent with the observation that reduced MTHFR activity contributes to impair survival and function of circulating endothelial progenitor cells [ ], whose inefficiency is important on stroke onset [ ]. Interestingly, ADMA levels are increased in subjects reporting migraines with aura [ ], and the L-Arg/ADMA ratio is accepted as an independent predictor of mortality [ ].

The lack of specificity in current classification confines cryptogenic strokes to an exclusion diagnosis, wherein multiple pathogenic factors coexist. While paradoxical embolism cannot explain strokes occurring in patients with no interatrial abnormality, or carrying a septal aneurysm not associated with a right-to-left shunt, the presence of endothelial dysfunction may help to unravel a potentially unrecognized contributor to cryptogenic stroke. Consistent with our hypothesis, lower values of flow-mediated dilation (indicating endothelial dysfunction) have been proposed as an independent risk factor for strokes, irrespective of PFO presence [ ].

## 5. Limitations of the Study

The following limitations should be taken into account when evaluating the overall message of our study: First of all, the narrow number of patients evaluated does not allow an authoritative indication of a direct cause–effect relationship between MTHFR genotype, IAS defects, and cryptogenic strokes. In this respect, the demographic characteristics of subjects enrolled might represent an important drawback: For example, although PFO and MTHFR-inherited thrombophilia share roughly the same prevalence worldwide [ , , ], ischemic strokes have been related to PFO with larger tunnels and a low frequency of MTHFR mutations in a black population; on the other hand, PFO with tighter tunnels and a high frequency of MTHFR mutations have been documented in Hispanic patients undergoing strokes [ , ]. More inclusive studies will hopefully help to ascertain the specific risk in a sub-population of patients.

One second point is related to the use of the L-Arg/ADMA ratio to indicate endothelial dysfunction. Although strongly suggestive of a relationship between impaired MTHFR activity and abnormal endothelial function, the L-Arg/ADMA ratio does not give information on the intracellular content and activity of key molecules or signaling cascades. One possibility to corroborate the link between the L-Arg/ADMA ratio and the degree of endothelial performance in patients with cryptogenic stroke could come by the characterization of pro-angiogenic molecular signaling from circulating Endothelial Progenitor Cells (EPCs). It has been proven that the level of circulating EPCs is an independent predictor of the prognosis for patients with an acute ischemic stroke, and that circulating EPCs are significantly impaired in patients with cerebro-cardiovascular diseases with respect to control subjects. Since EPCs can differentiate into endothelial cells, replacing or directly integrating with the damaged endothelial layer, it is likely that any alteration in their expression pattern of eNOS or caspases might reflect the impaired activity of mature endothelial cells. Unfortunately, because of the retrospective nature of our study, these experiments could not be carried out at present. Nevertheless, and consistent with literature data, impaired eNOS protein expression and NO production with concomitant increased ROS production and NF-kB activation were observed in human endothelial cells incubated in vitro under high homocysteine concentrations. If confirmed, these observations—too preliminary to be shown at present—might provide further support to our idea of a tight link between folate-related endothelial function and unbalanced L-Arg/homocysteine levels.

Moreover, several other possibilities exist: For example, the consequences of MTHFR defects might extend to abnormal function of other vascular cells types, such as smooth muscle cells. It is overly accepted that vascular cell proliferation may play an important role in the pathogenesis of cerebral vasospasm, and that both hyperhomocysteinemia and folate deficiency may influence key processes such as methylation and global gene expression patterns in smooth muscle cells. Finally, endothelial trans-differentiation process towards a more contractile phenotype, mostly referred as endothelial to mesenchymal transition (EndMT) could be jeopardized. In EndMT, endothelial cells adopt a mesenchymal phenotype displaying typical mesenchymal cell morphology and functions, including the acquisition of fiber deposition (myofibroblast) and contractile properties (smooth muscle cell).

In summary, considering the increasing recognition on the contribution that MTHFR plays in a myriad of physiological processes involved in the differentiation from endothelial progenitor cells->endothelial cells->vascular smooth cells or myofibroblasts, the lack of an established causative effect might represent the most significant limitation of this paper. Notwithstanding, findings provided here open a standpoint from which conceive novel perspectives. Altogether, the multifaceted and still largely incomplete knowledge on mechanisms underlying cryptogenic stroke highlight the critical importance of continued studies in this field.

## 6. Conclusions

From a clinical perspective, our results may contribute to clarify the current scenario of diagnostic and therapeutic uncertainty in patients with cryptogenic strokes. If validated, the L-Arg/ADMA ratio may represent a reliable marker of stroke susceptibility in carriers of IAS abnormalities implying that, in the near future, therapeutic strategies targeting endothelial dysfunction—in addition to antiplatelet and anticoagulant therapies—may reveal their importance in stroke primary prevention. Moreover, our findings may help to identify subgroups of subjects that would take full advantage from PFO surgical closure over medical therapy, as well as subjects that would instead obtain the maximal beneficial effects from folate administration to reduce stroke incidence [46,58].

**Supplementary Materials:** The following are available online at http://www.mdpi.com/2218-273X/10/6/861/s1, Figure S1: L-Arg/ADMA ratios across healthy volunteers, cryptogenic stroke patients, and acute myocardial infarction.

**Author Contributions:** Conceptualization, L.S., A.S.B., and M.M.; methodology, L.S., A.S.B., T.A., E.D.C., M.M.C., and M.G.; formal analysis, L.S., M.A.P., C.N. and M.A.D.S.; investigation, L.S., A.S.B., T.A., E.D.C., M.M.C., and M.G.; resources, A.S.B., M.M.C., M.G., C.N. and M.M.; writing—original draft preparation, L.S. and M.M.; writing—review and editing, M.M. All authors have read and agreed to the published version of the manuscript.

**Funding:** This work was supported, in part, by the University of Bari Research funds (CUP H96J15001610005 to M.M. and UPB:DIMO 102200201 to C.N.).

**Conflicts of Interest:** The authors declare no conflict of interest.

## Abbreviations

MTHFR     methylene tetrahydrofolate reductase
PFO       patent foramen ovale
IAS       interatrial septum
OS        ostium secundum
ADMA      asymmetric dimethylarginine

## References

1. Schulz, U.G.R.; Rothwell, P.M. Differences in Vascular Risk Factors between Etiological Subtypes of Ischemic Stroke. *Stroke* **2003**, *34*, 2050–2059. [CrossRef]
2. Marelli, A.; Mackie, A.S.; Ionescu-Ittu, R.; Rahme, E.; Pilote, L. Congenital heart disease in the general population: Changing prevalence and age distribution. *Circulation* **2007**, *115*, 163–172. [CrossRef] [PubMed]
3. Homma, S.; Sacco, R.L. Patent foramen ovale and stroke. *Circulation* **2005**, *112*, 1063–1072. [CrossRef]
4. Furlan, A.; Reisman, M.; Massaro, J.M.; Mauri, L.; Adams, H.; Albers, G.W.; Felberg, R.; Herrmann, H.; Kar, S.; Landzberg, M.; et al. Closure or Medical Therapy for Cryptogenic Stroke with Patent Foramen Ovale. *N. Engl. J. Med.* **2012**, *366*, 991–999. [CrossRef] [PubMed]
5. Carroll, J.D.; Saver, J.L.; Thaler, D.E.; Smalling, R.W.; Berry, S.; Macdonald, L.A.; Marks, D.S.; Tirschwell, D.L. Closure of Patent Foramen Ovale versus Medical Therapy after Cryptogenic Stroke. *N. Engl. J. Med.* **2013**, *368*, 1092–1100. [CrossRef] [PubMed]
6. Meier, B.; Kalesan, B.; Mattle, H.P.; Khattab, A.A.; Hildick-Smith, D.; Dudek, D.; Andersen, G.; Ibrahim, R.; Schuler, G.; Walton, A.S.; et al. Percutaneous Closure of Patent Foramen Ovale in Cryptogenic Embolism. *N. Engl. J. Med.* **2013**, *368*, 1083–1091. [CrossRef]
7. Kent, D.; Dahabreh, I.J.; Ruthazer, R.; Furlan, A.J.; Reisman, M.; Carroll, J.D.; Saver, J.L.; Smalling, R.W.; Jüni, P.; Mattle, H.P.; et al. Device Closure of Patent Foramen Ovale After Stroke: Pooled Analysis of Completed Randomized Trials. *J. Am. Coll. Cardiol.* **2016**, *67*, 907–917. [CrossRef]
8. Kitsios, G.D.; Thaler, D.E.; Kent, D. Potentially large yet uncertain benefits: A meta-analysis of patent foramen ovale closure trials. *Stroke* **2013**, *44*, 2640–2643. [CrossRef]
9. Homma, S.; Sacco, R.; Tullio, M.; Sciacca, R.; Mohr, J. Effect of medical treatment in stroke patients with patent foramen ovale. patent foramen ovale in cryptogenic stroke study. *ACC Curr. J. Rev.* **2002**, *11*, 46. [CrossRef]
10. Goel, S.S.; Tuzcu, E.M.; Shishehbor, M.H.; De Oliveira, E.I.; Borek, P.P.; Krasuski, R.A.; Rodriguez, L.L.; Kapadia, S.R. Morphology of the Patent Foramen Ovale in Asymptomatic Versus Symptomatic (Stroke or Transient Ischemic Attack) Patients. *Am. J. Cardiol.* **2009**, *103*, 124–129. [CrossRef]
11. Wessler, B.S.; Thaler, D.E.; Ruthazer, R.; Weimar, C.; Di Tullio, M.R.; Elkind, M.S.V.; Homma, S.; Lutz, J.S.; Mas, J.-L.; Mattle, H.P.; et al. Response to letter regarding article, "Transesophageal echocardiography in cryptogenic stroke and patent foramen ovale analysis of putative high-risk features from the risk of paradoxical embolism database". *Circ. Cardiovasc. Imaging* **2014**, *7*, 125–131. [CrossRef] [PubMed]
12. Serena, J.; Marti-Fabregas, J.; Santamarina, E.; Rodriguez, J.J.; Perez-Ayuso, M.J.; Masjuan, J.; Segura, T.; Gallego, J.; Davalos, A. Recurrent stroke and massive right-to-left shunt: Results from the prospective Spanish multicenter (CODICIA) study. *Stroke* **2008**, *39*, 3131–3136. [CrossRef]
13. Katsanos, A.H.; Spence, J.D.; Bogiatzi, C.; Parissis, J.; Giannopoulos, S.; Frogoudaki, A.; Safouris, A.; Voumvourakis, K.; Tsivgoulis, G. Recurrent Stroke and Patent Foramen Ovale. *Stroke* **2014**, *45*, 3352–3359. [CrossRef]
14. Pristipino, C.; Anzola, G.P.; Ballerini, L.; Bartorelli, A.; Cecconi, M.; Chessa, M.; Donti, A.; Gaspardone, A.; Neri, G.; Onorato, E. Multidisciplinary position paper on the management of patent foramen ovale in the presence of cryptogenic cerebral ischemia—Italian version 2013. *G. Ital. Cardiol. (Rome)* **2013**, *14*, 699–712. [CrossRef]
15. Giardini, A.; Donti, A.; Formigari, R.; Bronzetti, G.; Prandstraller, D.; Bonvicini, M.; Palareti, G.; Guidetti, D.; Gaddi, O.; Picchio, F.M. Comparison of results of percutaneous closure of patent foramen ovale for paradoxical embolism in patients with versus without thrombophilia. *Am. J. Cardiol.* **2004**, *94*, 1012–1016. [CrossRef] [PubMed]

16. Pezzini, A.; Del Zotto, E.; Magoni, M.; Costa, A.B.; Archetti, S.; Grassi, M.; Akkawi, N.M.; Albertini, A.; Assanelli, D.; Vignolo, L.A.; et al. Inherited Thrombophilic Disorders in Young Adults With Ischemic Stroke and Patent Foramen Ovale. *Stroke* **2003**, *34*, 28–33. [CrossRef] [PubMed]
17. Karttunen, V.; Hiltunen, L.; Rasi, V.; Vahtera, E.; Hillbom, M. Factor V Leiden and prothrombin gene mutation may predispose to paradoxical embolism in subjects with patent foramen ovale. *Blood Coagul. Fibrinolysis* **2003**, *14*, 261–268. [CrossRef]
18. Stover, P.J. Physiology of folate and vitamin B12 in health and disease. *Nutr. Rev.* **2004**, *62*, S3–S13. [CrossRef]
19. Linnebank, M.; Homberger, A.; Nowak-Göttl, U.; Marquardt, T.; Harms, E.; Koch, H.G. Linkage disequilibrium of the common mutations 677C > T and 1298A > C of the human methylenetetrahydrofolate reductase gene as proven by the novel polymorphisms 129C > T, 1068C > T. *Eur. J. Nucl. Med. Mol. Imaging* **2000**, *159*, 472–473. [CrossRef]
20. Moll, S.; Varga, E.A. Homocysteine and MTHFR Mutations. *Circulation* **2015**, *132*, e6–e9. [CrossRef] [PubMed]
21. Feng, C.; Bai, X.; Xu, Y.; Hua, T.; Huang, J.; Liu, X.-Y. Hyperhomocysteinemia Associates with Small Vessel Disease More Closely Than Large Vessel Disease. *Int. J. Med Sci.* **2013**, *10*, 408–412. [CrossRef]
22. Choi, B.; Kim, N.K.; Kang, M.; Lee, S.; Ahn, J.; Kim, O.; Oh, D.; Kim, S.; Kim, S. Homozygous C677T mutation in the MTHFR gene as an independent risk factor for multiple small-artery occlusions. *Thromb. Res.* **2003**, *111*, 39–44. [CrossRef] [PubMed]
23. Gerraty, R.P.; Parsons, M.W.; Barber, P.A.; Darby, D.G.; Desmond, P.M.; Tress, B.M.; Davis, S.M. Examining the lacunar hypothesis with diffusion and perfusion magnetic resonance imaging. *Stroke* **2002**, *33*, 2019–2024. [CrossRef] [PubMed]
24. Wessels, T.; Rottger, C.; Jauss, M.; Kaps, M.; Traupe, H.; Stolz, E. Identification of Embolic Stroke Patterns by Diffusion-Weighted MRI in Clinically Defined Lacunar Stroke Syndromes. *Stroke* **2005**, *36*, 757–761. [CrossRef] [PubMed]
25. Cotlarciuc, I.; Malik, R.; Holliday, E.G.; Ahmadi, K.R.; Pare, G.; Psaty, B.M.; Fornage, M.; Hasan, N.; Rinne, P.E.; Ikram, M.A. Effect of genetic variants associated with plasma homocysteine levels on stroke risk. *Stroke* **2014**, *45*, 1920–1924. [CrossRef]
26. Ozdemir, A.O.; Tamayo, A.; Muñoz, C.; Dias, B.; Spence, J.D. Cryptogenic stroke and patent foramen ovale: Clinical clues to paradoxical embolism. *J. Neurol. Sci.* **2008**, *275*, 121–127. [CrossRef]
27. Hart, R.G.; Diener, H.-C.; Coutts, S.B.; Easton, J.D.; Granger, C.B.; O'Donnell, M.; Sacco, R.L.; Connolly, S.J. Embolic strokes of undetermined source: The case for a new clinical construct. *Lancet Neurol.* **2014**, *13*, 429–438. [CrossRef]
28. Schwedhelm, E.; Maas, R.; Tan-Andresen, J.; Schulze, F.; Riederer, U.; Böger, R.H. High-throughput liquid chromatographic-tandem mass spectrometric determination of arginine and dimethylated arginine derivatives in human and mouse plasma. *J. Chromatogr. B* **2007**, *851*, 211–219. [CrossRef]
29. Kayacelebi, A.A.; Langen, J.; Weigt-Usinger, K.; Chobanyan-Jürgens, K.; Mariotti, F.; Schneider, J.Y.; Rothmann, S.; Frölich, J.C.; Atzler, R.; Choe, C.-U.; et al. Biosynthesis of homoarginine (hArg) and asymmetric dimethylarginine (ADMA) from acutely and chronically administered free l-arginine in humans. *Amino Acids* **2015**, *47*, 1893–1908. [CrossRef]
30. Chen, S.; Li, N.; Deb-Chatterji, M.; Dong, Q.; Kielstein, J.T.; Weissenborn, K.; Worthmann, H. Asymmetric Dimethylarginine as Marker and Mediator in Ischemic Stroke. *Int. J. Mol. Sci.* **2012**, *13*, 15983–16004. [CrossRef]
31. Teerlink, T.; Luo, Z.; Palm, F.; Wilcox, C.S. Cellular ADMA: Regulation and action. *Pharmacol. Res.* **2009**, *60*, 448–460. [CrossRef] [PubMed]
32. Stuhlinger, M.C.; Oka, R.K.; Graf, E.E.; Schmolzer, I.; Upson, B.M.; Kapoor, O.; Szuba, A.; Malinow, M.R.; Wascher, T.C.; Pachinger, O.; et al. Endothelial Dysfunction Induced by Hyperhomocyst(e)inemia. *Circulation* **2003**, *108*, 933–938. [CrossRef] [PubMed]
33. He, L.; Zeng, H.; Li, F.; Feng, J.; Liu, S.; Liu, J.; Yu, J.; Mao, J.; Hong, T.; Chen, A.F.; et al. Homocysteine impairs coronary artery endothelial function by inhibiting tetrahydrobiopterin in patients with hyperhomocysteinemia. *Am. J. Physiol. Metab.* **2010**, *299*, E1061–E1065. [CrossRef] [PubMed]
34. Dimitroulas, T.; Sandoo, A.; Hodson, J.; Smith, J.; Douglas, K.; Kitas, G.; Kitas, G.D. Associations between asymmetric dimethylarginine, homocysteine, and the methylenetetrahydrofolate reductase (MTHFR) C677T polymorphism (rs1801133) in rheumatoid arthritis. *Scand. J. Rheumatol.* **2016**, *45*, 267–273. [CrossRef]

35. Sniezawska, A.; Dorszewska, J.; Różycka, A.; Przedpelska-Ober, E.; Lianeri, M.; Jagodzinski, P.P.; Kozubski, W. MTHFR, MTR, and MTHFD1 gene polymorphisms compared to homocysteine and asymmetric dimethylarginine concentrations and their metabolites in epileptic patients treated with antiepileptic drugs. *Seizure* **2011**, *20*, 533–540. [CrossRef]
36. Scherbakov, N.; Sandek, A.; Martens-Lobenhoffer, J.; Kung, T.; Turhan, G.; Liman, T.; Ebinger, M.; Von Haehling, S.; Bode-Böger, S.; Endres, M.; et al. Endothelial Dysfunction of the Peripheral Vascular Bed in the Acute Phase after Ischemic Stroke. *Cerebrovasc. Dis.* **2012**, *33*, 37–46. [CrossRef]
37. Böger, R.H.; Sullivan, L.; Schwedhelm, E.; Wang, T.J.; Maas, R.; Benjamin, E.J.; Schulze, F.; Xanthakis, V.; Benndorf, R.A.; Vasan, R.S. Plasma Asymmetric Dimethylarginine and Incidence of Cardiovascular Disease and Death in the Community. *Circulation* **2009**, *119*, 1592–1600. [CrossRef]
38. Notsu, Y.; Nabika, T.; Bokura, H.; Suyama, Y.; Kobayashi, S.; Yamaguchi, S.; Masuda, J. Evaluation of Asymmetric Dimethylarginine and Homocysteine in Microangiopathy-Related Cerebral Damage. *Am. J. Hypertens.* **2009**, *22*, 257–262. [CrossRef] [PubMed]
39. Pikula, A.; Böger, R.H.; Beiser, A.; Maas, R.; DeCarli, C.; Schwedhelm, E.; Himali, J.J.; Schulze, F.; Au, R.; Kelly-Hayes, M.; et al. Association of plasma ADMA levels with MRI markers of vascular brain injury: Framingham offspring study. *Stroke* **2009**, *40*, 2959–2964. [CrossRef] [PubMed]
40. Bode-Boger, S.M.; Boger, R.H.; Kienke, S.; Junker, W.; Frolich, J.C. Elevated L-arginine/dimethylarginine ratio contributes to enhanced systemic NO production by dietary L-arginine in hypercholesterolemic rabbits. *Biochem. Biophys. Res. Commun.* **1996**, *219*, 598–603. [CrossRef]
41. Lepic, E.; Burger, D.; Lu, X.; Song, W.; Feng, Q. Lack of endothelial nitric oxide synthase decreases cardiomyocyte proliferation and delays cardiac maturation. *Am. J. Physiol. Physiol.* **2006**, *291*, C1240–C1246. [CrossRef] [PubMed]
42. Feng, Q.; Song, W.; Lu, X.; Hamilton, J.A.; Lei, M.; Peng, T.; Yee, S.-P. Development of heart failure and congenital septal defects in mice lacking endothelial nitric oxide synthase. *Circulation* **2002**, *106*, 873–879. [CrossRef]
43. Virdis, A.; Iglarz, M.; Neves, M.F.; Amiri, F.; Touyz, R.M.; Rozen, R.; Schiffrin, E.L. Effect of Hyperhomocystinemia and Hypertension on Endothelial Function in Methylenetetrahydrofolate Reductase–Deficient Mice. *Arter. Thromb. Vasc. Boil.* **2003**, *23*, 1352–1357. [CrossRef] [PubMed]
44. Prevention of neural tube defects: Results of the Medical Research Council Vitamin Study. *Lancet* **1991**, *338*, 131–137. [CrossRef]
45. Amorim, M.R.; Lima, M.A.; Castilla, E.E.; Orioli, I.M. Non-Latin European descent could be a requirement for association of NTDs and MTHFR variant 677C > T: A meta-analysis. *Am. J. Med. Genet. Part A* **2007**, *143*, 1726–1732. [CrossRef]
46. Zhao, M.; Wu, G.; Li, Y.; Wang, X.; Hou, F.F.; Xu, X.; Qin, X.; Cai, Y.-F. Meta-analysis of folic acid efficacy trials in stroke prevention. *Neurology* **2017**, *88*, 1830–1838. [CrossRef]
47. Zidan, H.E.; Rezk, N.A.; Mohammed, D. MTHFR C677T and A1298C gene polymorphisms and their relation to homocysteine level in Egyptian children with congenital heart diseases. *Gene* **2013**, *529*, 119–124. [CrossRef]
48. Zhu, W.; Yong, L.; Yan, L.; Dao, J.; Li, S. Maternal and offspring MTHFR gene C677T polymorphism as predictors of congenital atrial septal defect and patent ductus arteriosus. *Mol. Hum. Reprod.* **2006**, *12*, 51–54. [CrossRef]
49. Angeline, T.; Jeyaraj, N.; Granito, S.; Tsongalis, G.J. Prevalence of MTHFR gene polymorphisms (C677T and A1298C) among Tamilians. *Exp. Mol. Pathol.* **2004**, *77*, 85–88. [CrossRef]
50. Meissner, I.; Whisnant, J.P.; Khandheria, B.K.; Spittell, P.C.; O'Fallon, W.M.; Pascoe, R.D.; Enriquez-Sarano, M.; Seward, J.B.; Covalt, J.L.; Sicks, J.D.; et al. Prevalence of potential risk factors for stroke assessed by transesophageal echocardiography and carotid ultrasonography: The SPARC study. Stroke Prevention: Assessment of Risk in a Community. *Mayo Clin. Proc.* **1999**, *74*, 862–869. [CrossRef]
51. Rodriguez, C.J.; Homma, S.; Sacco, R.L.; Di Tullio, M.R.; Sciacca, R.R.; Mohr, J. Race-Ethnic Differences in Patent Foramen Ovale, Atrial Septal Aneurysm, and Right Atrial Anatomy Among Ischemic Stroke Patients. *Stroke* **2003**, *34*, 2097–2102. [CrossRef] [PubMed]
52. Daniel Leclerc, S.S.; Rozen, R. *Molecular Biology of Methylenetetrahydrofolate Reductase (MTHFR) and Overview of Mutations/Polymorphisms*; Database, M.C.B., Ed.; Landes Bioscience: Austin, TX, USA, 2013.

53. Hagen, P.T.; Scholz, D.G.; Edwards, W.D. Incidence and Size of Patent Foramen Ovale During the First 10 Decades of Life: An Autopsy Study of 965 Normal Hearts. *Mayo Clin. Proc.* **1984**, *59*, 17–20. [CrossRef]
54. Lemarié, C.A.; Shbat, L.; Marchesi, C.; Angulo, O.J.; Deschênes, M.-E.; Blostein, M.D.; Paradis, P.; Schiffrin, E.L. Mthfr deficiency induces endothelial progenitor cell senescence via uncoupling of eNOS and downregulation of SIRT1. *Am. J. Physiol. Circ. Physiol.* **2011**, *300*, H745–H753. [CrossRef]
55. Martí-Fàbregas, J.; Crespo, J.; Delgado-Mederos, R.; Martínez-Ramírez, S.; Peña, E.; Marín, R.; Dinia, L.; Jiménez-Xarrié, E.; Fernández-Arcos, A.; Pérez-Pérez, J.; et al. Endothelial progenitor cells in acute ischemic stroke. *Brain Behav.* **2013**, *3*, 649–655. [CrossRef] [PubMed]
56. Erdélyi-Bótor, S.; Deli, G.; Trauninger, A.; Komáromy, H.; Kamson, D.O.; Kovács, N.; Perlaki, G.; Orsi, G.; Molnar, T.; Illes, Z.; et al. Serum L-arginine and dimethylarginine levels in migraine patients with brain white matter lesions. *Cephalalgia* **2016**, *37*, 571–580. [CrossRef]
57. Sunbul, M.; Ozben, B.; Durmus, E.; Kepez, A.; Pehlivan, A.; Midi, I.; Mutlu, B. Endothelial dysfunction is an independent risk factor for stroke patients irrespective of the presence of patent foramen ovale. *Herz* **2013**, *38*, 671–676. [CrossRef]
58. Qin, X.; Li, J.; Spence, J.D.; Zhang, Y.; Li, Y.; Wang, X.; Wang, B.; Sun, N.; Chen, F.; Guo, J. Folic Acid Therapy Reduces the First Stroke Risk Associated With Hypercholesterolemia Among Hypertensive Patients. *Stroke* **2016**, *47*, 2805–2812. [CrossRef]

© 2020 by the authors. Licensee MDPI, Basel, Switzerland. This article is an open access article distributed under the terms and conditions of the Creative Commons Attribution (CC BY) license (http://creativecommons.org/licenses/by/4.0/).

MDPI  
St. Alban-Anlage 66  
4052 Basel  
Switzerland  
Tel. +41 61 683 77 34  
Fax +41 61 302 89 18  
www.mdpi.com

*Biomolecules* Editorial Office  
E-mail: biomolecules@mdpi.com  
www.mdpi.com/journal/biomolecules

www.ingramcontent.com/pod-product-compliance
Lightning Source LLC
LaVergne TN
LVHW070510100526
838202LV00014B/1824